W9-AYE-498

Praise for Laurie Garrett's *Betrayal of Trust*

"On a par with Rachel Carson's *Silent Spring*, this chilling exploration of the decline of public health should be taken seriously by leaders and policymakers around the world. Garrett, a Pulitzer Prize–winning journalist for *Newsday* (*The Coming Plague: Newly Emerging Diseases in a World Out of Balance*), has written an accessible and prodigiously researched analysis of disaster in the making in a world with no functioning public health infrastructure."

—*Publishers Weekly* (starred review)

"An IMAX of a book, with five gigantic screens playing sequentially, presenting pictures of moldering health systems. But it is Garrett's observations about the United States that are the most disturbing. Despite our extraordinary wealth and scientific capability, public health is supported in an erratic and underfinanced way in this country. Garrett is a journalist by profession and scholar by instinct."

—Dr. Fitzhugh Mullan, *The New York Times*

"The central message of this blockbuster of a book is simple and stark: Public health, Laurie Garrett tells us, must become global if local populations in the U.S. or anywhere else are to be spared exposure to lethal epidemics old or new. But administrative arrangements to safeguard public health are grossly inadequate everywhere and are decaying dangerously even in countries like ours, where antibiotics and other early 20th Century triumphs once promised to eliminate infectious disease as a serious threat to human life."

—William H. McNeill, *Chicago Tribune*

"In this spectacularly well-researched and well-argued book, [Garrett] details how poorly prepared the world's public health-care systems are to deal with these outbreaks of disease. . . . Garrett has done a masterful job of laying out the near-crisis state of public health."

—Catherine Arnst, *Business Week*

"Turning her attention to the frightening condition of public health throughout the world, Pulitzer Prize–winning science reporter Garrett repeats the call for action she initiated in her tremendously successful *The Coming Plague*. . . . Completely readable for general readers and experts alike, this reasonably priced book is highly recommended."

—*Library Journal*

"In plain language and with razor-sharp intelligence, Garrett chronicles the decline of public health capacity and responsibility in the USA, Africa, India, Russia, and around the world. Gapping and growing inequality between the rich and the poor, globalized trade, travel and microbes, rampant epidemic disease such as MDR-TB, AIDS, and hepatitis, rapacious neglect of a fragile environment, the disintegration of public health infrastructure, and the triumph of raw self-interest over public responsibility define this ever-growing web of failure and betrayal of trust for people's health. Who is looking to the future of public health? Apparently no one. If access to health care is a right for all, not a delusional privilege of the few, then global public health must be taken seriously by any responsible citizen, health specialist, or activist. This is their next 'must read.' Bravo to Garrett for a diagnosis and wake-up call that is both brilliant and prescient."

—Dr. James Orbinski, President, Médecins Sans Frontières, winner of the Nobel Peace Prize

"In *Betrayal of Trust*, Garrett's subject is public health itself: the desperate inadequacy of public health infrastructure in much of the developing world and the shocking neglect of that infrastructure in 'developed' nations."

—*Booklist* (starred review)

"With a compassionate heart and keen intellect, Laurie Garrett has toured the world to share with us her vision of public health in action and in failure in many climes. She reminds us that, 'The idea that the health of every nation depends on the health of all others is not an empty piety but an epidemiological fact.' Public health has become the stepchild of health care systems that exhaust the social budget in providing individualized care, and still leave fundamental problems of disease anticipation and control unsolved."

—Professor Joshua Lederberg, winner of the Nobel Prize in Physiology and Medicine

"If John Snow could have seen what Garrett has seen, he would have wept."

—Carl Zimmer, *Newsday*

For more reactions to *Betrayal of Trust* visit *www.lauriegarrett.com*.

Praise for *The Coming Plague*

"A Notable Book of 1994: A disturbing, meticulously researched medical alarm."

—*The New York Times Book Review*

"A fine and valuable work." —Bill Clinton

"Garrett brilliantly develops her theme that rapidly increasing dangers are being ignored. Her investigations have taken over a decade to complete, and her findings are meticulously discussed and distilled."

—*The New York Review of Books*

"Garrett has done a brilliant job of putting scientific work into layman's language, and the scariness of medical melodramas is offset by the excitement of scientific detection."

—*The New Yorker*

". . . Garrett has mastered an extraordinary amount of detail about the pathology, epidemiology, and human events surrounding dozens of complex diseases. She writes engagingly, carrying her themes as well as the reader's interest from outbreak to outbreak."

—*Los Angeles Times Book Review*

"A frightening vision of the future and a deeply unsettling one . . . a sober, scary book that not only limns the dangers posed by emerging diseases but also raises serious questions about two centuries' worth of Enlightenment beliefs in science and technology and progress."

—Michiko Kakutani, *The New York Times*

"Exciting, frightening, heartening, reassuring, and galvanizing . . . as up-to-date as tomorrow's newspapers . . . every literate American should read it."

—Leon Eisenberg, M.D., New York *Newsday*

"Garrett's stories are enthralling, like solid war reporting. But her book also offers the clearest, most detailed, and most impeccably researched description of the science of microbiology that lay readers have had in sixty years."

—David Perlman, *San Francisco Chronicle*

BETRAYAL OF TRUST

ALSO BY LAURIE GARRETT

The Coming Plague

BETRAYAL

OF TRUST

THE COLLAPSE OF GLOBAL PUBLIC HEALTH

LAURIE GARRETT

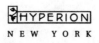

NEW YORK

To Dr. Jonathan Mann,
who dared to think boldly of a new public health in which
humanity held a place above technology.

Copyright © 2000 Laurie Garrett

Grateful acknowledgment is made to the following for permission to reprint material from: "Ghost Town" by Jerry Dammers. © 1981 Plangent Visions Music Limited. "Money's Too Tight" by Simply Red. Used with permission by The Otis Music Group. Poem by Aleksandr Galich. Used with permission by Ardis Publishers.

All rights reserved. No part of this book may be used or reproduced in any manner whatsoever without the written permission of the Publisher. Printed in the United States of America. For information address: Hyperion, 77 W. 66th Street, New York, New York 10023-6298.

LIBRARY OF CONGRESS CATALOGING-IN-PUBLICATION DATA

Garrett, Laurie.
    Betrayal of trust : the collapse of global public health / Laurie Garrett.—1st ed.
        p. cm.
    ISBN: 0-7868-6522-9
    1. World   health. 2. Medical   policy. 3. Epidemiology—Popular works.   I. Title.
RA441 .G37 2000
362.1—dc21   00-033425

Paperback ISBN 0-7868-8440-1

Book design by Richard Oriolo

FIRST PAPERBACK EDITION

10 9 8 7 6 5 4 3

CONTENTS

ACKNOWLEDGMENTS

A book of this magnitude obviously owes a lot of debts. So many people have generously offered their ideas, assistance, and support over the five years of research and preparation of *Betrayal of Trust* that I scarce know where to begin. I am overflowing with gratitude.

There are two groups of people without whose support this book would never have existed and so it is to them that I must express my most ardent thanks. I have had the pleasure of working for *Newsday* since 1988 where I have flourished under the editorial leadership of editor in chief Tony Marro and his management team of Charlotte Hall and Howard Schneider. I have been particularly fortunate in having uniquely supportive immediate editors and colleagues: Les Payne, Reg Gale, Marcy Kemen, Dele Olojede, Tim Phelps, Robert Cooke, Ridgley Ochs, Viorel Florescu, Delthia Ricks, Joe Dolman, and the staffs of 2 Park Avenue, the Washington Bureau, and the *Newsday* library. And while I'm on the subject of *Newsday*, thanks, Ray, for standing up to L.A.

I have a unique situation at *Newsday*, affording me—and my readers— opportunity to see firsthand plagues in India and Central Africa, declining life expectancies in Siberia, policy debates in Washington and Geneva, and dying tuberculosis patients on the wards of Bellevue. I know of no other news organization in the English-speaking world that sends reporters on as many far-flung journeys in pursuit of public health news. And I am grateful to the readers of *Newsday* who have over the years praised and circulated stories that described suffering not in their suburban communities, but in far-off countries where people struggled every day to survive. Many news organizations today mistakenly believe that Americans aren't interested in, and don't care about, the day-to-day struggles of Chinese farmers, Ugandan AIDS workers, Ukrainian prostitutes, or Indian truck drivers. Thank you, *Newsday* and our readers, for proving them wrong.

The other group I must thank in ardent terms is a trio of brilliant, hard-working women who formed the invisible team behind *Betrayal of Trust*: Amy

Benjamin, Jill Hannum, and Adi Gevins. Because I continue after ten years to suffer from repetitive strain injury, acquired through use of a lousy computer system, I cannot type. Hannum and Benjamin have been my fingers. But it would grossly understate their roles to label them transcribers, as both women have proven insightful, tireless editors whose feedback was invaluable every step of the way. Both faced tough personal challenges over the course of production of *Betrayal of Trust* and I thank them for their continued commitment to this project despite those diversions. In the final throes of production, Kathy Diamond lent her hands to the typing tasks, as well. Thanks, Kathy.

Gevins and I worked together as radio documentary producers (in former lives), and she has gone on to obtain a degree in library science and become one of the country's top researcher/archivists. I was, indeed, fortunate that her busy schedule allowed time for some digging for this book. Without her tireless tromping through obscure archives, most of the data that appears in Chapter 4 would never have been unearthed. Sad to say, public health archives in the United States are in shabby disarray. Gevins wishes to thank all of the librarians and staff that assisted her, particularly: Buddy Ferguson of the Minnesota Department of Health; the Reference staff of the School of Public Health at UC Berkeley; the Reference staff of the Bioscience and Natural Resources Library at UC Berkeley; The Urban Institute; Sandy Smith at the Centers for Disease Control.

I thank the families and significant others of Hannum, Benjamin, and Gevins for not squawking about how much of their time I was capitalizing. (And I thank FedEx for getting *nearly* all of our packages back and forth on time between New York, Oakland, Mendocino, Seattle, and Boulder.)

I gained additional research assistance from the staffs of the New York Academies of Science and Medicine, the New York City and State Departments of Health, the World Health Organization, the CDC, the NIH Office of AIDS Research, and the United Nations AIDS Programme. Particular thanks are owed to Peter Piot, David Heymann, Wendy Wertheimer, Malgorzata Grzemska, Anthony Fauci, Bill Paul, Jim LeDuc, Jim Hughes, and Bob Howard.

Chapters 3 and 5 and my work in the CIS and NIS owe tremendous debts of gratitude to a host of people, some of whom, for their own protection, I dare not name. Here in the United States I am grateful to Murray Feshbach; Jim Smith and his staff at the American International Health Alliance; Richard Stone at *Science*; Robert Steinglass of BASICS; Regina Napolitano and Howard Cohen of Coney Island Hospital; Ed O'Rourke of Children's Hospital in Boston; Lyle Conrad; and Alexis Shelokov. Overseas, I thank my marvelous translators: Irakli Gogorishvili in Tbilisi; Karin Keerdoo in Tallinn; Elena Frolova in St. Petersburg; Vadim Belogolovin in Kiev; Petra Francova in Prague; and many others. And among professionals in the region I am particularly grateful to Brigg Reilly (MSF);

Yuri Boshchenko (Odessa Plague Station); Archil Kobaladze (Atlanta-Tbilisi Health Partnership); Victor Aphanasiev (MOH, St. Petersburg); Grigory Latyshev (MdM); Alla Soloviova (UNICEF); Edward Korenberg (Ivanov. Institute); Boris Revich (Center of Demography and Human Ecology); Sona Strbanova (AIHA); Elena Gurvich (USAID-Moscow); Yuri Komarov (MEDSOCECONOMINFORM); and the staffs of AIHA Moscow and Kiev.

In Bombay, a special thanks to Subash Hira.

In the Democratic Republic of Congo, I am deeply indebted to several scientists, doctors, and translators, particularly Dr. Tamfum Muyembe. But because of the current civil war and repression in that country I fear that a kind word from me might do more harm than good for the rest of them. *Bonne chance, mes amis. Vous avez beaucoup de courage et j'espère qu'à l'avenir, la paix la justice règneront dans tout le Zaire.*

Thanks, of course, to Leigh Haber for her hard editing work on *Betrayal of Trust* at Hyperion.

And for ideas and encouragement, thanks to my family, close friends, and Joshua Lederberg, Peggy Hamburg, Steve Wolinsky, Phil Lee, Michael Osterholm, Mary Wilson, Doug Foster, D. A. Henderson, Jon Cohen, attorney Ed Burke, former student intern Robert Struckman, John Moore, and others who have generously shared their ideas and feedback.

Finally, there would be no book in your hands were it not for the tireless and energetic support of my good friend and agent, Charlotte Sheedy. Thanks for all of those soothing calls, Charlotte, that got me through the final phases of this mammoth project.

PREFACE

As a researcher and clinician specializing in AIDS and other infectious diseases, my daily work consists largely of staving off the myriad ailments that strike immunocompromised patients, transplant recipients, the elderly, and injection drug users. With the resources available to me at Northwestern University Medical School, I lead numerous studies using sophisticated techniques to learn how pathogens circumvent normal host defenses. It is a challenging job fraught with complexities, but technology and teamwork can produce positive results. Any frustrations I encounter usually involve such non–life-and-death issues as the inappropriate use of antibiotics by my colleagues, delays in the receipt of diagnostic test results from the laboratory, and perhaps, on a bad day, my mobile phone running out of battery power.

My peers in the developing world, however, don't have it quite so easy. Each day my colleagues confront the world's major microbial killers; the causes of acute respiratory infections and diarrheal diseases, tuberculosis, malaria, measles, pertussis, hepatitis B and C infections, neonatal tetanus, AIDS, and dengue fever. But critically, they do this without any of the resources that I consider essential for the diagnosis and treatment of such infections. The sheer volume of patients, the deteriorating facilities in which they are diagnosed and treated, and, more often than not, the limited resources available, all serve to prevent the heroic practitioners of the developing world from accomplishing what they would be able to in more ideal circumstances. Their daily frustrations are no doubt far greater than mine are. It is the paradox of our era that while they struggle, we are so privileged that we are frequently unaware that their struggle exists.

The only way to cope with the developing world's overwhelming problems is to build effective public health systems. Such services monitor the health and well-being of its citizens, identify problems in the environment and among the members of its community, and establish public health practices to address these problems, including the problem of whether proper health care is accessible to all, rich or poor.

The importance of public health elsewhere in the world to our own society may not be at first obvious. Our grandparents grew up in an era when infectious diseases were a frightening reality; when to survive infancy was an accomplishment; when giving birth in and of itself was an invitation to death. At times it seems we have forgotten all this. We now live in comfortable ignorance about the health and well-being of people in faraway places. But in truth we are never very far away from the experiences of our forebears.

We rely today on the effectiveness of medical science and our public health system to protect us. And yet, current medical science and public health practices, really because of their successes, have led to complacency and bureaucratic indifference and have helped to create the real biological peril in which we find ourselves. We live in a world in which new human pathogens emerge and old infectious diseases once thought conquered can resurface with a vengeance. It is bravado to believe that we are now immune to these killers.

Advances in public health and clinical medicine have reduced infant mortality and raised average life expectancy dramatically—at least for the people of the affluent nations of the world—but history also provides examples of public health measures that had an unforeseen catastrophic impact. In 1924, Albert Calmette and Camille Guerin developed a vaccine for tuberculosis that was widely distributed in developing countries. However, the vaccine was also associated with the death of seventy-seven infants in Lubeck, Germany, and vaccine recipients could no longer rely on the diagnostic tuberculin skin test for a diagnosis of tuberculosis infection. By lowering childhood exposure to what had been background microbes, water filtration systems and improvements in environmental sanitation actually left some people more vulnerable. The emergence of polio as an infectious epidemic disease occurred because children did not acquire immunity early in life.

The resurgence and spread of drug-resistant strains of disease-causing microbes represents yet another ongoing threat to our health and well-being. Microbes have the extraordinary capacity for generating genetic variation and growing to immense population sizes at incredible rates; for microbes, minutes are tantamount to years. Natural selection sorts out the best-adapted microbes, fueling an engine of rapid evolutionary change and improvement. Adaptation to a new environment is a potential outcome of this process, and the reason why some disease-causing microbes have developed antibiotic resistance so rapidly. Even now, continuously evolving microbes find their way comfortably into new hosts, and emerge triumphant after selective pressure is applied through drug therapies or vaccine-induced immunity, especially if these medical interventions are only partially effective. Resilient mutated strains of multidrug-resistant bacteria and tuberculosis-causing mycobacteria have evolved by this process and flourished, in part through ignorance of the need to complete a prescribed course of antibiotics and by the overuse and misuse of antimicrobial drugs. In the ungoverned world of biological terrorism, microbes have certainly responded, in a way that humans have yet to fully comprehend. The resurgence and spread of drug-resistant strains of disease-causing microbes once under control and now no longer curable demonstrates the power and productivity of microbial life. It also demonstrates the difficulty in deriving a durable defense against the microbial challenge.

The future of public health is to continue to make a difference in conditions in the broader international community. The challenge is to adapt our public health strategy to control environments and modify behaviors in a constantly changing world. Even with the expertise of modern medicine, people in the industrialized world may be surprised to find that they are woefully unprepared for the far-reaching challenges of an impending large-scale public health catastrophe. We need to develop new and continuing global partnerships with an ambitious, comprehensive agenda to readdress public health policies for the intervention and prevention of epidemic infectious disease. National health care policies should not languish and ultimately fail because politicians do not understand the difference between public health and curative medicine.

What is broken is fixable if the political will is there.

Laurie Garrett has written a provocative book on the global challenge for public health. In a world in which disparities in the health and well-being of populations in industrialized and developing countries are widening and the benefits of public health and disease prevention on life expectancy are not shared, the potential for a global health catastrophe looms large. The author takes us to the impoverished regions of the Indian subcontinent, where pneumonic plague ravages health and refuses to go away, despite readily available preventive measures and affordable curative medicines. In Zaire, outbreaks of Ebola hemorrhagic fever erupt upon disruption of local ecosystems. Curative medicine itself becomes a harbinger of public health calamity as outbreaks of Ebola hemorrhagic fever cluster in the health care setting. In the newly independent states of the former Soviet Union, economic and political instability, further deterioration of an already poor diet, increasing alcohol consumption, and the descent of a struggling medical system into chaos contribute to the resurgence of tuberculosis and a precipitous fall in life expectancy. The poor and vulnerable become oppressed by the ruthless and powerful as the organization of the Russian State disintegrates into a Dostoyevskian nightmare. In America, the public health system struggles to cope with threats to the health and well-being of the population because of inadequate regulatory staff to properly inspect and protect food and drinking water. Laurie Garrett's vision of this breakdown is indelible.

Albert Schweitzer wrote, "Man can hardly recognize the devils of his own creation." We need to take responsibility for our actions. It is a disturbing message and an urgent wake-up call for what must be done to avert a full-scale crisis. Laurie Garrett's plea demands our attention. She gives us a warning we dare not ignore. Our descendants may recall the latter half of the twentieth century as a lull in the gathering storm.

STEVEN M. WOLINSKY, M.D.
Professor of Medicine
Northwestern University Medical
School

INTRODUCTION

Act, before disease becomes
persistent through long delays.

—Ovid, 43 B.C. to A.D. 17

When I am not traveling on some distant continent, I walk across the Brooklyn Bridge at least once a day. Usually I'm in a hurry, racing to my office or an appointment, and the trek is executed at a dash, slowed only by the throngs of gawking tourists. There are days, however, when I am so overcome by the beauty of my adopted hometown, by its breathtaking skyscape and historic harbor that, like the tourists I sometimes disparage, I am compelled to stop cold in my tracks and stare. And in those moments, as I gaze over Wall Street, the ferry building, Ellis Island, and the Statue of Liberty, my imagination invariably rolls backward in time, to the mid-nineteenth-century days before the bridge anchorage upon which I stand was erected. In my mind's eye the harbor is packed, deck to deck with clippers and other sailing ships bearing cargo from all over the world. I can hear the shouting of stevedores and skippers. And I can see the great Brooklyn journalist Walt Whitman leaping from ship to ship as he crosses the East River from his *Brooklyn Eagle* offices, located just a few blocks from my home, to the bustling South Street Seaport of Manhattan. Nearly all of New York City was concentrated on that tiny tip of Manhattan Island, triangulated by the harbor, the Hudson River, and the misnamed East River—actually no river at all, but a tidal basin.

There are few places on earth where the populace races forward in time at a pace as furious as that pursued by New Yorkers. There's no time to look. Progress: it's a Manhattan mantra each new generation of immigrants has chanted. Not all progress was achieved in a deliberate, sagacious manner. Indeed, much simply sprung from catastrophe, as disasters gave birth to long-neglected or serendipitous change. Such certainly was the case for the health of New Yorkers. And, in many instances, for their general lifestyle. No matter how sorry their own lot, the immigrants dreamed that the fortunes of their children and grandchildren would be better. Progress.

I can almost see them when I pause on my bridge perch long enough to allow my imagination to slow. From that vantage point I can take in all that once was New York City back in the days when fewer than half of its children lived to blow out the candles on their eighteenth birthday cakes. I see Governors Island in front of me and visualize clipper ships held there in quarantine during hot, sticky summer weeks while the populace of Manhattan cowered in fear of yet another devastating epidemic of cholera, smallpox, or yellow fever. In dingy offices near City Hall scientists dutifully logged in the death tolls, using the latest statistical techniques to determine how many fewer, or more, New Yorkers succumbed in this year's plague, compared to the last. Progress then edged its way around the world at the pace of the winds in sails or of horses drawing wagons. Even so, its inexorable forward movement allowed spread of microbes to new continents with such devastating results as the obliteration of Native Americans and the introduction of smallpox to every human niche of the planet.

In this city of immigrants, nativists, and escaped slaves modern public health was invented. Sure, elements of the science and policies that form the core of public health also arose in London, Paris, Berlin, and Boston, but it was in Gotham at the dawn of the twentieth century that bands of sanitarians, germ theory zealots, and progressive political leaders created the world's first public health infrastructure. From its inception New Amsterdam, and later New York City, was a global trading post, its very survival dependent upon its multilingual, diverse population. While other colonial outposts also shipped goods, New York surpassed colonial competition by opening its harbor to ships and immigrants from all over the world. And in so doing, New York also opened itself up to the world's diseases. The city, from its earliest seventeenth-century days, had only two options: close itself off and suffer economically, or open its arms to the world while creating systems within the city to control disease. For two hundred years New Yorkers fought off epidemics and pestilence, learning by erring how to create an enormous metropolis that was, from at least a disease perspective, safe. Vital statistics, clean water, pasteurized milk, mass vaccination, less hazardous workplaces, public sewers—these were the hallmarks, achieved one agonizing step after another, of Gotham's public health system.

In the mid-1990s I wrote *The Coming Plague: Newly Emerging Diseases in a World Out of Balance*,[1] which looked at the reemergence of infectious diseases. It was clear to me then that the only dam that could effectively hold back the river of microbes and threatening pathogens was that very public health infrastructure.

To be effective, of course, a twenty-first-century infrastructure could no longer be confined to Gotham, or Los Angeles, or the United States of America:

it had to be global in scale. The very measures that ensured longer lives for New Yorkers at the dawn of the twentieth century would have to be implemented planetwide a century later if disease in one earthly ecosphere could be held at bay, away from the other towns, cities, and suburbs of the planet. Such a global public health infrastructure would have to embrace not just the essential elements of disease prevention and surveillance that were present in wealthy pockets of the planet during the twentieth century, but also new strategies and tactics capable of addressing global challenges.

To prevent the sorts of pandemics envisioned by scientists in *The Coming Plague* pharmaceutic, laboratory, government, and health forces worldwide would have to be marshaled as never before. The goal could not be a technological quick fix. Rather, society needed to take aim at a far more complex—and elusive—target, comprised not just of the fruits of scientific labor but also of politics, sociology, economics, and even elements of religion, philosophy, and psychology.

When *The Coming Plague* was published I was deluged with demands for solutions. As a journalist I felt uncomfortable: it wasn't my role to solve society's dilemmas, only to describe them. But as a global citizen I despaired. I could, indeed, see solutions, but they didn't fit into tidy sound bites—or bytes. And some of the answers appeared so complex that I felt inadequate to the task of elucidation.

I needed to know more.

To begin with, I had to understand what, exactly, was a public health infrastructure. I needed to see public health in action. I needed to fully comprehend how such an infrastructure worked—or, all too often—failed.

But how strong does such an infrastructure have to be? How much taxpayer money or international aid is needed to stave off disease? How vulnerable is the safety net that protects the health of New York City or any other society by providing for its most vulnerable and impoverished members?

To answer those questions, I went to the former Soviet Union in 1997, traveling across twelve time zones—from Western Europe to Eastern Siberia—for four months. I witnessed numerous epidemics, falling life expectancies, hospitals bereft of even the most fundamental supplies, physicians earning their livings as taxi drivers, and surging new health crises. It was abundantly clear that public health infrastructures were not terribly resilient; in the face of societal stress and economic difficulty they quickly collapsed. And the impact on human health was immediately observable.

It was also apparent that the Communist leaders of the Soviet Union had some bizarre notions of public health, based on ideologically inspired misinterpretations of biology. They rejected all notions of biological determinism, packing off to gulags and firing squads those geneticists who sought to prove that evolution was real, and that life began with the genetic molecules DNA and RNA. The staunch opposition to evolutionary theory of Joseph Stalin's reign left Soviet scientists and physicians intellectually crippled—a disability that still afflicted public health in that region of the world ten years after the collapse of communism.

In search of public health answers I also traveled extensively in sub-Saharan Africa and India, where public health crises abounded. Africa's struggle to catch up economically with the rest of the world was showing success in several countries, and public health improvements often—but not always—followed. But as the Ebola epidemic in Zaire illustrated, an unstable, corrupt society is inevitably a public health catastrophe. Many of the former Soviet nations shared with Zaire and other African nations deep-seated corruption that drained the life blood from their social sectors just as parasites suck the essence of life from the guts of infected children. The pandemics of drug-resistant tuberculosis and HIV further drained Africa's fragile economies, reversing their courses of progress and development, and commanding all of their public health resources. Every filled graveyard in Africa's plagued cities signaled another loss to the workforce and another step backward.

Progress: such an elusive pursuit.

In India's case economic progress brought worsening public health. The federal government, eager to spend its growing wealth on nuclear weapons and military efforts, relinquished all responsibility for the health of its one billion citizens. It turned public health over to the states, most of which lacked the resources and political will to do much more than create bloated, corrupt, inefficient bureaucracies. India had no real national public health infrastructure at the end of the twentieth century: no surveillance system, no reporting mechanism, barely a vital statistics registry.

But surely public health in the United States had witnessed bold progress during the twentieth century: as I stand on my beloved Brooklyn Bridge every day am I not gazing at a populace that is profoundly healthier than its great-grandparents?

To understand why America's public health leaders felt worried, cynical, and even besieged in the 1990s I focused on the history of the health of the peoples of New York City, the County of Los Angeles, and the State of Minnesota. The choice of New York City was an obvious one, as it had been the birthplace of modern public health.

Los Angeles County is where I and four generations of my ancestors grew up. When my grandmother, Evelyn MacKenzie Garrett, worked in the early twentieth century as a public health nurse in the Clara Barton Hospital in Los Angeles, the region had 875,000 residents, and the needs of those individuals—Californians and Mexicanos, alike—were, in the main, met. Occasional epidemics of scarlet fever, measles, and other infectious diseases claimed hundreds of lives. But Los Angeles County's sparsely populated expanse, temperate climate, and high employment rate guaranteed comparatively long lives for its citizenry.

By the time I finished college and graduate school, however, Los Angeles County boasted a 1980 population of 7.5 million people, and sharp political, cultural, and economic divides splintered the populace. A steady flow of Spanish-speaking immigrants from nations to its south ensured California a large, cheap labor force. But for Los Angeles County, which was responsible for the region's vast public health needs, the new Hispanic population only aggravated racial and economic tensions that already were high vis-à-vis the African-American population. During the aerospace industry boom of the early 1980s money flowed faster than Los Angeles water, for those fortunate enough to work in the proper economic sectors. And for the first time, amid wild real estate speculation, access to affordable housing reached crisis proportions. The public revolted, freezing property taxes.

And in the 1990s, with the county's population topping ten million and racial and class tensions genuinely explosive, the county struggled to pay public health bills with ever-decreasing property tax revenues. By 2001 Los Angeles County will have eleven million residents, half of whom speak Spanish in their homes, and the area's public health needs will increasingly reflect those of the regions where the new immigrants come from: Mexico, Central America, Indochina.

Under its constitution California placed responsibility for public health at the county level, and gargantuan Los Angeles County struggled to meet its mandate. In the 1990s it nearly went bankrupt doing so, and as the twenty-first century dawned the county's ability to pay its health bills was tenuous.

The prairie state of Minnesota approached the millennium wealthy, healthy, and sassy. After World War II it built the strongest public health infrastructure in the nation. In 1997 Minnesotans were among the ten longest-living populations in the world, and their public health system was internationally admired. But political winds shifted at the close of the 1990s, and Minnesota set to dismantling its social systems.

A sound public health system, it seems, is vital to societal stability and, conversely, may topple in the face of political or social instability or whim. Each affects the other: widespread political disorder or antigovernmentalism may weaken a public health system, and a crisis in the health of the citizenry can bring down a government.

The year 2000 found health in the old Superpowers endangered. And in the world's poor nations, where most of the planet's population resided, every improvement in health seemed to be smashed on the shores of underdevelopment. In 1996 Canadian scientist Joseph Decosas decried underdevelopment at a gathering of AIDS researchers in Vancouver.[2] Holding an imaginary glass of water in the air Decosas grimly said that "if the solution for AIDS would be to bring a glass of clean water to everybody in the world, we would *not* be able to bring that. We have not been able to stop children from dying from simple diarrhea by providing clean drinking water."

We have not, at the millennium, been able to bring clean water, food, or life's succor to the world's poor.

Every night in 1997 more than 200 million Indians went to bed hungry, officially malnourished—including half of the country's children. In China a smaller percentage of the nation's children—one out of every five—was malnourished, but 164 million Chinese went to sleep with hunger gnawing at their stomachs. As did some 25 million Pakistanis, 15 million Brazilians, and more than a third of all Africans.[3] In the Democratic Republic of the Congo (formerly Zaire) and central Africa half the population was malnourished, and globally in the 1990s nearly 800 million people on any given day were starving, or a population roughly two and a half times the size of that of the United States of America.[4]

No wonder that AIDS researchers moaned about the seemingly impossible requirements for a viable HIV vaccine: 100 percent efficacy, 100 percent safety, stability in tropical heat, and a price of less than one dollar a dose. Even at that price such a vaccine might be as elusive for the world's poor as Decosas's clean glass of water. While science searched for technological solutions, what really stymied most of the world was frighteningly basic.

In Eastern Europe the 1990s saw a rocky road to economic recovery, but progress did, indeed, emerge in such countries as Poland, the old East Germany, and the Czech Republic, with average per capita incomes nearly doubling during the decade. Not so farther east in the Slavic, Baltic, and Central Asian nations of the former Soviet Union. There wealth concentrated in the hands of former Communist bosses, criminals, and bankers, leaving the populaces in despair. In 2000 Russia ranked as the number one riskiest economy for foreign investment.[5]

Progress for public health seemed at the millennium chained to economics. Nations could not advance so long as their populaces were debilitated by illness. And they lacked the financial abilities to build health infrastructures. Still, optimists drew satisfaction from the World Bank's strong commitment to public health and its increasing global recognition that healthy nations developed more rapidly than those impeded by an ailing populace. That message was the World Health Organization Director-General Gro Harlem Brundtland's battle cry in 1999.

But the new century finds experts at odds over the mission of public health. No two deans of the West's major schools of public health agree on a definition of its goals and missions. While one school—the University of California, Berkeley—selected a biotechnology executive in 1998 as its dean, another—Harvard—opted that year for a leader whose battle was against the most ancient—even traditional—scourge, tuberculosis. A schism appeared and widened in academia, pitting technologists and health managers against the more traditional advocates of disease prevention and epidemiology.

Regardless of the mission statements of academic centers, it was clear by the 1990s that public health, as a discipline, was changing radically. Whether its practitioners were running family planning clinics in Cairo, antibiotic import and distribution for Sri Lanka, drinking water surveillance in Moscow, or multibillion-dollar Medicaid programs for the United States, their political clout was diminishing and cost-effectiveness was the watchword of the day. It was no longer sufficient to prove that a given intervention prevented disease and saved lives: now it had to do so *affordably*.

If an arsonist torches an office building the roles of the fire department and police are obvious. When they do their jobs—stop the fire and apprehend the arsonist—the community recognizes their achievements and applauds their actions. Because of this it is politically difficult-to-impossible to slash a police or fire department budget except in times of municipal bankruptcy.[6]

If, in contrast, the workers in that office building are strong, healthy, and long-lived, it is next to impossible to prove that the efforts of local public health officials are responsible.

Public health is a negative. When it is at its best, nothing happens: there are no epidemics, food and water are safe to consume, the citizens are well-informed regarding personal habits that affect their health, children are immunized, the air is breathable, factories obey worker safety standards, there is little class-based disparity in disease or life expectancy, and few members of the citizenry go untreated when they develop addictions to alcoholic or narcotic substances. In the absence of failures in these areas, politicians faced with budgetary crises, or dictators eager to expand their local and regional power, may feel justified in hacking away at government health budgets. Even if epidemics emerge, such as those of HIV, Ebola, pneumonic plague, or drug-resistant tuberculosis, national leadership is often insulated from the danger, as they typically are far more wealthy than the imperiled citizens and have access to elite health coverage.

And public health advocates, fearing for their jobs or programs, may be tempted to bend to political whims of the day, veering away from the voice of Science to back ideological or religious trends. Such was the case in the Soviet Union, where rational genetics and the medical social practices flowing from Darwinian evolutionary understandings were abandoned in favor of the absurd anti-genetics belief system of Lysenkoism. Only those Soviet scientists bent on perverting public health's mission, concocting ghastly biological weapons of mass destruction, were spared the shackles of Lysenkoism in favor of genocidal weapons based on the central dogma of DNA.

The scope of activities that fell under the rubric of public health was by the end of the twentieth century quite broad. In 1988 the U.S. Institute of Medicine (IOM) struggled for a definition of public health,[7] arriving at the following: "The committee defines the mission of public health as fulfilling society's interest in assuring conditions in which people can be healthy."

Elsewhere in their report, the Institute of Medicine committee tried to justify their overbroad definition:

> Knowledge and values today remain decisive elements in the shaping of public health practice. But they blend less harmoniously than they once did. On the surface there appears to be widespread agreement on the overall mission of public health, as reflected in such comments to the committee as "public health does things that benefit everybody," or "public health prevents illness and educates the population." But when it comes to translating broad statements into effective action, little consensus can be found. Neither among the providers nor the beneficiaries of public health programs is there a shared sense of what the citizenry should expect in the way of services, and both the mix and the intensity of services vary widely from place to place.[8]

In other words, there was no agreement about what constituted "public health" other than assuring that people were healthy. In the absence of a coherent definition of the discipline it was no wonder its advocates were struggling to defend their budgets and policies. During the 1980s, the IOM found that every state lost funding and personnel in all areas except provision of clinical health care. Such vital services as drinking water and food quality control, environmental and occupational health, laboratories and disease control all lost money and personnel.[9]

Even the prestigious Institute of Medicine found it difficult to distinguish medicine from public health. Though the two pursuits classically shared few interests and often were in direct conflict, political pressures over the course of the last half of the twentieth century had blurred the borders between the two. In the United States "public health" had become—incorrectly—synonymous with medicine for poor people. Few Americans at the millennium thought of "public health" as a system that functioned in their interests. Rather, it was viewed as a government handout for impoverished people.

When Congress and the White House set out in 1990 to retire the national debt public health suffered and the loss of federal funds was felt all the way down to the level of neighborhood clinics. In its first term the Clinton administration tried to map out a new national health care system, tightly linked with public health and able to absorb the then thirty-seven million uninsured Americans. Unable to find common ground with the Congress and the health insurance industry, the White House was soundly defeated.

By the end of the decade, more than forty-four million Americans were uninsured, the nation had no coherent health care system, and the numbers of uninsured was swelling by 100,000 people each month.[10]

In lieu of a national medical infrastructure, public health and curative medicine were provided by a hodgepodge of for-profit insurers, physician organizations (PPOs), county, state, and federal insurers, health maintenance organizations (HMOs), and managed care companies. With every passing day it became more difficult to decipher who, if anyone, was protecting the public's health. And government public health budgets continued to plummet, dropping 25 percent between 1981 and 1993.[11] While the federal and some state overall health budgets increased between 1994 and 1998, the bulk of those funds were directed to provision of medical care. Most key public health programs took substantial hits.[12]

By 1998 the states with the most people enrolled in HMOs and managed care plans had the weakest safety nets. In California, for example, which led the nation in HMO enrollment, one out of every four citizens was uninsured and the state's largest county health system repeatedly faced bankruptcy.

The health management perspective also found adherents in Europe, Latin America, and the developing world. Managed care advocates marched across Russia, the Baltics, Eastern Europe, and the Caucasus preaching the gospel of cost controls and team care. Western European governments, long the prime health providers in their societies, glommed on to the managed care miracle in hopes of slimming down their budgets, a key component at play in the new global capitalism.

And the World Health Organization, once the conscience of global health, lost its way in the 1990s. Demoralized, rife with rumors of corruption, and lacking in leadership, WHO floundered. Other international agencies—notably the World Bank and UNICEF—stepped up to the plate. By 1997 the World Bank was the biggest public health funder in the world, bankrolling $13.5 billion worth of projects, primarily in developing countries.[13]

"The health of the world stands at a crossroads," wrote an august group of international health leaders.[14] "For half a century, most countries have achieved impressive progress in their health conditions. Yet the causes of ill-health do not stand still—humanity's very progress changes them. The past decade has witnessed a profound transformation in the challenges to global health; persistent problems have been joined by new scourges in a world that is ever more complex and interdependent. The idea that the health of every nation depends on the health of all others is not an empty piety but an epidemiological fact."

It was time to face reality: as the vital statistics of the human race appeared to be improving, the threat, even materialization, of reversal was ever present.

It begs the question: what is public health?

It is not curative medicine. CT scans, open heart surgery, hormone treatments, fiber optic visualizations—these are all great boons for medicine, but they are not public health. And, perhaps surprisingly, they have not been responsible for the vast improvements in the public's health. Even vaccines and antibiotics—both of them vital tools of the modern public health arsenal—have contributed comparatively little to population-based improvements in such key indicators of public health as life expectancy, infant mortality, and infectious disease deaths.

Vital statistics data from England, Wales, and Sweden show that in 1700 the average male in those countries lived just twenty-seven to thirty years. By 1971 male life expectancy reached seventy-five years. More than half that improvement occurred before 1900; even the bulk of the twentieth-century increases in life expectancy were due to conditions that existed prior to 1936. In all, 86 percent of the increased life expectancy was due to decreases in infectious diseases.[15] And the bulk of the decline in infectious disease deaths occurred *prior* to the age of antibiotics. In the United Kingdom, for example, tuberculosis deaths dropped from nearly 4,000 per million people to 500 per million between 1838 and 1949, when antibiotic treatment was introduced. That's an 87 percent decline. Between 1949 and 1969 the TB death rate fell only another forty million cases to 460 cases per million, or 9 percent.

The same can be said for the United States, where less than 4 percent of the total improvement in life expectancy since the 1700s can be credited to twentieth century advances in medical care.[16]

It is a matter of considerable academic debate which factors were most responsible for the spectacular improvements seen in life expectancy and infant mortality in the United States and Western Europe between 1700 and 1900. A constellation of the following were key: nutrition, housing, urban sewage and water systems, government epidemic control measures, swamp drainage and river control engineering, road construction and paving, public education and literacy, access to prenatal and maternity care, smaller families, and overall improvements in society's standards of living and working. In the early twentieth century elimination of urban, overcrowded slums that lacked plumbing and toilet facilities clearly improved the health of tens of thousands of Americans and Europeans.

The critical dilemma for the twenty-first century was embedded in the disparity between the rich and poor, both within and among nations. In the wealthy world the twenty-first century was greeted by stock markets ebullient about biotechnology and protein-based public health—the alleged pharmacopeia of future disease prevention. But in much of the world the core advances in public health pioneered between 1890 and 1920 in New York City had yet, a century later, to take hold. Drinking water remained contaminated; human waste was dumped untreated; children went unvaccinated and malnourished; hygiene was ignored in hospitals and precious antibiotics were dispensed like candy in black markets worldwide.

What New York public health pioneer Hermann Biggs and his colleagues demonstrated before World War I in Gotham was that public health not only had little to do with organized medicine, but that it might often be antagonistic to physicians. It would oppose schemes that placed individual health in primacy over the good of the public, as a whole. Biggs battled doctors over the naming of tuberculosis patients, for example: doctors wanted discretion for wealthy clients while Biggs demanded safety for all New Yorkers. Public health fought on behalf of the community, placing special attention on the poorest, least advantaged elements of that community, for it was amid conditions of poverty that disease usually arose.

Public health is not an ideology, religion, or political perspective—indeed, history demonstrates that whenever such forces interfere with or influence public health activities a general worsening of the populace's well-being usually followed. As envisioned by its American pioneers public health was a practical system, or infrastructure, rooted in two fundamental scientific tenets: the germ theory of disease and the understanding that preventing disease in the weakest elements of society ensured protection for the strongest (and richest) in the larger community.

As infectious diseases became less of a concern in the wealthy world, in the mid-twentieth century public health leaders struggled to apply those basic tenets, and the infrastructure upon which they were based, to nonmicrobial collective health issues, such as cancer and heart disease. The translation was not easy, and in some arenas it clearly failed. It proceeded most coherently where the cause of disease—the culprit—had an outside, threatening nature similar to the fear invoked by mysterious microbes. In the world of fin de siècle New York City in the 1890s germs were sufficiently fearful to members of all social classes and ethnic groups as to readily drive communitywide solutions and support for public health. Similarly, in the second half of the twentieth century public health benefited by characterizing the tobacco industry and polluters as sources of cancer threat to the community, fast-food distributors as heart disease promoters, and radiation emitters as creators of deformed babies.

But the links were never as strong, either scientifically or politically, as those Biggs, France's Louis Pasteur, and their contemporaries made between germs and infectious diseases.

Public health in the wealthy world, therefore, struggled to maintain respect, funding, and self-definition in the late twentieth century.

It was no coincidence that one hundred years previously the precious concept of public health arose in New York City, as it was the world's center of nineteenth- and twentieth-century globalization. The public health leaders of Biggs's day weren't uniformly progressive individuals—indeed, many were flat-out bigots. But they were a practical lot. They understood that the economy of Gotham thrived on globalism, and that such a vast economic reach necessarily held risks. Chief among those risks were the microbial hitchhikers carried inside the immigrants, travelers, and cargo from all over the world. When the immigrants settled into horrible, crowded tenements lacking toilets and running water, the risk to the community was compounded, as even rare and latent diseases could be amplified in such environs into terrible epidemics. Thus, they reasoned, it was in the interests of the community as a whole to address the health needs of those tenement dwellers, providing milk to the children, disease surveillance and epidemic control for all, food inspections, pure water, clean streets, shorter and safer work hours, and improved housing.

In the newly globalized economy of the twenty-first century no part of the planet is too remote, too exotic, or too forbidding for travelers or business development. The whole world is becoming New York City—a polyglot of multiple language-babbling traders, artists, social classes, religions, and tensions.

Even hatreds and community conflicts have globalized. A group of alienated individuals might fight its battles on home turf or, quite frequently, choose symbolic sites thousands of miles away to target with weapons of terrorism. A confrontation in Asia might play out in a series of bombings in Paris, Berlin, and Chicago. By the 1990s the U.S. government was fixated on terrorism, recognizing not only foreign but also domestic forces capable and willing to resort to the use of deadly force against innocent civilians. Deadliest of all options—frightening beyond words—was the specter of deliberate release of supergerms that would sweep around the world claiming tens of thousands of lives in man-made epidemics.

The U.S. government once again turned to technology for answers, hoping some device could be invented that would sense such weapons of bioterrorism before their release. Once again public health—the *only* viable protection against epidemics, whether natural or man-made—was given short shrift.

If anthrax were released in Grand Central Station one morning, who would be the first in New York City to realize such a dastardly act had been committed?

Surely it would not be some mythical sensory device, nor the law enforcement officials wielding the contraption. It would be members of the public health infrastructure, alerted by hospital reports of unusual illnesses cropping up from Brooklyn to the Bronx.

In the absence of such an infrastructure, Gotham would be doomed to an anthrax epidemic that could not be stanched by millions of dollars of high-tech military and FBI interventions. The saviors of the city could only be her public health warriors.

From my perch on the Brooklyn Bridge, I can see jet after jet circle out of John F. Kennedy International Airport: the ships are gone, and the new globalism is airborne. Time has collapsed, bringing risks and opportunities to every community within days. Tomorrow it will be hours. Perhaps by 2050 it will be minutes. Progress.

The challenges of public health have never been greater, either in counties like Los Angeles, prosperous states such as Minnesota, or former superpowers like the Russian Federation. Each is now linked to the other. The community has expanded. Its membership is six billion human beings, more than five billion of whom live in the global equivalent of New York City's 1890s tenements.

For most of the world's population in 2000, the public health essentials mapped out in New York before World War I have never existed: progress, in the form of safe water, food, housing, sewage, and hospitals, has never come. An essential trust, between government and its people, in pursuit of health for all has never been established. In other parts of the world—notably the former Soviet Union—the trust was long ago betrayed.

Yes, scientific and medical tools invented in the twentieth century will form a vital basis to global public health efforts in the twenty-first century, as will bold innovations based on altering human and microbial genetics. But the basic factors essential to a population's health are ancient and nontechnological: clear water; plentiful, nutritious, uncontaminated food; decent housing; appropriate water and waste disposal; correct social and medical control of epidemics; widespread—or universal—access to maternal and child health care; clean air; knowledge of personal health needs administered to a population sufficiently educated to be able to comprehend and use the information in their daily lives; and, finally, a health care system that follows the primary maxim of medicine— *do no harm*.

In the days of Biggs and Pasteur public health was local, manageable enough if backed with sufficient political support. Its infrastructure provided, first and foremost, communitywide prophylaxis against disease.

Now the community is an entire world. It watches, and squirms, as plague strikes Surat, Ebola hits Kikwit, tuberculosis overwhelms Siberian prisons, and

HIV vanquishes a generation of Africans. The community grows anxious. Though it empathizes, it fears that what is "over there" could come "here." Worse, as it bites into bananas grown "over there," the community collectively worries: what microbes or pesticides am I consuming?

Public health needs to be—must be—global prevention.

Now that would be genuine progress.

CHAPTER ONE

FILTH AND DECAY

**Pneumonic plague hits India
and the world ill responds.**

*This town is coming like
     a ghost town
No job to be found
     in this country.
Can't go on no more,
          people getting angry.
This town is coming like
     a ghost town.
This town is coming like
     a ghost town.
This town is coming like
     a ghost town.
This town is coming like
     a ghost town.
This town is coming like
     a ghost town.*

From "Ghost Town"
—The Specials, 1981

No one else got off the train. Thousands got on.

Even before the aging Indian locomotive lumbered its way into Surat passengers began scouring their sacks and suitcases in search of rags or scarves to wrap around their faces. Protesting children wailed, but mothers, speaking Hindi, Tamil, Punjabi, Bengali, or English, sharply insisted.

"You must wear this, child. It will protect you," they said. And as the train approached the city the children's dark eyes widened above their impromptu masks and the rocking passengers grew silent.

The only Westerner aboard gathered her bags and, to the obvious astonishment of fellow passengers, exited the train, stepping into the torrid September heat of Surat. Throngs of masked Suratis, encumbered with bags and infants, elbowed their ways onto the train, shouting and jostling for seats. Though they had tickets, most would gladly stand for hours if need be, relieved to get far away from the monsoon-soaked city.

Far away from the plague.

In less than a week 500,000 residents of Surat had fled, forming a diaspora of Suratis that, thanks to India's vast train system, now stretched from the Himalayas to Sri Lanka. An estimated 600,000 day workers and business travelers who normally visited the gem and fabric districts of Surat stayed away. Thus, less than half of Surat's typical daily census of 2.2 million remained. They were the poorest of the Gujarat State's poor: lower caste citizens who could no more conjure the seventy rupees (or $2.50) for a lower class train ticket than $500 for a seat on a jet.

As the chugging sound of the departing train dissipated, a near silence, punctuated by occasional motorbike rickshaws, reigned. Four train cars remained, painted with large red crosses and signs saying ACCIDENT MEDICAL RELIEF. The grounds around the cars were chalk white with thick layers of DDT pesticide powder.

Trash and garbage blew about the streets, inspected by foraging cows sacred to the largely Hindu population. Roads that usually resonated with the high frequencies of diamond polishing devices and 300,000 power textile looms were silent. Boards, loosely hammered in place, sealed shut the pharmacies, private medical clinics, and nongovernmental hospitals. Those citizens who remained moved quickly, rags or masks wrapped about their noses and mouths.

Only the prostitutes near Ved Road flaunted their faces (as well as their figures), calling out from brothel balconies to would-be customers. And, perhaps surprisingly, there were customers, despite the plague.

"This came as a sudden grip, a blow from the sky," declared Gujarat's Minister for Health Subash Shelad. "I wish there weren't so much panic."

But panic had, indeed, taken hold, and Surat was a ghost town. At the sprawling new Holiday Inn a visitor could have any room she pleased, as all of the rest were empty. Meals were a bit limited, as farmers were afraid to bring their goods into the plague-ridden city. And it took some time for the turbaned Sikh doorman to find a rickshaw taxi willing, even for the equivalent of a normal month's wages, to take a visitor about town.

Amid the squalor of open sewers, ramshackle crowded houses, and roaming livestock emerged a cluster of poor Surati men shouting, "Plague! Plague! Plague!" The terrified men raced about madly, waving wooden clubs and shouting for all the world to hear. Kicking up a cloud of dust they settled into a tight circle, staring at the ground. And cowering in terror, trapped between human feet, was a brown rat, its beady eyes blinking in the bright sunlight.

"Plague," a man reiterated, waving his club menacingly at the rat. Yet so great was the collective fear that the men of Ved Road dared not hit the sorry rat lest it might give its assailant a retaliatory bite. After a moment the rodent made its escape, scurrying down a garbage-strewn hillside and disappearing into a DDT-coated hole.

The men looked sheepish. When told that the fleas that may carry *Yersinia pestis* plague-causing bacteria usually inhabit *Ratus ratus*—black rats—the cluster feels its manhood restored, each man puffing up his chest and sternly vowing to kill the first ebony-colored rat he sees.[1]

In September 1994 all of India resonated with plague panic, coupled with a near universal condemnation of a filthy Surat.

"Surat is perhaps the most decrepit, unlivable, and unmanageable Indian city of its size," wrote the *Telegraph*.[2] The Calcutta newspaper was typical of India's major media as it decried the Surati "bankruptcy of administration, the decadence of society and the collapse of basic civic amenities."

Nothing shamed the nation's commentators and intellectuals as deeply as world attention to India's rats, and the urban filth in which they thrived. While politicians wagged their fingers scoldingly at Surat's local government, the nation's intellectual elite found in the symbolic rat reason to denounce the most fundamental aspects of Indian economics and politics. Typical of the perspective were the views expressed by Nikhil Chakravartty, who noted that the vast Indian nation was ruled by a strong federal hand during the decades of colonialism.[3] But since independence, Chakravartty continued, the centralized federal government had weakened and local administrations had taken over rule of every aspect of Indian life, with disastrous results.

"In short, a fearsome underworld has surfaced in all the metropolitan centres and larger municipalities. The plague menace, we are warned now, spreads through garbage piling up on which rats thrive," Chakravartty wrote. "Come to the best of our urban centres and you will see garbage-piling has become a common feature. In Calcutta, garbage reaches mountainous proportions before it is touched by municipal authorities. Bombay may be better off in the posh super-rich pockets, but things are no better in the densely populated areas.

"It is fashionable nowadays to talk of globalisation, of getting into the world currents. But if our municipalities and district boards are in a state of disuse and become the inevitable breeding ground of epidemics, what sort of economic miracle are we going to bring about?"

Like their American and European counterparts in the late nineteenth century, India's intellectuals in 1994 cried out for sanitation and hygiene, the absence of which they blamed not only for the plague, but also for every imaginable failure in their society.

On such a note of hand-wringing, J. N. Dixit wrote that "this crisis should impel us to ruminate on the economic and social implications of such an epidemic. Speaking of crises, at times, one is pushed to superstitious apprehension, even para-psychological paranoia about India's fate!"[4]

But the focus of plague paranoia was nothing as surreal as parapsychology but rather the mundane, eyesore-inflicting, nose-offending filth that filled the streets and alleys of India, having long since become the single most familiar and reliable feature of her urban landscapes.

"It's as if a medieval curse is upon us. But the hex is self-inflicted. We are our own worst murderers. Because we are the practitioners of filth. The emperors of garbage," read one editorial in *India Today*.[5] "As in all societies that have made progress, a groundswell of public opinion against dirt and disease has been the backbone of fundamental reform because it is a simultaneous upheaval against endemic corruption and fatalism. Ultimately, the health of a nation is also its wealth. There are dramatic movements in this country in the fields of entrepreneurship, economic modernization, science and technology. But unless this collective lurch toward progress is accompanied by a vision of a cleaner and more hygienic life, India will never quite qualify in the eyes of the international community as a modernising nation. Nobody wants to invest in the dark ages."

And so by the fourth week of the epidemic, fires burned in every city in the nation, filling the air with the putrid smell of flaming garbage. Herds of day workers built mountains of awesome height made entirely of filth, doused them in gasoline, and with these pyres hoped to set India on a course from Plague to Progress. In perhaps the most vivid symbolism of the day, city administrators in Bombay hired Irula tribesmen from the southernmost state of Tamil Nadu to hunt rats in the city of some fourteen million humans crammed so densely that an average of 130,000 souls lived in each square mile. Famed for their rodent-catching skills, the Irula tribesmen had for centuries eaten rats, which comprised their major daily source of protein. Bombay told the Irula they could eat all they wanted, and actually get paid for their feasting.

But, despicable as Surat's verminous filth was, the stench, garbage, and rodents of the city played little, if any, role in the start or spread of the nation's plague epidemic. While it may have sparked a long overdue urban beautification campaign, the plague in Surat had much more to do with horrid housing, human panic, and bereft health care than *Ratus ratus*.

It didn't even start in Surat. And flea-ridden rats in the Gujarati city weren't responsible for its spread.

The epidemic began hundreds of miles to the southeast in a rural part of Maharashtra State, the capital of which is Bombay.

The earthquake hit while villagers slept, striking with a Richter force of 6.4: not enough to topple well-constructed freeway overpasses in Los Angeles, but quite sufficient power to level the mud and brick homes of the Beed and Osmanabad Districts. The September 30, 1993, earthquake's epicenter was the eastern Maharashtra city of Latur, in which tens of thousands of homes were leveled. Surrounding Latur some ten thousand villages were obliterated, one million homes destroyed, and more than ten thousand people killed.

For days afterward aftershocks of up to Richter scale 5.0 rocked the Osmanabad and Beed Districts, prompting a human exodus of survivors who fled the earth's rage. The peasants of Beed, being practical sorts, hastily harvested their crops and locked the food inside whatever structures had outlasted the earthquake before decamping the region.

The Indian government, with about $30 million in financial aid from the World Bank, erected prefabricated houses, sprinkling the structures where Latur's villages once had stood. And the residents trickled back into the region during the summer of 1994.[6]

No one in India had seen a case of plague in more than thirty years. During the 1980s, convinced that *Yersinia pestis* bacteria had disappeared from India, state governments one by one shut down their plague stations, stopped looking for cases, and eventually even ceased random rat and flea checks.

On August 26, 1994, Yashitha Langhe, a man from the village of Mamala, located near Beed, returned to his earthquake-ruined home. He opened doors sealed for months behind which he had hastily stored harvested grains before fleeing the tremors eleven months previously. And he was overwhelmed by a cloud of black fleas that seemed to leap from the decrepit storeroom, biting at every millimeter of his body. When he looked down it seemed that the very ground on which he stood was moving.

At his feet, and all about the Mamala man, were black rats, grown fat and populous, thriving on the stored grain bounty. The Mamala man's experience was repeated that week in village after village, in Beed, outside Latur, as earthquake refugees returned to their hamlets to lay claim to new government-built houses and retrieve their caches of grains.

Yersinia pestis is a bacterium that can survive for extended periods of time in an apparently dormant state in soil. This capacity was overlooked when Indian officials decided to abandon all plague surveillance programs. In Maharashtra State, plague public health programs were eliminated in 1987; the last officially certified human case appeared in nearby Karnataka State in 1966.

The bacteria can also hide in the guts of fleas, causing no harm to the insects, quietly reproducing and passing their offspring off to subsequent generations of fleas.

But when conditions change—in ways no one clearly understood even by the end of the twentieth century—a genetic signal is triggered in the bacteria's DNA. A gene called *hms* (for hemin storage) switches on, causing the secretion of proteins that essentially shift the *Yersinia pestis* population from acting as a benign commensal thriving in the gut of a flea into a superdangerous bacterial collective that invades the insect's foregut. There, the microbes block the movement of food, and the flea begins to starve.[7]

The starving flea shifts its diet and, frantic, becomes far more aggressive. It will then in a frenzy assertively attack any warm-blooded creature, living off the blood that it extracts from the animal's body. Rats, particularly those of the black *Ratus ratus* species, are primary targets. And aboard the rats the fleas are protected by the rodent's fur and are highly mobile, carried energy-free by the scurrying creatures.

When humans come in proximity of the rats the plague-carrying fleas are capable of leaping distances that are orders of magnitude greater than their own size, landing on *Homo sapiens* skin to feast on 98.6°F blood.[8]

Yersinia pestis then has other tricks in its genetic bag. The bacteria have a slew of special genes—at least twenty of them—that give the organism unique powers over the cells of humans and other animals. The instant *Yersinia* come in contact with human cells these genes switch on, causing production of a lethal cascade of chemicals.

The first set of chemicals drill a microscopic hole in the protective membrane of the human cell.[9] Then another set of genetically coded proteins becomes a transport tube carrying chemicals from *Yersinia* into the victimized cell. These chemicals swiftly incapacitate the targeted cell.

Meanwhile, *Yersinia* also secretes a set of proteins into its immediate environment that blocks defensive efforts of the human's immune system. Mighty macrophages—large immune system cells that usually gobble up invading microbes—are rendered impotent by the *Yersinia* chemicals. The effectiveness of this stunning and complex system of attack lies in the fact that these genes, and the proteins they encode, are not originally of bacterial origin. They are animal genes, stolen millenia ago through unknown means and put to deadly, effective purpose by the bacteria. Thus, a protein system originally intended to serve an entirely different purpose—a benign role—in animal cells has evolved into one of the most complicated and efficient offensive weapons apparatuses in the microbial world.

If *Yersinia* takes hold in cells of the skin and lymphatic system a disease called bubonic plague results. As colonies of *Yersinia* grow, the human's lymph nodes swell, often to enormous sizes, and ugly pustules form on the skin, oozing yellow, viscous liquid.

In the villages around Beed people began by late August to develop precisely these symptoms. And on September 14, 1994, Indian Union Health Secretary M. S. Dayal confirmed that there were four cases of bubonic plague in Mamala, Beed District, Maharashtra State.

Two days later the Maharashtra State authorities announced that 10 percent of the village population of Mamala were suffering bubonic plague, and India's National Institute of Communicable Diseases issued laboratory confirmation that the ailments of the Beed District were caused by *Yersinia pestis*.

While even a handful of cases of bubonic plague would have been justified cause for mass panic in India or anywhere else in the world six decades earlier, there shouldn't have been serious alarm in 1994. After all, *Yersinia* could be defeated with the cheapest and simplest of antibiotics: tetracycline and doxycycline. If administered in the first stages of illness, or simply after suspected exposure to infected fleas, these drugs were usually 100 percent curative.

Once illness was established, however, treatment became more problematic. *Yersinia* could move into the red bloodstream, causing septicemia and ravaging the heart and liver. Or it could colonize the lungs, producing pneumonic plague. That was the most contagious and dangerous form of the disease, for once *Yersinia* inhabited the convulsed, coughing lungs of a human being it no longer required rodents or fleas to spread, creating contagion. A microscopic mist of exhaled droplets was sufficient to pass the bacteria from one person to the next.

Untreated, or improperly treated, *Yersinia* easily claimed 50 percent of all infected human beings. But it was inconceivable that any nation in the world at the end of the twentieth century would fail to stop a bubonic plague outbreak, preventing the less easily controlled pneumonic form from emerging.

So on September 16, the Beed District's Health Secretary R. Tiwari told local reporters that "there is no need to panic." Help, he insisted, was on its way. Maharashtra State Health Minister Subash Salunke further insisted that all Beed District plague reports were "wildly exaggerated." But he admitted that *Yersinia* might have surfaced after its long hiatus, because the bacilli, he said, "could live in the soil for ten to fifteen years."

In Bombay, Dr. V. L. Yemul of the Haffkine Institute opined that the region's earthquake had disrupted the ecological niches of long-hidden *Yersinia* colonies, opening up previously hidden soils. Further, he said, in the aftermath of the quake populations of rival rat species grew and fought over the stores of grain left by frightened villagers. Their blood fights attracted fleas, allowing for a surge in that insect population. Thus, he argued, what was seen in the tiny village of Mamala, population 375, was likely to also be occurring in earthquake-ravaged villages throughout the region.

The earthquake had disrupted the health care infrastructure of the region, leveling clinics and driving physicians and nurses from their homes. So local authorities were hard-pressed to identify and treat all the bubonic plague cases.

And further exacerbating the problem was the monsoon, which in 1994 was the most powerful one anyone could recall. Roads were washed out, turning even a short distance into a severe, lengthy journey. A reporter who attempted to travel the roughly 400 kilometers (or 240 miles) of roads from Bombay to Latur had to give up after fourteen grueling hours of dodging elephants, diesel trucks, sacred cows, and other vehicles on a road frequently narrowed to less than a truck's width of passable pavement.

But in truth, India would have had difficulties no matter where *Yersinia* had surfaced, for the country's public health infrastructure was stretched beyond limits. At a time of record-breaking economic growth, India was slashing its public health expenditures, shifting responsibilities from the federal to state levels, and seemingly washing its hands of all responsibility for the people's health. By 1991 to 1992, federal public health spending, which included hospital services, was a mere 0.04 percent of the national budget, or more than tenfold less than was spent in the previous decade.

Bad as that might have been, the 1992 to 1993 federal budget saw a 20 percent further reduction in public spending. And few states compensated by increasing their local public health expenditures. None increased spending by more than 5 percent.

In 1992 only three nations—Brazil, Mexico, and the Russian Federation—were carrying more than India's astounding external debt of $77 billion.[10] Foreign investors had steadily increased their confidence in India, but even with annual growths during the 1990s, private foreign investment in the country was less than $1.5 billion in 1994.[11] The Indian economy grew steadily in the early 1990s by a rate of 4 percent a year—a genuine speed demon pace for India, but a crawl by regional standards. Pakistan in contrast grew by 9 percent annually, South Korea by 10 percent.[12]

Despite its massive external debt and comparatively slow economic growth, India was considered a promising financial state, heading toward a free market and rapidly eliminating former laws that rigidly controlled its industries and limited outside investment. With an estimated 1994 population of 900 to 950 million people and a gross national product (GNP) per capita of $310 per year, every sector of the Indian economy was growing in the early 1990s at rates well above those seen in most of Africa, Eastern Europe, or the Americas. Value-added manufacturing in 1991 was an impressive $40 billion—one of the largest seen in the third world. So the country was easily able to service its national debt and still meet its annual expenditure needs.

The boom was felt especially strongly in India's southern and western states, where trade deregulation prompted entrepreneurial zeal. In Bangalore, for example, industrious Karnatakans created a vast computer software manufacturing empire. Bombay swiftly became the core of capitalistic enthusiasm in India. And to its north Surat almost overnight was transformed.

Between 1971 to 1991, the population of Surat grew by an astounding 151.61 percent, with most of that increase representing impoverished migrant workers who toiled in the $600 million textile or $1 billion diamond industries. As the population grew, so did the number of horrendous slums—up from ninety in the 1960s to three hundred by 1994, inhabited by some 450,000 people. There were no formal sewage or water systems in these slums; housing was slapdash lean-tos, even tents; malaria and hepatitis were epidemic; and no one apparently enforced even India's weak labor and safety regulations in the businesses along Ved Road.

What drew industry to Surat was precisely the weakness of its government, lack of health and pollution enforcement, eager, unskilled labor force, and a virtual tax-free environment. By 1994, one out of every three diamonds mined in the world were polished in Surat.[13]

"Perhaps the greatest irony," wrote the conservative *Business Standard* of Bombay, "is that the epidemic has hit one of the economically most active areas of the country in a state which is considered to be the most business friendly. . . . What is more, the Gujarat government has gone out of its way to be more accommodating to business than most and has in turn been able to reap the benefits of a rapid industrialization which is not the case with the rest of the country. But somehow down the line, the need for good municipal services was forgotten. Businessmen who were busy making money cared little about minimum civic services or the basic quality of life that says no filth, mosquitoes, flies, fleas, and rats. And when the epidemic hit, they were the first to pack their Maruti 1000s and run. India today has clearly got its priorities wrong."[14]

The problem, indeed, was priorities. In 1992 India spent twenty times more on its military than on health. And for a decade, India secretly toiled on a massive, hugely expensive effort to create nuclear weapons. The public health sector was at its lowest rank of any major spending category. Just ahead of it was education, which was so poor in India that only 50 percent of adult males and less than a third of females were able to read, placing India below not just the global literacy average, but subaverage for the poorest nations on earth.[15]

In 1994 nearly a quarter of all Indian children hadn't received their full battery of UNICEF-recommended vaccinations, infant mortality rates were more than ten times those seen in Europe and North America, life expectancy was about fifty-nine years, and more than three humans were born annually for every one that died, guaranteeing that the nation's population explosion would persist well into the twenty-first century.[16]

Meanwhile, India was eager to move swiftly toward a free market and away from its formerly state-regulated socialist economy. It was privatizing many sectors, including health. More than 75 percent of all care was, by the mid-1990s, provided by private physicians, and the essential public health infrastructure was rapidly disappearing.

"Instead of moving forward to meet the newer health challenges, the situation is sliding backwards," Dr. Alok Mukhopadhyay, chair of the Independent Medical Commission on Health in India, said, noting that public health in his country was in a state of "gradual but sure decay."[17]

Against that backdrop, compounded by earthquake and monsoon, Maharashtra's key official, Salunke, and local Beed and Latur health officials struggled in mid-September to keep the bubonic plague epidemic under control. Quick surveys revealed a twentyfold increase in the Latur rat population, with similar rodent explosions counted in Osmanabad. A scouring of local records found that the first complaint of flea infestation was filed, but unheeded, on August 5, and the first human plague case occurred on August 26. Even more disturbing were national plague data released to the media: though India saw no human plague cases from 1966 to 1988, *Yersinia* did, despite prior claims to the contrary, make its comeback in 1989 with three human cases. And in 1991 with fifty. And in 1992 with 135 plague cases nationwide.

Given India's history with plague it seemed a substantial oversight to have dismissed this upward trend in cases. Plague broke out in Calcutta in 1895 and raged across India until 1918, killing more than ten million people.[18] After that *Yersinia* was endemic in India for five decades, claiming more than two and a half million additional lives between 1919 and 1968.

Yet the state governments had all ignored plague surveillance for years. And amid the outbreak in Maharashtra State, officials continued to downplay the situation, telling inquiring journalists that everything was under control.

A key exception was Dr. Syamal Biswas of the Plague Surveillance Unit in distant Bangalore. After investigating the situation around the Beed District of Maharashtra, he pronounced conditions "extremely favorable" for a pneumonic plague epidemic. His warning was ignored.

By that time 317 human bubonic plague cases had been identified in six districts of Maharashtra State. Though officials, including India's Minister of Health G. Shankaranard, continued to insist that there was "no cause for concern," newspapers in Bombay began attacking Maharashtra Governor Sharad Pawar and his government, accusing them of neglect.

"But now that it has happened I say don't worry," Maharashtra's Salunke insisted. "We have beautiful antibiotics. This is not the Middle Ages. We have pesticides. We have surveillance. I promise you, there will not be one death in Maharashtra. Not one."

But plague had already spread and was quietly erupting with lethal impact some six hundred kilometers to the northwest in Surat.

Filthy, ramshackle Surat reeled from the monsoon of 1994. For eighty-seven days rain poured on the city, dropping a record eighty-one inches. The Tapti River swelled and overflowed its banks, flooding the ghettos and slums of the city. Along the notorious Ved Road, considered Surat's most abominable slum, Tapti floodwaters rose perilously, reaching rooftops by the end of August. Tens of thousands of Suratis fled during early August, seeking housing in dry parts of the city. It was not uncommon during August to find a dozen people crammed into a shack that normally housed four, or to espy migrant workers sleeping on the floors between the textile looms or diamond polishing machines on which they toiled during the days.

Even during the dry season Ved Road was a horror. Most of its residents were migrant workers, 10 to 20 percent of them were usually from the Beed and Latur districts of Maharashtra. They crowded into houses and shared a handful of toilet facilities. There were 150 people per toilet, open sewers, and a constant stench.

Thanks to the August monsoon the Tapti waters didn't recede from Ved Road until the second week in September. As if to validate the miracle of Ganesh Chaturthi, the rains stopped on September 10, the Tapti receded below its banks, and the mud of Surat began to dry by September 15. It was cause for genuine joy and celebration, as befits the Festival of Ganesh.

Ganesh, the elephant-headed Hindu god, was a favorite of the poor and disadvantaged, for he had heroically overcome tragedy. Reunited after years of forced separation Ganesh greeted his mother, showering her with hugs and kisses. Upon seeing and mistaking the intent of their warm embraces, the mother's new husband flew into a rage, grabbed his sword, and sliced off Ganesh's head.

"What have you done," cried the mother. "You have killed my son!"

Shamed, the slayer searched frantically for a way to bring Ganesh back to life. Spotting a passing elephant, he chopped off the animal's head and placed it upon Ganesh's neck. And Ganesh became one of the greatest of gods, fun-loving, filled with great fortune, concerned about the poor.

Traditionally Ganesh's saga is celebrated on September 18 with jubilant festivals. Neighborhoods and households compete, each trying to outdo the other with their elephant statues of Ganesh. Amid dancing, singing, and drinking, the statues are paraded about for hours, eventually dumped into a body of water. In Surat, the Ganesh statuary found itself in the Tapti River.

Weeks of monsoon had left much of the Tapti's banks unstable, so the usually spread-out celebrations were concentrated, the crowds of festive poor jam-packed into small spaces. They carried their elephant god high, his four arms and trunk waving to the masses.

Somewhere in those crowds was at least one person from Maharashtra. A plague carrier whose infection had gone untreated and moved into his lungs. He coughed as he celebrated.

And three days later, seven feverish, pneumonic celebrants sought help from Dr. Pradeep Gupta and his staff in the emergency room of Surat Civil Hospital.

"By twelve-thirty we found that seven had been admitted," an exhausted Gupta recalled three days later. "Two had died. They all had bilateral pneumonia and blood in their sputum. And their history of illness was short—certainly less than four days. Then there were other admissions and by Thursday [September 22] by 11:00 A.M. we had thirteen. And seven of the first thirteen were dead."

The first wave of patients all came from the slums of Ved Road.

By then, six weeks after Yashitha Langhe had come down with bubonic plague in far-off Mamala village in Maharashtra, the federal government was insisting that less than seventy people in India had plague, all of them suffering the easily treated bubonic form.

Gupta, a young, energetic civil service physician, suspected instantly that his dead and dying patients were victims of pneumonic plague, a disease he knew only from textbooks. He took his suspicions to Dr. B. D. Parmar, who examined sputum samples from the dead under a microscope. A professor of medicine at the Medical College of Surat, Parmar was typically consulted when Civil Hospital physicians found puzzling infectious disease cases.

"I diagnosed the first case here on September 20," Parmar recalled. "The patient was admitted for malaria that developed suddenly. I ordered an X ray which showed bilateral pneumonia. We treated that case as pneumonic plague, since there are some cases reported from Beed District of bubonic plague. We suspected pneumonic plague since the symptoms were fast-developing over a period of six hours. And the patients developed blood in the sputum and respiratory failure within no time, with bilateral pneumonia."

Parmar's first case was a thirty-five-year-old migrant worker from Maharashtra.

"He had an X ray done at a private hospital," Gupta said of that first patient. "That was at 8 P.M. It looked completely normal. Then he developed a high fever at midnight. On taking his X ray here an hour later, we saw violent signs of pneumonic plague. Violent. He died that night. That indicates the virulence of the organism."

"Was that frightening to you?" a visitor asked.

"Definitely!" Gupta exclaimed, his voice muffled by the three respiratory masks he wore, one of which was designed to protect workmen from chemicals.

"Definitely," he repeated, shuddering.

On September 20, Parmar and Gupta cornered their new boss, the recently appointed medical supervisor of Civil Hospital, Dr. Dinesh Shah. A middle-aged man accustomed to the reins of authority, Shah wanted to see the lab work himself. After examining under the microscope smear samples from the patients, he said, "Yes, looks like pneumonic plague."

Shah ordered smears sent to the National Center for Infectious Diseases in New Delhi and contacted local authorities. But privately he was troubled by seemingly odd aspects of Surat's outbreak. There were no plague-dead rats in the city; all of the first cases were adult men, which seemed strange; there were no initial pediatric cases, which violated patterns seen historically.

"It's very surprising," Shah told his staff. "No ratfall. This just came in straight to the city in pneumonic form. Did someone from Beed come here? Maybe.

"Or maybe," he continued with a chill, "*Yersinia* has mutated."

Professor Parmar was also concerned about the apparent oddities in Surat's epidemic. And he told Shah that without help from the city's 137 private physicians, "This will spread like wildfire. It's a Black Death."

The civil doctors, fully supported by the Gujarat State Minister of Health Subash Shelad, did their level best to calmly spread word of the apparent plague outbreak, hoping to solicit assistance from the city's private physicians.

They were totally unprepared for what followed.

The private doctors panicked. Eighty percent of them fled the city, closing their clinics and hospitals and abandoning their patients. The fear in those physicians' eyes did not go unnoticed by the populace, and rumors of a great impending disaster spread swiftly among the largely illiterate masses. Surat's middle class discreetly packed their bags and slipped out of town.

Then, on September 22, Surati and Bombay newspapers carried banner headlines declaring, "Surat Fever!"

"Over eighty people are feared to have died following the outbreak of a mysterious fever here last night," read the lead of a typical Bombay newspaper article that morning.[19] "Dr. Mahendra Gandhi, a private practitioner in the city, has confirmed forty-five deaths and said the toll is likely to cross eighty."

It was only the opening salvo of a barrage of wildly exaggerated reports that would hit the world's media, most of them relying on panicked private physicians for their information. The BBC, which is hugely popular in India, echoed these reports, saying on September 22 that a mysterious deadly fever had broken out in Surat.

The exodus began.

Within twelve hours of the BBC broadcast an estimated 100,000 Suratis boarded trains headed in every imaginable direction across the Indian subcontinent. Because Surat had no unemployment it had attracted workers from as far away as Bangladesh, Tamil Nadu, Delhi, Uttar Pradesh, Punjab, even Nepal. Now they fled homeward, potentially taking with them infectious microbes.

Friday, September 23, found an estimated 300,000 more Suratis, handkerchiefs wrapped about their faces, queued up for trains. By then the Civil Hospital had seen thirty-one pneumonic plague deaths and its wards were packed with plague and with the worried well. Officials declared Surat a "ghost town," and five states, including Gujarat and Maharashtra, went on emergency health alert status.

News reports across India ran the gamut from the *Times of India*'s calming headline that day ("Disease is infectious, but curable") to the *Daily*'s claim that more than 250 Suratis were dead, and 10,000 had the plague. One report had it that half the population of tiny Kattar village in rural Gujarat were dead, all plague victims. Still another account had it that *all* of Surat was "disease affected."

Bombay was in a frenzy. Most of the Surati exodus came south to India's huge Arabic Sea metropolis, and local radio, television, and newspapers buzzed with rumors of dead rats and people within the city limits. It was said that eight people had died of plague the previous night in the Bombay suburbs of Borivili and Dadar.

So far the only clear casualty of the epidemic was truth. So expansive was the misinformation, government prevarication, and media frenzy that Indians from the Himalayas to the islands of Goa were almost to a one convinced the plague was among them. The reality would later seem disappointingly mundane as most of the ailing were, at least at first, lying in Surat's Civil Hospital.

But the federal government took no actions, made no effort to slow the Surati exodus, and did not offer any concrete assistance to the beleaguered medical staff of Civil Hospital. At the Bombay end of the Maharashtra State government similarly lacked a clear strategy. It seemed helpless to stem the monumental flow of Suratis who poured out of Bombay's several train stations in enormous human herds, quickly disappearing into the suburban and slum crowds of the densely-packed metropolis.

Hysteria was further fueled by India's unique perspective on medicine. Few societies on earth in the late twentieth century were as culturally complex as India. Outsiders often noted that India was like an onion: one peeled layer after layer, often finding cause to weep in the process, but upon reaching the core discovered another onion inside. Each of India's many religions demanded all-encompassing devotion from its followers, affecting every aspect of their lives. And India's experiments with democracy had to avoid granting dominance to any particular religious view. Failure to walk that delicate balancing act usually resulted in mass outpourings of violence.

Medicine and health are, in Western tradition, based primarily in a scientific tradition that requires proof not only of logical theorem but also of practice. The body is a concrete set of molecular and organismic systems. Illness is reversed through a host of interventions which seek to repair failing systems or obliterate invading microorganisms.

That Western medical discipline was widely practiced throughout India, and the Indian Medical Association adhered to scientific traditions that roughly mirrored those professional standards in place in England.

But on official, equal footing under Indian law were ayurvedism, homeopathy, yoga, Tibetan treatments, and a host of other health care traditions that viewed the human body and its illnesses in fundamentally different, usually spiritual, ways. While plague might in 1994 be easily treated with tetracycline under Western allopathic care, antibiotics played little or no role in ayurvedic or other ancient Indian practices.

The result was that nearly anyone could hang up a shingle, declaring himself a physician, and the nation's medical providers represented a mind-boggling blend of genuine healers, crackpots, and exploitative charlatans. More than 75 percent of all health care in India was delivered by "private" physicians, most of whom lacked serious training in either allopathic or other healing traditions and were likely to offer treatments that would certainly be illegal in nations that practiced Western medicine. The new free market atmosphere that reigned over health care in 1994 only exacerbated the problem, pitting charlatans with no medical training in any tradition against legitimate physicians who had devoted more than a decade of their lives to the vigorous study of either allopathic or traditional medicine.

The competition was fierce, and the hardest-fought battles took place in India's largest cities, where physicians practicing all traditions of health care went after the hearts, minds, and rupees of the growing middle class. By 1994 it was glamorous to be an antigovernment physician who decried the stupidities and corruption of state and federal authorities. It was fashionable to declare as lies most government public health declarations. And intra-physician competition often echoed this antiestablishment theme, making the most outrageous of "physicians" chic among the middle and upper castes.

Indeed, India's Minister of Health B. Shankaranand was not a physician, but a businessman who faced indictments on mishandling of public funds during his previous service as petroleum minister. Shankaranand and his predecessor in the Ministry of Health supported an unusual medical paradigm: daily consumption of one's own urine as treatment for cancer or AIDS.[20]

So from the first moments of Surat's epidemic the Indian public was deluged with at least as much misinformation as actual facts. And while it was tempting to blame the media for its lack of accuracy and for yellow journalism,

India's health care establishment had to share credit. The information schism—between truth and fantasy, accuracy and exaggeration—would prove disastrous for India in coming days.[21]

But in Surat itself there were few citizens left who could be misinformed, and nearly the entire medical profession, save the dedicated nurses and physicians of Civil Hospital, had flown the coop.

One exception was Dr. Lalgibai Patel, who on the morning of Thursday, September 22, anxiously paced the halls of Civil Hospital, distraught. His wife, Durga Watideri, had come down during the night with a nasal drip. That seemed pretty minor, Patel said, but rapidly worse symptoms appeared as the night wore on. Her throat began to burn so badly she couldn't swallow.

"And then I discovered she had a serious problem," Patel, who was at his wits' end, recalled. "She had chest pain, vomiting. I took her to a hospital for treatment, a private hospital. But the hospital was closed. By then she was vomiting blood. So then I brought her here." No sooner had twenty-eight-year-old Watideri taken to bed on the Civil Hospital plague ward than Patel's seven-year-old son and twenty-two-year-old brother also came down with the disease.

"Being a man of medicine I was confident of recovery," Patel said. "But then when I saw the horror of it I was terrified."

It would be weeks before Patel's family would recover, though all would, thankfully, live to tell tales of the Plague of '94.

Throughout the hospital nervous families related similar stories, describing sudden illness marked by vomited blood, loss of breath, chest pains, stomach pains, and high fevers. They spoke from behind masks, careful to stay out of the way of exhausted medical personnel. Occasionally tempers flared among the small remaining staff of sleep-deprived doctors and nurses: loud shouts of disagreement rang out in sporadic, brief bursts of rage.

Along the hallway leading to the plague ward masked lower-caste women, dressed in colorful saris, swept the floor and scrubbed the walls as if such cleanliness would prevent spread of *Yersinia* inside the hospital. The ward, separated in half by a long curtain, contained about eighty steel beds, white paint peeling off their rusty frames. Female patients were on the left side of the curtain, males on the right. With all the beds full, additional patients lay upon gurneys. Despite the crowd, there was little sound, as most of the patients were too sick to talk or even moan.

Behind thick isolation doors in two sealed chambers were the most dangerous patients—those who were actively coughing up *Yersinia*-contaminated blood and sputum. The nervous Dr. Gupta, still wearing three masks at a time, moved among the patients, checking their antibiotics, fevers, and pains. His manner betrayed three sleepless days as he stumbled and slogged his way from bed to bed.

The following Friday India began to pay what would eventually be an enormous price for its epidemic. The United Nations Security Council demanded a full accounting of India's plague control efforts amid quiet threats of boycotts of Indian goods. That put the plague on Prime Minister Narasimha Rao's agenda. He dispatched Health Secretary M. S. Dayal to Surat. Dayal, a graying, bespectacled civil servant, was the top bureaucrat in the Ministry of Health. He flew into Surat Friday morning, returning that afternoon to Delhi, and telling journalists and Prime Minister Rao that 44 Suratis had died of pneumonic plague and another 174 cases were in treatment.

"The situation in the affected area is well under control," Dayal claimed, adding that Surat health officials were commencing door-to-door surveys throughout the city, searching for additional cases.[22]

But Dayal's pronouncement did little to vanquish public—and world—fear. All over India sales of tetracycline soared and pharmaceutical supplies were swiftly depleted by a public convinced that the danger was great in every corner of the nation. To assure adequate doses for genuine treatment use, India's Food and Drug Administration was compelled to warehouse caches of tetracycline.

On Saturday morning accurate newspaper headlines told the Indian people that Rao's government had officially declared Surat "plague-hit" and dispatched the army's Rapid Action Force to the city in order to maintain quarantines and stop the exodus of potential *Yersinia* carriers to other parts of the nation.

By the time the bereted Rapid Action Force, clad in blue camouflage combat gear, arrived Saturday afternoon, Surat had already lost three-quarters of its population, or an estimated 450,000 to 600,000 people. Critics attacked the federal government for failing to act sooner. Railroad authorities, also drawing in a torrent of criticism, began to seal shut all trains as they passed through Surat, declining to stop in the city except to off-load medical supplies.

International concern rose. The World Health Organization called India's outbreak "the most serious" seen anywhere in decades. Authorities all over the world called out for plague expertise and advice.

They were greeted by an embarrassed silence. India wasn't the only nation that had shut down its plague programs, confident that *Yersinia* no longer posed a threat. The once vast plague infrastructure of the former Soviet Union was, three years after the collapse of the USSR, in complete disarray. Few European scientists studied *Yersinia* anymore. And representatives of the U.S. Centers for Disease Control and Prevention nearly choked with embarrassment as they conceded that only one employee—a half-time scientist based in Fort Collins, Colorado—had expertise in plague. No one had sizable stockpiles of plague vaccine, nor could any be manufactured on a time scale of less than six months.

World Health Organization Director-General Dr. Hiroshi Nakajima was silent. The world, left on its own to decide how to react to India's calamity, joined in the panic. Airports began to screen incoming Indian jets, and talk of more restrictive policies was in the air. In Delhi officials thought such drastic international reaction could be forestalled so long as plague remained confined to remote Beed and the city of Surat.

But no such luck.

Over the weekend alleged plague cases surfaced in Delhi and Baroda. A patient who appeared to suffer from plague fled hospital captivity, prompting a hysterical search of the ancient slums of the capital. He would never be found.

As international pressure mounted, Minister of Health Shankaranand himself journeyed to Surat on Saturday. With an entourage of Delhi officials, Shankaranand toured Civil Hospital only to be mobbed outside the facility by an angry group of Suratis and journalists demanding to know what the federal government was going to do to save the city. Belligerent, Shankaranand shouted angrily at the mob, ordered protection from army troops, and fled the city.

Meanwhile, abandoned Surat reeled under the stench of uncollected garbage, unfed, dying animals, and rotting shipments of food. There were too few workers remaining in Surat to take care of business. With an estimated forty-five thousand diamond polishing units idle, in the city notorious for profit priorities, it was little wonder that basic civil needs went unmet.

Monday morning found the situation out of control. Nationwide use of tetracycline was so widespread that the World Health Organization issued warnings that India might breed tetracycline-resistant microbes, of all sorts. More than ten million doses of the drug were distributed in Gujarat State alone.[23]

"We are trying," complained Gujarat State Minister of Health Subash Shelad. "We are telling people that only those should take tetracycline who come into contact with a known plague case. Only if there are symptoms. That is the continuous statement of the government. We are very clear about that."

Shelad, who had set up a command post inside Surat's Civil Hospital and worked round-the-clock coordinating the emergency plague response, patted the pocket of his tunic. "I've got mine in my pocket. I've not taken it."

But the public would continue to ignore such protestations from the government. Within a week Surat's much-depleted population consumed fifteen million doses of tetracycline. And drug companies, including American and European manufacturers, filled pages of newspapers advertising not just tetracycline, but also a long list of antibiotics, cleansers, pesticides, and rat poisons that people living in Indian towns hundreds of miles from Surat would clamor to purchase.[24]

India marked Tuesday's World Tourism Day with the most drastic decline in tourist visits seen in more than a decade. Twenty percent of all tour packages to India scheduled for October were canceled. Tourists already in country cut short their trips and fled. Such usually crowded landmarks as the Taj Mahal, Goa's beaches, Jaipur's "pink city," and the mountain Buddha of Bodhgaya were deserted. Hardest hit were resorts and hotels that catered to high-end tourists and business travelers: luxury hotels were suddenly emptied.[25]

As economic ministers sweated over how best to compensate for these losses, ten states, spread over a vast distance, declared that they had all identified suspected plague cases.

And that brought dire calamity: complete economic collapse. On Wednesday, September 28, the Gulf State Nations (Kuwait, Saudi Arabia, Qatar, Oman, and the UAE) banned all flights, goods, and citizens from India. Pakistan and Sri Lanka—both eager for long-standing political reasons to cripple India—immediately followed suit.

The Bombay stock market crashed, experiencing its worst one-day decline since the 1989 assassination of Rajiv Gandhi. Annually trade between the Gulf States and India usually amounted to $3 billion. Further, some 400,000 Indians worked in the Gulf, sending home hard currency remittances to support their families. This cash flow ceased abruptly because the Gulf States banned all postal communications to and from India—a move that certainly could not have any biological credibility for plague control but did succeed in striking another critical Moslem blow against the Hindu-dominated Indian economy. Air flights between the Gulf and India, usually carrying twelve thousand passengers a day, were canceled. All Indian-produced goods and electronic goods were banned in the boycotting Islamic countries.

Within forty-eight hours other critical trading partners and sources of valuable tourism dollars would close all connections to India: the Russian Federation, China, Egypt, Malaysia, and Bangladesh. And most nations that did not go so far as to completely ban Indian personnel, flights, and goods, did insist upon inspection of Indian travelers.

On September 29 Nobel Laureate Mother Teresa was compelled to submit to a medical checkup at Rome's Leonardo da Vinci Airport. Before departing the aircraft en route to her meeting with Pope John Paul II the hunchbacked, tiny nun smiled at her fellow passengers and told them that they had nothing to fear from the plague.

WHO did little to stop this international stigmatization of India, save issuing press releases: "There is no need for fear nor panic. . . . This is a treatable disease and the measures taken in India are considered to be wholly adequate." All reasonable boundaries between sound public health and globalized panic had been crossed. WHO did little to slow the stampede toward hysteria or stifle the opportunistic shouts of boycott calls from India's ancient nemesis, the Islamic states. The worldwide community reeled under the weight of fear that dated to the fourteenth century, and few authoritative voices sought to remind the terrified humanity that science had long since conquered *Yersinia pestis.*

The Indian cabinet met hastily on September 29, including the country's United Nations delegate. By then there were 1,463 suspected plague cases in the country and forty-seven deaths—all in Surat. Surat's Civil Hospital alone held 659 suspected plague cases. States reporting unconfirmed additional cases included Delhi, West Bengal, Rajasthan, Maharashtra, Gujarat—areas that spanned virtually the length and breadth of the nation. In Delhi, where suspected plague cases filled the beds of the All India Institute of Medical Sciences, panic drove closure of all public schools. Local authorities said that two people had died of plague in Delhi, one in Bombay.

The Ministers issued an assurance to the nation: "India will be free of plague epidemic in three weeks."

The Bombay stock market responded by dropping another 77.3 points in a single day's trading. States with no reported plague cases were, nevertheless, facing ruin. The southern state of Kerala, for example, witnessed cancellation of virtually every October tourist group.[26]

In Europe and North America trade and travel with India remained open, though passengers were asked to submit to medical inspections. On October 1 an Indian traveler aboard Air India flight 101 was detained at London's Heathrow airport on suspicion of having plague.[27] The man was locked for hours in a windowless room at the airport while authorities scrambled to find appropriate quarantine facilities. But England no longer had quarantine rooms at its airports, having long since abandoned such procedures. The man's isolation sparked political outcry both in New Delhi and in England's House of Commons. After five hours the man—who did not, after all, have plague—was transported from Heathrow in a special airtight infectious diseases ambulance and placed in isolation at Northwick Parks Hospital pending laboratory analysis of his blood and sputum.[28] Members of the Indian expatriate community in London decried the British action as racist. Whether racism, indeed, motivated the response, it remains impossible to justify such extreme measures on the basis of biology. Even if the unfortunate traveler had been infected with the bacteria, dispensing of antibiotics to his fellow passengers would have proven sound public health policy—*not* incarceration.

In Washington the plague drew considerable interest and concern. Though the U.S. State Department issued repeated pleas for calm, there was quiet concern that a plague carrier might disappear into an urban center, go untreated, and spark an American outbreak of the usually curable disease. Plague could easily be treated with antibiotics, but officials had little confidence that typical

American emergency room physicians could properly diagnose the pneumonic disease, prescribing appropriate curative and preventive measures. A quick survey revealed that more than 90 percent of all flights from India, arriving either directly or via a European city, landed at John F. Kennedy International Airport in New York City. Every day some 2,000 to 3,000 passengers from India arrived at the airport, many of them relatives of the estimated 100,000 Indian immigrants living in New York.

On September 27, the U.S. Centers for Disease Control and Prevention and the New York City Department of Health devised a strategy aimed at spotting plague cases swiftly and preventing spread within New York.[29] The plan hatched in New York and Atlanta was also implemented in six other American cities that served as lower volume ports of call for travelers from the Indian subcontinent.

The CDC set up a plague hot line which, between September 27 and October 31 received 2,692 calls from concerned, sometimes hysterical, citizens.

In New York responsibility fell to the city's new chief of infectious diseases, Dr. Marcelle Layton. The young, curly-haired Layton was a coolheaded individual widely respected by colleagues nationwide.

A month earlier (August 27, 1994) Layton had received a communication from the CDC concerning the outbreak of bubonic plague in the Beed District of Maharashtra State in India. As director of the New York City Department of Health's Bureau of Communicable Disease Layton routinely received such notifications of unusual outbreaks. And most overseas reports prompted only minor interest, posing no real threat to New York.

But by September, as word spread of the pneumonic cases of the disease in Surat, American concern heightened. Of particular interest to Layton was word from the CDC that "screening is not occurring of [airline] passengers in India." That meant it would be up to authorities at passengers' destinations to identify possible plague carriers.

As Layton's staff prepared an ambitious surveillance effort to monitor all thirty-one flights from India daily at JFK Airport, and alert the metropolis's medical personnel, Health Commissioner Dr. Margaret Hamburg met with Mayor Rudolph Giuliani. Hamburg convinced New York's mayor that, distant as India was, New York City health safety was at issue because JFK was America's major port of entry for visitors, tourists, and immigrants from the Indian subcontinent. Giuliani asked why planes from India couldn't simply be stopped—barred entirely from entry. And Hamburg laid out the biological and logistic reasons why such a politically sensitive measure would provide only false security: an estimated half million residents of the plagued city of Surat had already fled their city, reaching destinations all over the subcontinent—not just India; most passengers from India actually changed planes in Frankfurt, Amsterdam, Paris, and

London and would still get into the United States one way or the other. More-over, plague was completely curable with modern antibiotics, Hamburg re-minded the mayor. Giuliani lent Hamburg's health department his support.

On September 27 Layton's plan of action went into effect. Working closely with scientists at the CDC's plague lab in Fort Collins, Colorado, she mapped out a three-pronged strategy. First, her staff set out to alert the health providers of greater New York City. A special fact sheet, detailing the signs and symptoms of plague, was faxed to the emergency rooms and infection control offices of 102 hospitals in the city and dozens of facilities in neighboring Westchester, Suffolk, and Nassau counties. In addition, bulletins were sent to twenty thousand doctors practicing in New York City, and a Hindi-language flyer was distributed at an October 8 Indian festival in the borough of Queens.

Key to the city's efforts were activities at JFK Airport. The CDC gave all of the airlines pamphlets concerning plague, and airline personnel were expected to recognize symptoms of the disease. The CDC similarly informed represen-tatives of the Immigration and Naturalization Service and U.S. Customs, as it was employees of those agencies—not health officials—who routinely saw all international passengers. Thus, responsibility for spotting possible plague cases fell to employees of private airlines, the INS, and U.S. Customs: none of them medically trained.

"If there were a suspect case, a New York City medical officer would go to the runway," Layton later explained, "and remove the suspect. All the other passengers would remain on the plane until diagnosis was confirmed."

Under U.S. law, if a plague case were confirmed aboard such a flight, all passengers would then be required to submit to an examination, provide officials with details regarding their future destinations, and make themselves available for a full week's follow-up medical surveillance.

"If plague cases weren't spotted until the passengers had disembarked, finding those people would be very problematic," Layton said.

One suspected plague case was, indeed, identified aboard a flight from India, and Layton's plan was effectively put into action. But all the remaining nine suspect cases were spotted after the passengers had deplaned; two were noted by observant U.S. Customs officials; one by a JFK ticketing agent, and the remainder by emergency room physicians in the New York City area.

One Customs agent looked up from an Indian passenger's bags to see red fluid dripping from the individual's mouth. Alarmed, and convinced the Indian was bleeding, the Customs agent triggered the plague alert to health officials at the airport. It turned out that the Indian was simply chewing betel nuts, which exude a bright red juice and stain the consumer's mouth and teeth with a fiery crimson color.

But the other suspect plague victims were not so fortunate—all were suffering from serious illnesses; one died of malaria. Two others had malaria, four were ailing due to viral infections, one had chronic liver disease, and the last had typhoid fever.

It was fortunate, Hamburg said, that none of the cases were plague, as the exercise pointed up a number of deficiencies in America's disease safety net, some of which would be difficult, if not impossible, to correct.

Foremost, said Nobel Laureate Joshua Lederberg of Rockefeller University, was the vague and often contradictory nature of information from overseas. Typically, outbreaks that occurred in poor countries were inadequately characterized, even misdiagnosed. In the case of India's plague, valid laboratory confirmation that *Yersinia pestis* was the cause of the epidemic did not materialize until February, nearly six months *after* the outbreak. Diagnostic uncertainty overseas made Layton and her associates nervous. What if their entire alert system was directed toward the wrong microbial scourge, she asked, and some other disease managed to slip unnoticed into JFK? What if India was wrong, *Yersinia* wasn't the problem, and while all of Layton's resources were diverted some dangerous virus slipped into New York?

While it was easy to point up failures in a poor country, Drs. Ruth Berkelman, Jim Hughes, and Grant Campbell of the CDC retrospectively acknowledged severe shortfalls on the U.S. side. Physicians in the United States were largely unable to differentiate between plague and other ailments. Most American medical schools had long since abandoned public health and infectious diseases training, confining such subjects to elective courses or advanced classes for would-be specialists. The links between medicine and public health in America were, at best, weak. And there were large lags between the times of recognition of those possible New York City cases and the isolation of pneumonically diseased individuals, thus potentially allowing large numbers of people to be exposed.

Containing exposure and tracking down secondary cases—particularly deplaned fellow passengers—proved daunting for New York City.

"The bottom line is we had a gigantic protocol based on recognizing people on board planes," Layton said. "But most potential cases weren't recognized until they were already in the community." Even a single bona fide case of plague, spotted after the passenger deplaned, would have severely taxed the city's health resources and forced Hamburg to divert personnel from most other programs. Had there been multiple cases, or if the ailment had been viral (and therefore untreatable) the situation would have quickly overwhelmed the health department's resources. Such had not always been the case in Gotham: in the early twentieth century plague control had been routine, and successful.

Nationwide, the U.S. public health safety net caught thirteen potential plague cases related to the India outbreak: ten in New York City; one in Albany,

New York; and two elsewhere in the country. Overwhelmed as the New York City Department of Health might have been, it did prove the most vigilant and efficient local agency in the country, CDC officials insisted.

"The recent plague experience in India provides a clear example of the high price of ignoring global microbial threats," Hughes and Campbell concluded, noting that the U.S. public health system had long since lost any sense of vigilance over outbreaks occurring overseas.[30]

But those conclusions would be reached in hindsight. During the first week of October 1994 every nation in the world was on some form of plague alert and India was a pariah.

All of India was suddenly in October overcome with a fit of mass hygiene hysteria. Rats were caught; streets were scrubbed; garbage was piled high and set afire, thereby exuding eye-tearing stenches and a putrid smoke. Surat, alone, would burn up three thousand tons of garbage during the next weeks, and spread hundreds of pounds of probably unneeded DDT. (As there was no ratfall or flea-carried bacteria in Surat there could be no logical need for the pesticide.) Someone put a huge surgical mask over the mouth of Mahatma Gandhi's colossal statue in New Delhi. In the town of Thane in Maharashtra State a terrified man denounced visitors from Gujarat who came to his village as plague carriers: on the night of October 2 he murdered all three of them, the youngest being a seven-year-old girl.

The Bombay stock market continued to plummet, falling a total of 213 points, or 5 percent of its total value, since plague had struck Surat a month earlier. Stock market jitters reflected growing anxiety in circles of commerce about the government's ability to—frankly—*govern* in a crisis.

"Too many people in India, and abroad, are in near-panic," complained the *Times of India.* "Too few of our national and state leaders appear to be sufficiently agitated. It should be the other way around. To put it starkly: India's future is at stake."[31]

On October 2 New Delhi federal officials released startling new plague numbers: nationwide, they said, there were 4,059 cases, 1,297 in Gujarat State and 2,105 in Maharashtra. With the release of those numbers came yet another plea for international calm.

But Oman responded by conducting an emergency airlift of all its citizens then in Bombay. By Tuesday October 4 there were, officially, 4,780 suspect plague cases and forty-eight deaths. A five-year-old child in Old Delhi died: plague was blamed.

And then a sort of intellectual warfare broke out, pitting some of India's leading biologists and physicians against one another and fueling ancient suspicions and hatreds.

First, India's National Institute of Communicable Diseases—the nation's large federal research center in New Delhi—had possession of alleged plague samples from the nation's suspected patients. But the All India Institute of Medical Sciences also had samples. And the institutes locked horns in a seemingly bizarre turf battle. The AIIMS, which was handling all the suspected cases identified in Delhi, refused to release its blood and sputum samples to NICD on the grounds that the materials should remain within AIIMS labs and NICD microbiologists ought to come to AIIMS, rather than the samples leaving the hospital's grounds.

NICD, for its part, insisted it should act as the clearinghouse for all *Yersinia* samples. And in a case of possibly misplaced pride it declined laboratory assistance offered by the U.S. Centers for Disease Control and Prevention, London School of Hygiene and Tropical Medicine, and Plague Laboratory in Odessa, Ukraine.[32]

At the NICD an ad hoc plague laboratory was erected on the top floor of an old cinder block building. Amid the blistering October heat of New Delhi lab workers from the Zoonosis Division toiled round-the-clock under humbling conditions. Well-trained microbiologists, some of whom had studied in the best universities in the West, worked with equipment that might be found in an American high school teaching laboratory. No air-conditioning relieved their discomfort as they sweated beneath protective plastic gear, gloves, and goggles. Samples of sputum and blood cooked on lab benches in the tropical heat.

At the plague control room Dr. D. C. Jain and a team of epidemiologists struggled to keep track of the plague reports that were then pouring in from every corner of the country. Clearly sleep deprived, Jain nervously responded to a steady stream of phone calls, staff queries, and official interruptions. The exhausted epidemiologist could barely complete a sentence before another question was fired his way. To each he seemed to respond physically, recoiling, squinting, and tensing from head to toe. The key question leveled at Jain hourly by Ministry of Health officials was, "Is this an epidemic of *Yersinia pestis*, and are all these illnesses nationwide due to plague?"

"The molecular epidemiology has not been done," Jain sputtered, acknowledging that the sort of detective work that is essential in an epidemic hadn't been initiated in the Surat outbreak. "We still do not say it is plague because our laboratory is finding the bacteria has morphology similar to plague bacilli. They do not say it *is* plague, they say it's *similar*. The basic thing is whether it's plague or not: it's not possible at this juncture for me to say. It is yet to be confirmed."

But at New Delhi's Infectious Disease Hospital, Dr. K. N. Tewari was swamped with supposed plague cases. Most of the 749 people he tested were simply the worried well or individuals suffering from other, milder infectious diseases. Tewari placed those cases in general wards of the hospital.

But there were a few cases Tewari was convinced were genuinely caused by *Yersinia pestis*. His laboratory confirmed them.

"We have got definitely three cases without any history of going out of Delhi for that [plague] period," Tewari insisted. "All are from the slums of Delhi. And they have no history of contact with a person with plague. It *is* pneumonic plague. And we have thirteen more that need to be investigated."

One of Tewari's confirmed cases was four-year-old Vijay Kumar, who for four days had been suffering from a high fever, respiratory difficulties, and a sharp pain in his neck. Skinny Kumar stared with wild, terror-struck eyes over the edge of his mask.

Near Kumar on the plague isolation ward lay twenty-two-year-old Harish. For five days he had been suffering fever and uncontrollable coughing. From behind his mask, worn to protect a visitor to the plague ward, Harish spoke between fits of coughing.

"I had a sudden onset of fever," he related in Hindi. "And I have no recall of being around anybody who was sick."

Across the hall from the nearly empty plague ward was the crowded ward Tewari called "the plague phobia room," full of patients whom the doctor felt were fine. But the patients refused to leave, convinced that they had the dreaded disease.

Tewari was joined by a cluster of young colleagues who insisted that fear of plague was "silly," and horribly exaggerated.

"There must be a uniform global policy on these plagues," Dr. Dinesh Gupta insisted loudly, out-shouting the rest of the physician cluster. "No bans! No closed borders!"

While Delhi's Infectious Disease Hospital and the staff of Surat's Civil Hospital were absolutely convinced that they had lab-confirmed *Yersinia* cases on their hands, NICD officially vacillated, unable to produce definitive epidemiological or laboratory proof. Over at AIIMS doctors continued to hold on to samples. But they were in no position to settle the controversy. They were preoccupied with their own mysterious outbreak of hepatitis E, which was spreading through the facility, so far claiming sixty employees.

In Surat a group of four private physicians announced on October 1 that they had proof there was no *Yersinia* in the city. The epidemic, they said, was due to "hantana virus," a misstatement of a class of rodent-borne microbes called hantaviruses. Their claim drew rage from the hard-working physicians of Civil Hospital who on October 3 offered a substantial reward to anyone who could prove that their *Yersinia* diagnosis was invalid.

The critical quartet (Drs. Bipin Desai, Sudhir Marfatia, Nainesh Parikh, and Balwant Mistry) had to back off from their "hantana virus" claim in the face of overwhelming evidence that the ailing patients recovered when treated with antibiotics, which are only effective against bacteria. So on October 6 the group offered a new hypothesis: there was no plague; there was melioidosis. Admitting that "we do not have any patient or his sputum" from which to draw samples in evidence, the quartet said, "we request the doctors concerned to look into this theory and give the right solution of this disease to Surat, Gujarat, and the country."

Another group of physicians from B. J. Medical College in Pune, Maharashtra, said their alleged bubonic plague cases actually suffered from *Burkholderia pseudomallei*, a bacterium that rarely causes illnesses in otherwise healthy individuals.[33]

Scientists from AIIMS eventually weighed in, further roiling the waters. They announced in late October that their "attempts to culture *Yersinia pestis* from patients have failed so far, although it is not a difficult organism to grow."

They went on to suggest that the hantaviruses, melioidosis or another bacteria—leptospirosis—might be causes of the epidemic. However, they failed to note a critical detail: they hadn't isolated any of these organisms from their samples.

Digging further into the obscure possibilities the same group of Pune physicians that originally proposed *Burkholderia* was the problem switched their bets, backing the species *Pseudomonas pseudomallei* as the epidemic's agent. The group claimed to have cultured the melioidosis-causing bacteria from lymph nodes drawn from 30 percent of the patients diagnosed with bubonic plague.

The stakes in this fight, both medical and political, were high. If the critics were correct, physicians in Surat—*government employees*—had erred shamefully, bringing disgrace and economic ruin to the nation. If the critics were incorrect, the federal government could claim credit for alerting the world to the epidemic, and get off the hook for its public health failures in response to the outbreak. Either way the Civil Hospital physicians were too busy battling their epidemic, and too powerless—far too lowly in the government hierarchy—to effectively leap into the fray. And scientists in Delhi seemed unable to conjure convincing data rapidly enough to nip the debate in the bud.

Melioidosis is a disease rarely seen on the Indian subcontinent; it is more typically found in Southeast Asia. The bacteria are usually transmitted through skin wounds via exposure to contaminated water. There were no known epidemics of melioidosis ever reported, even in Southeast Asia. The microbe was never known to be passed from person to person. And most carriers of *Pseudomonas pseudomallei* never took ill, but became lifelong carriers of the generally harmless bacteria. It might not, therefore, seem surprising that 30 percent of the residents of an earthquake-torn rural area had the microbes in their lymph nodes. It would, based on known history of human melioidosis cases, be nothing short of medically astounding if upwards of 10 percent of a village population developed acute symptoms analogous to bubonic plague as a result of exposure to the agent.

Tularemia—another suggested explanation for the epidemic—was a more severe bacterial disease whose symptoms more closely resembled those of pneumonic plague, including fevers and enlarged lymph nodes. But most tularemic patients also developed terrible skin ulcers, which were not seen on the Beed or Surat patients. Further, the bacteria were not endemic to the Indian subcontinent and were usually carried by species of ticks found only in much colder climates such as the North American plains and the Russian Steppes.

"I wish these so-called Senior Scientists had taken the time to talk to the lab at NICD," an exasperated Health Secretary Dayal exclaimed. "In Beed there is *no doubt* it's plague. We saw antibodies in serology. There was no doubt it was bubonic—the symptoms were clear and distinct. We have cultured samples from the blood! We have isolated the bacteria! True, the molecular epidemiology has not yet been done. But combined with all this evidence—sputum, PHA, high titers, antibody responses—we do *strongly* suggest it's *Yersinia pestis*."

But the common people of India were all too willing to believe virtually anything except the government's position. In Bombay they spoke on street corners of a Pakistani conspiracy.

"Look who was first to call for a boycott of India," they would knowingly tell a visitor. "Pakistan! There is no plague. It's all a big lie Pakistan used to bring down our economy."

Conversely, in Calcutta they spoke of a government cover-up: "Thousands are dying of plague every day, but they are hiding it! And now they say it's something else. It's a lie."

With each day the distrust grew, NICD's credibility fell, and more nations carried out punitive actions against India. The Dutch airline KLM sprayed pesticides throughout its plane cabins as they disembarked India. North Korea denied docking privileges to all ships, of any nationality, that had previously been in Indian waters. Sudan placed all travelers from India in jailed quarantine for six days. China barred all Indians, period. Hong Kong informed all Indians that they would face two days mandatory quarantine or immediate deportation. The Ukraine placed one hundred passengers from India under armed guard, refusing to allow them to disembark from their aircraft.

The world was behaving in an utterly irrational manner over an entirely preventable and curable bacterial disease whose greatest threat was from the historic collective memory of the human species. India's domestic responses were obviously confused, contradictory, and inadequate. Yet the World Health Organization took no strong action on India's behalf until October 7, nearly two months after the Beed outbreak began. That morning, WHO Director-General

Hiroshi Nakajima flew with an Indian government entourage to Surat, examined cases at Civil Hospital, and then returned to New Delhi to face the Indian media. Citing article 11, paragraph 3 of the International Health Regulations, Nakajima said he had come at the request of the Gulf State Nations to assess India's epidemic.

Speaking with a thick Japanese accent that Indian journalists were at pains to decipher, Nakajima criticized the "very large gap between so-called suspect cases and confirmed cases" in Surat, but said that there were, indeed, "a large number of pneumonic plague cases."

And then he added a puzzling statement: "Concerning Surat I would say today there is a plague in Surat. But if you compare the number of confirmed cases—192—in a city of I think 1.8 million population we cannot say there is an epidemic. I prefer to say there is a plague in Surat. But I'm not prepared to say there is an epidemic in Surat."

As Nakajima spoke tension and whispers spread among the journalists. Not knowing the cause of the Indian media's agitation Nakajima nervously continued, his accent thickening and the press corps' inability to comprehend growing worse.

"As for laboratory work," Nakajima began, obviously flustered, "NICD technology is good. But working conditions are so bad that I recommended to the minister of health to provide better working conditions. The lab is oversaturated. I'm a little afraid the NICD laboratory isn't able to perform in such a way."

The WHO director-general severely condemned the quality of laboratory facilities in Surat, recommended large-scale epidemiology and rat surveillance, and called upon the Indian government to conduct serious scientific studies.

As for international boycotts, Nakajima was evasive. Official WHO policy called for no such action, he said, but article 7 of the International Health Regulations stipulated that an epidemic couldn't be declared over until twice the organism's average incubation time, or twelve days in the case of plague. Therefore, India's epidemic—an "epidemic" he'd already refused to grant even existed—would officially persist until November.

The room erupted.

"You are coming here like Caesar to judge!" shouted one reporter.

"You are reaching hasty conclusions!" another cried.

"What will you tell the Gulf States about this boycott?" asked another.

"There is no plague in India! You are a liar," shouted a chorus of reporters. Chaos replaced order and the distressed WHO entourage left in haste.

It would be another two weeks before India's international woes would cease. By then the outbreak would have proven disastrously expensive. Dr. Ann Marie Kimball of the University of Washington in Seattle estimates tourism and trade losses, alone, amounted to $1.3 billion.[34] That is close to other published estimates for tourism and trade losses.[35] None of the published estimates of the cost of India's plague factored in the nearly two-week-long cessation of textile and diamond industrial activity in Surat, loss of agricultural production in Maharashtra, panic purchasing of antibiotics, or direct medical costs.

Certainly when these issues are factored a toll approaching $2 billion seems reasonable: an extraordinary price to pay for what eventually was a total of fifty-six deaths and fewer than 6,500 cases of an antibiotic-susceptible infection.[36]

India continued to pay a political price for its epidemic long after all the plague wards were closed and the last *Yersinia*-carrying rat was exterminated. It was the cost of inadequate government attention to public health.

The lack of rapid, definitive evidence of *Yersinia pestis* infection in the sick and dying patients and a clear epidemiological explanation for the two separate outbreaks of bubonic and pneumonic diseases left wide open a door for the entry of fanaticism, conspiracy theories, crackpot ideas, and general antigovernment sentiments. Though the U.S. Centers for Disease Control and Prevention was eventually invited to examine available Surat samples and confirmed the presence of *Yersinia*, most of the sputum and blood extracted from the initial flurry of cases in September was destroyed through lack of proper handling and refrigeration in either Surat or Delhi. Thus, it wasn't possible to match case by case the presence of symptoms with laboratory evidence of *Yersinia* infection. That left plenty of room for other, often conspiratorial, interpretations.

The CDC did a full genetic analysis of the Surat strain, concluding it was a *Yersinia* strain not previously seen. Similar conclusions were reached by scientists at the Pasteur Institute in Paris and the Plague Laboratory in Stavropol, Russia. Though the agency meant simply that it didn't match any strains in their archives, the finding fueled a new slew of conspiracy theories. In particular, the *Hindustan Times* claimed that the strain was manufactured in a biological warfare laboratory in Kazakhstan and sold to a Kashmir rebel group called the Ultras.[37] That was enough to prompt the Ministry of Defense to lay claim to all remaining *Yersinia* samples, thus removing them forever from public health analysis.

Before the Ultra theory hit newsstands in mid-1995, WHO and the Indian government had requested epidemiology assistance from the U.S. Centers for Disease Control and Prevention. Dr. David Dennis, the only plague expert on the U.S. payroll, led a small team of investigators that examined cases in Surat, Delhi, and the Beed District during the last two weeks of November 1994. They concluded that the epidemic was genuine, but were unable to isolate *Yersinia* from most samples, partly because mass use of antibiotics was widespread and may have eliminated some evidence of the bacteria. Nevertheless, in March of 1995, with assistance from the CDC, the NICD published definitive evidence of *Yersinia pestis* in samples from both Beed and Surat. A few months later re-searchers from the Central Public Health Laboratory in London would publish evidence that the microbe responsible for melioidosis absolutely was *not* present in disease victims, utterly refuting claims made in October 1994 by the doctors in Pune.

But just as it seemed controversy over *Yersinia*'s culpability in the outbreak was settled and the book might be closed on India's epidemic, PCR (polymerase chain reaction) genetic sequencing reports released by the United States, France, and Russia fueled an entirely new set of accusations aimed directly at the United States. PCR sequencing revealed that the Surat *Yersinia* strain was of compara-tively low virulence and contained a unique set of genes not previously seen with plague. The role of these genes was unclear, but not thought to be worri-some, as Russian tests showed the strain to be highly susceptible to a broad range of readily available antibiotics. Within days of the release of these reports the U.S. embassy in New Delhi found itself under siege, as local scientists and reporters claimed that the mysterious extra gene segment in the Surat *Yersinia* could only have been man-made. It was, they said, a product of genetic engi-neering. And the engineers were either Americans, or, in an alternative theory, Kazakh scientists working at the behest of the U.S. government. U.S. Ambassador Frank Wisner came under personal attack, accused of crafting the entire scheme.

The logic was deeply conspiratorial and ultimately U.S.-paranoid.[38]

That the logic defied basic tenets of microbial evolution and was patently incorrect made no difference. And conspiracy theorists insisted that only the U.S. government possessed adequate technology to create such superbugs. Some Indian news publications during the summer of 1995 claimed that the United States had a massive biowarfare program under way. To back up their allegations they pointed to $300 million allocated by Congress that year for pro-duction of defensive bioweapons measures such as development of vaccines.

The unfolding diplomatic crisis pointed up a crucial, and previously un-seen, problem for public health: bioweapons technology. As technological ad-vances made in the 1980s allowed the possibility of formerly unthinkable forms of terrorism in the 1990s, governments had to distinguish natural microbial events from those that were man-made. This put the United States in a partic-ularly dicey catch-22 situation, as its government employees were among the few scientists in the world capable of both making such horrible bioweapons and proving whether or not an outbreak was man-made. In the case of the Surat strain, Indian accusers charged that it was either manufactured at the army's old Dugway Proving Grounds or in the Kazakh lab of Dr. I. L. Martinevsky, a

Russian BW expert. His lab, the Indian press claimed, had been visited by U.S. Secretary of Defense William Perry, and Martinevsky now worked for the U.S. Defense Department making offensive BW agents.

What was the motivation, and how did the alleged BW weapon get to Surat? It was claimed that the United States used Suratis as guinea pigs, testing new biosensing devices in the city. That such devices were never seen in Surat, and are so enormous that they could hardly go unnoticed, was not mentioned. The release was allegedly conducted by none other than the CDC's David Dennis— the very individual who, two months after the epidemic began, led a team of investigations to Surat at the request of the Indian government.

Ambassador Wisner's role in the conspiracy was "proven" because he had played a key role in treaty negotiations with China and India, trying to persuade the two massive nations to sign the 1972 Biological Weapons Convention. In other words, because he tried to broker peace, he must have actually been the kingpin in a horrible scheme to inflict plague on India.

The accusations proved embarrassing to the United States, and conveniently deflected anger away from the failed policies and negligence of Indian authorities. When plague first broke out in Surat the Indian press had loudly declaimed the lack of essential public health services, the filth, the squalor, the lack of plague surveillance, and the slow pace of government response. Now, with national elections approaching and Prime Minister Rao's leadership wildly unpopular even within his own Congress Party, it was convenient to point the finger at another nation.

But Indian public health authorities had much for which to answer.

"Let our nation learn the lesson: economic advancement requires adequate investment in human health," said Dr. Jacob John.[39] "Second lesson: infectious diseases are the major causes of morbidity and mortality. Well-informed tourists coming to India take immunizations against Japanese encephalitis, hepatitis A, typhoid fever, and chemoprophylaxis against malaria; they carry with them drugs against giardiasis and cholera. Some even carry a few doses of rabies vaccine. And we want rich tourists to come and see India, risking their health? Third lesson: infectious diseases must be diagnosed by laboratory methods and not by government decree. Fourth lesson: microbiology laboratories and microbiologists should be available in all districts. . . . Fifth lesson: there should be continuous monitoring of causes of diseases and of death in order to detect epidemics of diseases."

Indian expatriate researcher Dr. Vikram Chand felt the most appalling event was the mass exodus of physicians away from Surat during the plague.[40]

The gross disparity between the health status and care of India's poor versus her tiny elite of wealthy, upper-caste members formed the basis of the most sweeping critiques of the country's response to plague. In a nation where

53 percent of all children under five are officially underweight and growth stunted, and 21 percent are severely so, basic health needs were clearly unmet.[41] Perhaps the clearest illustration of the nation's public health weakness lay in its exploding *true* plague of HIV. Recognizing that India had all the social ingredients necessary for rapid spread of the almost 100 percent lethal virus, the World Bank in 1992 awarded the country an $84 million grant for AIDS prevention efforts. Six years later Indian authorities were still trying to figure out how to spend that money, and the United Nations AIDS Programme (UNAIDS) was convinced that India's HIV population outnumbered that of Mexico, the United States, and Canada, combined. In 1998 the World Bank sadly estimated that India's failure to respond swiftly to the initial spread of HIV among prostitutes and IV drug users in the early 1990s would, by 2000, cost her $11 billion, or 5 percent of her GDP, in direct medical care and lost worker productivity due to death and illness.[42] And by 1999 the UNAIDS Programme was convinced that more than 1.5 million Indians were infected. As with *Yersinia* plague, India's HIV epidemic spread primarily among its poorest citizens—a fact critics charged fully explained the country's inadequate public health response to both HIV and the plague.

"The chances of being rich and getting plague, in India or anywhere else in the world, are about as remote as the ability of the rat flea to jump from its slum habitat to the distant electronically protected environment of the rich," wrote the *Lancet* in an editorial.[43] "The distance between a slum environment and five-star comfort is rather more than an inch."

The British medical journal labeled plague a disease of poverty, and concluded: "Is it chance, or nemesis, that this revenge is taking place at a time when India, indeed the whole planet, is moving towards a 'free market' economy that benefits some but not all. The epidemic of plague has meant that instead of being marginalised in their socially distant slums, the existence of the poor has abruptly impinged on the consciousness of the rich."

Critics within India were less likely to beat the drum of international guilt, and more apt to aim their anger squarely at their nation's economic elite and inept leaders.

"If India can afford an aircraft carrier," wrote Dr. Eswar Krishnan, for example, "she can very well afford more epidemiologists and the resources they need. It is merely a question of priorities."[44]

In Bombay the press devoted November 1994 to dissecting blow by blow Maharashtra's response to the Beed and Surat outbreaks. It wasn't a pretty sight. By name, public health officials were accused of negligence, folly, and laziness. But the Indian media could hardly be considered guilt-free, as some of its less reputable members had wildly exaggerated the original threat of plague, whipped up national hysteria, and then, months later, joined in conspiracy fever.

Meanwhile, in Surat, poor women, one hand clutching their saris in place, spread white DDT powder with their bare hands along Ved Road. At an empty lot Kamlesh Patel supervised another crew of women who under orders plunged ungloved hands into piles of putrid garbage, tossing animal carcasses and debris into a massive bonfire.

The poor were doing as they always had in India: taking care of themselves.

Four days before the first of November WHO finally recommended that all boycotts and travel restrictions against India be lifted. There had been no more deaths reported for twelve days. The epidemic had, officially, stopped.

WHO had by then allowed India to be treated as a global pariah for more than two months.

Shortly before WHO's declaration, but with the epidemic clearly under control, a weary reporter boarded a British Airways jet in Bombay, headed for London. The cabin was redolent with insecticides aerosolized over every inch of the place. And more were then sprayed upon the seated passengers and their carry-on bags.

For hours the chemical stench reminded passengers that Britain feared they might be carrying *Yersinia*-infected fleas. It was, to say the least, an unpleasant thought.

Upon landing outside London the aircraft stopped just off the runway, not at a gate. Passengers were ordered to remain seated. A pair of public health service personnel in uniform boarded, flanking a robust, buxom blond physician in her sixties.

"Is anyone feeling unwell," she called out as she slowly made her way down the aircraft aisles, studying each passenger closely. "Anybody have a fever? Hmmm? Headache? Touch of delirium? Speak up, please. Fever?"

A smartly dressed Bombay businessman commented in the physician's wake, "Only a bloody fool would answer yes," and the passengers burst out in uproarious laughter. Clearly nobody aboard the jet trusted such measures would stop plague, were it present.

In every possible way the essential public health trusts between authorities, science, medicine, and the global populace were violated during the 1994 plague outbreak in India. Indian citizens trusted that their governments—both local and federal—would respond swiftly to a disease crisis, reach sound scientific conclusions, and act rapidly in a manner that both staunched the outbreak and quelled panic. Indian authorities failed to reach timely and irrefutable diagnoses, to assist beleaguered plague responders in Surat, to calm the public, or to offer accurate information as the epidemic unfolded. The plague tiger was well out of his cage, causing havoc across the countryside, before the hunters and trainers set out in search of the beast.

Global authorities also failed in their responses. The World Health Organization's only real power rests with its credibility as a voice of scientific reason that can rise above international politics to give timely guidance the global community can trust. But WHO's press releases and statements were weak, late, and politically influenced. Rather than decry all forms of international hysteria and punishment of India WHO fell under the influence of politically motivated rival nations. The agency dragged its feet, seemingly lending credibility to such inanity as Gulf State boycotts of such outrageously misnamed plague-carrying items as Indian postage stamps, oranges, Madras bolts of silk, and Bangalore computer chips.

The very word *plague* still conjures fear decades after both its prevention and cure have been developed and globally distributed. No new technology is needed to conquer *Yersinia pestis*, just implementation of very basic public health measures. Nevertheless, WHO and health authorities worldwide failed to consider the historic, almost visceral, impact the word *plague* arouses. Perhaps in their offices chatting by telephone with colleagues around the world they dismissed word of *Yersinia* on the grounds that, well, it was a controllable, harmless agent. But in so doing they utterly failed to recognize that while the organism may be easily vanquished with modern tools of medicine, the panic it sparks cannot possibly be addressed in a technological or dismissive manner.

In the end it was that very panic which proved most costly during the plague outbreak. And in the months that followed, panic gave way to its close cousin, conspiratorial thinking. Cloak-and-dagger explanations for epidemics have always proven attractive in the absence of unambiguous, timely, scientifically validated public health pronouncements. And conspiracy thinking undermines the credibility of the very health authorities in whom the public ought to place its trust.

That trust would soon be tested again in one of the remotest locations on earth.

CHAPTER TWO

LANDA-LANDA

**An Ebola virus epidemic in Zaire proves
public health is imperiled by corruption.**

*One is always alert, protecting oneself against the objects
that can steal your soul, the* landa-landa *that can inflict all
forms of ill fortune, illness, and, frequently, death. Death,
in such cases, is the sober thief that comes.*

—Kibari N'sanga and Lungazi Mulala[1]

*We are the ones who first bring life, but we never believed
in such powerful disease. Now it is true: we have lost the
brothers and sisters with whom we worked. In the name of
our ancestors I say: remove this evil spirit from amongst us
or we cannot work in peace*

—Twela Say Ntun, chief nurse of Kikwit Maternity Hospital No. 2[2]

The night air was, as always, redolent with the smells of burning cook fires
fueled by wood, wax, propane, or cheap gasoline. The distorted sounds of
overmodulated 1995 hit *ramba* music echoed from the few bars along Boulevard
Mobutu that had electric generators or well-charged car batteries. Fully dilated
pupils struggled to decipher shapes in the pitch darkness, spotting the pinpoint
lights of millions of dancing fireflies. Gentle footsteps betrayed what the eye on
a moonless night could not see; the constant movement of people, their dark
skin hiding them in the unlit night.

From a distance a woman's voice rang sharply, calling out in KiCongo, "*Afwaka!* Someone has died! Someone has died! He was my husband! He was my husband."

As she continued her call to heaven, detailing the virtues of the just-deceased, the woman's eerie cry was joined by a succession of her relatives' voices.

"Someone has died! Someone has died! He was my father!"

"Someone has died! Someone has died! He was my son!"

The padding of feet on Kikwit's mud paths paused as people turned their ears to catch the name of the latest *landa-landa* victim. In a city without newspapers, radio, television, telephones, or electricity, such cries in the night constituted local broadcast news. And no sooner had the flow of pedestrians resumed than another voice rang out from the opposite side of the emotionally electrified city-without-electricity.

"Someone has died!"

Landa-landa. Foreigners. Something called a virus. Something called Ebola. These things gripped the estimated 400,000 people of Kikwit with a terror unlike any they had ever felt. Fear was no stranger to them: hadn't they lived under the brutal Mobutu Sese Seko regime for more than thirty years? Wasn't death already a steady companion, fueled by malaria, measles, HIV, TB, and malnutrition?

But this *landa-landa* was different, more terrifying than all the other diseases that had taken the lives of Kikwit's children and young adults. The victims died fast. But first, they bled, had long fits of hiccups, cried out in agonizing pain, even went mad, and screamed incoherent phrases of apparent devilish origin. They seemed possessed.

There were ancient ceremonies handed down by the ancestors that could purge evil spirits—they usually lifted the *landa-landa*. But not this time. The magic was too powerful. Surely it must be the work of an exceptionally evil one.[3] Who was the potent fount of Satanism?

The rumors were numerous, and were spread in hushed tones so as not to be overheard by the evil ones. Only the Christian leaders, imbued with the strength of Jesus, dared decry the evil out loud. Pentecostal preacher Eloi Mulengamungu declared it the work of Satan, himself, allowed to roam freely over doomed Kikwit by God, in punishment. Kikwit, the preacher declared, had become a modern Sodom replete with prostitutes, corruption, illegitimate children, abandoned elderly parents, and other wages of sin.

From the Baptist Community of West Africa (CBCO) the people also heard of Satan's mischief. As members of CBCO fell ill and died of the strange new malady their leader declared that Kikwit had lost sight of God. In the absence of a large core of true believers Satan could claim even a tiny pool of the pious. As his congregants also fell ill, Pastor Kutesa Mayele of the Assembly of God Church reached a similar conclusion: it was God's punishment for Kikwit's sins.

Only the Catholic church's Monseigneur Alexandre Mbuka Nzundu accepted the outsiders' verdict that there was no *landa-landa*, just a terrible virus that was passed by the loving touch one person gave another: a virus that exploited moments when a husband might daub the forehead of his ailing, feverish wife; a child might hand wash the bloodied sheets upon which his ailing brother slept; a mother might spoon-feed her delirious son; and a grieving family would reverentially wash down the body of their deceased relative, rinsing off the sweat and blood of his hemorrhagic demise.

It was not *landa-landa*; it was a mortal pestilence that passed from one human to another through acts of kindness and love.

The virus was named for the Ebola river in Northern Zaire, which passes near the site of the microbe's first known epidemic in Yambuku, in 1976.[4] Though the 1976 death toll in Yambuku was less than four hundred villagers and Catholic Belgian missionaries, those members of the international scientific team who were deployed to the region to conquer the mysterious outbreak still held Ebola in awe in 1995. In their meetings with other public health officials for years after the 1976 outbreak, surviving members of the Yambuku crew always placed the deadly filovirus in a special, particularly fearsome category: a small assemblage of hemorrhagic fever viruses that included Lassa, yellow river, Marburg Disease, and a handful of others, most of which were discovered only in the last three decades of the twentieth century.

The fear evoked by Ebola among Westerners was largely a matter of enigma: in classic European and American tradition, that which could be understood, even if still dangerous, was no longer fearsome. The act of explanation diminished Western terror. But nineteen years after the virus's last outbreak in Zaire Western science still could not answer the most basic questions about Ebola: where did it come from? In what animal or plant species did it normally reside, when not infecting the human species? Exactly how was it transmitted from person to person? Could it, under any circumstances, pass through the air, infecting people who had no physical contact with patients? Precisely how lethal was the virus? Was it treatable with any drugs or methods available to 1995 physicians?

At the close of the century these issues would largely remain enigmatic. And in the absence of clear understanding of the elusive Ebola virus public health responses would rely on classic measures, practiced by scientists, physicians, and nurses during epidemics for a hundred years.

For the Zairois Ebola's presence raised horror for very different reasons. The inexplicable nature of an event, or lack thereof, was rarely a primary cause for consternation among the people of Kikwit, as more than three decades of an increasingly brutal dictatorship had left few individuals with a sense of power over their own fates. The major shocks in their lives rarely involved circumstances of their own making or full comprehension, but might well result from an offhand remark made by the dictator the previous day in the faraway capital of Kinshasa. Besides, *landa-landa* served as the all-purpose explanation for otherwise mysterious horrors, deaths, pains, and traumas in life.

Nor could disease, alone, be the source of their collective trepidation. The United Nations Children's Fund (or UNICEF) ranked Zaire number twelve in child mortality, meaning only eleven nations in the world witnessed higher proportional death rates among their under-five-year-olds.[5] Every year the mothers of Zaire gave birth to just over two million babies. And 442,000 of them didn't live to see their fifth birthdays. Nearly half of the nation's children were, by strict medical definition, malnourished, 45 percent of them growth-stunted as a result. The major causes of child death were malaria (increasing due to drug resistance among the parasites), malnutrition, measles, and HIV.

If a child survived to age five, odds were good he or she would reach adolescence. Then the youngster would face a new series of threats: AIDS, tuberculosis, murder, maternal death in childbirth.[6] Malarial episodes were frequent, as were the pains of syphilis, gonorrhea, and chlamydia. The main road of Kikwit—Boulevard Mobutu, named after the dictator—was lined with mud hut pharmacies offering everything from, literally, snake oil to out-of-date antibiotics as remedies to the long list of ailments that formed an assumed, seemingly normal, part of life atop the equator.

No, death and disease were not, in and of themselves, the causes of Kikwitians grave fear in the face of Ebola.

The terror grew from the horror evoked by the illness itself and its rapid progression to death.

"I dare to say that anyone who has seen a case of Ebola will never forget it," Dr. Tamfum Muyembe said.[7] Recalling his first encounter with the virus in September 1976 Muyembe said that he'd worked barehanded on patients who were drenched in blood.

"I had never before seen blood continue to flow at the site of injection," Muyembe recalled, describing Ebola as "strange, a fever that responded neither to antibiotics or antimalarials."

Muyembe spoke as a scientist and physician, finding concern in details similar to those that worried his Western counterparts. But in Kikwit's central marketplace, where all manner of rain forest meat and plants were sold, Ebola raised different fears.

"I pray most of the time now in order to get protection from God," fishmonger Kieghilamga said, holding her palms upright beside her tattooed cheeks and raising her eyes to the clouded day. Those people who died, she insisted, "were poisoned. I don't know who poisoned them. It makes me afraid."

Brigitte Mwalanga sadly rearranged her display of smoked caterpillars, which because of their crunchy flavorfulness usually sold quickly. But there were few buyers now, she said, because, "everybody is afraid. I'm very afraid."

The usually bustling market was oddly quiet and bereft of its typical mob of morning buyers. Sugar seller Pascaline waved at fellow traders, all of whom, like her, were having trouble moving the goods that they displayed upon make-shift wooden tables of crate boxes. Usually the plump woman drew crowds who admired her humorous banter and jolly mood. But Pascaline's outlook was cool now, and, "Salutation is forbidden. I don't greet people and I don't like to eat with others or share food."

Pascaline's usually gregarious behavior was reined in by Ebola, which "instantly," she says, killed her good friend Willy Ndumba, a nurse at Kikwit General Hospital.

As Pascaline speaks, young groundnut vendor Brigitte nods sadly, then ticks off a list of those she knows who have died suddenly of the dreaded disease. When asked how she copes with her fears Catholic Brigitte looks down at her feet and whispers, "I just pray."

Far away from the quarantined Bandundu Province, accessible only by chartered plane or a drive of three and a half days over the potholed Mobutu Highway, a warlike state of siege reigned in the Zairois capital, Kinshasa. The rooftops of her few hotels are dotted with portable satellite dishes, impromptu news bureaus fill the hotels' suites, multilingual hustlers find ready employment as translators for the media, and cell phones beep in the hallways. A horde of journalists, most of them shell-shocked after previous weeks of bearing witness to the horrors of civil war in Rwanda, set up camp in Kinshasa. With the same aggressive verve that had kept them alive during one of Africa's most brutal conflicts, a media corps from all over the world clamored and competed for news from the front of humanity's battle with a microbe. If the reporters feared the virus they did not show it, for missing deadlines or being trounced by their competitors were paramount concerns.

Not far from the media encampments another frenzied horde was gathered around Health Secretary Lonyangela Bompenda. Bureaucrats, generals, and the dictator's cadres struggled to guess Mobutu's whims while preventing panic in the capital. All too aware of the satellite dishes atop the Hotel Intercontinental, the government leaders struggled to keep the nation's face while maintaining access to Zaire's oil and diamond reserves.

Reading the tea leaves to surmise the dictator's will was something of an art in Kinshasa. No one survived, either politically or in material reality, for long if Mobutu's ire was raised. But the sixty-five-year-old dictator offered little guidance. Indeed, he seldom set foot any longer in the capital, preferring the security and solitude of Gbadolite, some 750 miles to the northeast of Kinshasa. There he was surrounded by Mouvement Populaire de la Révolution cronies and leaders of the seventy-thousand-strong Zairois Army. The sycophants bowed to their "democratically elected leader," who held court seated upon a throne, clutching the staff traditionally given to tribal chieftains and wearing the royal skins of leopards. With his eyes always invisible behind pitch dark glasses Mobutu had held sway since 1964.

Back then Zaire was called Belgian Congo and had suffered nearly four hundred years of brutal colonialism, slavery, and exploitation. Though it was seventy-seven times the size of tiny Belgium, the Congo was ruled from 1876 to 1908 by a white king enthroned in Brussels. Africa's largest nation was controlled by the Belgian Parliament from 1908 to 1960. A bold leader emerged named Patrice Lumumba who espoused African nationalism and vaguely socialist ideals. In 1960, after only months on the job, Lumumba threatened continued Western access to the vast natural resources of Congo, including cobalt and uranium, then in demand for nuclear weapons production.

Convinced Lumumba would open the African door to Soviet communism, CIA director Allen Dulles ordered Congo's head of state assassinated.[8] Driving Dulles's decision were a series of cables from Leopoldville (the colonial name of Kinshasa) sent by Congo CIA station chief Lawrence Devlin. In a key cable Devlin claimed that "embassy and station believe the Congo experiencing classic communist effort takeover government. . . . Whether or not Lumumba actually Commie or just playing Commie game to assist his solidifying power, anti-West forces rapidly increasing power Congo, and there may be little time left in which take action to avoid another Cuba."

Under direct orders from Dulles and President Eisenhower's National Security Council the CIA created violent riots in Kinshasa and selected thirty-one-year-old Colonel Joseph Mobutu as the heir apparent, pending assassination of Lumumba.

Two attempts to kill Lumumba using CIA-developed biological weapons failed. The CIA deliberately leaked word of Lumumba's pending murder, causing the legally elected head of state to flee the capital for distant Lumbumbashi. There, with CIA assistance, Mobutu's troops surrounded and murdered unarmed Lumumba on January 13, 1961, placing his body in the trunk of a car, much as a gang of Mafiosi might dispose of their enemies in a gangster hit.

Mobutu seized power but was immediately opposed in armed insurrections in the Katanga and Shaba provinces. To ensure the political survival of the Mobutu regime during the tempestuous years of 1961 to 1967 the CIA flew in Cuban anti-Communist mercenaries, trained an elite corps of 243 Zairois soldiers in Israel, and occasionally dropped top units of the U.S. Special Forces into hotly contested areas. Belgium also bolstered Mobutu's climb to power, deploying commando units to lead his troops in combat in rebellious Katanga.

From the beginning Mobutu proved a wily leader. Outwardly he donned all the appearances of classic African nationalism. He wore the attire of traditional chiefs, mixed with his own version of business jackets—a stifling cross between Nehru jackets worn in India, Chinese Mao jackets, and thick European business suits. The nation's name was changed to Zaire, a wholly concocted amalgam of Bantu names. All Zairois were commanded in 1971 to also change their names, dropping the Christian appellations that had been used for more than two centuries. The new leader changed his own name from Joseph to Sese Seko Kuku Ngbendu wa za Banga, or "the all-conquering warrior who triumphs over all obstacles."

The nationalistic veneer fooled many pan-Africanists, who thought Mobutu the equal of such contemporaries on the continent as Kwame Nkrumah in Ghana, Nelson Mandela in South Africa, and Tanzania's Julius Nyerere.

Prophetically, on his cancer deathbed in 1961, the Algerian intellectual Franz Fanon warned, "Our mistake is to have believed that the [Western] enemy had lost his combativeness and his harmfulness. If Lumumba is in the way, Lumumba disappears. . . . Let us be sure never to forget it: the fate of all of us is at stake in the Congo."

Throughout the 1970s and 1980s Mobutu proved a ready ally for Europe and the United States, offering his country as a staging and training ground for counterinsurgency forces bent on toppling governments and guerrilla fronts considered hostile to the apartheid state of South Africa: Angolan troops fighting in opposition to the MPLA (the Popular Movement for the Liberation of Angola); mercenaries and South African Special Forces troops battling Namibia's SWAPO (Southwest African People's Organization); Frelimo (Mozambique's anticolonial organization); and all presences of Cuban troops in Africa. That all of these organizations eventually attained power in their respective countries—and in some cases still retained that power at the close of the twentieth century—is indication of the failure of the West's Zaire strategy.

Nevertheless, the Zaire engagement stratagem remained in place throughout the Cold War and well into the 1980s. It was not until the arrival of the Clinton administration in the United States that Mobutu felt the slightest chill in his warm alliance with the West.

In exchange for Mobutu's willingness to act as Africa's proxy for Western anti-Soviet interests the dictator gained tremendous power and personal wealth. From 1963 to 1984 France, Belgium, South Africa, and the United States provided the dictator with astounding amounts of foreign aid—often in the form of zero-interest, no-strings-attached loans—and direct military assistance.[9]

Perhaps even more valuable to the dictator than the West's military support was its willingness to ignore Mobutu's obscene greed and corruption. As the Western governments poured cash into Zaire's coffers, everyone knew that the Mobutu regime couldn't provide legitimate receipts, for the funds rarely found their way to the programs for which they were designated. A massive General Electric–built Congo river dam, sufficient to power the electrical needs of all sub-Saharan Africa, fell to ruin because U.S. foreign aid funds for maintenance mysteriously never reached the electric power authority's bank account. Roads were never built. Hospitals and schools fell to ruin, most faring worse under Mobutu than they had when a Belgian colonial missionary system handled the bulk of Congo's health and education needs. Only 42 percent of the nation had access to anything vaguely resembling safe drinking water, and sanitation and garbage services were available to just 15 percent of the population. Nothing in the nation—from telephones to airports—functioned reliably. Agricultural production was poor, but distribution of foodstuffs even worse. The 42.3 million Zairois suffered in a country almost entirely lacking in infrastructure, their complaints met with brutal repression, torture, and military assault.

Meanwhile, North American and European companies routinely paid hefty "fees" to Mobutu and his cronies in exchange for access to Zaire's genuine wealth: her cobalt (60 percent of the world's reserves, and a strategic metal), copper, cadmium, gold, silver, uranium, tin, germanium, zinc, manganese, oil, diamonds, ivory, and rubber.[10] While per capita income stagnated for twenty years, never exceeding $180 per year, Mobutu became one of the world's wealthiest men, Belgium's biggest property owner, and a key real estate player in France and Switzerland.

As early as 1977, after just twelve years of such graft and corruption, Mobutu is estimated to have amassed a personal fortune equal to Zaire's official foreign debt—$5 billion. To ensure the loyalty of his cronies, as well as his personal safety, Mobutu allowed graft to flow to a tiny coterie of fellow gangsters, most of whom resided near him in Gbadolite. His uncle, Litho, for example, died leaving assets in excess of $1 billion. His second wife was arrested in Belgium in 1977 trying to smuggle $6 million worth of diamonds into the country.

By the time Ebola struck Kikwit the dictator and his friends had stolen at least $11 billion from the Zairois people.[11] The national bank had been shut down since 1991, when soldiers looted Kinshasa having learned that the currency in which they were paid carried no value. There was no cash in the bank, and no legal exchange of currency. The black market was Zaire's only monetary system, and there a $100 bill could fetch two twenty-five-pound satchels full of 100- and 500-Zaire notes, each of which bore the portrait of the nation's greatest thief, Mobutu. Even at that exchange rate it was hard to see the worth of the Zaire note, given that a tankful of gasoline required an inch-thick stack of the nation's highest denomination Z500 notes. For the seasoned traveler accustomed to the currency crises of developing countries the Zaire stood out as a "funny money" challenge that defied space afforded by pockets, purses, wallets, and money belts. Zairois businessmen routinely carried foot-thick stacks of Z100 and Z500 notes, arranged in rubber-band-held bundles valued at Z5,000 or Z20,000. Payments were usually negotiated by bundle, and only the most paltry of goods—such as Brigitte Mwalanga's smoked caterpillars—could be purchased with individual Z100 or Z500 notes.

It was in this national climate of corruption and currency fraud that the Ebola virus flourished in 1995. By the time it surfaced in Kikwit after a nineteen-year hiatus the nation's public health and medical infrastructure existed in name only. There were twenty-four thousand Zairois for every hospital bed in the nation. The majority of the population was under eighteen years of age in a nation almost bereft of condoms and contraceptives. HIV was rampant, afflicting an estimated 10 percent of the adult population. The multinational Project SIDA, once the most productive AIDS research center in all of Africa, was shut down, its equipment looted during the 1991 soldiers' riots.

And, most importantly, the nation's civil servants, including more than 95 percent of Zaire's physicians and nurses, had gone unpaid since the 1991 riots. The dictator, having grown smug in his old age, ceased even pretending to maintain national cash reserves to back civil service paychecks: Mobutu and his cronies were by 1995 overtly siphoning every penny of foreign exchange directly into their personal bank accounts.

When a Zairois became ill in 1995 his or her family had three choices: ignore the ailment and pray the individual muddled through somehow; carry or transport the ailing relative to a missionary hospital and there beg for free treatment; or, most often, get the relative to one of Zaire's government clinics or hospitals. In a foreign-funded mission facility Western-trained physicians offered good care, using reasonable equipment and drugs. But in the civil facilities the physician or nurse would make a diagnosis, usually without the use of such nonexistent or long-since-broken-down medicinal tools as X rays, laboratory tests, CT scans, or blood pressure devices. Even thermometers were in short supply.

Once a diagnosis was reached, the government health care worker would tell the family what was needed to ensure their relative's recovery, and the Zairois family would dutifully pool their resources and search their homes and local stores for the prescribed essentials: bedsheets, anesthesia, sterile equipment, antibiotics, food, bandages, and the like. More often than not sterile equipment was the lowest priority and, frankly, unavailable. In contrast, the black market and private pharmacies were chock-full of medicines of all kinds, even state-of-the-art broad-spectrum antibiotics.

The market was well supplied because doctors and nurses, lacking paychecks or other means to support their own families, simply sold off whatever medical supplies reached their facilities, either doled out by the Ministry of Health or, more commonly, donated by foreign nongovernmental charities and religious organizations. Everything that was saleable, from latex gloves to X-ray film, had disappeared from the nation's hospitals and clinics since 1991, and by 1995 the Zairois people had grown begrudgingly accustomed to bartering their worldly goods and services in exchange for medical supplies and the skills of local health care workers.[12]

Two things are clear: Ebola spread in Kikwit because the most basic, essential elements of public health were nonexistent. And those exigencies were lacking in Kikwit—indeed, throughout Zaire—because Mobutu Sese Seko and his cronies had for three decades looted the national treasuries. Ebola haunted Zaire because of corruption and political repression. The virus had no secret powers, nor was it unusually contagious. For centuries Ebola had lurked somewhere in the jungles of central Africa. Its emergence into human populations required the special assistance of humanity's greatest vices: greed, corruption, arrogance, tyranny, and callousness. What unfolded in Zaire in 1995 was not so much the rain forest terror widely depicted then in popular media worldwide as an inevitable outcome of disgraceful disconcern—even disdain—for the health of the Zairois public.

Gaspard Menga Kitambala was a forty-three-year-old charcoal maker, Jehovah's Witness, husband, and father of five small children. Those were his vital statistics, along with the fact that he resided near Ndala Avenue in a modest mud-and-brick house located along a precarious, steep muddy pathway that was alternately engulfed by rain forest vegetation or transformed into a waterfall during equatorial monsoons. By all accounts Menga was a hardworking fellow, devout Jehovah's Witness Christian, and devoted father.

Menga's strong, muscular body bespoke the tough physicality of his profession. The making and transport of charcoal was arduous and phenomenally labor intensive, given the low cash return. Menga regularly bicycled or walked to the rain forest, which until the 1970s engulfed most of modern-day Kikwit, but each year retreated farther and farther away, yielding to the axes of firewood-hungry Kikwitians. After two decades of hacking at the forest the periphery was more than a full day's walk away. And reaching the denser regions where Menga toiled took up to three days.

Once there, Menga would make camp, dig large pits, and fill them with the wood of felled trees. Then he would set the wood afire, lightly bury it, and allow the smoldering heat to char the trees down to hefty chunks of charcoal. After two weeks of such labor Menga would haul his heavy cargo back to Kikwit, selling it to fuel-starved neighbors.

It was never difficult to sell charcoal at a comparatively decent price, for

Kikwit had few other sources of cooking fuel. Propane and gasoline were far more expensive, and in such short supply that idled vehicles awaiting petrol frequently lined the road. Most so-called gas stations were little more than crates atop which sat a haphazard selection of gasoline-filled bottles and plastic jugs, thirty of which were usually needed to fill an automobile tank. Not surprisingly, there were few cars or trucks in Kikwit, and most people—Menga, included—walked everywhere, carrying their burdens atop their heads.

In December 1994 Menga was camped deep in the forest, not far from the Lwemi River. It was a verdant place, redolent with well-mulched soil and fragrant flowers. Butterflies danced in the areas penetrated by the sun. Tall trees, laced with lianas, protruded from the dense undergrowth. In some spots a plant locally called "quatre-vingt," or "eighty," choked all rival growth, leaving patches where nothing but the local weed grew. No one knew from whence "quatre-vingt" had come, but its name signified the year, 1980, when the alien vegetation suddenly sprung up all over Bandundu province. The tall weed crowded out all indigenous growth, much as kudzu had long ago taken over the untended areas of America's Deep South. In place of growth that was once diverse and filled with edible plants and animals, sprouted the poisonous "quatre-vingt."[13] Wherever stands of the tall weeds appeared the Bandundu wildlife was forced elsewhere, crowding into dwindling sites of indigenous growth.

In his own very small way Menga was contributing to the region's deforestation, knocking down trees and creating spaces into which the opportunistic "quatre-vingt" could grow.[14] The terrible weed, which choked manioc and corn crops as well as the forest, was just one of a long list of ecological changes Bandundu's forests had undergone since local human populations grew to their 1995 proportions. The so-called city of Kikwit with its 400,000 residents was little more than a gigantic village, as it lacked even a modicum of an urban infrastructure. A key missing item was employment: Kikwit had no industry or large businesses. If the people had stayed in their villages they might have lived off the land, growing cassava, manioc, and corn. But in Kikwit their village-style wattle huts were jammed one against the other, leaving no room for cultivation. In the absence of an urban employer Kikwitians had little choice but to arise with the dawn and trek to the forest in search of animals to sell as bushmeat, caterpillars, snakes, medicinal herbs, and other saleable items. Every year the people made their task more difficult as they chopped and pushed the forest's periphery, extending the distance of their periodic treks.

The fortunate, resourceful few laid claim to the newly timbered lands, planting small plots of corn, manioc, or cassava. They fought daily battles with encroaching "quatre-vingt" weeds, but usually could eke out a subsistence from decent-size plots. Gaspard Menga had such a plot, located along his route to the rain forest. It was a source not of income but of food for the large, hungry Menga clan.

For Menga the long journeys to the forest signaled time away from his family, and hours of lonely work surrounded by enormous black and red ants, malarial mosquitoes, venomous snakes, spiders larger than a human hand, flying squirrels, mongoose, small antelopes, bats, and, rarely, monkeys. That which he caught, Menga ate. And at night he slept in a makeshift hut, where he was undoubtedly tormented by insects.

Shortly after Christmas 1994 Menga loaded up another batch of charcoal and headed back to Kikwit. No one knows when the fever, sore throat, fatigue, and achy muscles first hit the hardworking man. No matter how sick he felt Menga had little choice but to push on for Kikwit, as there were no refuges nor medical aid along his route.

By the time he reached his humble home on Ndala Avenue Menga had a fever and was exhausted. His wife, Bébé Ando, tended to him and shooed away their youngest boys, seven-year-old Judo and Michael, age two. But by January 6, 1995, his fever had soared, and Menga had bloody diarrhea. Alarmed, Bébé Ando took Menga to a local clinic where he began vomiting blood, becoming so weak he could not walk. The clinic transferred Menga to Kikwit General Hospital, where he was placed in Pavilion No. 3. The doctors who cared for Menga were understandably alarmed by their patient's rapid deterioration, and on the assumption he was suffering from Shigella-induced dysentery, filled him with locally available antibiotics.

On January 13 Gaspard Menga died, and the family brought his body home. There Bébé Ando and Gaspard's younger brothers, Pierre and Bilolo, lovingly washed down the dead man and dressed him in his church clothes. Menga family members from faraway villages came to the open-casket funeral and, as was customary among local Catholics, touched or kissed the body, bidding Gaspard speedy admittance into heaven. Photographs of the mourning depict a family deeply distraught by their loss, with some draping themselves in grief over Gaspard's body.

A few days later Gaspard's brother Bilolo fell ill, exhibiting symptoms the family knew were the same as those that had devastated Gaspard. On February 3 he died in the Kikwit General Hospital emergency room.

Sensing that she, too, was falling ill to some terrible *landa-landa*, Bébé Ando sent her children off with their aunt, Marie-José Nseke, to the care of their grandparents in the village of Ndobo. And then she, too, began to bleed uncontrollably from her anus and nose. At a local infirmary her condition was mistakenly diagnosed as malaria and, when she vomited blood, pneumonia. Like her brother-in-law before her, Bébé Ando died in the ER of Kikwit General Hospital.

Meanwhile, in the village of Ndobo, a day's drive away, Bébé Ando's youngest son, Michael Jackson Menga (named after the family's favorite pop star) took ill, suffering the now-familiar litany of Menga family symptoms: headache, fever, fatigue, depression, anorexia, muscle aches, sharp stomach pains, inability to swallow, bloody diarrhea, bloody nose, bloody vomitus, hiccups, reddened eyes, and red urine. In short, he bled to death on February 11. His older brother, Judo, followed suit, five days later.

Ndobo was one of six villages affected by the tragedy unfurling for the Mengas. Located across the Kwilu River from Kikwit, the villages were connected by a spider's web of dirt roads barely traversable with a four-wheel-drive vehicle. In some stretches the roads were little more than meter-wide paths beaten out of stands of savannah grass by the steady treading of feet.

Every village had its own character, often dictated by its chief. Ndobo's chief, Santu, was a white-bearded, bald man who appeared to be elderly, though he was probably less than fifty years old. When visitors arrived Santu struggled to silence Ndobo's mobs of unruly children, which outnumbered the adults fifteen-to-one. Only by swinging his staff sharply, occasionally connecting with a youngster's backside, could Santu maintain a semblance of order.

In the center of the village was a large, rectangular thatched building in which Michael Jackson, Judo, their Aunt Marie-José, and their three sisters Lenza, Asinta, and Gizelle stayed with their grandparents following Gaspard's funeral. By March 1, both grandparents had died of Ebola.[15]

Nobody in Ndobo understood the terrible *landa-landa* that struck the Menga relatives. It would be months before explanations would come from distant Kikwit. For village chief Santu and the unruly herds of children that raced about the place the Menga clan's suffering was simply a more mysterious and frightening version of the death toll that haunted their lives. Some of the children were AIDS orphans, after all. But AIDS killed slowly—this *landa-landa* destroyed bodies and minds in a week's time. So the villagers ordered the family's bodies buried well outside of their tiny town, where the fearsome *landa-landa* could not reach them as they slept at night.

When the Menga death toll was counted, in Kikwit and the various villages, sixteen of the twenty-three who either had attended Gaspard's funeral or tended to those who contracted Ebola from Gaspard died of the disease. Amazingly, every Menga who developed symptoms eventually perished—an astounding 100 percent kill rate. Perhaps equally amazing were the cases of Mengas who apparently never did get the disease. Twenty-six-year-old Pierre, for example, washed his brother's body which, unbeknownst to him, was drenched in virus-rich blood and fluids. And he tended to his other dying brother, Bilolo, and sister-in-law, Bébé Ando. Yet Pierre said he never suffered as much as a headache. Neither did Pierre and Gaspard's father, Innocent, who participated in several

Menga funerals. Most startling was elderly Innocent's survival. Having long suffered from tuberculosis, Innocent was a frail, weak man. He helped bury three of his sons, three daughters-in-law, and several grandchildren. Yet he never caught Ebola.

Similarly, Lenza, Asinta, and Gizelle touched their father's corpse and cared for their dying brothers, Judo and Michael Jackson. When the boys succumbed the sisters prepared the bodies for burial in Ndobo. And when their grandparents subsequently developed Ebola disease the three little girls were again exposed to the virus. Yet they never took ill. Nor did the members of the Mbelo family who helped the three little orphans and buried all of the Mengas who succumbed in Ndobo.

After the Menga grandparents died Ebola simply stopped in the village of Ndobo. Why? No one knows. But Ndobo's confrontation with the dreaded virus was long over before the people knew the cause of their tragedy or the world knew that Ebola had broken out in Zaire.

A similar pattern played out in other villages where Menga relatives resided following Gaspard's funeral. In the neat, orderly village of Kimputu-Nseke, for example, thirty-five-year-old Romaine Mawita—wife of Gaspard's brother Nico Menga—and her two small children died in mid-February. And though the villagers helped care for the ailing trio, and buried their bodies, no other residents of Kimputu-Nseke came down with the virus. By March the villages' struggles with the virus were over. When Ebola would rage months later in Kikwit the people of Kimputu-Nseke would be untouched, both by the virus and by panic. While fear would grip most of the region, Kimputu-Nseke residents still greeted strangers with the palms-up gesture of friendship and salutations of *Mbote*.

By mid-March this cycle of death had passed, allowing the villages of Ndobo, Kimputu-Nseke, Nkara, Mukolo, Bulunga, and Ikubi to return to normal life—and death.

Such was not the case back in Kikwit. In the villages, where the only medical care available were the ministrations of friends and relatives, Ebola failed to pass beyond its initial chain of infections. But in Kikwit, where public health was a shambles, but medical clinics abounded, the virus would find grand opportunity.

Gaspard, Bilolo, and Bébé Ando all died in the decrepit emergency room of Kikwit General Hospital. So did Gaspard's aunt, Rosalie Sandrala, on February 14, 1995.

A wide dirt road, accessible from a back alleyway, met the ramp up to Kikwit's Salle d'Urgence. Rusted, heavy steel gurneys covered with thin, worn-out plastic pads, were strewn haphazardly about the area, some nestled among the weeds and mud of the hospital grounds, exposed to the equatorial heat and daily downpours, while others sat just at the top of the ramp under the cinder block turquoise veranda entryway to the ER. On any given day dozens of family members milled about the area, using the gurneys as benches and beds while they awaited word on the status of an ailing relative.

An officious ward clerk barred entry to the ER, using his table to create an obstacle that prevented the anxious families from mobbing the already crowded medical facility. Names and symptoms were dutifully entered into his logbook in a mix of KiCongo and French when one ER bed was vacated and another patient was allowed to come in. Protected from the tropical rain, usually lying on the concrete floor of the veranda, were the desperately ill waiting to see a doctor. Most were malnourished children—toddlers, really—whose eyes stared out vacantly from feverish heads. Malaria, measles, bacterial infections, and meningitis were among their predators.

The adult infirm were also largely victims of microbes, which caused them variously to spit up blood from tuberculosis-infested lungs; walk on stick-thin legs wasted by years of HIV infection; fight malarial fevers of more than 103°F; or, most commonly, combat some mysterious *landa-landa* that produced sudden fatigue, fevers, headaches, and malaise.

These patients could wait. That was what the clerk was taught. First priority was the comparatively rare case of trauma, a bleeding accident victim. Second priority were feverish babies, for everyone in Kikwit had seen how rapidly little ones could die: one day they seemed like normal babies, and the next day they were cadavers.

Inside the dark ER only indirect sunlight could guide the physicians' and nurses' activities by day, kerosene lamps by night. Decades-old steel-framed beds lined two walls of the ER, leaving a narrow walkway between. So crowded was the place that health care workers stumbled into one another as they moved among patients. Most patients stared out from pain or fever, an IV drip delivered through recycled needles silently passing into their bloodstreams saline, antibiotics, or antimalarial drugs, along with whatever microbes might be on the needle.

Next door in a tiny chamber was the transfusion table, set diagonally toward an eastern window. When malarial parasites overwhelmed the oxygen-carrying red blood cells of an individual's body, minutes counted. Death could occur in the blink of an eye if the suffering one didn't immediately receive millions of healthy, oxygen-rich red blood cells. These, of course, had to come from a genetically matched relative or the victim's immune system would reject the transfusion, and death due to anaphylaxis would swiftly follow.

More often than not a child less than five years of age lay upon the transfusion table receiving blood drawn from a parent or older sibling. Encrusted with dried blood and rust, the transfusion table loomed like some medieval torture rack. And though it was a site for short-term cures, the old steel slab was also a daily source of infection where, through either nonsterile needles or directly from the contaminated donor's blood, the transfused received doses of HIV, hepatitis B, *Plasmodium falciparum* parasites, and assorted other microbes.

The health care workers did the best they could, given their nearly complete lack of resources. There were syringes and surgical supplies which, when the electrical generator worked, could be sterilized in an autoclave. A small supply of latex gloves were washed and recycled after a day's use. The hospital lab performed rapid tests to determine that transfusions involved matched blood types. But they lacked kits that could as rapidly test the blood for HIV, hepatitis, or other infections.

The surgical pavilions were similarly sparsely supplied. The sorts of massive, round overhead lights used in surgical theaters in Europe four or five decades previously loomed over the operating tables but were rarely powered, as electricity was a precious commodity. Sunlight pouring in through screenless windows typically guided the surgeons' hands. The patients, nurses, anesthesiologists, and surgeons were protected from one another's germs by a thin veneer of hygiene: cloth tie-up masks, recycled latex gloves, cotton surgical gowns. These items, as well as the surgical equipment, were washed every day in local water. The hospital had no tap water, nor any source of sterile liquid. Instead, physicians scrubbed in tubs of toted river water, often unable to obtain soap that might offer a modicum of hygiene. When electricity could not be generated, surgical instruments were boiled over a wood or charcoal fire—thus, the Bandundu forests offered both fuel for sterilization and refuge for the very microbes responsible for much of Kikwit's *landa-landa.*

Patients that were hospitalized ended up on designated one-story cinder block wards, lying upon bare steel-framed beds. Only a wafer-thin plastic pad shielded their bodies from jutting steel, and any amenities such as food, pillows, and sheets were provided by visiting relatives. The wards, or pavilions, were designated according to Kikwit's greatest health needs. The largest was pediatric, where mothers often slept with their ailing children. As those youngsters confronted death new babies were born in the hospital's most densely packed ward, maternity. There expectant mothers frequently had to share a twin hospital bed, lying diagonally head-to-foot alongside a stranger, their newborns jostling for space. Babies were delivered by gloveless midwives who toiled amidst maternal and neonatal blood, usually with only the faint flicker of a single kerosene lamp to guide their efforts as they slit episiotomies, cut umbilical cords, performed C-sections, or corrected breech births.

Off to the side, disconnected from the rest of the hospital, was the Salle du tuberculose et de la SIDA where adult AIDS and TB patients languished.

And in two tiny chambers at the end of the long, blue open-air hallway that connected the pavilions were the hospital's laboratories and statistics office. There technicians hunched over one of two available light microscopes, usable only by sunlight. Their laboratory samples sat in unpowered refrigerators. Glass tubes, stoppered with rags or cotton balls, rested in racks awaiting analysis. And, as was the case with most of their hospital colleagues, the laboratory personnel lacked any protective gear to prevent their infection in the event contaminated samples spilled onto their hands, eyes, noses, or cut into their bloodstreams.

Even worse conditions reigned at Kikwit Maternity Hospital No. 2, where most of the city's babies were born. On March 2 Pauline Kabala, Rosalie Sandrala's best friend, checked into Kikwit Maternity Hospital No. 2 suffering bloody diarrhea and vomiting blood. Eight nurses and several friends attended to Kabala, who was dying; within days all of them came down with the same bloody illness. Six of the eight hospital employees died of it in March. Before they died— indeed before they even realized that they were ill—these nurses and friends passed their infections on to still more hospital employees, family members, and patients, starting a chain of death that would in April spiral out of the maternity hospital and into the general community. Kikwit's mysterious *landa-landa* was getting out of control.

Meanwhile at Kikwit General Hospital doctors had their hands full in March with cases of what looked like shigella bacterial infection, the leading cause of bloody diarrhea. True, it was rare to see shigella patients also vomit blood, bleed from their noses and gums, and have bloodied eyes. Shigella didn't usually cause such things. But in 1995 a new type of shigella had emerged in the world, in the far east of the country in a rocky, volcanic place called Goma. There, tens of thousands of refugees had taken haven from the civil war slaughter in neighboring Rwanda, living without viable shelter, food, or safe drinking water. Cholera and shigella broke out among the refugees, claiming thousands of lives.[16] And due to widespread misuse of antibiotics the strain of shigella rampant in the region became resistant to all available drugs. Only one drug in the entire world had any effect against the new superbug, and it was at least ten times more expensive than anything in use in the region. Ciprofloxacin, a German-made powerful, third-generation antibiotic was the last, completely unaffordable hope for Central African shigella sufferers.[17]

It seemed a logical conclusion, then, that the wave of bloody deaths in Kikwit General Hospital and Maternity Hospital No. 2 were caused by the new supershigella. Or so Dr. Mungala Kipassa thought. To be certain, the young M.D., who had a master's in public health, ordered Maternity Hospital No. 2 lab technician Kakesa Kimfumu to take blood samples from several of the patients.[18] If shigella were in those samples Kipassa knew that steps would have to be taken to decontaminate Kikwit's water supplies lest a full-fledged dysentery epidemic might erupt.

Kimfumu, age thirty-six, did his job in early April, drawing samples from several patients, including hospital administrator Kimbambu. Somehow Kimfumu became infected, probably through an accidental poke with the needle drawn from Kimbambu (who died on March 27), and Kimfumu went from being a hospital employee to patient.

On April 10 Kimfumu was transferred to Kikwit General Hospital where Kipassa's team struggled to understand what had happened to the laboratory worker. Kimfumu had some of the same symptoms seen in the other suspected shigella patients, with two key exceptions: he didn't have bloody diarrhea, but he did have a hugely protruding, distended belly. In the eyes of his physicians it looked like Kimfumu was suffering from appendicitis.

That day he underwent an appendectomy, conducted by surgeon Nyembe. But the removal of his appendix failed to improve Kimfumu's status. Indeed, in subsequent hours he became delirious and the distension of his belly worsened. The physicians concluded that their first diagnosis had been incorrect: Kimfumu had not appendicitis but an intestinal perforation caused by the bacterial infection typhoid fever.

So on April 12 Kimfumu underwent a second round of surgery intended to mend his perforated intestines. Present in the OR were anesthesiologist Willy Mubiala and nurses Mingweni Lakamoyo and Sister Floralba, a European nun with the Sisters of the Poor of Bengame. The surgeons were Drs. Nkuku and Bwaka, who were watched closely by local medical student Pila Puskas. As they prepared their patient for surgery the group was well aware that Kimfumu was one of their own—a fellow medical worker.

Things began to go wrong as soon as Nkuku made his incision, for Kimfumu's distension was full of blood, which spewed all over the unprotected surgical team. As they tried frantically to comprehend what was happening and save their colleague, the team members became drenched by Kimfumu's blood. Unable to find a single source of Kimfumu's bleeding or distension the surgeons had no choice but to sew the lab technician back up and return him to the postop ward. There, on April 14, Kimfumu died.

On the same day as he performed Kimfumu's appendectomy surgeon Nyembe also operated on Géraldine Katadi, the wife of prominent Pentecostal Pastor Kabanga, a follower of the evangelical faith Nzambe Malamu, or God is God.[19] Katadi had suffered placenta previa during a C-section of her baby and now required emergency surgery. Nyembe operated on Katadi immediately after completing Kimfumu's appendectomy. Nurses Anne Lusilu Manikasa and Jean Kingangi assisted Nyembe while Raymond Katima stood guard over the procedure.

And they would die: all but one person present during those three operations would perish, suffering the same litany of bloody symptoms as had tormented the Menga clan. But first they would travel, attend to other patients, and spend time with their families. The first to take ill would be Dr. Nyembe, who died on April 20, ten days after performing surgery on Kimfumu and Katadi. His cause of death was recorded as unknown etiology.

Two days later in Kikwit medical student Puskas, too, succumbed, as did scrub nurse Lakamoyo.

So when seventy-year-old Sister Floralba took ill the members of her order placed the ailing nun in the care of people who were told to take her to Sister Daniella. A nurse, Sister Daniella worked in a Catholic-run hospital located 120 kilometers away in the town of Mosango. Funded by the U.S.-based Catholic Relief Services, the Mosango 590-bed facility was larger, cleaner, and better supplied than Kikwit General.

The road to Mosango was in decent shape, even paved most of the way. Lined with jacarandas and palms the drive afforded a magnificent view, taking in verdant hillsides, tall monkeypod trees, red clay soil, and steady streams of colorfully dressed pedestrians toting on their heads baskets full of bananas, breadfruit, corn, and fish. The road crossed the Nko River to vast grasslands that reached up to open blue skies. The Mosango mission and hospital, perched atop a hill at the end of the grasslands, offered solace from the tropical, sweltering heat.

It's doubtful the sister noticed the view, as Floralba was deathly ill. By the time Belgian-born Dr. Marie-Jo Bonnet saw the Italian nun the sister was suffering "the worst hemorrhaging I've ever seen. She was elderly. And there was a huge amount of blood coming from her mouth. Her tongue was thick, covered with lesions and bleeding. Her gums, tongue, and lips . . . they all were bleeding," Bonnet grimly recalled days later.

Upon her arrival in Monsango on April 23 Floralba could only speak in monosyllables, and her fever exceeded more than 103°F. During the night, while Sister Daniella looked on, Sister Floralba's status worsened. Red, pinprick blood spots appeared all over her body, along with bruiselike splotches indicating uncontrolled bleeding under the skin. Wherever the doctors injected fluids and antibiotics bleeding started, and then never stopped.

By then Bonnet's group had tried five different antibiotic cocktails on Sister Floralba, with absolutely no effect.

The following day, on April 24, with Floralba's condition appearing hopeless and pressing matters awaiting her at another, distant clinic, Sister Daniella left. She'd only been in contact with Floralba for a few hours. After Daniella's departure, Bonnet tried desperately to stop Floralba's hemorrhaging, giving the nun high doses of vitamin K coagulant. "It was incredible," Bonnet recalled later. "The blood simply would not coagulate. Anything we did, it just kept bleeding, . . . the hemorrhage was so profound."

On April 25 Sister Floralba fell unconscious, her blood pressure plummeted, and at 10 A.M. she died.

Bonnet, who had worked in the Mosango hospital for a decade, was stunned. The sheer amount of the hemorrhaging, and no indications that Sister Floralba had contracted her illness from a patient in Kikwit General Hospital were both disturbing. Bonnet and physician colleagues Drs. Anicet Mazaya and Philippe Akamituna discussed the case, speculating as to whether Sister Floralba's death was caused by the same agent that had claimed four previous patients in Monsango.

Akamituna, a tall, young Zairois physician, noted the case of Pila Kikapindu, a male student nurse from Kikwit General Hospital. He'd arrived in Mosango on April 3, after being ill in Kikwit for four days.

"His brother-in-law said, 'Oh, it's AIDS,' " Akamituna remembered. "But his sister, who cared for him, came down with the same symptoms."

As Sister Floralba lay dying, so did Kikapindu's sister. And his mother. Their only connection to the horrible disease was the care they gave to Pila, who, despite the hospital's best efforts, died on April 14. (The mother and sister would also soon succumb.) And the same day that Pila Kikapindu bled to death another diseased refugee from Kikwit had arrived: Sambubanda Wagona. He died, suffering similar symptoms, three days later.

The doctors debated every aspect of these cases: were they connected? What caused their deaths? Was there danger for the rest of the hospital, given Mosango had no more gloves, masks, or sterile gowns for the health care workers?

Hours before Sister Floralba died another ailing nurse from Kikwit General Hospital arrived, seeking a cure that he knew could not be had in the far poorer government hospital. Twenty-five-year-old Ekara Mpolo had the now-classic set of hemorrhagic symptoms, and died a few hours after his arrival. His death sparked a chain of eight more cases, all among Mosango health care workers. Sister Daniella died. So did nurse Nzaka Munsango, who had cared for Mpolo. A lab technician, more nurses, the wife of one of these men—all died in rapid succession between April 26 and May 11.

Watching Munsango's deterioration proved particularly difficult for the hospital staff, as the illness affected his brain. He became a wild man, shouting deranged thoughts, accusing his colleagues of all manner of evils, flailing his arms wildly. Panic started to set in among the hospital staff and rumors of strange goings-on spread to the nearby villages.

Then something truly fearful happened. The wife of one of the deceased lab technicians died of the mysterious disease. Her room was scrubbed down, the mattress cleansed, and no one entered the room for more than two weeks. Then twenty-year-old Mupangi, hospitalized for unrelated reasons, was placed in that room, on the dead woman's bed. When Mupangi developed the symptoms of the now-terrifying disease, Bonnet faced panicked insurrection among her staff.

Mupangi's situation was analyzed thoroughly. It was clear the young woman had no other possible source of infection, Bonnet insisted. She could only have caught the disease from the plastic-and-foam padding that was her mattress. And the agent of death had somehow survived on that surface for fifteen days.

Bonnet's staff threatened to abandon the hospital, but top doctors staved off desertion by creating true isolation rooms for the remaining patients, and personally caring for Munsango and the rest. One, thirty-nine-year-old nurse Jean-Pierre Sabkuti, was caring for Munsango. When, at the end of April, he died, "no one here agreed to deal with the body," Bonnet said. "I did it, wearing a mask and gown and so on that I had. I, and Akamituna and Mazaya. We took the body for burial."

As the trio of physicians carried the body of their nurse down the hill to the cemetery, terrified Mosango villagers grabbed up their children and fled into their homes, hiding from the *landa-landa*. When the grieving doctors returned to the hospital the staff announced it would not enter Sabkuti's room to clean it. One nurse, when directly ordered to do so, quit. The three doctors thereafter had to perform all the saddest tasks themselves: placing the dead in coffins, hauling the bodies to the cemetery, burial, and the cleansing of the deceased's rooms.

On May 11 Nzaka Munsango died. And that afternoon shortwave radio reports broadcast from France informed the doctors that the culprit responsible for so many deaths in their hospital was a virus called Ebola.

That conclusion had not been reached swiftly. Indeed, the cause of the Bandundu *landa-landa* crisis was not determined until May, five months after the first Ebola death, that of Gaspard Menga. And the diagnosis was reached as much by luck and fate as by science.

In April other regional hospitals, like Mosango, experienced outbreaks of the bizarre, frightening disease, always commencing with a visitor from Kikwit. And nearly all the deaths in these facilities were among health care workers.

One such case turned out to be crucial. In the Yasa-Bonga hospital, located about 180 kilometers away from Kikwit, nurse Jean Kingangi underwent treatment, and there died of massive hemorrhaging sixteen days after becoming infected during Géraldine Katadi's surgery at Kikwit General Hospital. The doctors of Yasa-Bonga had tried every imaginable treatment on Kingangi, including attempts to clot his blood and antibiotic therapy to halt his presumed bacterial dysentery. Numerous blood and urine tests were done on Kingangi: his was the most extensively documented case.

And it would prove fortunate that a Zairois military surgeon, Dr. Kongolo, who specialized in tropical medicine, happened to pass through and personally see Kingangi's death. Kongolo speculated that the cause could be Ebola virus, about which he had read a great deal. Kongolo was the first person to reach that hypothesis, which he voiced shortly after Kingangi's death on April 26.

There were no telephones in Yasa-Bonga and therefore it was at first impossible for Kongolo to notify authorities or scientists who might confirm his dire suspicions. His only choice was to make the arduous 420-kilometer journey to Kinshasa and search for Professor Tamfum Muyembe, the famed veteran of the Yambuku outbreak of 1976.

Meanwhile, in Kikwit Dr. Kipassa was worried sick. His hospital seemed full of this bizarre, bloody disease, and most of the ill were members of his own staff. He was desperate. Convinced the supershigella had arrived in Kikwit, Kipassa sent pleas for better antibiotics to UNICEF and Muyembe, both in Kinshasa.

By the end of April Muyembe was, as a result, well aware that something terrible was afoot in Zaire. Zaire's leading scientist, Muyembe was a thoughtful, multilingual University of Kinshasa virologist whose serious nature was nicely counterbalanced by his warmth and strong sense of humor. One minute Muyembe would wrinkle his brow in deep thought over a dangerous conundrum, and the next his eyes would sparkle mischievously and he'd let loose with a loud guffaw.

His first action upon receiving Kipassa's desperate plea was to fire off a cable to Sister Agnes, a Catholic nun who had once served as a regional pharmacist in Bandundu. She had long since retired and now lived in a convent outside Antwerp, Belgium.

After hearing the military surgeon's conclusion that the Yasa-Banga case could have been caused by his old nemesis, Ebola, Muyembe packed his bags and grabbed the first charter plane to Kikwit.[20]

Meanwhile, in Belgium Sister Agnes was in a quandary. Muyembe's cable asked for thousands of doses of ciprofloxacin, an antishigella drug far more expensive than anything her poor order could handle. She estimated that she would need more than one million Belgian francs (or $37,000) to fill Muyembe's request: an impossible sum. Uncertain where or how to rapidly obtain the life-saving drugs, eighty-year-old Sister Agnes visited Dr. Simon van Nieuwenhove, showed him Muyembe's missive, and asked for advice.

Van Nieuwenhove worked in the tropical research institute in Antwerp, Belgium, and had done work in Zaire. What disturbed the middle-aged Flemish scientist was not the almost prohibitively expensive drug request, but a postscript Muyembe had hastily tagged onto the message: this could be not shigella, but Ebola. Muyembe had added that postscript after speaking to Kongolo, though the Zairois virologist hadn't yet tested blood samples from Kikwit patients. The word *Ebola* gave van Nieuwenhove a shudder, for his entire life had been influenced by that virus. While still a young scientist he had been part of the international team that investigated the Yambuku Ebola outbreak in 1976. He knew Muyembe, and respected the Zairois scientist's hunches.

So van Nieuwenhove told Sister Agnes to delay her search for ciprofloxacin. And he called up another veteran of the 1976 epidemic, American Dr. David Heymann. On loan from the CDC to the World Health Organization Heymann was working in Geneva at the WHO Global Programme on AIDS. His colleague had barely whispered the word *Ebola* when Heymann mentally packed his bags, considered which WHO and CDC people he'd like on his team, and visualized what needed to be done.

But first, he said, they needed laboratory samples for analysis. Nobody at WHO wanted to utter out loud the word *Ebola* unless they were certain that the virus had, indeed, reappeared after its nineteen-year hiatus. Having watched the global panic a few months earlier over India's plague outbreak, Heymann realized that a new era had dawned for public health. Back in 1976 when genuine fear had gripped the scientific team in Yambuku their terror had not been reflected in media coverage: fewer than ten wire stories had reported on the events, and there was no broadcast coverage. The scientists back then had toiled only under the watchful eyes of the Zairois soldiers and the terrified people of Yambuku. Frankly, back then nobody outside of Zaire seemed to take note of the event.

But times had changed. The avalanche of global media attention that greeted India's epidemic signaled a warning to Heymann. And there was more: the number one best-selling book in the English language at the time was *The Hot Zone*, by Richard Preston. A gripping account of an Ebola outbreak inside a monkey colony in Reston, Virginia, *The Hot Zone* had captured international attention, focusing a vague sense of public phobia on a virus of which few had previously heard. The book caught Hollywood's interest, and as Heymann pondered the Kikwit situation from his vantage point in Switzerland movie audiences from Rio de Janeiro to Tokyo were queuing up to see *Outbreak*, a Dustin Hoffman thriller about an imaginary Ebola epidemic.

So Heymann was discreet. He packed his bags, bought tickets to Kinshasa, and quietly informed only a handful of colleagues of Muyembe's suspicion.

Meanwhile, on May 1 Muyembe and his technical staff arrived in Kikwit, examined the patients, and collected blood samples. They were immediately able, based on laboratory analysis, to rule out shigella. And by the time he left Kikwit that day Muyembe was convinced that the Ebola virus had resurfaced. Muyembe on May 6 would send samples to Antwerp, which would then be rerouted immediately to the CDC's Biohazard Level 4 laboratory in Atlanta, Georgia.

On May 9 C. J. Peters, director of the Special Pathogens Laboratory, received the samples and within less than ten hours his team was able to confirm that the disease was, indeed, Ebola. Within two days the lab was able to say not only that it was Ebola, but also that the viral strain in Kikwit was almost genetically identical to that seen nineteen years earlier in faraway Yambuku.

A skeleton crew of just six scientists would toil round-the-clock in rotating shifts throughout the Ebola crisis inside the CDC's Biohazard Level-4 (BL-4) laboratory. The agency was overwhelmed by the deluge of human and animal blood and tissue samples that from May 9 onward arrived from Kikwit and neighboring villages. Though many—perhaps most—of the samples came up negative for Ebola infection, all had to be handled with the same level of care and caution a scientist might exercise while working with a container of weapons-grade plutonium. Because nobody knew precisely how the virus was transmitted, but did know that Ebola infection was incurable, all lab work was performed by scientists who wore full-body space suits that were attached to respiratory umbilical cords that pumped fresh air into their protective gear. The people living outside the Atlanta laboratory were protected by a system similar to nesting Russian dolls: the BL-4 lab was inside another, larger building which, in turn, was inside yet another. Each of these structures was airtight, maintained under tight security and accessible to fewer than a hundred people. The innermost, highest security chambers were verboten to all but a dozen human beings and a host of research animals.

Inside their respiratory suits C. J. Peters's team toiled with great care. Each one knew that any slipup could be immediately lethal to the scientist, and pose a significant risk to society as a whole should the organism have escaped its BL-4 containment.

Shortly after the CDC's Special Pathogens Laboratory confirmed on May 9 that blood samples from Kikwit General Hospital contained the Ebola hemorrhagic fever virus, lab director Peters issued memos to higher-ups at CDC warning that there was a distinct possibility that exhaustion, due to overwork among his downsized scientific crew, could result in a serious accident.

Because of the extremely highly skilled nature of BL-4 work it was not possible for the agency to simply draft personnel from other sections of the CDC to temporarily fill in gaps left by the budget cuts and congressionally mandated downsizing that had rendered the lab's seven scientists short of its former staffing level. His staff was too small, and the scientists were exhausted. Twenty years previously the CDC had been able to respond in such crises by shifting some laboratory work in two directions: non–BL-4 samples could go to its next security tiered Biohazard Level-3 facility and some of the extremely dangerous BL-4 load could be shared with one of the four other maximum security laboratories in the world.

But in the spring of 1995 some of the other BL-4 options simply were no longer reasonable. For example, there was a BL-4 lab in Siberia—a holdover from the heydays of Soviet science—but its security and safety had deteriorated considerably along with every other aspect of Russian public health and scientific research. Britain's Porton Down biological warfare facility was once considered suitable, and had played a role in the 1976 Ebola crisis. But due to changing political considerations vis-à-vis biowarfare and several rounds of budget cuts, Porton Down did not meet 1995 BL-4 standards.

For decades the leading backup to the CDC was France's Institut Pasteur in Paris. But WHO officials were reluctant to direct "hot" samples to the French laboratory because a scientist studying Ebola-contaminated blood there in the fall of 1994 had come down with the disease, indicating a security breach.

That left only one alternative BL-4 facility: the U.S. Army's Fort Detrick laboratory in Maryland. There, too, downsizing and budget cuts had taken a toll, as the Department of Defense sought to reduce its share of the national debt. However, the CDC's C. J. Peters, who had once worked at the Fort Detrick lab and maintained close contact with colleagues there, was unable to convince the army facility to help the CDC with analysis of Ebola samples.[21]

Meanwhile, the CDC was reluctant to pass non-Ebola work down the security tier to its two BL-3 facilities because the forty-year-old lab buildings had so deteriorated that a team of inspectors from outside the federal government had urged their condemnation more than five years previously.

So serious was the decay that air ducts meant to draw biological hazards away from lab benches and into safety filters actually did the reverse: they blew microbes right into scientists' faces. On at least three occasions in the last eighteen months scientists had, as a result, caught the very diseases they were studying.

In 1993, the U.S. Public Health Service had requested funds from Congress to construct a new BL-3 laboratory, and in the interim Congress had appropriated $88 million of the more than $110 million that was needed to build the facility. All but $1 million of this had been accumulating in an earmarked federal account, awaiting a time when sufficient additional funds were available to purchase land in the Atlanta area and construct the lab.[22]

Shortly after the world learned of the Kikwit Ebola outbreak Congress voted to rescind $40 million of that accumulated fund, and apply it toward retirement of the national debt. The Senate voted to rescind all $87 million remaining in the fund. President Clinton vetoed the two budget proposals, hoping to salvage at least $47 million of the BL-3 funds.

Republican staffers for the committees on Capitol Hill that oversaw HHS and CDC budgets said that the funding situation for all aspects of public health was "very fluid." As one staffer put it, "It's all a moving target—difficult to predict."[23]

Perhaps the strangest twist in funding events concerned WHO. Long reliant upon largesse from the United States, WHO initially faced the Ebola crisis with a budget of less than $10,000. But on May 19 a handful of private European corporations and foundations came up with $2 million in special aid to support Ebola control efforts. For most Americans and Europeans an outbreak of an exotic disease in a far-off African country seemed none of their business—particularly during post–Cold War national budget crises. Thus, the governments that traditionally underwrote such public health efforts initially demurred in the face of resurgent Ebola.

"The CDC is the only ball game in town," Dr. James LeDuc, head of WHO's special virus division, insisted, underscoring the world's complete, utter dependence on the American facility.[24]

On May 10 Heymann's tiny WHO team of three Ebola-fighters left Geneva, bound for Zaire. That same day the U.S. government officially declared the Kikwit epidemic a disaster. Over the following five days additional epidemic-fighters would stream in from France, Belgium, the Netherlands, the United States, Sweden, Ghana, Zimbabwe, and South Africa. Laying the groundwork for all these foreigners were Muyembe, Kipassa, and a team of Zairois health care workers that included local medical school students and the Kikwit Red Cross. Together these people, speaking more than ten different languages and representing the cultures and worldviews of three different continents, would face the toughest challenge of public health: stopping an epidemic firestorm and the panic it produces. In the coming six weeks, 2,793 English-language media reports on Ebola would be stored in the LEXIS/NEXIS computer system,[25] and media in every one of the world's major languages would be filing daily reports on the unfolding epidemic. Heymann's media hunch would almost immediately prove correct: things truly had changed for public health.

But that wasn't obvious when Muyembe and Heymann first sat down on May 10 on beat-up vinyl chairs in an abandoned Kikwit VD clinic to assess the city's situation and map out a public health strategy.

Cries of *"Afwaka! Afwaka!"* or "They died!" filled the air in Kikwit. At Kikwit General Hospital those staff members who hadn't caught Ebola or died were hysterical: terrified and grief-stricken. Rumors of deadly *landa-landa* at the hospital had nearly closed the facility. Kikwitians, perhaps rightly, had begun to prefer remaining ill at home rather than dying in Kikwit General Hospital. Only twenty patients, most suffering from Ebola, remained in the hospital.

In town the people concluded that the facts spoke for themselves: everybody who'd died had been in one of the local hospitals. In each outbreak surgery was directly or indirectly involved. Doctors are corrupt, the townspeople said. Therefore, the doctors were killing people. The dominant explanation for this apparent raft of nosocomial homicides was diamonds.

Much of the world's diamond reservoir is located in northern Angola and Zaire. To prevent theft diamond workers were routinely strip-searched at the end of their shifts. The only way a worker might smuggle a promising gem out of the mines was by swallowing the diamond. Some physicians earned handsome sums of cash by performing surgical removals of diamonds that became lodged somewhere in the individual's gastrointestinal tract rather than finding their way "naturally" out of the smuggler's body.

The rumor that was all over Kikwit during the second week of May was that Kikwit General Hospital physicians, no longer satisfied with their customary payments for such smuggler surgery, were now killing the patients, and taking the diamonds for themselves. There was no *landa-landa* in the hospital, people said, just greed.

The diamond story didn't carry any currency with those who had actually seen the agonized, bleeding Ebola patients. But it was a hugely popular myth in Kikwit that terribly undermined the credibility not only of Kipassa's staff but also of physicians in general.

Faced with demoralized, even hysterical local health care workers, a public rife with panic and suspicion, a virtual absence of all essential public health and medical resources, and, at that point, no cash from outside the country, Muyembe and Heymann confronted a daunting challenge.

Exhausted from their long journeys, Heymann and WHO's Mark Szczeniowski were shell-shocked by what they saw. The usually open-faced Heymann wore a strained, emotionless mask, overwhelmed as he was by the horror. It was Heymann's practiced way of confronting chaotic disasters: with stony calm. Szczeniowski, who had for years in the 1970s lived in Zaire working on WHO monkeypox surveys, was no less ashen. Even the ever-gregarious Muyembe was at an emotional loss.

"There was blood everywhere," Heymann later recalled. "Blood on the mattresses, on the floors, on the walls. Vomit, diarrhea . . . When we got here it was really awful. Apocalyptic. There were people dying everywhere. And the women were wailing. It was surreal. They were filling up the graves and we realized that this was not like Yambuku."

Heymann and Muyembe, the Yambuku veterans, knew that by the time an international team of scientists had gotten to Zaire in 1976 that original Ebola epidemic was already winding down. Some of the international team members back in 1976 never saw an Ebola case, and even Muyembe—first on the scene in Yambuku—came after that outbreak's zenith. In Yambuku, it turned out, nearly every case was spread by one of three syringes that Belgian nuns used over and over again in a tiny mission hospital. Once the nuns succumbed and the hospital closed, the Yambuku epidemic wound down. All this was determined retrospectively by the international scientific team in 1976, which reached Yambuku after the nuns had self-imposed a quarantine on their mission and clinic.

But this time, in Kikwit, Heymann recalled, "I said to Muyembe, 'We're right in the middle of it.' The women sat here, family after family, wailing, facing the morgue. And the Red Cross truck was right here," he continued, just days later, pointing at locals on the grounds of Kikwit General Hospital, "taking the bodies straight to the cemetery. The volunteers were doing it with only surgical masks on."

The stunned trio watched as Ebola-contaminated blood dripped from cadavers onto the brave Red Cross volunteers. Heymann then turned to Muyembe and said, "Our number one priority is to stop the epidemic. Number two is everything else."

Heymann, Szczeniowski, and Muyembe sat down immediately to map out their plan. Szczeniowski's role was the most obvious, for it was one he had played brilliantly in countless previous epidemics: logistics. The athletic forty-something American moved swiftly in the sweltering, 90 percent humidity torpidity, rarely seeming to break a sweat or smudge his spotless wire-rimmed glasses. A walking polyglot, Szczeniowski was an American-born man of Polish descent who grew up in a peripatetic family and was multilingual before even setting foot in college. His facility with languages—which included Zaire-dialect French and KiCongo—was a valuable asset, especially when coupled with his easygoing manner and efficient ease with complex logistic concerns. It would be Szczeniowski's job to ensure that all the material necessities were in place: satellite telephones and fax machines, four-wheel-drive vehicles, gallon upon gallon of safe drinking water, housing, local maps, translators, paper, pens, food—each and every item scarce or unavailable in Kikwit. It was a testament to Szczeniowski's past stellar performances in epidemics all over the world that Heymann and Muyembe simply assumed the resourceful WHO point man could handle his end of things, and after Szczeniowski took charge they had no concerns about dwindling gasoline supplies, choleral water, or lack of bedding for the large crew of scientists that was en route. If lack of sleep and the tremendous pressure ever got to Szczeniowski he never showed it.

Muyembe, the noted Zarois scientist, of course, would be the leader. He would set the priorities, deal with the Zairois government, and act as the team's general.

Heymann, who for nearly all of his adult life had worked for the CDC, had recently had a spell of bad luck. Assigned by CDC to work at WHO in Geneva, Heymann had for the last two years been ensconced in a tiny, windowless office inside the AIDS program. There he had fallen out of favor, finding himself on the losing side of too many political arguments. So completely had his star fallen that there was talk in Atlanta of terminating Heymann's employment before he could qualify for significant government retirement funds. Just weeks before he learned of the Kikwit epidemic Heymann had felt desperate about his career future.

Yet there could be no doubt, even among his detractors in Geneva, that Heymann was the right man—the *only* man—for the Ebola problem. Though American, he spoke perfect French. The slim, boyish-looking scientist had a reputation for being cool under fire and not cracking under pressure. Heymann had faced Ebola before and spent time in Zaire, as well as other central African nations. Finally, he was trained in epidemic control and surveillance. That the forty-nine-year-old Heymann hadn't been compelled to resign his WHO post was a stroke of luck for the people of Kikwit.

Under the leadership of Director-General Hiroshi Nakajima many once-vital WHO capacities fell into ruin amid changing budget priorities, staff purges, and the generally poor morale that marked the mood in the Geneva headquarters. Heymann was hardly the only scientist whose status was precarious. By 1995 WHO had no emergency response office and only one employee—funded entirely by the CDC—who monitored typically tropical epidemics. The CDC's Dr. James LeDuc held that position in 1995, primarily overseeing the laboratory capacities of WHO's far-flung string of affiliated surveillance sites. LeDuc's research career had focused on animal-and insect-carried microbes such as yellow fever and hantaviral diseases, and he had never supervised response to an emergency epidemic.

Nearly all of the disease cowboys who faced down epidemics during the 1960s, 1970s, and early 1980s had long gone, disillusioned and dispirited by the Nakajima regime. Donors were also giving up on the World Health Organization, no longer convinced the once-vital agency had the vision, will, or resources to fulfill its mission. Nakajima, who had recently claimed diplomatic immunity when arrested trying to smuggle religious icons out of Russia, was the object of much disdain.

So it fell to a disgruntled employee to wave the WHO flag in the crisis. Heymann's role was to function as a combination diplomat, attaché, colonel, and chief epidemiologist. Keeping all the various physicians and scientists, as well as the institutions for which they worked, functioning as a unit would be a monumenal challenge. Initially limited to a handful, the team would grow to more than a hundred scientists and volunteers. Egos, language differences, institutional power struggles, and legitimate cultural and scientific variations in how individuals pursued their respective jobs all had to be carefully smoothed over. Egos had to be massaged.

Heymann told Muyembe that it was preferable to have a small but well-coordinated team in place. Large numbers of loose-cannon scientists would surely spell disaster. Muyembe agreed, and the pair set about mapping the most crucial tasks ahead. Muyembe would prove deft at mobilizing local volunteers and abating potential rivalries among African scientists. Together, Heymann and Muyembe formed a strong leadership team.

The fourth key player in the team's leadership arrived the next day from Amsterdam: Dr. Barbara Kiersteins of Médecins Sans Frontières (MSF), or Doctors Without Borders. The humanitarian, European-based organization had offered crucial support in hundreds of crises all over the world, with a track record dating back more than twenty-five years. Formed in response to another African crisis—the famine of civil war–torn Nigeria in 1968—MSF's doctors and volunteers were deployed all over the world to health crises spawned by war, famine, tyranny, or epidemics. From its outset MSF was committed to principles atypical for international relief organizations: its staff did not seek governments' permission to assist in civilian crises; doctors were encouraged to publicly denounce political or economic conditions they felt contributed to such catastrophes; and nobody in MSF was expected to make a lifelong career of such work. The organization strongly believed that career relief workers tended to make too many compromises with corrupt governments or use local disasters as rungs on their personal ladders of prestige ascendancy.

Though only in her early thirties, Kiersteins had already seen more of humanity's horrors than most people glimpse in a lifetime. Just two weeks before arriving in Kikwit MSF's Kiersteins had wrapped up her extensive tenure battling cholera and shigella in the refugee camps of Goma. Like most educated Europeans, Kiersteins spoke several languages, including Dutch, French, and English. If she appeared humorless under pressure, she also stayed emotionally cool and focused. Kiersteins was indefatigable: even the rivers of tropical sweat that seemed perpetually dripping from her body failed to slow her down.

Kiersteins's arrival on May 11 was a welcome sight for the Heymann/Muyembe/Szczeniowski trio. They all respected the organization she worked for and were in desperate need of the supplies, vehicles, and volunteer MSF logicians that Kiersteins brought with her on a chartered plane from Kinshasa. Wasting no time, Kiersteins drove straight to Kikwit General Hospital to assess the situation and determine how best MSF might help.

"The hospital was in a sorry state," she said a few days later when, for the first time, she allowed herself a moment of reflective relaxation. "The patients were in a sorrier state. The staff had no protection and they hadn't been paid for risking their lives. So we decided to focus on hospital sanitation and establishment of an isolation ward."

The MSF crew began by trying to repair the hospital's ancient, long-unused water system but gave up after a few futile hours. The pipes were choked with weeds, eroded, rusty, and irreparable. So they switched to plan B, erecting a plastic rainwater collector attached to a filtration cache.

Across the central courtyard of Kikwit General Hospital the MSF team stretched bright yellow plastic tape, demarking a cordon sanitaire line that only authorized medical personnel could cross.

Muyembe ordered all non-Ebola patients sent away from Kikwit General Hospital, and he decreed that all suspected Ebola cases in any other clinic, or in people's homes, be collected by the local Red Cross and brought immediately to Pavilion No. 3, the hastily designated isolation ward.

Barely had the cordons sanitaires been stretched around the pillars of the hospital's arcaded central hallway than dozens of family members gathered at its edge, anxiously staring at Pavilion No. 3. To one side of the cordons was the morgue, and for days to come a ghastly ritual would repeat itself: as nurses carried a deceased patient to the morgue all of the family members would strain to see who had died, often calling out, "Who is it?" Once the identity was known, that individual's family would commence their wailing to heaven, crying, "Someone has died! Someone has died," often in a loud huddle beside another family still mourning their own recently deceased kin. This wailing would persist for hours. And it could be heard by the staff and ailing Ebola victims in Pavilion No. 3. Kiersteins realized immediately that the deaths, wailing, and stress had taken a terrible toll on the medical staff, most of whom continued to toil away in the hospital despite their lack of pay and tremendous dismay over the demise of their colleagues. The staff was scared, sleep deprived, and grieving. A steady stream of local Red Cross volunteers carried in ailing patients and hauled away the dead for burial. None of these brave Kikwitians possessed protective gear, and all were terrified and exhausted. At least three had become infected performing their heroic deeds. Remarkably, as volunteers died others eagerly took their places, displaying levels of courage that Kiersteins and Heymann found truly awe-inspiring.

But none of them need have died. Muyembe ordered that all of the staff and volunteers brought under MSF's wings receive immediate training in infection control, and Kiersteins ensured that every one of them was outfitted with scrub gowns, rubber galoshes, long rubber aprons, latex gloves, goggles, masks, and hair coverings. Though the team didn't know whether or not Ebola could be transmitted through the air, it was obvious to them that contact with the blood or bodily fluids of the sick or dead was extremely dangerous. Heymann and Muyembe reasoned that any measures that placed barriers—such as latex gloves—between infected patients and health providers would block transmission.

Kiersteins also knew from experience that exhausted, frightened health care workers make mistakes: needles slip, bottles break, hands tremble, all creating opportunities for spread of the virus. When she spoke to the Kikwit crew she could see that they had all long since exceeded reasonable levels of sleep deprivation and exhaustion. A first prority had to be the professionalization of the volunteers' work routines.

Making matters worse, the physicians and nurses had to pass a small cemetery every day on their way to the hospital, which by now was full of their colleagues' bodies. Nestled among weeds and monkeypod trees were rows of wooden crosses, marked with the names of Kikwit's Ebola victims.

"I have seen many African countries, and this is, by comparison, shocking," Kiersteins told Heymann. Strong words from a woman who had just been in the deadly Rwandan refugee camps. But Kiersteins could plainly see that infection control practices in Kikwit were even worse than those executed in emergency medical tents in Goma. Supplies were nonexistent, and the medical facilities of Kikwit were in states of fatigued chaos.

Kipassa chastised Kiersteins, urging her to look at the poverty of the hospital, the lack of resources: "The only thing we have to work with is our brains," he complained.

And your brains, Kiersteins responded, can't think properly. You all need a rest.

MSF erected a series of tents on a small lawn space in the interior of the cordons sanitaires, positioning beds and chairs for the staff inside. She set up work schedules, making sure that all hospital personnel had breaks, naps, and far shorter shifts. No more all-nighters were allowed. Meals and safe water were provided to the staff for the first time. And, perhaps oddly crucial, paychecks. In order to normalize the situation Kiersteins used MSF resources and made every person on the Pavilion No. 3 and morgue staffs employees of her organization, clocking hours for which they were paid. With the imposition of a routine came a calming normalization. As a result the hospital spread of Ebola came to an immediate and grinding halt.

Similarly, MSF put the Red Cross burial crews on modest salaries and helped their leaders create manageable schedules for their grim tasks. Trucks and a bulldozer were found, applied to the horrible job of creating enormous mass graves on the edge of town, in which the plastic-wrapped bodies of the dead were stacked.

But MSF's supplies were limited: enough protective gear and sterile equipment to match Kikwit's needs did not arrive until May 27. In the meantime, everyone simply made do. On Friday, May 12, Kiersteins spent the morning on her satellite telephone talking to MSF headquarters in Brussels: "Send respirator masks, latex gloves, protective gowns, disinfectant, hospital linens and plastic mattress covers, plastic aprons, basic cleaning supplies and cleansers, water pumps and filters, galoshes, tents . . ."

It was not the high-tech equipment popularized in science fiction movies that would halt Ebola's spread, Kiersteins knew. What Kikwit needed were the basics: soap, gear, and safe water.

Between Friday afternoon and Monday, May 15, the vital members of Heymann's crew arrived. Dr. Philipe Calain, a Swiss physician attached to the U.S. CDC, was given command of Pavilion No. 3 and put in charge of the Ebola isolation ward. Belgian Dr. Bob Colebunders took over the hospital's emergency room and screened incoming patients, sending all new Ebola cases to Calain and the rest to alternative hospitals. The CDC's Drs. Pierre Rollin and Ali Khan worked with WHO's Dr. Güenal Rodier to track down all of the region's Ebola cases and figure out how the virus was spreading. South Africa's Robert Swanepoel of the National Virology Institute, located outside Johannesburg, set up an on-site Ebola laboratory, carved out of the hospital's tuberculosis center. From WHO's Zimbabwe office came veterinarian Oyewale Tomori, whose task was to investigate whether any animals within Kikwit were carrying—and possibly spreading—the virus. His samples were hastily analyzed by Swanepoel. Their efforts were supplemented by dozens of volunteers drafted from a local medical school, as well as a host of research institutes in the United States, Europe, and Africa.

Heymann and Muyembe had made rough counts of the Ebola toll, and realized that the numbers of dead were quadrupling daily. In his conversations with Kipassa, Muyembe learned of the Ebola-spreading operations performed on Kimfumu and Katadi, and subsequent illnesses in the medical staff. When he tallied it all up on Friday Muyembe estimated that 73 percent of the dead were health care workers.

More alarming, Muyembe told Heymann, "This epidemic has been going on since March,"—for three full months—and clearly had spread well beyond Kikwit General Hospital. He didn't yet know about Mosango and all of the nearby villages—that would be learned over the next week—but Muyembe already realized that Kikwit's epidemic was more explosive than what he had seen nineteen years earlier in Yambuku. Though many pieces of the Kikwit puzzle were yet to fall in place, Muyembe could see that unlike in Yambuku (where most cases traced to those reused missionary syringes) this epidemic was bursting out from many different directions. In Yambuku the epidemic chain of transmission from one person to another had flowed from a single stem, with only tiny branches extending along the way. But in Kikwit in May there seemed to be several apparently unrelated sprouting outbreaks. The links among them—and the Menga family roots of the epidemic—had yet to be unearthed.

Heymann immediately set to work with Rollin and Khan, training a cadre of medical students in basic epidemiology and planning a schedule of surveillance. Teams were dispatched on Sunday and Monday to every neighborhood in Kikwit, where they went door to door in search of Ebola cases. As they returned to headquarters the team members brought news of active cases, sending the Red Cross to pick up the ailing. The mounting data they amassed help fill in a rapidly expanding tree of infections Muyembe was sketching out, depicting who transmitted Ebola to whom. It all seemed to trace back to those March operating procedures in Kikwit General and the maternity hospital, particularly the operations performed on lab tech Kimfumu. At Heymann's request the sketch was faxed to WHO and the Ministry of Health offices in Kinshasa.

Trusting to Kinshasa's discretion would later prove to have been a mistake.

As the team interacted they were careful not to embrace, shake hands, share food or water. A novel form of greeting was invented to prevent passage of Ebola: in salutation friends tapped the backs of their forearms against one another, carefully keeping their hands pointed toward their own chests, palms away from the friend. Team members worked closely without wearing masks or protective gear, but avoided touching one another. Blood and tissue samples were drawn and handled with well-gloved hands. And all of the team members exclusively imbibed bottled water that Szczeniowski had flown into the city from Kinshasa.

Based on their first, cursory examination of the city the team relayed their primary field report via satellite telephone to Geneva on May 11, and daily thereafter. The Zairois government placed Kikwit under quarantine, halting all trade and transport to and from the city, save airlifts of medical supplies and personnel. Almost immediately the canned foods, sacks of rice, batteries, tools, and other goods usually sold in Kikwit markets disappeared and store shelves became barren.

By that time Kikwit authorities had identified twenty lab-confirmed Ebola deaths and sixty-one hemorrhagic cases assumed to be caused by the virus. Many more suspected cases awaited laboratory confirmation.

On May 13, team members returned from Mosango and a sweep of the villages, unfortunately confirming that Muyembe's fears were well founded: the virus had spread well beyond the confines of Kikwit. Heymann decided that the surveillance net needed to be widened, and team members embarked on long journeys over bumpy dirt roads in search of Ebola cases.

Meanwhile, cases continued to pour into Kikwit General Hospital's ER, usually carried in by Red Cross volunteers, wailing relatives in tow. Belgian physician Colebunders saw immediately that conditions in the chaotic ER were outrageous.

"People were moving in and out, Ebola cases and other emergencies were all mixed together and six ER nurses had died of Ebola," Colebunders explained a few days later. "I said, 'I can't keep aseptic conditions here if people are just wandering about,' and the Red Cross had walked off with all the protective gear. So we went around with the protection leftovers. All of the best equipment went to Pavilion No. 3."

Colebunders, who wasn't able to reach Kikwit until Tuesday, May 16, discovered that all of the supplies had already been claimed by Calain for Pavilion No. 3 or by MSF. And the ER staff were examining bleeding, delirious patients without even the basics—masks and gloves—to protect themselves. The tall, nervous Belgian pleaded for supplies, but it would be ten days before more protective equipment would arrive.

Nevertheless, the ER served as the screening and triage site for every case of diarrhea and fever found in Kikwit. Colebunders tried to minimize the risks for himself and the hospital ER staff, but he knew that they were all in considerable danger. And he struggled to hide a terror that would build within him over subsequent days.

Colebunders was perhaps ill-suited to the task. The very day that the CDC laboratory confirmed that Ebola was the cause of Kikwit's crisis Colebunders had attended the funeral in Antwerp of a longtime friend and colleague. This death had come close on the heels of his father-in-law's demise. Despite his grief, when Colebunders learned of the CDC's lab results he rushed to volunteer. He had never before worked under such desperate third world conditions. But having devoted his career to AIDS research at Antwerp's Institute of Tropical Medicine, Colebunders seized upon the opportunity to participate in a great adventure, and, in the process, advance his status within the claustrophobic Belgian scientific community.

Now he was doing his best to hold down a fear that was welling up from his viscera, threatening to push him over the brink into hysteria. As patients arrived in the emergency room Colebunders anxiously examined their bleeding noses, bloody diarrhea, fever-ridden faces—always careful to minimize how much he actually touched them. He developed a case definition of Ebola—a way to diagnose patients in the absence of confirmatory laboratory findings. He tried desperately to stay focused on his tasks, to not let the horror of the situation overcome him.

Nevertheless, after six nearly sleepless days of the greatest stress he had ever experienced the forty-seven-year-old doctor suddenly collapsed on a gurney. His body felt leaden. His mind was spinning. He struggled to gather his thoughts, reaching the diagnosis that he was having a nervous breakdown.

Each of the team members had come to do battle with the notorious virus for their own reasons and fought internal battles with competing emotions of duty, fear, compassion, ambition, and scientific curiosity. Though Colebunders was the only team member who completely broke down under the pressure, each of the scientists had moments of high temper, sharp words, exhausted malaise, or self-doubt.

On Sunday, May 14, a group of twenty-three reporters pooled their resources, chartering a hulking old airplane for a flight from Kinshasa to Kikwit. Upon landing on the cracked tarmac at the tiny Kikwit airport the reporters immediately fanned out across the city in search of Ebola cases and scientists. With the skilled guile and instincts of seasoned Africa-based journalists the horde, though unfamiliar with Kikwit, soon found Heymann's team and the hospital's Pavilion No. 3.

The scientific team was caught completely off guard. No one among them had given a thought to the media, largely because Africa's many epidemics and health crises rarely rated more than a few minutes per year of broadcast news time in North America, Western Europe, or any of the non-African world. Only a handful of foreign reporters had traveled to Surat during India's plague epidemic: media coverage had largely come from government sources in far-off Delhi. And Ebola was certainly more dangerous than plague, the scientists reasoned. Therefore, it seemed unlikely that more than an easily ignored number of reporters would turn up in Kikwit, or so they had reasoned.

They were, of course, forgetting that since *The Hot Zone, Outbreak,* and other TV movies and documentaries Ebola now carried a certain cachet among diseases. The public had become fascinated by the hemorrhagic fever virus and the special fearsome status Ebola had among microbe fighters. Every major news organization in the world either dispatched a reporter to the site or bought stories and film from freelancers who had made their way to Kinshasa. The Italian media, in particular, were well represented because of the deaths of their countrywomen, the Sisters.

On May 14 the scientists, physicians, and people of Kikwit got a small taste of what major political candidates and celebrities went through in the West at that time, when confronted by camera crews, photographers, and reporters.

Three other reporters had already been in Kikwit for two days, filing their stories overseas and causing little consternation within the Ebola control team.[26] Heymann had added the role of press secretary onto his long list of tasks, showing the three the lay of the land and ensuring that they got the tape, stories, and photos that were needed to document the unfolding epidemic.

But even Heymann was taken aback by the additional twenty-three reporters and photographers who showed up on May 14. His agitation grew as cameras shot the new cemetery plots, Red Cross teams gathering bodies, the hospital, and the epidemic command post.

Brooklyn-born Ali Khan stood to the side and watched, aghast, as camera crews filmed a chart he had made, listing the names of the dead and dying.

"Outrageous!" Khan cried. "We posted those lists for the team so we could keep track. They're never supposed to be public. What about patient confidentiality? These people have the same rights to privacy as Americans."

Khan, the son of Pakistani immigrants, took propriety so seriously that despite the stifling Kikwit heat he always wore a dress shirt and tie: "a sign of respect," Khan said, for the people of Kikwit. If such attire had been appropriate in New Mexico in 1993 when he investigated the hantavirus epidemic, Khan reasoned, then it should also be correct in Kikwit. He expected similar ethics and propriety from everyone else, including journalists.

So it was with outrage that he helplessly stood by watching the photographers and TV camera people shoot his precious chart of death, and hours later saw patients and weeping funeral participants filmed without their consent. These things, he shouted, were not right.

And then and there Khan started to hate the media. As did Pierre Rollin, a French scientist on loan from the Institute Pasteur to the CDC.

"I detest reporters!" Rollin hissed. "I will never again give another interview. You are a member of the lowest, most vile profession on earth."

The most demonstrative expression of antipathy toward the pack of reporters came from Switzerland's Calain. The photographers, not surprisingly, wanted to take pictures of the patients inside Pavilion No. 3. Given that the ward was intended as an isolation area and most of the patients were too ill to grant consent, Calain demurred. Tempers rose, shouts were heard, and Calain threw a punch at a female photographer on assignment for Reuters. Witnesses later insisted that both parties were out of line. Regardless, the photographer apparently scraped her knee on the possibly contaminated floor during the fracas. At the very least this constituted a break in infection protocols, and the photographer, who would soon return to Kinshasa, could have been an unwitting vehicle for spread of the virus.[27] (Fortunately, the photographer was not infected, though nobody knew that when she departed Kikwit.)

Some member of the enraged medical team radioed word of the reporters to Kinshasa, and when the group of twenty-three landed at dusk back in the capital later that day Zairois soldiers surrounded the plane. Held inside the aircraft in the blistering equatorial heat, the reporters were first informed that they would be confined indefinitely under quarantine. After an hour's standoff diplomats from several embassies intervened, convincing Zairois officials that the reporters could safely be released.[28]

The incident prompted greater attention to accreditation details on the part of Zaire's Ministry of Information. The agency, which might better have been termed the Ministry of Bribery and Disinformation, welcomed money in exchange for accreditations for foreigners and rarely provided anyone—foreigner or citizen—with accurate news about anything, especially public health.

Located in one of several decrepit, thirty-year-old government buildings at con-siderable distance form Kinshasa's hub, the Ministry was on the nineteenth floor of a decaying structure with only one remaining, marginally functional elevator.

Though the Ministry officials emphasized the grand panoramas afforded from their windows of Kinshasa and the Congo River, it was the offices, them-selves, that offered the clearest views of the Mobutu regime. Water stains and creeping fungi on the walls and ceilings betrayed the building's inability to with-stand Zaire's equatorial downpours. Exposed, rusted pipes explained why no water ran from the nineteenth-floor faucets. A collapsed ceiling spoke to the generally shoddy workmanship and poor maintenance of the building. And look-ing down from every wall was the dictator, scowling from photographs shot during his youth, postured arrogantly, attired in his trademark mix of Pierre Cardin glasses, Rolex watch, leopard skin hat, and Western-style jacket. Without meaning to the Ministry of Information staff thus presented a perfectly realistic image of modern Zaire.

The information officers were at a loss when it came to providing an ac-counting of Zaire's epidemic. Genuine information was not their forte; con-cealment was. But while hiding the truth might ward off the dictator's domestic critics, such action only further provoked foreign journalists.

So epidemic information control fell to the Ministry of Health. On May 15, with Minister of Health Mbumb Musong oddly out of the country during his nation's most significant international medical fiasco, the Ministry staff mud-dled through. Secretary-General Lonyangela Bompenda derided the large for-eign press corps in a briefing in Kinshasa, saying that they "are putting people in danger" by their movements.

"If the quarantine cannot be held the country will be closed. *Voici la verité!* You—if you go to Kikwit, you break the quarantine," Bompenda said, adding ominously, "so I will repeat: if we have to detain some people it will be the police that will detain them."

Meantime, a virtual industry sprang up in Kinshasa, focused on obtaining as much of the foreign journalists' currency as possible. Taxis raised their rates, phone calls out of local hotels suddenly required $20 and even $50 bribes to switchboard operators, room rates skyrocketed, and the price of meals at the local eateries soared. As competition among the journalists escalated—partic-ularly among rival television networks—basic bribery rates jumped to astonish-ing levels. Airport officials and local charter companies were negotiating prices in excess of $25,000 to cover transport and bribery fees for flights to Kikwit in violation of the cordons sanitaires. With the government obfuscating, even threatening, and rumors of deaths and disease rife in the capital both the inter-national media and local Zarois were at pains to separate fact from fiction.

Mobutu, who flew into Kinshasa to meet visiting American televangelist

Pat Robertson[29] and would hours later return to his distant retreat in northern Zaire, far from the Kikwit crisis, thanked Robertson "from the bottom of my heart."

Addressing his country's Ebola epidemic, Mobutu said, "I would have liked to go [to Kikwit] but my doctors have forbidden me to go to this area. The first responsibility of a chief is to show solidarity with his people and be strong for his people. My purpose is to help the people and cooperate with all international groups."

With that the dictator thanked the international team then toiling in Kikwit, expressed gushing gratitude to his political supporter Robertson, and disappeared. For the remainder of the epidemic the Zarois leader would stay secluded, never issuing another word of concern or condolence for his people.

In Kinshasa's enormous slum La Cité the dictator's brief appearance was greeted with open derision. One of the popular local newspapers, *Salongo*, brazenly asked in a bold headline, "EBOLA VIRUS. BLOODY DIARRHEA. WHO IS AT FAULT?" The rhetorical headline's answer: MOBUTU. The paper noted that the epidemic "is without a doubt" the result of widespread social and environmental "degradation" brought about by "demagogues" in the government who were clinging "to the old order" and blocking democracy. As the epidemic unfolded even the scientists toiling in Kikwit would be compelled to conclude that the etiology of Zaire's epidemic was at least as much political and economic as it was biological. Authoritarianism and corruption may not have spawned the Ebola virus, but they certainly created formidably fertile ground for its spread.

It had now been one week since the CDC had confirmed that Ebola had returned to Zaire. Unfounded rumors of cases loose in Kinshasa had finally been squelched with the apprehension of two suspected patients, both of whom proved to be well, and negative for the virus. On the streets of the capital vendors complained that they could not obtain fruits and vegetables from Bandundu Province, thanks to the quarantine. People along the boulevards and alleyways stopped white-skinned journalists, begging for news of the epidemic and asking their assessments of the regime's efforts to control Ebola.

"Are there enough scientists in Kikwit?" they asked.

"Is the government telling the truth—are there really no cases in Kinshasa?"

"Don't believe the government—it only lies!"

"Will the world save us?"

It was clear that the government hadn't a shred of credibility in La Cité, or perhaps anywhere else in the troubled nation. The populace was counting upon WHO and the foreigners, whose presence offered them the only consolation they could see in the unfolding crisis.

By then eighty-six people had died of laboratory-confirmed Ebola—numerous other suspected cases had surfaced or died. And in Kikwit a new wave of cases, results of spread not in the hospitals but within households, was sweeping through the community. The growing international team was watching what had begun primarily as a health care worker epidemic turn into a more generalized phenomenon.

Heymann's teams of local medical students and foreign scientists were finding what he dubbed "hot houses" in which whole families had contracted Ebola and most died.

For example, in one of Kikwit's barely accessible neighborhoods where no vehicles could manage the muddy, rutted roads, a young woman slowly rocked back and forth on her tiny porch, her baby nursing at her breast. She stared straight ahead, shell-shocked. She suddenly had found herself the sole support and caretaker of her baby, her teenage sister, and sixteen other children.

The horror started, she said, when in April her niece had a C-section at Kikwit General Hospital. Nine days later the new mother died of Ebola. Her newborn followed suit two days later. Then their mother, who had cared for the dying mother and child, suddenly developed a piercing headache at her daughter's funeral. The family rushed her to a local dispensary where a nurse diagnosed the problem as a tipped uterus and reached in, barehanded, to adjust the bereaved woman's womb.

A week later both she and the nurse were dead, victims of Ebola. And soon thereafter relatives at that funeral died: the shell-shocked woman's father and two more sisters.

"They hiccuped," the survivor said, seemingly stunned by the curiosity of it. As they neared death, the Ebola victims each had fallen into fits of uncontrollable hiccuping.

An international team member asked if he could take blood samples from the surviving woman and the pack of orphans that she now had in her charge. She leapt to her feet in horror, crying, "My sisters got needles in their arms! *Afwaka*—they died. My mother got needles. *Afwaka!* My father—*Afwaka!* No! I will not!"

The fear of Kikwit's hospitals, particularly their needles and surgical equipment, was, of course, quite rational, even wise. It was obvious to the international team that several of the Bandundu Provinces medical facilities had served as Ebola amplifiers: turning isolated cases that entered the facility into outbreaks, multiplied several times over as a result of poor hospital hygiene. Thus, the local health establishments performed roles in precise opposition to their mission: rather than preventing an epidemic, they had created one out of what previously had been a problem isolated within the Menga family.

But, thanks largely to the efforts of MSF, by mid-May hospital transmission had stopped and the team knew that Ebola was primarily continuing to spread within so-called hot houses. Though everyone agreed that Ebola was exploiting human altruism, spreading via acts of compassion among Kikwitians, the precise biology of that transmission wasn't clear.

In the evenings, exhausted and emotionally drained from their day's work, members of the international team gathered in one of Kikwit's few restaurants, located inside her only hotel, Kwilu—named after the river that bisected the city and until less than a decade earlier was the rain forest's border. Like soldiers at war the scientists tended to be boisterous and drink plenty of Primus beer on such occasions. And often they would speculate about what they had seen during their investigations that day. Inevitably they were drawn to one key question: are we sure that we are taking correct preventive precautions in this epidemic?

Over several meals of local fish, bananas, rice, and tough goat meat spiced with hot peppers, the men—and nearly all were men—ruminated over the vagaries of the deadly, hemorrhagic fever virus. The Mosango case, in particular, troubled them because it indicated that the virus could survive atop open-air surfaces in the tropical climate for days on end. But was Dr. Bonnet's observation correct? Was it the hospital room itself that was the source of that ill-fated patient's infection, or might there have been other possibilities? Perhaps, they agreed, the virus was on the hands of a health care worker who tended to the woman. Or on her dishes. Or in the drinking water.

WHO's Rodier voiced a shared concern: if the virus is in a well or on a glass of water is it safe to use that water? He reflected on lessons from Yambuku. Recalling the original laboratory work done in 1976 Rodier felt that there were grounds for such a suspicion because the original Yambuku samples were improperly packaged and arrived at the Institut Pasteur in Paris in a condition that, with most organisms, proved useless for analysis. The liquid nitrogen that was supposed to keep test tubes full of virally contaminated blood cold had long since melted and the viruses had been at room temperature for days. Nevertheless, Dr. Pierre Sureau had had no trouble isolating living Ebola viruses from those containers.

That, Rodier concluded, dictated that scientists take a conservative course in Kikwit, assuming that the virus thrived in tropical heat and could live in food and water. Muyembe didn't like that idea one bit: it might be all right for the foreigners to take such precautions as drinking and washing in bottled water hauled at considerable expense from Kinshasa, but such measures were impossible for Kikwitians. Any talk of virally contaminated food or water would only exacerbate the already near-hysterical public panic.[30]

Back in America Fort Detrick researchers at the U.S. Army Medical Research Institute for Infectious Diseases, or USAMRID, and at the CDC were studying the Ebola transmission question closely. Perhaps fortunately, for the sake of limiting panic, their findings would not be known until the Kikwit epidemic was over. Dr. Nancy Jaax of USAMRID, for example, would demonstrate using monkeys that inhalation of aerosolized Ebola viruses could cause infection and death.[31] And the BL-4 group at the CDC would discover evidence of secreted Ebola viruses in cells of human skin, indicating that mere touch might lead to infection.[32] Taken together, these two discoveries might have raised fears in the international team about casual inhalation or skin contact and transmission of the terrifying virus.

Based on what they did know at the time, however, the team felt American provisions for universal precautions, modified to include goggles and rubber boots, were probably adequate for the Red Cross and health care workers. For Swanepoel and his tiny group of on-site lab workers full-body space suits were, despite the stifling heat and humidity, deemed wise.

And for the people of Kikwit door-to-door education efforts advised two modes of protection: do not care for people suffering from high fevers or diarrhea, and do not perform mortuary procedures, washing down the dead and having open-casket funeral rites. Rather, they advised, send a runner to the Red Cross as soon as a family member falls ill. In a city bereft of mortuaries and funeral parlors this meant that the families should abandon ailing loved ones and allow their bodies to be buried unclean and without Catholic ritual. Though such measures were emotionally wrenching for family members, they were, Muyembe insisted, the precautions most likely to successfully stop the epidemic.

"Someone has died! He was my papa!" screamed a teenage girl. Surrounded by her six younger, grieving siblings the girl's face and blouse were drenched in tears. "He was my papa," she cried again, pushing a photograph of the deceased into the hands of a passing stranger. While her brothers and sisters wailed, sometimes jerking in spasmodic death dances, the distraught girl told a foreigner what tragedy had befallen her family.

"Mama got the Ebola," she explained, foisting a photo of a plump woman in her thirties at the visitor. "They took her from us. They took her to the hospital. Then Papa took ill, and they took him away. And today he died there! He died in the hospital. *Afwaka!*"

On hearing the fatal *Afwaka* the other children escalated their wailing, one boy, appearing to be about five years old, collapsed facedown on their small dirt yard, lost in his screams.

"Mama had a headache. And she had a high fever," the eldest child continued. "She is still at the hospital. Oh, Mama! Oh, Papa! Who will care for us?"

For days the children had fended for themselves and watched the steady flow of Red Cross trucks that lumbered past their tidy home, en route to the mass graves at the top of the hill. With each passing truck they had worried: is this one carrying Mama? Papa? And just now the eerie caravan had, indeed, passed by, its cargo including the white plastic wrapped body of their father, they were told.

The children's tragic cries faded and were eventually drowned out by the grinding noise of a large Red Cross truck mired in a muddy rut on the hilltop. A cluster of men and women, dressed in their colorful protective attire, held a row of body bags laid out on the truck bed, lest the lurches of the vehicle send one shooting out onto the roadside. Such a thing would be ghastly and undignified— certain to provoke anxiety among the crowds of people who stared from a safe distance at the sorry sight. At last freed from the rut, the truck maneuvered to the edge of a deep trench some thirty feet wide, and already layered with dirt-covered bodies. Two Red Cross volunteers adjusted their big, knee-high, European rubber boots and jumped off the truck bed, into the pit. The others handed down the heavy, ominous white body bags: one tall one here, a baby-size one there, a medium-size adult shape . . . the corpse of the father of the wailing children down the road.

Carefully, the two volunteers in the pit received the bodies, some of which still bled Ebola-rich fluids, and placed them side by side along the pit floor. Then a third man, wearing a large metal backpack tank, leaped into the pit, pointed a nozzle at the bodies, and doused them with a veneer of DDT. Their job nearly complete, the DDT was sprayed on all of the volunteers, a second layer of dirt was added to the pit, and the crew headed back to the hospital in search of another grim cargo.

Each crew, or *equipe*, included seven volunteers and there were fourteen *equipes* toiling around the clock in Kikwit, finding the ill and taking them to the hospital and hauling the dead in trucks for burial. Three of the volunteers had died of Ebola before Kiersteins doled out protective gear, and two were fighting for their lives in Pavilion No. 3.

"They are volunteers who are doing this of their own free will," Red Cross Secretary-General Kadiata Vunga said. "No one from government has told them to. They are willing to die for others. They will do what God says to relieve suffering."

Neither the International Committees of Red Cross and Red Crescent, nor any wealthy nation's sister organizations (such as the American Red Cross) offered assistance to the heroic Kikwit group. Indeed, volunteers canvassed local businesses for stacks of nearly worthless Zaires currency with which to buy gasoline and spare tires for their trucks and bulldozers. When donations ran out, the volunteers reached into their own near-empty pockets.

"There is no help from anyone," Vunga said, barely hiding his anger. "We do it all ourselves. . . . If the American Red Cross can see our situation here—we

are suffering a lot! We need money and resources. They should see the conditions we are working under here in Zaire."

Perhaps equally vital to their grim task of shuttling bodies was mass education, as it was the Red Cross volunteers who canvassed the community, warning of the deadly disease. Their protective gear, Vunga said, frightened people. So volunteers also traveled about in their normal clothing, telling Kikwitians, "See? We are just like you! Don't be afraid."

But suspicions, superstitions, and fears persisted. The crowds that witnessed the by now regular burials spread word of the DDT sprayings, suggesting that the Red Cross was keeping a magic potion from them. Ten days after Heymann, Muyembe, and their team arrived a runner came to the hospital, announcing that his neighbor had just died of Ebola. Because the name was not on any surveillance list Khan and Heymann followed the Red Cross to the site.

A funeral was in progress. An older, thin man stared, bewildered, beside the open casket of his deceased wife. He had, unfortunately, cared for her himself, never sending her to the hospital for treatment. Like most Kikwitians the widower feared the hospitals. He had also prepared his wife's body for burial. She was the second family member to die of Ebola, the first having been their adult son.

The old man appeared dazed, uncomprehending when Red Cross volunteers, dressed in protective gear, asked if they could remove the body. He silently nodded, and the horde of wailers screeched and cried when the casket was covered and Red Cross volunteers carried it to their truck. As the truck slowly departed the old man beseeched Heymann for an explanation. Dutifully, in perfect French, the angular American explained how the virus spread from one person to another, in the loving ministrations the well gave to the sick. He then asked the old man if he would provide a sample of his blood. As medical student Norbert Lafulu inserted a needle in the old man's arm he did not wince nor take his eyes off Heymann's deliberately emotionless, calm face.

"Can you give me a drug now?" the old man asked as the realization that he might be infected dawned. Heymann shook his head sadly. The man—who though only fifty looked quite old—turned plaintively to the more than one hundred mourners gathered around him, and one shouted, "Look at the Red Cross—Le Croix Rouge! *Regardez!*"

Those volunteers who hadn't followed the truck were busily scrubbing the site in the house where the coffin had lain, and spraying the area with DDT pesticides.

"Why did you spray the house?" the old man asked. And then, raising his arms and preparing for a mist he pled, "Spray me, too! Spray me! Why not me, too?"

Heymann patiently explained that the DDT was a precaution, in case insects could carry the virus. Nobody knew, Heymann added, whether or not insects played a role in the spread of Ebola. But such sprays could not protect him if the virus was already in the old man's body.

An American photographer, without asking his permission, shot the old man's stunned face. Ali Khan quietly cursed the photographer. Heymann thanked the old man for his blood. And the outsiders departed, leaving the widower agape, amid a throng of tear-soaked friends and family.

In another misunderstanding between the populace and epidemic control efforts an entire neighborhood rose up in a near riot. It began when a man and woman drove up to a house located on a street near the University of Bandundu. The exhausted, frail woman waited in the car while the man called out for her brother. No one responded, so the man returned to the vehicle and ordered the woman out. She stood silently, clutching her cloth-tied parcels, as the man sped off. With great difficulty she hobbled toward the house, collapsing on the road. Neighbors ran to her aid, finding her to be feverish, weak, and semilucid. She explained that her husband had died of the new disease at their home in Mosango village, and now she was searching for help from her brother.

But no one in the swelling neighborhood crowd had ever heard of her brother. She was delirious. She had come to the wrong address. Hearing the word *Ebola* a local teenager took off on a full sprint for the Red Cross. And when the Red Cross volunteers loaded the woman onto a stretcher shouts and fights broke out.

"Why are you taking her away," cried a woman, demanding that, instead, the Red Cross bring the ailing stranger into her home. "I must take care of her! They will kill her because of this disease! Everybody who suffers from this Ebola, they [the Red Cross] destroy him forever!"

A robust, authoritative man—the neighborhood political chief—stomped up to his neighbor, shouting at the top of his lungs, "If someone wants to debate this thing I will accuse him!"

"You are crying with your politics here in order to destroy people," countered another large female of the neighborhood. "You know this town is dangerous! You are the chief of the area, it's your duty to protect people. Why don't you?"

"I'm not sure she will ever come back alive," screamed the first woman, brandishing her fist at the chief. "Most of the time when someone is taken from here, he dies! Maybe he gets the disease at the hospital."

The chief waved at the Red Cross to depart swiftly, and turned on his accuser, asking the woman, "Are you afraid to go to the hospital?"

"Everybody is running away," she retorted. "How can you ask me such a question?"

As dusk darkened the neighbors shouted and threatened one another, each convinced of one of two positions: either the sick and dead were the sources of contamination and therefore had to be removed for the sake of the community, or malevolent doctors were gathering up sick people and murdering them—intentionally or accidentally—with the virus.

The first woman continued: "As I'm not a doctor, I haven't heard anything about this virus. But I have heard that it is a virus that kills. And so I am afraid to go to the hospital because we have seen the source is there."

While the shouting escalated and fists flew in that neighborhood Heymann and Muyembe burned the midnight oil at their impromptu offices, discussing what to do about other communities that were overreaching, going too far, putting virtually every ailing person out on the road for Red Cross pickup, regardless of the nature or cause of their illnesses. And Vunga was outraged because some Kikwitians were using the Red Cross as a way to get free burials for relatives they knew had died of AIDS, malaria, or other non-Ebola causes.

Outside of Kikwit even greater difficulties were arising. In the village of Kimbinga, for example, Chief Justin Muntunu ruled with an iron fist and was determined to use his own brand of public health to stop Ebola. There had been cases in Kimbinga, the lanky chief told a visitor, "of the disease which in Kikwit is called Ebola."

In Kimbinga it seemed to have begun when a village woman went to Kikwit to care for her ailing brother. After he died of Ebola, Muntunu said, this woman returned to her home in Kimbinga. Muntunu visited the woman in her thatched hut and, upon discovering that she was ailing, commanded her to depart immediately to her family's nearby village of Insomi, which she did. Under local tradition women can always be ordered to return to the village of their birth if they in any way displease their chiefs, husbands, mothers-in-law, or eldest sons. Two days later she died in Insomi.

And for the last four days, by order of Chief Muntunu, the two young men who had carried the ailing woman to her parents' village had been incarcerated in a sort of makeshift village quarantine.

"I have heard that the virus can take twenty-one days to cause disease," said the chief accurately, "so they will remain there for seventeen more days."

Pointing to a thatched building some hundred yards away, Muntunu gestured with authority. A young girl busy pounding manioc near the quarantine site started to giggle, as did other children near the building. Angrily Muntunu strode to the building, finding it empty.

"They went into the forest," a village woman defiantly told the chief.

"You should not have let them go," Muntunu cried. "If they die it's your problem, not mine!"

A fight ensued among the villagers, fists flew, and in the scuffle a huge cloud of dust arose, enveloping the participants. The chief's son, a tall, strapping young man, raced into the dust storm shouting, "My father is the chief of the village! When he tells you to take care of these boys you must do it! People are dying in Kikwit. You have to respect the chief and pay attention to the lives of all of the people!"

Back in Kikwit the international team doggedly pursued information about Ebola cases, their surveillance net now firmly in place. By May 19—ten days after the first members of the team had arrived—Heymann had begun to feel confident that the epidemic control effort was working well. His troops were deployed, all known Ebola cases were in Pavilion No. 3, and investigators were scouring nearby villages. So, he said, the epidemiologists could return to "hot houses," gather blood samples from survivors, and pursue larger scientific issues. For example, he pointed out, nothing was really known about healthy Ebola carriers: did such people exist? Could they spread the virus to others? And it was clear some people survived Ebola—why? How had they outwitted the virus, given there was no treatment for the disease?

Heymann and Khan decided to go back to what appeared to be the epidemic's origin in the hospitals: the case of lab technician Kimfumu. Walking through hills not accessible by vehicles or bicycles, the duo reached Kimfumu's pretty, young widow. Seated outside a wattle house next to her sister the widow calmly answered the scientists' questions. No one in her family had acquired the disease, even though they'd attended to Kimfumu during the first days of his illness.

Suddenly the widow's brother-in-law stormed in, angrily demanding to know what Khan and Heymann were up to.

"We are all well," he insisted, "why are you here?"

Heymann calmly began to respond, but the brother-in-law interrupted, shouting, "Why is all of the world saying Kimfumu started this epidemic? I heard it on the radio—on Radio France and VOA!"

Heymann knew that it was true—that poor Kimfumu's name was broadcast worldwide. And Heymann knew he was helpless to stop it. He shook his head sadly, trying to gain the brother-in-law's confidence. But it was useless. Heymann and Khan learned nothing from the visit except that their patient's confidentiality had been betrayed.

The betrayal originated in Kinshasa, where government officials were still trying to fight off panic.

The capital city, with its run-down, tawdry buildings and pot-holed roads, was abuzz with rumors. District Governor Bernadin Mungul Diaka declared that whatever was necessary should be done to protect the estimated six million urbanites: "If the disease penetrates to Kinshasa, that will be a catastrophe," he cried, noting grimly that the city's morgue only had room for 150 corpses.

Secretary-general of the Ministry of Health Loyangela Bonkuma Bompenda, acknowledging rumors on Tuesday, May 16, that at least two Ebola-infected individuals were "on the loose in Kinshasa," decreed that the army would protect the city—at all costs.

Muyembe's hastily drafted chart, depicting Kimfumu at the center of Kikwit's epidemic, was mysteriously, anonymously distributed all over Kinshasa. No one ever took credit for its release, but obviously somebody had violated a basic tenet of public health: patient confidentiality. Muyembe's chart noted all of the patients involved in the original hospital outbreak, and had arrows pointing from "Kimfumu" to several names. Within hours poor Kimfumu was the Typhoid Mary of Kikwit, named in media accounts from Hong Kong to Buenos Aires as the source of Africa's latest disaster.

That boomeranged on his grieving family. Neighbors attacked the widow, accusing her of spreading disease, and she had been forced to flee with her children to her sister's family home in a remote part of Kikwit. In his blind rage the brother-in-law accused Heymann and Khan not only of libeling Kimfumu, but of misdiagnosis. The lab tech did not die of Ebola, he claimed, but of a sliced artery, cut by a murderous doctor at Kikwit General Hospital.

There would be no further discourse and certainly no blood samples from Kimfumu's survivors. Heymann and Khan trudged back to their vehicle, enraged at authorities in Kinshasa, who they assumed had released Muyembe's chart to the media. Khan sneered and cursed in the car. Heymann, who was equally angry but less demonstrative by nature, simply shook his head and quietly said, "We didn't have that problem in Yambuku. No press came. Now they bring their satellite uplink and set up shop. And we can't control it."

It was dawning on Heymann that public health had entered a new era in which at times of crisis scientists' every move would be scrutinized. Live television coverage of unfolding epidemics was now, and in the future, inevitable. He pondered what this could mean for the future of public health: it worried him deeply.

Meanwhile Nigerian veterinarian Oyewale Tomori, a veteran of Lassa fever epidemics in his home country, wanted to be sure that animals within Kikwit weren't spreading the virus. He began by combing the city for monkeys, chimps, and gorillas, which were kept in homes all over the town, as pets or possible sources of future revenue. Many of the animals—particularly the gorillas and chimps—were in alarming shape, clearly suffering from a variety of bacterial infections. But none appeared to have Ebola symptoms.

At considerable personal risk Tomori, assisted by the pets' owners and the CDC's Scott Dowell, held the strong animals down and drew blood samples. This was not, of course, a procedure the cousins of *Homo sapiens* enjoy; teeth were bared and struggles ensued. Clearly, Tomori's latex gloves would have proven useless if one of the animals had managed to sink its teeth into the veterinarian. Fortunately, Tomori escaped unscathed, loaded with monkey and ape blood samples.

Analysis fell to Swanepoel, who worked in just ten-minute shifts, the brevity necessitated by the sweat and torpor produced by working inside a space suit in the tropics. He swiftly ruled out Ebola infection in the primates, and set about searching for other possible Ebola-carrying animals. The amiable South African managed to recruit local volunteers who helped snare bats from Kikwit's trees and church belfries. In coming days he would capture dozens of species of birds, bats, rodents, and insects in the Forêt Pont Mwembe, or Mwembe Forest.

By May 20, with the epidemic slowing but still under way, Kikwit's mayor, Ignace Gata Mavita, felt thoroughly overwhelmed. The problems and petitioners just kept piling up at the Hotel du Ville, the town's one-story cinder block city hall, nestled in a weedy, run-down former park. Deeply grateful for the international assistance, Mavita felt that, at long last, the epidemic was coming under control, but now new problems were proving invulnerable to his best efforts.

"The town is in isolation," the handsome young politician explained. "It is difficult for people to get goods at decent prices. Those traders in other regions are afraid to come here. And those who have goods are increasing their prices. And you can imagine how the people are suffering, because they are so poor. It's good to issue a quarantine, but they have to find a solution or we will have dire economic consequences. If not, the world may have its solution, but we will starve . . . and they will create another crisis here in Kikwit."

Mavita noted sadly that Ebola was creating hundreds of orphans, and Kikwit had no orphanages.

"This is the greatest challenge that Kikwit has ever faced," he concluded.

While Mavita pressured officials in Kinshasa to lift Kikwit's crippling quarantine Heymann and Muyembe felt that they were soon going to complete their primary mission: stop the epidemic. Heymann sent word to CDC and WHO that relief crews should come soon, allowing the crisis team to head home after two grueling weeks for well-deserved rests. As the numbers of new cases slowed to a daily trickle the team concentrated on setting in place two key scientific efforts. The first, using the far-flung surveillance system they'd created, would focus on mapping out the epidemic's history, from Gaspard Menga to the end, noting who had gotten the virus from whom and how it had been transmitted. Further, that mission would search for evidence of uninfected Ebola carriers.

The second mission, already begun by Tomori, Swanepoel, and Dowell, would hunt for whatever animal, plant, or insect normally carries the mysterious virus. To accomplish that, they reasoned, a large team of ecology experts would have to comb Mwembe Forest, gather thousands of samples, and ship the carefully cataloged material back to the CDC for BL-4 lab analysis.

But before any such activities could be undertaken in earnest Kikwit desperately needed more supplies, particularly protective gear for use in the hospitals and by the Red Cross. For seemingly the millionth time, on May 23 Szczeniowski telephoned via satellite requests to Geneva. WHO, short on cash and lacking any genuine emergency response capability, simply passed the request along to various North American and Western European governments.

On May 26, with a fresh scientific team on its way and no new Ebola cases in the previous forty-eight hours, Heymann decided to head home. His one concern was that vital supplies *still* had not arrived, and if doctors performed procedures without infection protection the epidemic could start all over again. And then, of course, all of their heroic efforts would come to nothing.

The next morning Heymann stood in the blistering heat on Kikwit's tiny tarmac, awaiting a chartered plane to Kinshasa. In vain he scoured the skies for signs of his oft-requested supplies. But the only plane he saw was that which flew him to Kinshasa.

Several hours after Heymann departed, however, a huge Hercules transport plane lumbered down the Kikwit tarmac, loaded with supplies and scientists from Sweden. Among the much-needed syringes, gloves, masks, and such were a few supersuits, designed with built-in air-conditioning units. These were the suits Hollywood expected to see. And they arrived after the epidemic was nearly over.

At the Hotel Intercontinental in Kinshasa later that evening Heymann savored his first shower in sixteen days, as well as news of the Swedish supplies, which he celebrated with an ice cold Primus beer.

"We did it !" he cried jubilantly. "We beat the virus!"

A month later the CDC and WHO reported that 296 people had died of Ebola during the Kikwit epidemic, and 79 percent of all identified infections had proved lethal. A third of the dead were health care workers. The epidemic had waxed and waned several times between February and June; it had peaked exactly when Heymann first arrived. In August, with all possible incubation periods—the hypothesized lengthiest being twenty-one days—long past since the last Ebola case was seen, WHO officially declared the epidemic over.

Barely had the world issued a sigh of relief when the virus resurfaced, hundreds of miles away in the West African nation of Côte d'Ivoire. Twenty-five-year-old Jaster Chea traveled from nearby Liberia to Côte d'Ivoire, taking ill on December 8, 1995. A WHO team led by Dr. Deo Barakanfitiye—who had been part of Muyembe's group in Kikwit—discovered within a few hours that Chea was from the Liberian village of Plibo, where three other men were suffering from the disease. In short order a fifth case—a woman, also from Plibo—was found in Abidjan, the capital of Côte d'Ivoire.[33]

The government of Côte d'Ivoire immediately shut down its border with Liberia, suspending all trade between the two nations. And the WHO investigators found themselves entangled in ongoing civil war disputes, as Plibo was located in a region controlled by the guerrilla National Patriotic Front of Liberia, led by rebel warlord Charles Taylor. The rebels cooperated with WHO, allowing an investigation. The team concluded that the outbreak was limited to the Chea family.

But that incident prompted a review of two previous Ebola incidents in the same rain forest region. In November 1994 a miniepidemic broke out in gold mining camps that were deep in the forests of Gabon.[34] Accessible only by canoe, the camps were particularly remote, located in a region called Makokou. The suspected Ebola cases were transferred by canoe to a Gabonese military hospital where they were immediately placed under quarantine and treated exclusively by physicians and nurses attired in basic protective gear. Blood samples were analyzed in Paris, at the Institut Pasteur, where four of the first eight cases were confirmed as Ebola.

After three years of analysis French researchers concluded that forty-four people had contracted Ebola in the camps, twenty-eight of whom died of the disease. And the military hospital, thanks to appropriate infection control efforts, prevented any further spread of the virus.

The outbreak caught the interest of local chimpanzee researchers who had noted die-offs among the animals in the 4,200-square-kilometer Tai rain forest that spans parts of Liberia, Gabon, Côte d'Ivoire, and Cameroon. A few months before the mining camp outbreak a team led by Swiss Institute of Zoology scientist Cristophe Boesch had collected twelve dead chimps (out of forty in a colony) and discovered on autopsy that the animals' blood wasn't coagulating, and there was evidence of internal bleeding. The scientists feared that a terrible new disease had surfaced.

Eight days after those chimp autopsies were performed one of the Swiss scientists fell ill and was evacuated to Institut Pasteur. Though diagnosed with Ebola, she survived, and standard infection control procedures prevented any further spread. No one was able to determine how the veterinarian had gotten infected in the first place, however, as she'd worn protective gear throughout the autopsies.

The two Tai Forest outbreaks sparked widespread speculation among scientists that whatever creature normally harbored the Ebola virus was located in abundance in the area and had close contact with human beings. That, they said, was exciting news, as it might mean they were close to finding the source, the Ebola reservoir.

Eight weeks after the Liberian Chea incident, Ebola surfaced again, this time in Gabon, in villages located in the same Makokou region in which the prior mining camp incidents had occurred.[35] At least nineteen villagers from the remote Mayibout settlement were infected; all were immediately placed under quarantine in the Makokou Hospital, where infection control standards were elevated to minimize spread. The diagnosis of Ebola was made in the Centre International de Recherches Médicales de Franceville, a local state-of-the-art laboratory built by the French government.

Teams of internationally known scientists poured into Gabon, taking the arduous ninety-three-mile canoe journey to remote Mayibout, population 150 people. By late February it appeared that one-fifth of the village's population was infected with the terrifying virus.

The Gabonese government swiftly rounded up everybody who might have had contact with the initial Mayibout cases, placing them under observation.

In the village, researchers discovered that children had found a dead chimpanzee on January 26, and all of the original ten deaths were among people who had feasted that night on the chimp. The Gabonese government, on learning of the chimp connection, issued radio bulletins nationwide warning citizens not to touch or eat dead chimps or monkeys.

By February 19 twenty cases had been confirmed: thirteen were dead. WHO intervened successfully to prevent international airlines and bordering nations from placing sanctions on Gabon, and the military imposed a strict quarantine on Makokou district. Given the area's inaccessibility such a quarantine was easily enforced, even when it came to keeping the media out. WHO officially praised the Gabonese efforts, saying that the government had taken "all appropriate measures . . . to limit the outbreak."

By the end of February, 20 percent of the Mayibout had fallen ill: 9 percent had died. But the rapid control measures taken by the Gabonese government and local hospitals prevented any further spread. Twelve of the dead had helped butcher and consume the chimpanzee. The remainder were relatives who had cared for the original group of Ebola sufferers.

And then Ebola broke out again in Gabon, nine months later in an area called Boué.

The WHO team, which included Kikwit veteran Rodier and the CDC's Mike Ryan, identified some fifty possible cases and eight Ebola deaths in Boué during October 1996. And though Boué was relatively close to Makokou district, Ryan and Rodier felt certain that the new epidemic was unconnected to the earlier Mayibout outbreak.

Reviews of local medical records revealed that for at least a decade the villagers living around the periphery of the Tai Forest in Gabon suffered three to nine apparent Ebola deaths every year.

Suspicions mounted that the notorious virus's natural habitat was in that rain forest. Heymann, who had been in the process of creating a new emerging diseases unit inside WHO ever since his triumphant return from Kikwit, started hunting for funds for construction of an Ebola station in the Tai Forest.

A year after the 1996 Boué outbreak an ailing Gabonese doctor flew to Johannesburg, South Africa, for treatment at the exclusive Morningside Clinic in the posh Sandton suburb of the city. The patient found himself, said Dr. Adrian Dusé, "in an urbanized setting in a first-class hospital."

Physicians did not then diagnose Ebola but did impose isolation care on the Gabonese, who recovered fully within two weeks. On November 11 his case was still officially undiagnosed, and the doctor was released from the hospital.

But on November 2, 1997, Morningside Clinic nurse Marilyn Lehana, age forty-six, came down with a sharp headache, spiking fever, and elevated white blood cell count. Initially, no one suspected a link between Lehana's case and that of the Gabonese doctor. And it would only be in retrospect that Dusé and infection control nurse Gerry Sharpe would recall that Lehana had been poked with a needle while trying to insert a blood line into the Gabonese.

As Lehana steadily deteriorated her medical colleagues struggled to understand: What was ailing her? How should it be treated? The hospital laboratory tested for every organism ever previously seen in South Africa, finding Lehana negative for all. Then on November 11 Lehana developed petechia, or pinhole bleeding spots all over her body, which appeared something like a measles rash. And the laboratory reported seeing microscopically the classic question mark form of the Ebola virus in Lehana's blood.

As word of her diagnosis spread within the hospital one doctor cried out, "We are all going to die!" Sharpe recalled emotionally. Panic set in, and soon local radio stations were spreading the news. The following day hundreds of parents kept their children home from schools, while others put masks on their youngsters, instructing them to keep the coverings on in class. Attendance at Johannesburg sporting and cultural events plummeted, and even the enormously popular rugby games were sparsely attended.

Lehana's illness drew particular attention because her husband was a celebrated lawn bowler, a popular sport in South Africa. Her illness became a national obsession, updated live from Morningside Clinic every morning on Johannesburg's top station, Radio 702. Throughout her illness local newspapers carried detailed accounts of her progress along with letters and prayers penned by Lehana's thousands of supporters.

Meanwhile, Dusé and Sharpe set to work tracking down every hospital worker who had had contact with the Gabonese doctor, Lehana, or their blood and tissue samples. "The number was mind-boggling," Sharpe said: 360. Every one of them was tested for antibodies to Ebola and counseled.

Meanwhile, despite their Ebola fears, Lehana's colleagues found it hard to constantly wear gloves and masks while tending to the popular nurse. Many admitted removing their gear and spending time chatting at Lehana's bedside, trying to cheer up their ailing colleague. Similarly, Dusé and Sharpe discovered countless cases of lax infection control in the hospital: lab accidents, people eating or smoking in the lab, nurses tending to patients ungloved, inappropriate waste disposal. Even in the obviously dangerous crisis health care workers found it difficult to adhere to strict infection control guidelines.

Fortunately, none of Lehana's 360 contacts tested positive for Ebola infection. But on November 24 Lehana died, her brain filled with Ebola-saturated blood.

"So even in a top-of-the-line modern hospital you can get spread of Ebola," Dr. Neil Cameron, secretary-general of communicable diseases for the South African Ministry of Health, said. "Morningside is the best private hospital in Africa. It is better than many of your American hospitals—certainly better than your urban, public hospitals."[36]

The South African incident hadn't yet occurred when most of the world's Ebola virus experts gathered in Antwerp, Belgium, to compare notes, in September 1996. It had been thirteen months since WHO officially declared the Kikwit epidemic over, and at least three small outbreaks had occurred in West Africa's Tai Forest region. Enough time had elapsed to allow the scientists to assemble laboratory and field data, in hopes of making sense of the hemorrhagic filovirus. Yambuku outbreak veteran Guido van der Groen organized the International Colloquium on Ebola Virus Research, convened at his Institute of Tropical Medicine.

Nearly all of the Ebola veterans were there—the elder statesmen who'd witnessed Yambuku, the Kikwit team, and a host of young Turks who were working on sophisticated molecular biology or blanketing the Tai Forest in search of Ebola's reservoir. One excited participant pronounced it "The Ebola Woodstock." Missing, however, were most of Africa's Ebola experts, with the exception of Muyembe. The Zairois virologist bitterly explained that the Belgian government had refused visas for his colleagues because it feared the Africans would not return to their home countries. It was, Muyembe explained, typical of how Belgium prevented African immigration to its little piece of the European continent.[37]

Heymann set the meeting's tone, telling the scientists that there was little about which they could gloat. Ebola broke out in January 1995 in Kikwit: the world didn't hear of it until May 9. He ticked off a long list of public health catastrophes of the 1990s, noting a consistent trend. The crises occurred in poor countries, largely because of essential public health failures.[38] The outside world didn't learn of the problems until things had spread beyond easy control. And resources from the wealthy world were scarce. All told, he said, $3.5 million was spent on Kikwit's epidemic efforts, more than $2 million of which came from European companies and humanitarian aid groups. Only $1 million had come from the U.S. CDC. To prepare the world for the twenty-first century, Heymann insisted, "We need a whole new vision of the function of the World Health Organization."

In the absence of genuine infrastructures of public health, separate from but in tandem to medical treatment systems, episodes such as the Kikwit Ebola epidemic would repeat, and repeat, and repeat—well into the twenty-first century. Few of the world's poor nations at the close of the twentieth century had a genuine public health infrastructure. Instead, they had a poorly funded medical care system and small offices located in large cities, inside of which bureaucrats tallied up the nation's annual death counts.

But numbers alone could not a public health infrastructure make. Indeed, they could offer little more than false reflections used to justify bad policies.

At the time of the Antwerp meeting 92 of 193 nations surveyed by UNICEF spent less than 10 percent of their budgets on health-related services.[39] That's 48 percent of the countries, providing services to well over four billion human beings. In contrast 12 percent of the budget of industrialized nations—19 percent of the U.S. budget—were directed to health spending.

At the bottom of the bottom was the Democratic Republic of the Congo, formerly Zaire, which spent less than 1 percent of its budget on health. Globally, 16 percent of all governments devoted less than 5 percent of their budgets to protecting and improving the health of their citizenries.

The Ebola virus and innumerable other less exotic organisms would always be part of the global ecology, Heymann warned. And they would always have opportunities to infect *Homo sapiens.*

It was a sentiment echoed by the CDC's Dr. Reva Khabbaz, who noted that hemorrhagic fever viruses had broken out at least thirteen times in Africa since 1986, in almost every case noted only after epidemics were well under way. Better disease surveillance was essential, she declared.

"Ah, but you cannot establish a surveillance system if there is no public health system at all," Michel Pletschette of the European Commission countered, noting that the fifteen nations of the European Union reacted poorly to Kikwit's outbreak. Lack of public health infrastructure created Zaire's crisis, Pletschette insisted, but the inability of Europe to respond wisely was indicative of those wealthy nations' public health inadequacies, as well. For example, during the epidemic some European governments banned all African primate imports—a measure Pletschette labeled "dumb." After all, there was no evidence Ebola was transmitted from monkeys to humans except, perhaps, when people ate chimps which, of course, was a practice Europeans condemned. Four countries stopped all flights from Zaire—also a move he considered "dumb." No European nation had a laboratory any longer that WHO would certify BL-4. And nearly all Europeans who took part in epidemic control in Kikwit did so under the aegis of the American CDC, Medécins Sans Frontières, or WHO—not under their own country's sponsorship. In general, he concluded, European governments did not want to spend money on an African problem and lacked clear, scientifically based public health leadership to guide their domestic Ebola-prevention policies.

Veterinary researcher Frederick Murphy of the University of California, Davis, was even blunter; funding to date in North America and Western Europe was merely "tokenism; token funds to get us scientists out of [politicians'] offices. . . . Who is to pay? Today for lack of funds the infrastructure of tropical diseases is a mere skeleton of what it was twenty years ago. That says something about the political acumen of those involved.

"So who is to be the world's public health doctor?" he asked. Who, indeed, was the leader? As colonial interests in Africa had waned after World War II, so had all North American and European commitment to tropical diseases research and control. England, France, and the United States, once the clear leaders in the arena, had stepped back, leaving no nation or institution in charge. Funding had all but disappeared for most "tropical diseases"—better termed "diseases of poor nations." Murphy bemoaned the absence of a powerful leadership voice.

The list of unknowns regarding Kikwit's epidemic remained enormous, despite hundreds of hours of research and collection of more than fifty thousand samples of human blood, and animals, plants, and insects of the Mwembe Rain Forest. South Africa's Swanepoel said that transmission was still an open question, as the CDC team was unable to explain how 5 percent of Kikwit's sufferers were exposed to Ebola: could it have been airborne contagion? Or, perhaps, utensils and food? In support of the latter hypothesis Swanepoel revealed that he had analyzed a set of contaminated syringes he'd collected at Kikwit General Hospital. More than a month after he'd collected them, and left them sitting on a desktop at 90°F the whole time, Swanepoel harvested living Ebola viruses off the needles.

The South African criticized the international team's medical efforts, noting that very little data existed on the immunological responses of Ebola survivors, "so we have *no* idea what is an effective immune response," the bombastic South African insisted. Further, he had found upon return to Kikwit after the epidemic that patient samples were mislabeled, virtually all were collected only between May 14 to 29 of the epidemic, and nothing of substance could be conjured regarding the Menga cases or any of the other pre-May 14 infections.

Murphy also bemoaned the lack of reliable immunological data, noting that the "level of destruction by this virus, the speed, begs the question why did

12 percent of the infected people of Yambuku survive? And 21 percent in Kikwit? It's one of the most overwhelming pathological images of any acute disease you can imagine."

After the international team had left, doctors in Kikwit transfused blood from Ebola survivors into eight still-ailing patients in hopes that it would prove curative. One of the patients died, seven survived. Did the experiment work? Muyembe argued no, noting that all of an additional five acute Ebola cases who were later given similar transfusions died. It was possible, therefore, that the seven transfused survivors, all of whom were less acute cases to begin with, would have survived regardless. But in the absence of reliable antibody and immune system data on any of the Kikwit cases it was impossible to judge.

Animal studies done by Peter Jahrling at USAMRIID suggested that such antibody transfusion can't succeed once monkeys or guinea pigs have developed Ebola-like symptoms.

Science similarly remained in the dark regarding the elusive source of Ebola. Researchers throughout the summer of 1995 combed Mwembe Forest, searching for anything that might have infected Gaspard Menga. Around Menga's campsite, "everything that crawled, we collected," a British expert said. Scientists from Belgium, France, the United States, England, and Zaire combed the area. And CDC and USAMRIID dedicated tremendous human resources to analyzing those samples.

"It was a lot of work," the CDC's BL-4 lab analyst Tom Ksiazcek said. "But so far the Holy Grail is still out there and up for grabs."

Privately several scientists complained of turf battles among the Institut Pasteur, CDC, and USAMRIID, each of which hoped to find that Holy Grail. One researcher complained that each of these three institutes were hoarding their samples and reagents, forbidding access to other scientists. Another griped that discoveries, when made, were never shared with African scientists who reside in Ebola-endemic areas.

And then Dr. Karl Johnson, the retired CDC officer who led the international response in Yambuku, rose and took the microphone. Renowned for decades of ground-breaking hemorrhagic fever research, Johnson was a sort of senior statesman of the field. Now living outside Bozeman, Montana, Johnson felt no need to pull his punches. He ran down the list of scientific failures in the Kikwit investigation, concluding with a sharp attack on the searches in Mwembe Forest: "I would like to ask you, number one, whether you were working under *any* kind of hypothesis at all. And number two, do you think you can even eliminate any species," as possible reservoirs, based on your investigation?

The CDC's Paul Reiter was chagrined. "I felt the same way as Karl. The fact is we went out there to do the best we could. I'm afraid that it was just a fishing expedition."

Further, the teams had tromped all over Mwembe a full six months after Menga's original infection. It was a different season, Reiter said, and probably unrealistic to think any reservoir could be found at that late date.

"There wasn't a lot of good planning," the CDC's C. J. Peters conceded.

The most tantalizing revelation came not from the heart of Africa, but via a little-known plant researcher in the Danish Royal Veterinary and Agriculture University in Copenhagen. Dr. Thorben Lundsgaard had spent years studying the festuca leaf streak virus, which attacks grasses used to feed livestock in Europe and North America. He had a hunch that the virus was carried to grasses by tiny flying insects called leafhoppers. So he grew a batch of leafhoppers, mashed them up, and scoured cell samples, using a powerful electron microscope. He never found his leaf streak virus.

"But I did find something else," the shy Danish scientist recalled. "And it was by chance. I see something and then I go, of course, in more detail. I look and it looks like a filovirus. And I was very excited, in fact."

Old Ebola hands at the colloquium were stunned by Lundsgaard's photographs, and most agreed that the microbe looked remarkably similar—but not identical—to Ebola. Still, it caught the CDC's Jim LeDuc's excited attention, because he had taken part in a 1981 U.S. Army search for Ebola's sources in northern Zaire.

"Everybody in the villages was raising guinea pigs to eat," LeDuc recalled. "And they feed the animals these grasses that are loaded with leafhoppers."

In 1981, Dr. Joseph McCormick ran the top-security Special Pathogens Laboratory at the U.S. Centers for Disease Control, where he conducted tests on guinea pig blood and tissue samples LeDuc sent from Zaire.

"Those animals did test positive for Ebola," said McCormick. But the test methods used to verify Ebola infection fifteen years ago often provided false positives, so the reliability of such findings was questionable.

Dr. Elena Ryabchikova of the State Research Center of Virology (or VECTOR) in Novosibirsk, Russia, infected laboratory guinea pigs with Ebola. First, she said, they seemed resistant. But when she passed the virus through eight generations of guinea pigs, a strain of Ebola surfaced that was 100 percent lethal to them. This probably meant, Ryabchikova said, that guinea pigs rarely got sick with Ebola in nature, though they might carry the virus.

The leafhopper/guinea pig connection was pure speculation, of course. And no one was suggesting that Euro-American leafhoppers carried the virus. Only a handful of tests had been performed on African leafhoppers, all by Robert Swanepoel of the National Institute of Virology in South Africa. Swanepoel was unable to infect the insects, but he was able to infect three species of bats found only in the so-called Ebola Belt of Central Africa.[40] The virus quickly replicated in the bats, with no deleterious effects on them. Most disturbing, Swanepoel said, was the discovery of large amounts of Ebola in the salivary glands and lungs of the bats, pointing at a possible respiratory route of Ebola transmission from the winged rodents to other animals or human beings.

An entirely different line of observation was offered by French researchers working in the Tai Forest. WHO's Dr. Pierre Formenty was studying wild chimpanzees, which had experienced die-offs due to Ebola. Most of the chimp deaths seemed to have occurred during the rainy season, when male apes hunt for Colobus monkeys. Chimpanzees who ate the Colobus, Formenty said, were five times more likely to develop Ebola than were those who avoided monkey meat.

Dr. Tom Monath of Oravax in Boston said that he had discovered that another deadly hemorrhagic virus, Lassa, was carried by the brown *Mastomys* rats in West Africa and passed to humans via inhalation of dust contaminated with rat urine. Monath told the Antwerp gathering that the Ebola puzzle was likely to be complex, possibly involving insects that were eaten by animals. Those animals were, in turn, eaten by people. Or Ebola was passed via a bite to another animal species, which were eaten by yet another animal or by people.

"I'd be very surprised if this doesn't turn out to be a complicated story," Monath concluded.

"Ah, yes," Swanepoel said with considerable gusto, "but a damned fascinating one!"

Throughout 1997 and 1998 researchers continued their efforts in the Tai Forest, erecting elaborate networks of observation stations high in the jungle canopy from whence they could observe chimpanzee activities. It was, perhaps, a long shot, but the scientists thought they might witness something that could finally solve not only the Ebola mystery but also the larger question of how viruses jump from one target species to another, and eventually to human beings.

In five Tai Forest countries (Central African Republic, Cameroon, Congo, Gabon, and Equatorial Guinea) an Institut Pasteur team led by Jean-Paul Gonzalez ran blood tests on a variety of animals, as well as local Pygmy tribes people, looking for the presence of antibodies against Ebola. Nearly 8 percent of the *Mastomys* rats tested positive, meaning that they had at some time been infected with the virus. More striking were antibody-positive rates in wild pigs, guinea pigs, and dogs in the 16 to 18 percent range.

The human results were particularly intriguing and clearly demonstrated that the Ebola virus frequently infected *Homo sapiens* who lived their lives in the Tai/Congolese rain forest. Further, it appeared that infection rates varied year by year, indicating that exposure to the virus was, for people, erratic. In Pygmy blood samples taken in 1979, for example, about 5 percent proved positive. In 1985 it spiked at 35 percent seropositive blood samples.[41]

It seemed, then, that Ebola epidemics were a rarity among the human and

animal denizens of the Congo Basin and Tai Forest, but individuals were frequently exposed to the virus, perhaps infected, and probably more commonly
than anyone realized, killed by the virus.

Ebola was hardly the only relatively recently discovered virus toward which
the region's animals and peoples had antibodies. HTLV types I and II, Marburg
virus, and HIV types 1 and 2 were also present and infected several species
besides human beings. In the early 1990s several research groups showed that
the less pathogenic AIDS virus, HIV-2, was a monkey microbe. So closely did
HIV-2 strains resemble those found in monkey populations in any given West
African area that scientists concluded the two primate populations were being
exposed over and over again.[42] That meant that people in the region were in
contact with monkey blood—probably while butchering animals for consumption—so often that the monkey SIV-2 viruses were reintroduced over and over
again into the human population, becoming HIV-2.[43]

In 1999 two separate teams of scientists, led by Beatrice Hahn of the
University of Alabama in Birmingham and Francoise Barré-Sinoussi of the Institut Pasteur, discovered that the same might be true for the far more dangerous
HIV-1. The virus was exclusively seen in one of four subspecies of chimpanzees,
the *Pan troglodytes troglodytes*, which live in the Tai and Congo Basin rain forest
area. Based on observations of only a handful of the infected animals it appeared
that the virus was harmless for the chimps, though lethal to more than 95 percent of all infected *Homo sapiens*.

Given that chimpanzees and *Homo sapiens* differ genetically in only 1.5
percent of their total genetic makeup this seemed startling. It suggested to Hahn
that study of wild *Pan troglodytes troglodytes* might reveal immunological secrets
vital to finding effective treatments or a vaccine for AIDS.[44]

But since 1991, Hahn learned, chimpanzees in the region have grown
scarce, their ecologies and very existence thrown upside down. It was a turn of
events with implications for not only the future of HIV-1 but also of all Central
African animal viruses.

Prior to 1991 the government of France had subsidized the currency of all
of its former West African colonies, artificially bolstering its value. But in 1991
France dropped the subsidy, allowing the African currencies to plummet to their
"natural" values. Overnight the resources of those countries—which included
Central African Republic, Equatorial Guinea, Côte d'Ivoire, Cameroon, and Gabon—became highly desirous for European investors. The costs of resource development and transport, labor, and goods fell so far that even comparatively
low value items, such as scrub trees, were profitably exploited. By 1992 dozens
of European companies were logging the region's rain forests at a feverish pace.[45]

In their zeal the loggers were slicing roads deep into previously inaccessible rain forest regions. And a new industry arose across the region: bushmeat

hunting. In its novel incarnation the exploits varied, both in quantity and form, from the traditional hunter-gatherer search for subsistence. The new hunters came from cities in the region, wielded rifles and automatic weapons, and sold the meat in urban marketplaces for tidy profits. The actual rate of bushmeat kill, its impact on the local ecology, and the numbers of primates hunted were all matters of considerable controversy, due largely to their powerful political repercussions.[46]

While controversy and the bushmeat trade swelled in tandem, so silently did the risk of transmission of monkey and ape diseases to human beings, as the slaughter and butchering of these animals exposed hunters and cooks to tremendous amounts of primate blood.

It only took exposure to one dead chimp to spark Mayibout's 1996 Ebola outbreak. Escalating the primate hunt obviously increased the odds that such viruses as simian forms of HIV, HTLV, Ebola, Marburg, and monkeypox—as well as microbes not previously known to human beings—would make the cross-species jump, infecting *Homo sapiens.*

In Zaire the bushmeat trade was driven not so much by foreign logging operations as starvation. Without the animal meat of Mwembe Forest, for example, the children of Kikwit would no doubt have suffered even worse kwashiorkor, malnutrition. The dictator's greed was their burden, and the tax upon their ecology. It was also the focus of their collective rage, which had risen steadily as Mobutu's reign wore on.

Not long after the Kikwit epidemic ended, old, simmering civil war activities in Zaire heated up. Sensing that aging Mobutu was losing his grip upon the Zairois Army, and having formed an advantageous pact with the neighboring Rwandan government, rebels took bold steps. For years rival rebel groups had waged tiny battles from isolated parts of Shaba, Katanga, and the Mitumba regions, sparring with Zairois troops. But from the Mitumba Mountains that border Lakes Kivu and Tanganyika, and Rwanda and Burundi, arose a new organization, the alliance of Democratic Forces for the Liberation of Congo-Zaire. It was an amalgam, made up of a host of different anti-Mobutu forces and tough, seasoned killers drawn from the Tutsi population that had been living in exile in Zaire since conflicts heated up in their home countries of Burundi and Rwanda.[47]

At an extraordinary pace the new movement, led by long-obscure rebel Laurent Kabila, captured Zaire's towns and cities in its drive from the country's eastern-most border to the Atlantic Ocean. So great was the populace's hatred of the dictator that rebels barely had to engage in genuine conflict as Zairois troops fled, steadily westward, looting everything in sight in their hasty retreats. Hailed by jubilant, cheering throngs, Kabila's army entered towns from Lumbumbashi to Mbuji-Mayi. As Kabila's forces closed on the capital in May 1997 the dictator was fighting his own battle in France with malignant cancer. Realizing that Mobutu could, after thirty-one years in power, no longer command fear and respect in his army and general Zairois populace, the coterie of his cronies who had so benefited from the dictator's greed-fest fled Kinshasa, and took anything of value that they could grab with them to European hideaways.

Kabila's march into Kinshasa was greeted by enormous, cheering crowds from La Cité ghetto, and hailed by Western officials and businesses that had long before grown weary of the Mobutu regime. The dictator's corruption had made business dealings and investment nearly suicidal.

Kabila took control of a capital that bore little resemblance to beautiful Leopoldville, the colonial name of Kinshasa. Gone were the lazy palms and bougainvillaeas, the well-swept boulevards and quiet bistros. Gone, too, were the promising commercial buildings that during the first years of Mobutu's reign had housed representatives of foreign banks, businesses, and diplomatic corps. In their place were stench, decay, rot, garbage heaps, potholes big enough to destroy a chassis, street beggars, barefoot gangs of starving children, and rain-soaked buildings covered in fungus.

The jungle was reclaiming the capital, as lianas, mildew, weeds, and rain forest shrubs overgrew the streets and buildings. Like a postapocalyptic vision from 1950s science fiction, sidewalks were splintered by aggressive roots and weeds, trees sprouted through rooftops, turning whole buildings into seeming multistory flowerpots, waves of mud rolled with the afternoon rains through the dirt roads, and human waste visible in open sewer lines filled the tropical air with an eye-stinging redolence.

The day Laurent Kabila took power Zaire's external debt was $14 billion. The national bank vaults were, literally, empty. And the World Bank estimated that repairing the country's essential infrastructure—key roads, telephone system, power generators, and the like—would cost $4.5 billion. Overall, Africa's gross domestic product grew a promising 4.6 percent in 1996, and 3.3 percent in 1997. But Zaire's *shrank*, went backward, by 8 percent from 1990 to 1995 and 6 percent in 1997 alone.[48]

In June Mobutu was on his French deathbed and Kabila was surrounded in Kinshasa by petitioners, foreign advisers, and businessmen eager to cut deals for access to Zaire's vast oil, mineral, and gem wealth. It was a moment of optimism. Western leaders, the World Bank, and the International Monetary Fund paid homage to Kabila but cautiously avoided offers of cash until the new leader's intentions were clear. At the close of 1997 U.S. Secretary of State Madeleine Albright paid Kabila a visit, calling the new leader "a friend of democracy."

But if it was democracy Kabila intended his approach was unusual. The robust, bald leader who, ominously, dressed in the famous Mobutu suits declined to name a date for national elections. Much-needed funds for repairing

Zaire's decay—including her clinics, hospitals, and public health infrastructure—weren't forthcoming from United Nations agencies because Kabila, amid reports of genocide in eastern Congo, refused their access to the country's eastern regions for human rights investigations.

When the New Year of 1998 dawned euphoria had vanished from Zaire, replaced by disquiet amid fears that one dictator had simply been replaced by another. Worse yet, the new one seemed more beholden to African foreigners than to his own people.

Amid the military and political chaos another monkey disease made the leap from rain forest animals to human beings: monkeypox. Though the first human cases of the disease surfaced in the Katako-Kombe region in February 1996—almost exactly one year after Ebola had made its way out of the Mwembe Forest—notification of WHO and field investigations were severely hampered by the war. It would be a year before WHO scientists got a look at the problem firsthand, and that investigation was aborted because of guerrilla military operations in the region. In October 1998 WHO returned to the area, discovering that the epidemic was still under way and could well constitute the largest known human monkeypox outbreak.[49]

The single biggest killer of the twentieth century was the smallpox virus which, before its 1977 eradication, claimed more lives than all of the century's wars, combined. The smallpox virus only infected *Homo sapiens*, and was spread through casual contact and in the air.

The monkey form of the virus was similar enough to smallpox that many scientists had protested WHO's declaration of eradicating smallpox, insisting that as long as monkeypox existed in the jungles of Africa the threat of reemergent smallpox remained.[50]

The new monkeypox epidemic worried WHO because it seemed that the virus was spreading among people, rather than merely from monkey-to-person. During seventeen years of prior investigation in the entire Central African rain forest region only 476 human monkeypox cases were found, and few were more than two rounds of transmission away from a monkey source.

But in this new epidemic at least 511 human cases of the disease had occurred between February 1996 and October 1998, and some appeared to be more than twelve generations of transmission away from the original monkey source.

Though the connection to smallpox made monkeypox worrisome, it was not a terribly dangerous disease to humans, and only eight people had died in the latest epidemic. It did illustrate to WHO, however, that the political and ecological crises in the region were increasing the probability of epidemics that could have implications well beyond the country Kabila had renamed the Democratic Republic of the Congo, or DROC. Local WHO representative Dr. Abdou

Moudi warned that there were an "alarming" number of epidemics in the country, and information systems were rapidly breaking down.

The story wasn't over.

By March 1998 the already abominable conditions in Kikwit under which its 400,000 residents survived had, amazingly, worsened. The Hotel Kwilu's kitchen and power generator had been looted by soldiers, as had its water pump, doorknobs, curtains, mosquito nets, bedsheets, and even pencils and paper. That paucity of valuables was echoed in every sector of Kikwit society, rendering cast-off beer cans and shipping crates treasured replacements for stolen pots, pans, baskets, and totes. Even fewer cars crawled the streets, as spare parts for the aging vehicles no longer could be found, and soldiers had stolen everything from steering wheels to spark plugs.

In 1995 the largest denomination bill had been the 500-Zaire note, large stacks of which were needed to purchase even one banana. In 1998 the largest currencies were the 500,000-and one-million-Zaire notes, which still carried the profile of Mobutu Sese Seko. The size of the stacks needed for rudimentary purchases were thinner, but it remained Monopoly money, so worthless as to be laughable. A 100,000-Zaire note was worth $1.10. A bottle of Primus beer cost 600,000 Zaires.

As was the case in most of DROC, roads connecting Kikwit to other major cities were destroyed during the war. Trade never had a chance to recover from the Ebola-required quarantine of 1995. For most of the now-dubbed "Congolese" traders, overhead had become almost prohibitively high, as all goods had to be transmitted either by boat or air. In the case of Kikwit, river transport didn't carry goods in profitable directions. Only chartered airplanes carried goods in 1998, along with paying passengers who sat atop the cargo, sipping colas that flight attendants distributed as they carefully maneuvered among packing crates inside old Soviet cargo planes.

Though the configuration of the army and the flag under which it served had changed, soldiers holding M-16 rifles still stood guard in the same positions in 1998 as in 1995. More than two hundred drugstores still lined Boulevard Mobutu, and no one had gotten around to changing the name of Kikwit's only paved street. In Kikwit's markets the usual paltry display of smuggled plastic goods and packed foods was presented, along with the plants and animals gathered from Mwembe Forest.

But among government officials only Makarios Manikasa, chief of the National Security Services' Bandundu office, retained his job. The rest of the Mobutu-era officials were swept away, replaced by those loyal to Laurent Kabila.

"There is little peace in the country now," Manikasa said sadly, seated behind his large wooden desk in a small office bathed in sun, sweltering heat, and mosquitoes. The security chief never removed his black sunglasses, nor would he permit photographs, because, he explained, "I don't want the CIA to know what I look like. As you know I am an agent and must remain under cover."

Manikasa took his area's safety seriously, seeing his role as one that extended well beyond the usual security concerns of intrigue, rebels, smuggling, and insurgency. That was because, he explained, "As I am responsible for security, I don't see security just in terms of weapons but in all things."

Including disease.

In 1995 Manikasa's wife, Lusilu, was a nurse at Kikwit General Hospital. She was in the operating room when hapless Kimfumu's abdomen was cut open releasing Ebola-rich blood that spattered over everyone, herself included.

"She got it in that first surgical case in that cluster after the orderly took ill," Manikasa said, still stiffening when he recalled those events three years later. "She was sick for three weeks. Nobody could touch her. Everybody was afraid. Even myself, in the hospital, could not touch her. Especially when we learned it was a deadly virus."

It took Lusilu Manikasa many more weeks to recover all of her physical health. But after three years the pretty thirty-year-old nurse still had not bounced back emotionally. For reasons she could not fathom, but troubled her deeply, Manikasa alone survived that first cluster of cases. As she had lain in Pavilion No. 3 during April and May of 1995 Manikasa watched each of her colleagues die around her, listened to the seemingly nonstop wailing of grieving families standing in front of the nearby morgue, and felt certain that at any moment the virus would claim her life, too.

"For four days I didn't eat anything," Lusilu Manikasa recalled, relaxing under a shade tree on a steamy, equatorial afternoon. "My throat burned and my gums hurt. I had bloody spots on my thighs. And bloody diarrhea. I felt weak."

Manikasa patted her multicolored full-length cotton skirt, touching her thighs, and said, "One more thing. I don't understand. Every now and then those bloody spots on my thighs return. They're like . . . you know, when you hit something. Like big bruises. What could that be?"

Manikasa's relatives gathered around the corner of their cinder block ramshackle home, peering at the white woman who had come to speak to their cousin. Nervous about her life in Kikwit, Manikasa was spending most of her days far from her husband and two children, living with relatives in Kinshasa. Though she missed her family, Manikasa explained, it was frightening to return to Kikwit and her nursing job.

"It takes courage to go to work," she insisted. "The conditions are not good!"

A forty-minute airplane ride away in Kikwit Manikasa's security chief husband said that his wife had *"beaucoups de courage."* Every time she returned to the Kikwit General Hospital he worried. By mutual agreement she rarely came to Kikwit anymore.

"It is certain that we will have another epidemic because conditions are unchanged," Manikasa insisted.

"And when the international response came we were happy. We knew WHO came here to save our lives. A good part of Zaire at that time, now the Congo, could have been decimated," Manikasa continued. "In that time the entire world community was organized to come here to Kikwit, and Kikwit became the center of the world. The population believed that because of the terrible disease a health infrastructure would be developed. Some even believed the hospital here would become the reference facility for the whole country. The hospital believed that from then on Kikwit would develop a genuine health infrastructure."

Manikasa lowered his voice and spat out his words bitterly as he concluded, "But everything has returned to square one, where people are suffering to find medicine and medical support. Everything is forgotten. Could it happen again? For sure! There are no changes!"

Well, that wasn't exactly true. There had been changes: for the worse.

In 1997 Kabila appointed Marc Katshunga to be the Bandundu Province's governor, which, among other things, meant that the plump politician and his wife, Cornelie, could move into the sprawling two-story governor's mansion in Kikwit and maintain a staff of servants and gardeners who kept the lace tablecloths well ironed and the colorful, tropical garden well weeded. A similar well-staffed mansion was at his disposal in Bandundu City. And among his entourage were several advisers and a video cameraman who documented the governor's every move. Puffing up for the camera the politician explained that, in the long run, the Ebola epidemic had little—if any—lasting impact on Kikwit and its neighboring villages. He credited "aggressive political mobilization," engineered by himself, with "almost annihilating the fear."

Apparently confident that Kikwit no longer needed to be prepared for such emergencies Governor Katshunga confiscated the region's only ambulance, had it painted and outfitted with sofas, and pressed it into the service of his office. In 1998 the ambulance that had previously carried Ebola patients to Kikwit General Hospital functioned as Katshunga's chauffeur-driven limousine.

For Kikwitians poverty had become a constant. A local Catholic nun put it in perspective by noting that her order found the resources to supply one pen to each family every school term. When siblings took exams in school, they shared their family's sole writing implement.

It was, of course, the utter lack of infection control and hygiene in Kikwit's hospitals that the Ebola virus had exploited, turning an isolated chain of cases occurring in the community into a profound epidemic. Once the virus had entered a hospital that lacked even the most minimal elements of infection control—soap and clear water—it raced through the patients and medical staff like fire burning its way up a hillside of dry grass.

WHO's David Heymann said that "this epidemic was driven by hospital workers who did not respect the most minimal health standards."

It was a "lack of respect" driven largely by the paucity of options.

But in 1998 conditions in Kikwit's frail health infrastructure were, remarkably, even worse.

What few medical supplies reached cut-off Kikwit in 1998 cost far more than they had in 1995 because the only remaining form of transport was a network of private airplanes. Flying post–World War II Russian cargo planes, three newly created companies carried passengers and shipments daily to and from Kikwit. Every now and then a plane bore X-ray film for tuberculosis diagnosis, antibiotics to treat bacterial infections, chloroquine for malaria, surgical gloves or other life-and-death supplies.

In 1997 Dr. Pius Kongolo had moved from Bomba some two hundred kilometers away to become the new chief of Kikwit General Hospital. Though his colleagues warned him against moving for fear he would encounter Ebola in Kikwit, Kongolo, a handsome Kinshasa-trained internist, decided the job "represented a certain amount of risk, but it was a calculated risk."

A big part of Kongolo's calculus that led him to accept the Kikwit job was word that the international response to the Ebola epidemic brought "a lot of equipment here. But my surprise was huge when I discovered it was not here."

Every microscope, water purifier, specialized protective gear, laboratory instrument, test kit, and piece of lab equipment that scientists from the CDC, WHO, Institut Pasteur, and Medécins Sans Frontières had brought in May 1995 were gone by September of that year.

Kikwit's primary medical facility by 1998 had only the same two microscopes that were there before the Ebola epidemic, both of which could only be used with the aid of sunlight. It had one aging X-ray machine. One of the diagnostic labs had a forty-year-old centrifuge—a device essential for preparing blood samples for analysis. The hospital's ancient, rusted generator provided only sporadic electricity, so there were no freezers to hold blood and tissue samples, or refrigerators for safe storage of transfusion blood or temperature-sensitive drugs and vaccines. Unless boiled on coal fires, the hospital's water was unsafe for human consumption. Nighttime labors and deliveries—including emergency C-sections—were performed with the aid of one of the three kerosene lamps on the OB-GYN ward.

In the surgical theater—the same operating room in which Lusilu Manikasa had been infected with Ebola three years before—every piece of equipment was recycled, from gloves to masks, scalpels to hemostats. And the equipment that was inserted in one body after another was usually not sterile, Kongolo said, "because we lack the fuel to run our generator and therefore have no power for the autoclaves," which would heat-sterilize surgical instruments.

For the previous fifteen months—since the civil war—the medical staff of Kikwit's hospital had not yet been paid. And Hospital Director Baudouin Ndulu had to lay off 30 percent of the staff, leaving 265 doctors, nurses, maintenance workers, and other essential personnel. It had been more than ten years since he had received federal funds for equipment, Ndulu said, and the hospital was so deeply in debt to medical suppliers that it technically was insolvent.

"Apart from the human factor, the infrastructure is demeaning," Kongolo insisted. "We always have to do makeshift things in order to achieve the minimum. There are times when we feel as if we've been sacrificed."

Ndulu—as well as every other Kikwit health care worker—insisted that were Ebola to hit the hospital then, "It would be worse! Because no preventative measures have been taken and nothing has come to this hospital."

Ndulu claimed promises were made by all the international agencies that responded to the 1995 epidemic, but none of the pledged supplies ever materialized.

"That's the usual behavior of international people," DROC's Health Minister Dr. Jean-Baptiste Sondji said dismissively. "They came when there is a lot of coverage in the media, then they leave as if nothing happened."[51]

But it was not just international health agencies that forgot poor Kikwit's plight. Her own officials, citizens, and health providers appeared to have shoved Ebola out of their minds, forgetting all the lessons of prevention they were taught three years earlier by the international team.

"I haven't noticed any change in Kikwit because people in Kikwit did not believe really that it was a virus that attacked," University of Bandundu history professor N'sanga Kibari explained. Kibari, whose twenty-seven-year-old brother, Mombolo, perished in the epidemic, wrote a detailed history of the crisis entitled, *The Ebola Virus in Kikwit: Myth, Mystery or Reality?* He concluded that despite all the obvious scientific evidence that the Ebola virus caused Kikwit's calamity, most of the populace, still in 1998, believed something else had been responsible for the 296 deaths.

"First people believed it was an experiment conducted by the Americans," Kibari recalled. Then the concept of *landa-landa* swept Kikwit. In nearby Vanga it was rumored that a local American missionary physician who had run a hospital in the village since 1960 was capable of transforming himself into a hippopotamus that trawled the Kwilu River, performing ominous spiritual acts. And because the first person to contract Ebola in January 1995 was Gaspard Menga, a Jehovah's Witness, it was widely suggested among the majority Catholic population that the epidemic constituted God's revenge for deviant beliefs and behaviors.

All these beliefs, coupled with the poverty of the health care system, conspired to create a profound level of postepidemic denial. The people returned to practices that spread Ebola in 1995, including cleansing bodies of dead family members and thus exposing themselves to infected fluids. At the hospitals all the infection control practices followed during the epidemic were swiftly abandoned.

At Kikwit Hospital statistician Ebwala Dambwala saw that fear ruled nearly all behaviors during the epidemic, particularly among health care workers. Nearly 22 percent of the deaths were hospital employees, he noted, pointing to stacks of charts and tables he had painstakingly hand-drawn, depicting the epidemic's toll. But by 1998 Dambwala asserted, "They don't think of it anymore. They have forgotten."

Most had put Ebola out of their minds, except the survivors. Like Lusilu Manikasa, the majority of the eighty-eight Ebola survivors now saw life through prisms of apprehension. In Kikwit they formed a club that met monthly to discuss their fears about future returns of the deadly virus.

Enery-Raphael Mikolo had a pile of photographs of his bout with Ebola in a drawer in the hospital's leprosy and tuberculosis laboratory. He had taken ill on April 29, three days after burying a friend who died of the disease. And when he got well doctors at the hospital used his blood as an antiserum for other Ebola patients.

Three years later Mikolo was still haunted by his battle with the virus. He ate constantly to stay strong and had a nervous manner. Despite his fears, Mikolo continued to work at the hospital, taking sputum and blood samples from TB and leprosy patients.

"We test saliva with no protection. We don't have the necessary gloves and equipment," Mikolo said, his voice high-strung. "We do all we can not to position ourselves in front of patients who are coughing. But for lepers there is no means of protection. You see, here washing hands is difficult because I don't have any soap."

When a visitor offered Mikolo a small container of antiseptic hand-wash liquid he grabbed it in an instant, immediately hiding it from the view of colleagues. For the next ten minutes Mikolo hovered around the soap's hiding place, eyeing his colleagues. Once certain they were unaware of his treasure Mikolo grinned broadly.

Pierre Menga still vividly recalled the January 1995 funeral of his brother Gaspard. He had photos of the funeral depicting the Menga family gathered around Gaspard's open casket.

Of all his siblings only Pierre was alive in 1998. He was saddled with a slew of small children—his, Gaspard's, and those of other deceased relatives. And he cared for his aging, tubercular father, Innocent. In all, Pierre cared for twelve people.

"We look and search every day," for food and money, Pierre, who was unemployed, said. "But everyone is kind to us in Kikwit."

Innocent glared through rheumy eyes at his son and retorted, "Don't sound as if we're all right—we're suffering!"

And indeed, they were. The Menga clan of thirteen people lived in a two-room wattle home located in an almost inaccessible gully well off Ndala Road. The densely crowded neighborhood resonated with the laughter and cries of small children. During heavy rains the clay grounds flooded. And after each downpour the humid, steamy air filled with malarial mosquitoes. The children were all barefoot, their clothes tattered and ill-fitting.

Pierre, who was unmarried, had his hands full caring for all of the children and hustling for work and money. During the Ebola epidemic Pierre set aside grief over the deaths in his family to assist WHO and the CDC in their investigations. For his services Menga received no money or compensation.

"Between that time and now there's no change at all," Menga said of Kikwit and of his family. "We've gone back to our old ways. We are suffering. Of course, now many of us are missing. We just wish that the international community would be aware of our suffering here."

The thirty-four-year-old man looked overwhelmed as he introduced the many children in his care.

"We have kept one child in school all along, but [because of the fees] we cannot afford to put the others, with all our losses, through school. And we are wondering what will be the future of our family."

Every morning Pierre awakened from a dream. Someone had given him enough money to start a business, and he had built a house large enough for all of the surviving Mengas to live in comfort, dry during storms and free of disease-carrying insects.

That, he said, "Would stop the pain and anguish."

In Kinshasa, meanwhile, it was hard to detect any action and effort to improve matters.

"The problem is they're overwhelmed," a Western gold developer said. "Mobutu left such a massive disaster that they just don't know where to start."

Congo's Health Minister Sondji added that the crisis in Kikwit's health care infrastructure was no better or worse than what was the current state of affairs "in hundreds of towns all over the nation. We estimate that minimally $530 million will be needed to address the problem. We are battling very hard to find those funds. But look, $700 million is just the entire national budget!"

Obviously, the tall, middle-aged Sondji said grimly, health must compete for every one of those $700 million against every other sector of the society. And Congo, just two years before the millennium, had few of the necessities of the twentieth century. Most Congolese had no electricity, running water, telephones, paved roads, or other essentials of life.

For Professor Muyembe the sorry state of affairs in his country was deeply painful. He grew up in Bandundu Province, not far from Kikwit, during colonial days when strict nuns sharply doled out lessons in Latin, classical Greek, French, and the Western humanities. A worldly father of five, Muyembe remained in Kinshasa despite invitations for appointments in Europe. But he used his European connections to fund research and clinical work in Kinshasa, and to keep a back door open should escape from his beloved Congo be necessary. Few, if any, of his colleagues were so fortunate.

The situation, even in April of 1998, was ominous enough. It soon worsened.

By May counterrevolutions were breaking out all over DROC as disenchantment with the seemingly paralyzed Kabila government grew. Political activists in Kinshasa who had courageously tolerated beatings and imprisonment under Mobutu found little improvement in the democratic climate. Opposition political parties, though officially legal, were harassed to such a degree that local newspapers called the era the Time of Darkness.

Rebel counterforces surrounded key Congolese cities, including the capital, by August 1998. An exodus of foreigners followed, bringing all mining, oil, and general large business operations to a halt. Even within his own ranks Kabila was finding dissent, as breakaway factions of his army seized airplanes, airports, and whole towns.

By the end of August Kabila's alliance had collapsed, and for all intents and purposes his rule extended only a few miles beyond Kinshasa. The already beleaguered economy went into a tailspin. All foreign investors disappeared. The Zaire/DROC war was threatening to expand, drawing in adversaries from all over Africa. Angola now backed Kabila. Uganda and Rwanda had switched their allegiances, supporting Tutsi dissidents that formerly were part of the Kabila alliance. Zimbabwe sent military "advisers" to Kinshasa. Namibia flew in twenty-one tons of military equipment, also backing Kabila. Water and electricity for Kinshasa were cut off by rebels.

From South Africa President Nelson Mandela pleaded for a peaceful resolution. He was ignored.

By September 1998 troops from at least five African countries were on the ground in DROC, fighting alongside either the Kabila government's soldiers or rebel forces. The entire east of the country was under rebel/Rwanda/Uganda control.

By October it seemed that, thanks to foreign troops, Kabila had driven the rebels back to the far east and maintained control. It had cost the government $5 billion, sinking the nation toward the $20 billion debt mark.[52] To the victors went the spoils: each of Kabila's supporting nations laid claim to various Congolese oil, mineral, and gem reserves.

As the last year of the twentieth century dawned the armies of Africa were mobilizing to decide the fate of the continent's massive equatorial nation.

And on November 13, 1998, armed soldiers, by order of Laurent Kabila, marched into Health Minister Sondji's office. He was removed from his office for "insufficient display of solidarity," having voiced concern that the new dictator had no intention of holding elections or creating a democracy. Sondji was arrested, leaving the nation—and the people of Kikwit—without any health leadership.

The public health implications of Ebola extended well beyond the dismissive notes that were usually struck by Westerners when discussing seemingly intractable African problems. Failure to take action guaranteed that such public health crises would recur, not only on the Congo Basin but also wherever there is a confluence of similar social and biological factors.

Clearly the Kikwit outbreak was nosocomial. The local hospitals functioned as amplification systems: a pianissimo stream of individual cases went in; a loud fortissimo din of epidemic proportions came out.

At the peak of the Ebola outbreak nothing more exotic than latex gloves and basic protective gear was needed, along with clearheaded planning, to bring the epidemic under control. The sorts of high-technology tools favored in North America and Europe not only would have been useless in Kikwit, but they might even have, in the long run, proven deleterious. If Kikwit's demoralized doctors toiled in fear in 1998 because they couldn't afford latex gloves, their paranoia could only have been compounded further if the control of Ebola had necessitated even costlier items, such as the air-conditioned space suits brought—too late to be used—by Swedish volunteers.

High-tech solutions are also unlikely to hasten diagnosis and notification of such crises in Kikwit or any other isolated, impoverished pocket of the earth. If Kikwit General Hospital had been left a $10,000 satellite telephone with which to call David Heymann in Geneva in the event of another epidemic, it would not now possess the device. More than likely the exotic phone would long since have been "liberated" for the use of a general in one or another of the armies now fighting over the future of DROC/Zaire. Or perhaps it would be used by Bandundu Province's governor, making phone calls from inside the ambulance he "liberated" from Kikwit General Hospital.

CHAPTER THREE

BOURGEOIS PHYSIOLOGY

**The collapse of all semblances of public health
in the former Soviet Socialist Republics.**

*Moscow meanwhile was empty. There were still people in the city; a fiftieth
part of all the former inhabitants still remained in it, but it was empty.*

    It was deserted as a dying, queenless hive is deserted. . . .

    *Almost all have died, unconscious of their coming end, sitting in the
holy place, which they had watched—now no more. They reek of death and
corruption. But a few of them stir still, rise up, fly languidly and settle on the
hand of the foe, without the spirit to die stinging him; the rest are dead and
easily brushed aside as fishes' scales. The beekeeper closes the partition, chalks
a mark on the hive, and choosing his own time, breaks it up and burns it.*

—Leo Tolstoy, *War and Peace*[1]

Either socialists defeat lice or lice will defeat Socialism!

—Joseph Stalin

*The public health situation worsened so much that at first it seemed unbeliev-
able. No country has ever exhibited such an abrupt change in peacetime.*

—Vladimir Shkolnikov, Moscow epidemiologist, 1994

What we face is unprecedented, colossal!

—Dr. Gerasimenko of the Russian Academy of Medical Sciences in a May 1997 address to the Duma

By the time Leonid Brezhnev died in the autumn of 1982 there wasn't much
left of his seventy-five-year-old cardiovascular system. The ironfisted dictator
who had served as Soviet premier and then president for eighteen years had
blood veins and arteries that were so clogged with atherosclerotic plaque that
blood cells could barely pass. In his abdomen the aorta had ballooned into a
massive aneurysm. His heart, scarred after innumerable heart attacks—the exact
number was a state secret—fluttered irregularly, struggling for years before finally giving up, felling the leader of the Union of Soviet Socialist Republics. The

all-powerful leader died as a result of decades of overeating, overdrinking, and chain-smoking.

Less than two years later his successor, Yuri Andropov, also succumbed. The once-feared leader of the KGB secret police, famed for always wearing sinister darkened glasses, was buried in the winter of 1984 alongside the KGB's notorious founder, Feliks E. Dzerzhinsky. Officially Andropov died of kidney failure. But like Brezhnev, it was a lousy diet, smoking, and alcohol that brought down the man once considered the most fearsome Soviet of his day.

And thirteen months later seventy-three-year-old Konstantin Chernenko was also buried in Red Square, having served as the last of the Soviet Union's Stalinist-style premiers. Years of smoking cigarettes and drinking massive quantities of vodka felled him as well, turning his lungs into emphysema-besieged, wheezing apparati and his liver into cirrhotic Jell-O.

In March 1985 the Politburo finally gave up on placing men who had served in Stalin's shadow in power, turning to Mikhail Gorbachev, comparatively youthful at age fifty-four.

It was the beginning of the great change.

Gorbachev would be the first leader of the Soviet Union—indeed, in Russian history dating back to A.D. 913—to survive his political tenure, not either dying in office or forced out, having been crippled by fatal physical or mental illness.

If Gorbachev's physical health signaled improvement for Soviet leadership it did not augur commensurate enhancement in the health of the Soviet masses. Indeed, it marked the beginning of the most astounding collapse in public health ever witnessed in peacetime in the industrialized world. For the Euro-Slavic world it would be the most radical reversal, in the absence of war, since the Black Death of the fourteenth century.

I

Then that frightening word demography *appears, and it is clear that Russia today is on the eve of a demographic catastrophe: the death rate is exceeding the birth rate, life expectancy is declining sharply, the number of suicides is rising, and there are 240 abortions per 100 live births.*

—Andrei Sinyavsky, 1997[2]

I f there was one thing the Soviet Union seemed justified in bragging about it was their health care system.

In a series of bold five-year plans executed from Moscow, the Soviets, and their counterparts in Eastern Europe, claimed one victory after another over disease and illness in the Communist world. By 1970, Russia had raised life expectancies from 1917 pre–Bolshevik Revolution levels of thirty-eight years of age for men and forty-three for women to sixty-five and seventy-four, respectively. And infant mortality plummeted from 250 deaths per 1,000 babies born in 1917 to about 20 per 1,000 in 1970.

Trumpeted globally as evidence of the human, caring face of communism, the successes were buttressed by a public health infrastructure so massive that the Soviets could honestly claim to have more doctors, nurses, and hospital beds per capita than anyone else in the world.[3] So it came as something of a shock to the global health establishment when a series of epidemics suddenly exploded across twelve time zones of the Communist world less than a year after the Soviet Union collapsed in 1991.[4]

Diphtheria infected 200,000 people regionally over this time period, killing 5,000; polio rolled into Azerbaijan in 1991, Uzbekistan in 1993, and Chechnya in 1995; and hepatitis was suddenly so commonplace as to be considered endemic, rather than epidemic. Flu hit so hard in 1995 that the Ukrainian government closed for more than a week; typhoid infected 20,000 in Tajikistan in 1996 and then stayed endemic; St. Petersburg coped with dual epidemics of cholera and dysentery four times from 1993 to 1998. AIDS grew exponentially, with 20,000 full-blown cases projected in Ukraine alone by the year 2001; TB, syphilis, and gonorrhea followed suit. And alcoholism, drug abuse, and suicide were by 1995 considered epidemic, according to international health standards.

Even childhood mumps became a major problem, rising 30 percent from 1992 to 1994 alone.

Life expectancy nose-dived—men's, for instance, dropped three years between 1992 and 1993. Suddenly, just eight years after the Soviet state ceased to exist, the grandest health care system known to man was spiraling into chaos.[5]

What had functioned as the "human, caring face" of communism became, instead, a vision of despair and disease.

In Moscow, that vision was personified by Konstantin, an emaciated, former Soviet soldier who was dying from drug-resistant TB, developed in a Russian prison, that had invaded his lungs, liver, kidneys, and heart. And in Tbilisi by frail, tiny Irakli Sherodzle, fifteen, huddled with his mother around an orange hot electric coil, suffering from the drug-resistant flesh-eating streptococci that was inexorably destroying his body.

In the Ukraine, it was most obvious in the killing field surrounding a neighborhood where drugs were sold openly, then injected by hundreds of teenagers and young adults who shared their needles while squatting on the ice-cold parkland. And on the streets of Odessa, where a pretty, fourteen-year-old prostitute said that she always used condoms, then laughed derisively and winked knowingly at a nearby friend.

The new face of health care in the former USSR could be seen at an AIDS clinic in Kyiv,[6] where a nurse took blood from an HIV-positive man without wearing protective latex gloves, using her bare forefinger to apply pressure to the site of injection. It could be seen in Georgia, at the Deserter's Bazaar in Tblisi, where Goga, an economics student with no medical training, sold antibiotics from an open-air booth, advising customers how to use the drugs, and which to take.

It was in Tskhinvali, Georgia, on the empty pediatric wing of Republican Hospital. Asked about the patients, a nurse—holding a log in her hand, as if it were a baby—was contemptuous: "Can't you feel the cold?" she asked. "We sent them home. It's safer for them, no matter how sick they are, to be home than to be here where we have no heat." And it was on the hospital's top floor, where a hernia operation was being conducted. The patient's respiratory ventilator was hand-pumped by a nurse, his anesthesia was dripped onto a cloth over his face. The surgeon was working quickly because the generator only provided fifteen minutes of electricity for the lights.

The depth of this public health catastrophe varied among the former Soviet and Eastern Bloc nations as the twentieth century reached its close. But it was undeniably grave regionwide.[7]

"No country in peacetime has ever exhibited such an abrupt change," said epidemiologists Vladimir Shkolnikov and France Meslé, of Russia's Center for Demography and Human Ecology and France's L'Institut National D'etudes Demographique, respectively, in a 1997 report to the Russian nation.[8]

In 1970 Soviet scientists were so impressed with their nation's health achievements that they forecast a population of 160 million people in Russia alone by the year 2000. But Russia's population was shrinking so rapidly during the 1990s that it was expected to dip to between 126 million and 140 million by 2010—its lowest level since the eve of the 1917 Bolshevik Revolution.[9]

But the prognosticators were fooled. In 1999 Russian homicide rates declined, yet premature death rates continued to soar. Somber forecasters predicted in revised 2000 projections that by 2050 Russia's population might be a mere 80–90 million, or the smallest number of people in more than two centuries. If such an abysmal foretelling proved correct, Russia's population would shrink in just sixty years by more than any Northern Hemisphere society had in known human history, including during wartime.[10] Even by 2016, American demographer Murray Feshbach predicted, Russia's population would decrease by up to 17 million people.[11]

The average male born somewhere between Vladivostock and St. Petersburg in 1917 could have expected to live to the age of thirty-eight years. His most likely cause of death would have been any of a number of infectious diseases that raged across the region with terrifying regularity. In the hot summers mosquitoes carried malaria, yellow fever, and encephalitis. Ticks passed local hemorrhagic fever viruses. Rats carried bubonic plague. In the winters influenza, bacterial pneumonias, scarlet fever, typhus, tuberculosis, and a host of other diseases swept through hovels high in the Caucasus, mansions in St. Petersburg, and cabins in the steppes.

Thanks to the creation of a vast public health infrastructure, provision of housing, and improved nutrition during the Communist years, however, the grandsons of those boys that had been born in the year of the October Revolution could live almost twice as long: Russian boys born in 1970 faced an average life expectancy of sixty-five years.

But by 1993 when the first post-Communist generation of Russian boys was born, life expectancy had plummeted to a grim fifty-eight years. And it kept declining, reaching fifty-seven in the fall of 1998, and fifty-six by that Christmas.[12]

Such a thing would have been utterly inconceivable to Soviet public health planners. With crusading zeal they had pursued the dream of a disease-free workers' state.

"There were huge, fantastic epidemics," recalled Dr. Sergei Pozorovskii, in 1997 the director of the Gamaleya Institute, considered Russia's most prestigious medical research center. "Then came World War I, the civil war, and by the end of the 1920s millions were dying of infectious diseases, especially typhus. So The Ruler [Stalin] came out with an eloquent slogan: either lice conquer socialism or socialists conquer lice."

With a chuckle Pozorovskii admitted that Stalin's command was followed vigorously, but "not quite democratic ways were used to accomplish this." The vaccine for typhus hadn't yet been invented, nor were effective antilice pesticides that could kill the insects that carried the deadly bacteria. So, by order of Stalin, every man, woman, and child in the Soviet Union was ordered to a bathhouse, their clothing and bedsheets deloused, and infested homes were often burnt to the ground.

What this first sweeping Soviet public health campaign lacked in scientific finesse it made up for in zeal and, where that failed, authoritarian action. The result was an astounding success that became an international propaganda bonanza. While typhus continued to rage in many capitalist nations the Communists could claim a victory for the proletariat.

Stalin, who had terrible scars all over his face that attested to his childhood battle with smallpox,[13] embraced the battle against infectious diseases. It was wholeheartedly enjoined by the new public health establishment—Stalin-style.

A vast network of sanitation and epidemiology was created, eventually reaching into nearly every village in the nation. Medical schools and sanitation training centers were constructed all over the Soviet Union during the 1920s, churning out specialists for the powerful Sanitation and Epidemiology Service, or SanEp. SanEp had powers akin to those of the KGB. It spied on doctors, looking for deviant behavior, both medical and political. SanEp agents rounded up infectious disease carriers and removed them from greater society until they either healed or died. Those who suffered so-called social diseases—such as tuberculosis, syphilis, gonorrhea, and alcoholism—were publicly named, denounced in their factories and schools, and made to list all other people with whom they might have had intimate contact.

As preventive treatments and vaccines were developed the masses were compelled to undergo immunizations and such at the hands of SanEp. The leaders of SanEp were always loyal Communist Party members, and eager Komsomol (Communist Youth League) volunteers were typically put to the task of rounding up the proletariat for its latest public health intervention.

With time the system of both SanEp and hospitals and clinics became so enormous that it was one of the three biggest lines of employment in the state.

At laboratories such as Gamaleya work focused on inventing and mass-producing antitoxins, vaccines, and eventually antibiotics. After World War II that role shifted to huge so-called biodefense factories—the Soviet equivalent of pharmaceutical plants in the capitalist world—which mass-produced materials for use by SanEp.

During the Khrushchev years of the 1950s the most prestigious biomedical laboratories, such as Gamaleya, became basic research centers, much as they had been before the revolution. The scientists functioned within an elaborate hierarchy, with academicians—equivalent to senior Ph.D.'s—atop. For them life was grand. Their offices were often plushly decorated with details taken from bourgeois homes and palaces; they had meals and tea services brought to them by a staff of state-employed servants, and chauffeurs drove their free automobiles.

In addition SanEp built five plague laboratories, dedicated to the control and eventual eradication of *Yersinia pestis* and its rat and flea carriers.

And by 1970 the goal set officially by the Politburo was nothing less than the complete eradication of all infectious disease in the Soviet Union.

"When we started working we realized that these tasks were hard, if not impossible, to fulfill," Pozorovskii admitted. "But for a time that goal was inspiring."

One by one diseases that had until quite recently devastated Soviet people were, indeed, nearly vanquished: diphtheria, smallpox, cholera, malaria, tuberculosis, typhus, polio, typhoid fever, whooping cough, measles, tick-borne encephalitis, tetanus—all brought under control by SanEp. And if the methods they used were a bit repressive, even cruel, to some people, well, Pozorovskii said, they worked—"and wasn't that what mattered?"

"Then came 1991," Pozorovskii said, his body visibly slumping, facial muscles sagging. "The change caused not only political crumbling, but also a crumbling of public health, medical care, and medical science."

First the Warsaw Pact nations and Baltic states broke away from Soviet influence and ousted their old Communist rulers. Then the Soviet nation ceased to exist, each of the former Socialist Republics splitting off to become fifteen separate nations. Thousands of scientists left the laboratories of Moscow and Siberia for their home countries.

"And starting from 1993 the [Russian] state stopped funding all research subsidies," Pozorovskii said. "Starting from 1994 the state stopped funding the overhead of the Institute. But salaries were still paid. It's a laughable salary— the head of a lab here receives less than $100 a month. . . . But then in 1996 we saw more change—no salaries, at all."

Pozorovskii sighed, nearly breaking down as he concluded, "The Gamaleya Institute is dying. I feel like I'm a watchman at a cemetery."

But the real graveyard sentries were those who counted the region's demographic numbers, tallying the grim reversals witnessed after the collapse of the Soviet Union. Among their numbers was Pozorovskii, who died a few weeks after welcoming his American visitor, suffering from, a colleague insisted, "a broken heart."

There was no category for broken hearts in the statistical tables of Russian, Ukrainian, Moldavian, and other ex-Soviet epidemiologists. But there were categories for cardiovascular diseases deaths, all of which soared after 1991, in populations from the shipyards of Poland's Gdansk to the ports of Vladivostock. The shift in the body politic was, it seemed, breaking the hearts of the masses.

In a May speech before the Russian Duma Dr. N. F. Gerasimenko of the Academy of Medical Sciences summarized the situation in exceptionally strong language. "We want to make it clear to everybody . . . that the national security of the country is threatened."[14]

Gerasimenko then listed a dramatic series of statistics: the Russian mortality rate, he said, was 1.6 times the birth rate in 1992, with about three million young men dying as a direct result of the health care crisis, or about ten times the number killed in the Afghan[15] and Chechnyan wars, combined. And he said that every third recruit for the army could not be accepted into the armed forces for health reasons in the last few years, as opposed to one in twenty in 1985.

"In other words, the situation is catastrophic," he said. "If it doesn't change, only 54 percent of the sixteen-year-olds [males] will live to pension age. It's even worse than it was in Russia a hundred years ago."

Gerasimenko turned on the Russian medical system, leveling at least part of the blame at state-supported care: "Article 41 of the Russian Constitution guarantees health protection and medical aid to the population," he continued. "But, in federal medical centers patients have to pay up to fifty million rubles for surgeries—and if they don't have these surgeries they die! But where can millions of our citizens get such money, especially when their salaries are delayed? . . . Further, federal centers in 1996 only received 46 percent of allocated funds. This is something between financial ischemia and fiscal infarction!"

In a report to President Boris Yeltsin from his Committee on Issues of Females, Family and Democracy in 1997, public health experts stated that between 1991 and 1996 the premature death rate for Russians grew by a ghastly 126 percent, with the most striking increases seen in alcohol-related mortality, accidents, suicides, trauma deaths, respiratory tract infections, infectious disease deaths generally, poisonings, homicides, and automobile injuries.[16]

Between 1990 and 1994 Russian men lost, on average, six years of their life expectancies; women lost three years according to a 1998 joint U.S./Russian study.[17] And death rates in that period soared 100 percent for men.

Russian epidemiologist Vladimir Shkolnikov and French scientists France Meslé and Jacques Vallin collaborated on a series of studies aimed at appreciating the enormity of Russia's gruesome statistics and when, exactly, the great decline commenced.[18] They discovered that the disintegration of Russian public health actually had begun in Soviet days, as early as 1966, and was partially covered up through a series of neat accounting tricks used by the statisticians of that time. For example the statisticians shifted the goalposts of the health field by adjusting data for the age of the subjects in ways considered completely unorthodox in the West.[19]

Nevertheless, the Russian/French team asserted that the dramatic escalation in the pace of public health collapse after 1991 was genuine and "express[es] unambiguously the failure of the health care system to make any headway in cardiovascular mortality and to contain the upsurge in 'man-made disease,' " such as alcoholism, drug abuse, and tuberculosis.

This failure to control heart disease, either through prevention or treatment, appeared even more significant when the researchers compared death trends in Russia to those in France, England, and Wales. During a period when those European areas witnessed fivefold decreases in heart disease death rates, Russia's rose threefold to fivefold from 1970 to 1995. And most of that death rate magnification had never appeared in Soviet official data tables.

Murray Feshbach had spotted it, though. Indeed Feshbach, who was approaching his seventh decade of life as the world neared its millennium, had devoted most of his life and career to finding truth amid Soviet—and after 1991, Russian—obfuscation and "damnable lies," as some labeled all statistics. Since

1956, working first for the U.S. Census Bureau and then as a professor at George-town University in Washington, D.C., Feshbach had successively uncovered one horrendous canard, prevarication, or deceit hidden in Soviet data after another. He was obsessed with the pursuit, driven by the same desire to command a field of information as guided his endless searches for rare postage stamps and obscure rocks.[20] A fluent speaker of Russian, Feshbach had been making data-hunting trips to the USSR since 1973. And make no mistake about it: Feshbach was relentless, if not ruthless, in his pursuit of numbers.

Long before the collapse of the Soviet Union occurred Feshbach uncovered evidence of public health failure hidden by the creative accountants in the Kremlin. For example, adult premature death rates started climbing in 1964 all across the USSR, jumping from 6.9 per 1,000 adults annually to 10.3 per 1,000 in 1980. And by 1980, he discovered, the life expectancy gap between Soviet men and women was more than eleven years—already the widest gender chasm in the world. Buried in 1979 data he found measles rates in Soviet children that were fifteen times those at the time in American youngsters, and typhoid fever rates that were twenty-nine times America's.

In 1980 Feshbach discovered that the Soviets used two creative statistics methods to cover up soaring infant mortality rates. First, beginning in 1975 they simply stopped publishing any infant mortality numbers at all, burying the toll of dead babies inside the broader category of deceased children. And then, sometime around 1976, the Soviets redefined "infant" to be a baby born maturely (after twenty-eight weeks gestation), weighing more than a thousand grams, being of more than thirty-five centimeters in length, and surviving at least seven days after birth. Thus, all premature births were neatly wiped out of the records, eliminating the very group of babies that accounted for the bulk of all American and Western European infant mortality.

The Bronx-born son of Ukrainian immigrant Jews discovered mountains more evidence of public health deterioration throughout the Brezhnev years, including extreme nutritional deficits in the region's children, tremendous shortages in medical equipment and supplies at state hospitals, an adult alcohol-associated death rate that by 1978 was one hundred times that of the United States, and hints of mounting cardiovascular disease problems in the population.

With the Gorbachev era came *glasnost*, or openness, a gold mine for Feshbach. While *pravda*—truth—didn't immediately surface, *glasnost* gave access to Russian colleagues and tantalizing clues, which in turn led to *pravda*.

What he then saw in the trail of tallies, noted in lengthy, boring columns of fudged data, prompted Feshbach to ask: "If it's so bad why isn't everybody dead?"

And in answer to his own question Feshbach answered, "My feeling is they are dead."

While most Westerners, including the U.S. government employees who had for decades relied on Feshbach's findings, celebrated the end of communism the plump, bespectacled Georgetown University professor declared that calamity had struck.[21] His office reflected the deluge of data suddenly available, stacked in precarious piles that nearly reached the ceiling. Miraculously, when prompted by an incredulous visitor, Feshbach could immediately locate and pull evidence from a seemingly random pile, without toppling the entire mass. As with everything else, Feshbach saw order in what to mere mortals seemed utter chaos. And the order he saw in the ruins of the Soviet Union was calamitous.

"You can look at these figures. See?" he demanded, punching a stubby digit at a Cyrillic column. "What can you make of these figures? I don't care how exaggerated they are, you have a disaster!"

Feshbach confronted stacks of grim data. "Look at this one. In the U.S. roughly two hundred to four hundred people in any given year die of alcohol poisoning, okay? Okay, so look. In 1994 fifty thousand Russians died of it. Okay? Okay, now this, syphilis. Incredible! A thirtyfold increase in ten-to-fourteen-year-old Russian girls between 1990 and 1994. See that? How about this. Look. It says—and this is an official document, you see. It says, '38 percent of babies are born normal.' Well what does that mean? It means 62 percent of all Russian babies born in 1991 were *abnormal!*"

According to Feshbach's crunching of Russia's population data 1992 marked a telltale turning point, from which few civilizations have ever historically recovered. That was the year more people died in the Russian Federation than were born. Every year since then the gap had widened.[22] By January 2000, the Russian death rate was two and a half times its birth rate, and in some regions of the country the death rate was a staggering four times the birth rate.

Of particular concern for the future, Feshbach predicted, was the observation that the bulk of all premature deaths were in men, aged fifteen to fifty. These were the productive workforce and would-be fathers of the region's future generation. These men were dying in the 1990s at four times the rate of their female peers, and Feshbach asked, "Where are the men?" He predicted that the 1996 life-expectancy gap of 13.1 years between men and women in Russia would widen by 2010 to 17 years.[23] Given that most of those deaths were among marriageable men, Feshbach predicted a second great crisis loomed as women, unable to find mates, all but stopped bearing children. In such a scenario even the grimmest of population forecasts for 2010—namely, that Russia's population will have fallen back to 1917 levels—would fall short of the eventual reality.

In 1994 UNICEF decried the regional situation as "a societal crisis of unexpected proportions, unknown implications and uncertain solutions. . . . The 'excess mortality' accumulated between 1989–93 is far greater than that wrought by the 'Great Depression' of 1929-33 in North America.[24] . . . the 'excess mortality' over the entire 1989–93 period amounts to approximately 800,000 people, a figure that reveals all too clearly the severity of the current crisis."[25]

Why was this nightmare occurring? Why had the world's largest public health safety net completely failed?

II

Around forty-three thousand people have died in Russia this year from drinking low-quality vodka, the Interior Ministry said today.

—Agence-France Presse, November 28, 1997

The recent upsurge in criminality, in synergy with alcoholism, is above all the aftermath of the sweeping economic reforms and accompanying lower standards of living and of the dismantling of the former political and administrative system.

—Shkolnikov, Meslé, and Vallin, 1996[26]

Drinking is the joy of the Rus. We cannot live without it.

—Vladimir of Kyiv, founder of the Russian state, tenth century

On a frigid, dank night in Moscow, beefy bodyguards, armed with automatic weapons, served as sentinels, eyeing the entrance to the posh eighteenth-century building that until recently housed the Writers' Union, and had been occupied at one time by famed Soviet author Maxim Gorky.

Known to Muscovites as the Griboyedov House, named after its original aristocratic owner, the mansion was a crucial location for all Soviet-era writers. It was here that judgments were passed: this writer deserves a free trip to the Crimean to give a lecture; this enemy-of-the-people author merits a trip to the gulag! And it was here that the proletariats' scribes—voices of the supposedly classless society—dined on meals available to precious few other Soviet citizens.[27]

With the fall of the Soviet Union and Communist Party the state no longer subsidized the grand, palatial writers' restaurant, so a private company took over its management. By the late 1990s the former hall of politically correct purveyors of prose was Moscow's most elegant restaurant, complete with waiters attired in formal tuxedos, sparkling crystal chandeliers, concert pianists, ample supplies of beluga caviar, and the best reserve supplies of Russian vodka, Georgian wines, and Armenian cognacs to be found anywhere in the world.

While the French embassy staff enjoyed a private party in the upstairs room that once had housed Gorky, diners quietly feasted in the main hall, sipping vodka while listening to the lilting tones of Chopin produced by a talented concert pianist.

One group of diners deviated. Dressed in black turtleneck sweaters and leather Gucci coats, signifying that the four men were gangsters, the quartet was accompanied by a younger, spandex-attired woman. The men drank heavily, growing collectively louder with each round of fiery Russian vodka and peppery Georgian wine, their language becoming increasingly vulgar. The plump leader of the group in a grandiose gesture withdrew a two-inch-thick wad of U.S. $100 bills from his pocket, waved it in the air for all to see, and called out for the check. An obedient waiter brought the bill, noting that it was illegal to accept payment in foreign money.

After glancing at the bill the head gangster sneered and in a movement so rapid that its details could not be discerned the gangsters had the waiter on the floor and were pummeling the poor man with clenched fists and stabbing forks. Little noise was produced, as the drunken mobsters were professionals and the waiter quickly went into shock. The pianist never missed a note, and most of the posh restaurant's clientele seemed unaware of what was transpiring.

A team of waiters, apparently accustomed to such drunken outbursts, formed a human wedge, plowing into the fray, rescuing their unconscious colleague and repairing to the kitchen. The gangsters gave chase; the kitchen door was bolted.

"So much for our dessert," muttered one of the few diners who had paid heed to the bout. Seamlessly the pianist switched to a Cole Porter tune, and the gangsters, puffed with victory, poured themselves another round of cognac and laughed loudly. The maître d' quietly approached the robust chief mobster, whispering a negotiation stance on behalf of the restaurant. And in an instance—*pow!*—he, too, was on the floor, showered with sharp jabs and fisted blows. As he crawled out in retreat, the pianist—who had yet to miss a note—began to sweat, her eyes widening in fear. The clientele, however, remained largely oblivious.

A triumphant gangster rolled the liquor tray to their table, and the criminal quintet happily served themselves vintage French cognac. The staff remained safely behind locked doors. The pianist segued to Gershwin's "Rhapsody in Blue."

One of the security guards that had been on post outside the restaurant entered, moving his hulking, muscular frame with deliberate nonchalance. He wore a suit that seemed to be bursting at the seams under the stress of his impressive musculature: a Russian Arnold Schwarzenegger. Recognizing a fellow-professional the gangsters stiffened and, after exchanging words, rose and headed toward the restaurant's exit. Peace, it seemed, was at hand.

But suddenly, standing at the pianist's back in the restaurant's threshold, the head gangster spun on his heels and swiftly slapped the security guard back and forth across his cheeks. In a microsecond the guard had an automatic magnum lodged against the chief mobster's left temple. And instantly a gang lieutenant had his arm stretched over his boss's shoulder, a pistol pointed back at the guard.

The pianist ceased playing Gershwin and crawled out of crossfire range. Some diners, finally taking notice of the escalating standoff, quietly moved their chairs out of the presumed line of fire and watched. Seconds passed, neither man lowering his weapon. Waiters, peering out of the kitchen, collectively held their breaths.

Suddenly a balalaika player performing for the upstairs French Embassy crowd shouted, "Hey! Hey! Hey!" and was greeted with a rousing stomping and cheering from his French audience. The performance was a classic tourist treat, the sort of thing Westerners who had seen *Dr. Zhivago* more than once savored. The guard and gangsters stifled a shared laugh and, having found a mutually face-saving way to stand down, lowered their weapons. Negotiations ensued, the chief mobster dismissed his sidekicks, grabbed his girlfriend, and returned to savor yet another round of cognac.

When the waiters returned, attending to their tables, the cause of what nearly was at least two homicides was clarified. The mobsters, it seemed, didn't like the exchange rate the restaurant was using to compute dollar-to-ruble values. They were willing to kill, in front of scores of witnesses, over what amounted to less than a ten-dollar dispute.

All over the former Communist region homicides, suicides, car accidents, and outright alcohol poisonings were occurring in record numbers, fueled by elegant cognac, run-of-the-mill vodka, and, more often, cheap rotgut moonshine.

Outside the Siberian city of Ulan Ude, a village has been created downwind of the municipal garbage dump. Fifty-two adults and eight children live in a pine grove that is covered in an artificial forest floor made of trash that blows off the ten-story-high, redolent garbage heaps. The loose group of otherwise homeless Siberians had dug holes in the earth, some twelve feet deep and ten feet wide, in which they live, even during the harsh, snowbound winters.

Wooden beams stabilize their underground homes, which are lined with items scavenged off the nearby trash heaps. The group lives without running water, electricity, heat, or fresh food, says Nikolai Constantinovich, the encampment's unofficial leader. Most of them were bilked out of their housing in the city, talked into selling when property was privatized but too naive—and eager for quick cash—to realize their apartments' true values. Unable, with the paltry sums they obtained, to buy new homes the three score Ulan Udeans had ended up homeless, Constantinovich explains.

Seventy-year-old Alexander pops his head above ground, sees strangers, and ducks back into his hovel. Constantinovich allays Alexander's fear that the police have arrived, and the aging pensioner, his breath thick with the smell of moonshine, emerges, greeting his visitors.

"We never, never could imagine that we would end up here," says Alexander. "We were supposedly living in a worker's paradise. Well, I was a worker—where is my paradise?"

During the day, the children's job is to search through the stinking dump for saleable items that can be rescued from the vicious rats that live there and can be converted into cash. It's a disgusting task, which, Alexander tearfully says, "breaks my heart," but the children obediently return each day with their sacks full of items.

Then, the adults take turns riding a bus into the city for supplies—including bread, to survive on, and alcohol.

"Don't think badly of us," cries Alexander's neighbor, middle-aged Lena, her face reddened by years of alcoholism. "We live underground, but we are not murderers. The drink has just got us."

At nine on a dreary Moscow morning homeless Nikolai Yelizarov, a thirty-four-year-old ex-convict, is in line, as he has been every weekday for twelve months, trying to get a work permit. He was robbed one day as he lay unconscious somewhere in Moscow, lost in an alcoholic stupor. The thief got Yelizarov's most valuable possessions—Moscow residency and work permits. Without these, Yelizarov says, his blue eyes tearing, "I cannot have a home, and I cannot have a job. Ever since [the robbery] I've been dealing with this damned bureaucracy."

Yelizarov "deals with the bureaucracy" by arising from whatever hovel he's shivered in the night before, downing a high-proof rotgut, and queuing up to beg, again, for new papers.

In Moscow's Pushkin Square metro station a middle-aged drunkard tries to enter an exit-only turnstile and bounces off the machinery, landing headfirst on the tiled floor. Stunned, he lays semiconscious for several minutes while a gang of fourteen-year-old boys, high on heroin-and-speed cocktails, loudly mock, "the filthy old drunk," kicking at the downed man. Unable to comprehend what has happened, the drunk pulls himself up onto his feet. The boys stand aside, laughing and shouting, "Come on, Old Man, you can do it. Walk!" Once again the man tries to enter the wrong way, is rebuffed, and lands on his head. The boys surround him, ready for another round of mockery, but lose interest when they realize that this time the drunk is truly unconscious.

By the mid-1990s public drunkenness was so common as to leave the visitor uncertain what was reality: the steady view seen by the sober eye, or the wavering, blurred perspective of the throngs of swaying fellow pedestrians. In devastated old industrial cities, from Bohemia to Vladivostock, unemployed men, no longer able to imagine their futures, simply pulled daily alcohol curtains over their presents.

Alcohol-inspired violence and self-destruction were not new to the Eastern European world. No. But after 1991 it was far more extreme and dangerous. As was the case with abortions and other basic public health indicators the rise of alcoholism and its associated catastrophes was the result of a trend dating to Soviet years that spiked dramatically after 1991.

In 1999 just over 1.2 million babies were born in Russia, for example, while more than 2.1 million people died. Any nation with such a profoundly greater death, versus birth, rate was bound to shrink dramatically. Some of the contraction was due to a plummeting birth rate, which, in turn, was driven regionally by astonishing abortion rates.

The trend began during the late 1970s in large part because of the very poor quality of Soviet-made contraceptives. Condoms,[28] diaphragms, and other safe forms of contraception were virtually unavailable, and Soviet-made birth control pills contained higher levels of hormones than were found in Western-made products—and, therefore, induced more horrendous side effects, including cardiac failure.

So women in the Soviet Union and Eastern Europe accepted abortion as their primary form of birth control. The numbers of abortions performed every year in Soviet state-run clinics rose steadily, reaching 7,228,000 in 1988, or 1.2 officially registered abortions for every one live birth.[29]

A survey conducted by the Zhordania Institute of Human Reproduction in Tblisi in 1995 revealed that the average Georgian woman had, by age twenty-six, undergone ten to twelve abortions, with dangerous illegal procedures outnumbering officially registered hospital ones by two-to-one. And though slight improvements in the Georgian economy subsequently lowered the abortion rate, in 1996 the country of 5.5 million people witnessed 25,000 legal abortions and at least 50,000 illegal ones, the institute found.

"I have met women who have had more than thirty abortions. The highest number I ever saw was a sixty-nine-year-old woman who told me she had sixty abortions," Institute director Dr. Archil Khomassuridze asserted. As the leading expert on family planning for Georgia and the Soviet Union, Khomassuridze was responsible for filing fertility and abortion data with the World Health Organization in Geneva. In the late 1980s the WHO computer rejected his reports because it wasn't programmed to believe data claiming any woman underwent more than twenty lifetime abortions.

As shocking as these figures may seem, Khomassuridze explained that he understood, and sympathized, with the women, for two reasons. First, "I am surprised how they can exist. How they can work. How they can have sexual lives. Why they don't hate their sexual partners. I still don't understand—not only for Georgian women but Russian women, too. I have deep sympathy."

Their lives were not only filled with finacial difficulty, Khomassuridze explained, but with abusive, often drunken, men. Not only was sex often involuntary for the women, they told Khomassuridze, it was rarely pleasurable even when mutually consenting. When asked how they abided the brutality of their lives as prostitutes, hookers in Russia, Estonia, and Ukraine typically said, "It's no worse than marriage."

While some women were heavy drinkers, alcoholism regionally was an overwhelmingly male phenomenon. And vodka, when consumed at Russian levels, drove men to astounding heights of violence and brutality committed against their wives, girlfriends, children, even suicidally against themselves.

In the six years Mikhail Gorbachev led the Soviet Union, he had saved, conservatively, more than a half million lives in the region—but not because of any military or political decision he made.

Startled to learn that Soviets were in 1983 consuming, on average, three liters a year of pure ethanol equivalent, Gorbachev waged an all-out war on alcoholism, using the classically repressive apparatus of the Soviet state. Warehouses were destroyed; illegal sellers were jailed; vodka prices were artificially hiked; and police were given free rein to arrest public drinkers.

But in 1988, the campaign collapsed, a surprise victim of Gorbachev's own political reforms, *perestroika* and *glasnost*. Overnight, alcohol so regained its high stature that Vladimir Zhirinovsky, an ultra-nationalist presidential hopeful, raised campaign funds selling his own brand of vodka, picturing himself on the label attired as Vladimir Lenin.

It is estimated that Gorbachev saved 600,000 lives over three years, dropping the combined incidence of alcohol poisoning, cirrhosis of the liver, and alcohol-induced violence and accidents to 179 deaths per 100,000 in 1988, a level not seen since 1965.[30]

But after the fall of the USSR per capita consumption jumped by 600 percent and incidences of alcohol-related deaths followed suit. Government figures from 1995 showed a rate approaching 500 per 100,000, in contrast to an American alcohol-associated death rate in 1995 of just 77.[31] Russia witnessed a 550 percent increase in alcohol psychosis cases between 1989 and 1993.

Regionally violence, particularly against women, rose in tandem with soaring male alcoholism. Up to ten percent of women in the region, according to UNICEF in 1999, reported experiencing at least one beating from a spouse that was severe enough to require hospitalization, and about a fifth of married women complained of regular beating.

Some estimates were that eighty percent of all Russian men were alcoholics, consuming in 1999—*on average*—600 grams of booze a day, or roughly three liters of vodka every week. The male alcohol poisoning death rate in Russia was about 200 times that of the United States.[32]

Murray Feshbach argued that Russians were not only drinking more than they had in the past, they were also drinking more dangerously. What was marketed as vodka or whiskey in Moscow could be anything from 100 proof genuine vodka to "rotgut moonshine," aftershave, or even—commonly—jet fuel. And much of the booze was sold in pop-top, nonresealable bottles that prompted the drinker to consume the entire contents in a single sitting.

"It's not just that consumption is high, although it is," Feshbach said. "It's the way they consume. It's chug-a-lug vodka drinking that starts at the office during the morning coffee break and goes right into the nighttime."

Drinking on the job was a practice that went across all levels of society in the region, even among health care workers.

At a Moscow hospital a visitor was invited to join a cognac party among doctors, held on a weekday at 10 A.M. In the Arctic city of Talnakh a group of four cardiac physicians downed a bottle of champagne and a couple of rounds of cognac over lunch—a routine break, they said. And in the physicians' lounge at a Kyiv hospital, surgeons relaxed between operations by sharing a bottle of vodka. A private doctor in Bohemia proudly displayed a large and diverse alcohol selection, spread out all over his office, most bottles having been given to the physician in lieu of monetary payment for medical services.

This form of abusive binge drinking was historic in the region, although not at the levels being evidenced in the post-USSR era. "Russians drink, essentially, to obliterate themselves, to blot out the tedium of life, to warm themselves from the winters," Hedrick Smith wrote during the Brezhnev years, "and they eagerly embrace the escapism it offers."[33]

Two Russian customs added to the problem: one, that a vodka bottle once opened must be finished, never recorked; and two, that a shot glass of vodka must be downed in one gulp. Violation of either custom within the male community in particular was roundly considered rude and insulting to one's host, and prima facie evidence of a lack of manhood.

Dr. Boris Logna had watched this alcohol trend closely over the years from his vantage point as chief of the largest poison control center in Estonia, located in the capital city of Tallinn. During the Gorbachev campaign, Logna said, the country had about 120 alcohol poisoning deaths per year. In 1995, there were 400 such deaths in Tallinn alone.

"There is no national alcohol policy here," Logna says, echoing complaints from his counterparts throughout the former Communist bloc. "As you see, everywhere alcohol is for sale—even in gas stations at night. More people go late to gas stations for a drink than to fill their tanks."

The problem also started early: teenage arrests for alcohol-related crimes more than tripled from 1991 to 1997, and suicide rates—which many health experts link directly to drinking—were also on the rise.[34]

For teens and adults alike, alcohol was a way of life that was easily available, legal, and remarkably cheap.

Because export-quality vodka, such as Stolichnaya Cristall, sold for about thirty dollars a liter in Moscow or Kyiv, few local people would dream of wasting their money on such a product. Most vodka was sold for less than eight dollars a liter, and some was available in street kiosks for a dollar.

"Between December 1990 and December 1994, consumer prices [in Russia] increased by 2,020 times for all goods and services, by 2,154 times for food products, but only 653 times for alcoholic beverages," stated a report issued jointly by the California-based Rand Corporation and Moscow's Center for Demography and Human Ecology.[35] "This means that over this period, in relative terms, alcohol became over three times cheaper than these other products."[36]

Adult alcohol consumption in 1996 was 18 liters a year of pure alcohol, or the rough equivalent of 38 liters of 100-proof vodka, according to the Russian Ministry of Health. That's the equal of consuming one and a half bottles of high-proof vodka weekly. The rate for other countries in the region was as high: in Estonia, for instance, it was 16.5 liters annually; in Ukraine, 17 liters.[37]

Bad as that was, it soon got much worse in Russia, Belarus, Ukraine, and other parts of the region. In the fall of 1998 Russia's President Yeltsin announced that Russia's populationwide average had reached more than 25 liters of pure ethanol equivalent a year. Adjusting for age, that implied that Russian adults were—*on average*—consuming an astonishing three bottles of high-proof vodka a week.

Another terrible trend emerged from the adult alcoholism upswing: child abuse and abandonment.

At Father Alexander's crisis center for children in Odessa, Ukraine, dozens of rag-clothed youngsters live together, abandoned by their parents or escapees from homes of poverty and alcoholism. Young Misha, for example, has lived in the sparsely decorated quarters of Father Alexander's haven—a converted nursery school—for two months. He sports a hip pierced ear and scratches his head absentmindedly while making conversation, probably because of the lice that infect his scalp. Admired by the younger children for his tough-guy swagger, the blue-eyed blond fourteen-year-old loses his cool when he tries to explain why he is now homeless.

"My parents drink a lot. And then they humiliate me and beat me. The problem is they don't like me," Misha says, tears drenching his pink cheeks, his voice cracking. "Even my grandmother doesn't like me. I often went to school hungry," Misha concludes.

Misha's story is echoed a thousand times over by the sorrowful tales of the ultimate victims of the alcoholism and drug abuse sweeping from Prague to Vladivostock: the children. Pyotor, for example, left his three sisters and brother when he was ten, moving into Alexander's haven because his parents drank themselves—and their children—into homelessness and, he concluded, "There is nothing to eat."

Eleven-year-old Andrei ended up in the center after his stepfather in a drunken rage poisoned Andrei's mother. Now his stepfather is on the run from the police and Andrei is alone in the world.

Since 1988, Catholic priest Father Alexander says, the number of abandoned children in Odessa has increased twentyfold. And for those who still have parents and homes, alcohol and poverty often makes abandonment seem preferable.

"Nowadays we have children living at home whose malnutrition is even worse than the street kids," Father Alexander says. "I know boys who weren't allowed to go to school in winter because they had no shoes. So one wrapped his feet in plastic bags. They eat once a day and work as cleaning boys."

When he was eighteen years old Father Alexander took the unusual step of getting baptized as a Catholic and undergoing training for the priesthood—political suicide during Communist days. He studied in Poland, Brussels, and Rome, ultimately returning to establish this ramshackle home for wayward and abandoned children. Plump, bearded, and bombastic Father Alexander has few friends in the Odessa power structure and is openly hated by the police, who suspect most Catholic clerics.

But, he claims, without him children like Misha, Pyotor, and Andrei would have nowhere to go.

In 1997 the Moscow Human Rights Research Center estimated that there were a million homeless children in Russia; the government said 700,000. No one knew how many more children had parents in homes but were left largely to survive on their own because of their parents' alcoholism. In Russia a term was coined to describe these kids: the Lost Generation.

In Moscow, Sapar Kulyanov runs a small charitably funded shelter for children, some 92 percent of whom come from families of drug or alcohol abuse.

Kulyanov, a gentle forty-five-year-old man, has witnessed "an avalanche," he says, of abandoned and abused children since the fall of communism.

"It's true that there was less openness in Soviet days and the problem existed before," Kulyanov says. "But I am absolutely sure the bulk of this is new, because of social change. . . . When *perestroika* started all the old links and ties broke. Families had to confront their problems. Some families started to drown their problems in drink, and children had to learn to live their own lives."

Most of the children in Kulyanov's center suffer classic symptoms of parental abuse: bed-wetting, crying out in their sleep, nightmares, inability to respond to direct questions. Eight-year-old Katia, for example, boldly approaches a stranger and responds to a smile with heartbreaking warmth, crawling into the adult's arms. But she cannot answer when asked about her parents' names or whereabouts. When asked, Katia's face, framed in a blue Russian scarf, takes on the innocent look of an angel, but all she can recall of her past is that "at home I was in school and I graduated from first grade."

She remembers nothing more, and stares blankly into the eyes of a stranger when asked, "And where was your home?"

Asked to tell his story eleven-year-old Vanya reluctantly jumps from a high perch to the floor and collects himself into a ball, sitting on his heels, his striped shirt–covered arms wrapped tightly around his knees. Vanya can't control the involuntary nervous tics in his face that make him blink and give his cheeks sudden ripples. But the tics are his only animation: he is otherwise almost without affect, seemingly emotionless.

When Vanya was just nine years old, he explains with utter lack of emotion, his parents' drinking escalated. His father—whom Vanya says he detests—beat the boy and his mother repeatedly. And his mother drowned her sorrows in moonshine purchased at local kiosks. The bad booze drove her insane, and escalated the violence in the household.

One day, after his father had committed a night of household bloodletting, Vanya's mother gathered the child's belongings into a small bag, hers in a larger one, and said, "We're leaving." She dragged little Vanya to the massive Belarus train station, located on the western end of Moscow. He had never been there before, and Vanya stared at all of the strange immigrants who seemed to be living in the station. There were the so-called Blacks from the Caucasus, the Orientals from southern Siberia and Central Asia, the White Siberians . . . packed so densely that the child and his mother could barely squeeze by.

And then it happened. As a train was about to leave the station Vanya's mother let go of his hand and jumped into the departing train, never looking back.

"I lost her at the railway station," Vanya says, taking blame for what Kulyanov says was a classic case of abandonment. For a full year—his tenth year of life—Vanya survived on the streets of Moscow, begging for food and sleeping in a telephone booth. He discovered hundreds of other similarly abandoned children, and they formed a gang to protect one another against the older bullies of the streets.

Now Vanya's only emotional moment comes when he thinks of the other street waifs: "I wish they would come here," to the shelter, he says.

Kulyanov's center was one of only five in all of Moscow—and that's five more than existed in virtually every other city in the region. There were, instead, old Soviet orphanages, famed for the abusive way in which they warehoused abandoned and "defective" children—those born with disabilities of one kind or another. Kulyanov was trying to build a Western-style network of halfway houses for children, focused on rehabilitating and reuniting Russian families. Until 1993 such activities, even shelters, were illegal in Russia, and it was illegal until 1996 to remove—under *any* circumstances—a child from his parents. Even when a child was hospitalized prior to 1996 with evidence of life-threatening beatings the youngsters would, if they survived, simply be returned to the home of their tormenters.

Seated in his office before a table coated with the photos of abused and neglected children, Kulyanov points out the stacks of stuffed animals and toys that clutter every other surface in the room. Such things, he said, were not found in the homes of these abused children. When they reached the shelter most of these children received the very first playthings they ever had.

"In the past we had many expenses covered by the state, greater egalitarianism in income without such extremes," forty-five-year-old Kulyanov softly continues. "I grew up in a safe society. After school we went to Young Pioneers clubs and lessons and sports, all available for free. . . . But now there are no children's clubs, no Young Pioneers, no puppet shows. . . .

"So now kids get their fun from criminals. From motley crews of thieves and drug dealers," Kulyanov said.

In Novosibirsk, Siberia, the Club 888 was a hip oasis filled with ironic Communist memorabilia displayed as kitsch, complete with an empty but bona fide nuclear bomb shell painted with a bright red star and CCCP, which is Cyrillic for USSR. Adolescent artists and college intellectuals huddled in niches throughout the labyrinthine nightclub, drinking, smoking, and debating their futures.

"I'm just a human, rolling through life," boasts twenty-year-old deejay Sevi. "I'm totally against drugs. My choice is vodka. I'm an alcoholic!"

Fyodor adjusts his black leather motorcycle jacket, denounces Moscow (as Siberians are frequently wont to do), and declares, "Heroin is an American drug! Our drugs are different. We take drugs as camouflage—we are only pretending to give up."

That said, he hoists his vodka and murmurs to twenty-two-year-old Sergei that perennial presidential candidate Zhirinovsky is trying to win over the youth with vodka—and may succeed.

Sergei shakes his head, reminding Fyodor that they have all experimented with shooting opium extracts and amphetamines. The group of young men grows momentarily quiet, the only sounds the background rock 'n' roll and the gentle sucking noises they make as they all simultaneously drag on their American cigarettes.

"What is a Russian?" they are asked.

"Drinking," eighteen-year-old Alex answers. "And loneliness. No one is lonelier than a Russian."

Later, when the discussion turns to alcohol's effects on their future, Sergei blurts out a bit of his past. "I tried to commit suicide," he says, pulling up his black leather sleeve to reveal the scars of slit wrists.

"Me too!" Alex says, displaying a similar set of scars, and quickly, all five of the young men in the group roll up their sleeves to the astonishment of a reporter, excitedly comparing suicide methods and scarred reminders.

Sergei then speaks up again, silencing the group when he takes a visitor's hand and raises it to his temple. "Here, feel this," he says as the visitor traces the outline of a bullet still lodged in his skull, left over from a failed attempt to blow out his brains. "I thought suicide was the best drug."

Psychologist Anna Terentjeva said that the feelings expressed by the young men of Novosibirsk were typical of what she's heard throughout the region. On the staff of the Moscow-based drug group NAN, which stands for "No to Alcoholism and Drug Addiction," she said she saw a steady daily stream of young men and women similar to those at Club 888.

The issues for many of these young men and women "has to do with recognizing oneself, one's identity," she says, adding, "they think they have nothing else" other than alcohol.

"What is self?" she asks. "Where are the borders of me versus us? This is all new. The [Soviet] state used to decide such things. The value of one's self was not supported. Individualism and personal reflection were discouraged, even penalized."

Terentjeva's staff had just completed surveys in Moscow colleges that revealed a startling 100 percent of the students have tried drugs; all drank hard liquor, and half of them said that they use heroin, other narcotics, or amphetamines regularly. In their survey responses most of the young Muscovites said that they saw no other alternative—no other way to face each day—except inebriated or stoned.

At Club 888 Sergei changed tables, plopping down under a speaker that blasted rock 'n' roll. For the first time since meeting the visiting foreigner Sergei smiles, content to hear his favorite tune: "Revolution in Paradise."

III

There are no conditions to which a man cannot become used, especially if he sees that all around him are living the same way.

—Leo Tolstoy, *Anna Karenina*

B eside a white concrete bandshell that protrudes into the Angara River, dozens of teenagers are dancing, dressed in outfits that imitate the looks of American rock videos. The lyrics to a techno-pop tune are blaring in the background: "Here we go, here we play! It's revolution in paradise!"

It is May Day, the traditional Communist day for celebrating the triumphs of the proletariat. But today, the teens celebrate nothing more, or less, than the end of winter. They couldn't care less about politics. The Siberian teens of Irkutsk flirt, frolic, and strut, as do adolescents the world over. One draws admiring throngs of girls as he strolls nonchalantly into the bandshell, dressed in a genuine Nike jacket and pants made from an American flag, one leg the stars, the other red and white stripes.

The first generation to come of age absent the social restrictions of the Soviet state, these teens seem healthy enough. But to hear their parents talk, there is a generational time bomb of cancer, genetic mutation, immune deficiency, and disease hidden beneath their youthful glow. These youngsters are damaged goods, they say, weakened to the genetic level by a dual legacy of environmental devastation and misanthropic social engineering.

"The Russian gene pool has been destroyed," Dr. Askold Maiboroda, dean of the Federal Medical University in Irkutsk, explained. "First there were Stalin's slaughters of millions of people, especially the Jews and the most creative and intelligent people. Then the Nazis slaughtered more of the strongest people in the Great Patriotic War. Then more perished in the gulags—our best minds: artists, writers, poets. And now we suffer this environmental assault.

"We have been weakened. Our genes are damaged," he said. "You cannot expect much from the Russian people—do not ask much of us."

It was a jarring view, to say the least. But it was a perspective widely shared by physicians and parents from Warsaw to Sakhalin—labeled Chernobyl Syndrome by those who believed it to be an example of mass psychosis. And no one—from the doctors toiling in the small cities throughout the former Soviet Union to the medical experts located in the region's grandest cities—knew whether this view was based on fact or fear fueled by regionwide feelings of helplessness.

Certainly there was strong anecdotal evidence of a link between cancer and the Chernobyl nuclear power plant explosion. And there was equally strong anecdotal evidence that the rape of the land in places like Noril'sk and Murmansk, key mining and industrial centers, contributed to rising incidences of cancer, cardiovascular disease, and the like.

But there were very few focused, well-planned general population studies that allowed these links to be viewed in either an historical or scientific context. Indeed, during Soviet days most key industrial centers, nuclear power plants, and military installations weren't even on official maps, and some seventy entire cities were classified as state secrets, their very names protected by a veil of KGB surveillance. In another sixty-some cities, where chemical weapons were manufactured, it was illegal during Soviet days to publish any scientific information regarding local pollution. It was, similarly, illegal to study the environmental impacts of the Soviet nuclear power or weapons industries, or even ask the question, "Where is the nuclear waste dumped?"[38]

Prior to 1991, therefore, no legitimate academic departments of toxicology, environmental sciences, human environmental epidemiology, or epidemiological oncology existed in the Soviet Union. There was no trained pool of scientists who could sift through the evidence, separating fact from fiction.

The first time the Soviet government tried to confront the pollution issue came in 1988. In a startling address to the nation, then-Soviet leader Mikhail Gorbachev said that fifty million Soviet citizens were living in 102 cities in which air pollution exceeded the USSR health standards by more than tenfold.

In the years since, the Yeltsin government determined that, minimally, two hundred cities in Russia alone posed "ecological danger to human health" due to toxic pollution of the air and/or water.

And the facts—the horrible ecological truths—didn't really begin to be revealed until 1994 when Article 7 of the Russian State Secrets Act was enacted, requiring publication of long-clandestine environmental data.

The result was a regional collective gasp of horror and a tendency among caregivers to simply throw up their hands in defeat, blaming all public health crises—even the staggering regional demographics—on pollution and radiation.

The Chernobyl incident was a good case in point. Precise figures on the number of people exposed to fallout from the Chernobyl meltdown don't exist. Most Moscow authorities have said it was fewer than ten thousand, while the Ukrainians say more than thirty-four million of their countrymen were exposed. Not a single aspect of the Chernobyl incident—from details of what occurred on April 26, 1986, to how many Ukrainians, Belarusans, Russians, and Moldavians have subsequently taken ill—is settled.

"For years after the explosion, physicians would just tell parents that every ailment in their children is related to Chernobyl," psychiatrist Semyon Gluzman, a member of the Joint Ukrainian/American Project to Study Post-Chernobyl Children, explained. "But this is not so. It's just an outsized reaction to all the lies we were told when Chernobyl occurred."

The April 25, 1986 Chernobyl nuclear power plant disaster ranked as the largest civilian nuclear contamination event in history. Radioactive fallout blanketed 17 million acres of Ukraine and then moved northwest to cover Belarus, St. Petersburg and western Russia, eastern Poland, eastern Germany, the Baltic States, and Scandinavia.

Hardest hit, of course, was a circular area of 30 kilometers around the Chernobyl complex. It is still officially dubbed the Alienation Zone.

Encircled by a security perimeter, the Alienation Zone was at the dawn of the twenty-first century closed to all but Chernobyl employees and government-approved visitors. Ghost towns dotted the zone. More than 135,000 former residents fled for their lives in April 1986, never returning to pull the sheets off their clotheslines: eleven years later shreds of fabric flapped in the wind, offering anthropological clues to the lives once lived here. Once-cultivated fields had gone fallow. Baby pine trees sprouted like weeds out of former potato fields.

Closer to the Chernobyl site, 100-foot-tall steel structures that looked like the Imperial Army's megatanks in *The Empire Strikes Back* stood rusted into rigid positions. Weeds surrounded their footings; the cables and pulleys that once were functional components of the hulking steel cranes dangled and creaked in the wind. The grounds were brown, trees few and far between.

Prypat City, which once housed most of the Chernobyl workforce, was, eleven years after the explosion, empty save for a few black crows and three Ukrainian army guards who lazily smoked cigarettes. The only sound in Prypat City, except for crows, was a vague hum from one of the still functioning reactors at the power plant, located more than a mile away.

The risk of protest actions by alienated workers is rising, claims Chernobyl information officer Mikhail Bogdonov. "The [Ukrainian] legislature now forbids the personnel to go on strike. I wouldn't talk of sabotage—it's practically impossible. The person who is normal, sane, it's unimaginable that he would do something harmful. But of course it's natural one who works at the controls and he's anxious about money for his family, his children, you can say his attitude is not what it should be," Bogdonov said, shrugging his shoulders.

Every day the 6,252 Chernobyl workers pass by a large silver bust of Lenin as they enter the building, then show their security passes and walk through metal detectors. There is little chatter or animation among the grim-faced nuclear workers. A visitor was not permitted to speak to workers inside the Chernobyl facility or to people spotted in the Alienation Zone.

The workers know that Ukrainian president Leonid Kuchma, eager to please future NATO allies, has agreed to shut down all the Chernobyl reactors by 2000, reinforce the concrete sarcophgus that currently enshrouds the damged reactor,[39] and remove the nuclear cores from the other reactors. But in mid-2000, decommissioning had yet to commence, and Ukrainian president Leonid Kuchma claimed that there wasn't adequate evidence of cancer in Chernobyl workers to warrant an immediate shutdown.

"My friend worked here since before the accident and he's still healthy," biologist Boris Oskolkov, chief of the Chernobyl Ecology Service, says dismissively, speaking broken English. "What concerns cancer and other long-term effects of radiation, weakened immunity, and increased morbidity—there are no reliable data to prove such increases. . . . The main factor affecting morbidity is the psychological effect of the stress of the accident. That psychological effect is in place. Definitely. But it doesn't have any physical foundation."

The blond, goateed Oskolkov discounts the infirmity and disability claims filed by hundreds of Chernobyl workers since 1986 as mere ploys to obtain early pensions and sick pay. Though it is illegal to eat hunted boars or wild mushrooms from the Alienation Zone, Oskolkov insists the food, water, soil, and air of the area are now completely safe. And due to reports from his staff the Ukrainian government has loosened up regulation of the Alienation Zone, allowing about one thousand people to move back into the outer perimeter area.

But scientists from Russia's Severtsov Institute of Ecological and Evolutionary Problems measured topsoil samples in villages both inside the Alienation Zone and up to one hundred kilometers northeast in Russia and Belarus. They found gamma radiation levels of 100 to 320 micro-Roentgens per hour.[40] That is, according to sources at Brookhaven National Laboratory, fourteen to forty-six times the amount of background radiation emanating from the soils of Long Island, New York, even in close proximity to that U.S. nuclear research facility.

In 1996 the Centre for Russian Environment Policy, an independent scientific group based in Moscow, published strong evidence of radioactive contamination and cellular mutations in plants and wild animals collected from the Bryansk oblast and eastern Belarus.

And Ukrainian physicist Valery Kukhar readily conceded that the Chernobyl ecology would never be the same. Extensive research indicated that the overall extent of biodiversity in plants and animals was unchanged after the 1986 radioactive catastrophe. But the comparative sizes of animal and plant populations, and therefore the overall balance of the ecology, changed radically. Concentrations of plutonium isotopes found in soil samples up to ten years after the accident exceeded those produced by *all* nuclear weapons tests that were conducted in 1960, combined—in some cases by a factor of 89.[41]

Invertebrate insects were decimated by the radiation, some species of spiders and worms nearing the local level of extinction.

Among small mammals, such as voles, rats, and mice, populations initially fell, then restored to pre-1986 levels. But the nuts and plant seeds these animals were consuming were radioactive, and there was evidence of declining photosynthesis rates in trees and other large flora, resulting in growth stunting.

Local fish were highly contaminated with Cs^{137} radionucliides, and several species showed signs of abnormal development. Frogs and other amphibians showed similar evidence of radiation-induced abnormality, and their immune systems—levels of functional lymphocytes and neutrophils—appeared to be weakened.

Mutation rates escalated, based on study of animal and plant chromosomes. And the mutation rates correlated perfectly with the amount of radiation that had fallen on any specific site, indicating what toxicologists referred to as a dose/response curve.

But Chernobyl's Oskolkov insists, "Everything, all of this fallout, now lies at the bottom of the water and doesn't make a problem. And there radiation is now measured in 10^{-11} cu/liter level, so it is not a problem, I tell you."

Psychiatrist Semyon Gluzman, an intense Ukrainian Jew who has studied regional psychosocial reactions to Chernobyl, says that to the degree that people suffer some post-Chernobyl hypochondria the nuclear authorities are entirely to blame.

"The former [Soviet] Ministry of Health said, 'A certain amount of radiation is good for you.' It's natural that the absence of precise information, accurate information, gives rise to anxiety."

For years after the accident the Gorbachev Soviet regime refused to extend *perestroika* and *glasnost* to Chernobyl, instead denying any possibility of a widespread deleterious health impact, Gluzman recalled. And people who expressed fear that Chernobyl's deadly isotopes were hurting them were labeled "radiophobic," meaning they suffered a psychiatric state of hysterical fear of radiation brought on by the traumatic event.

But since the fall of the USSR, Gluzman continued, "the same medical *nomenklatura* are shouting that 'everything is *so terrible*! People are just dying walking down the streets.' They can get Western grants and trips out of this, of course."

"Radiophobia," or "Chernobyl Syndrome"—whatever appellation it be given—swept the former Soviet Union and Eastern Bloc nations in the wake of the 1986 Chernobyl accident. And with each passing year it grew, affecting every aspect of how the region's adults viewed their health, and that of their children.

For example, at Novosibirsk Pediatric Infectious Disease Hospital No. 3, located a thirty-minute drive outside the Siberian city, Natalia Nikiforova, the chief physician, is convinced that the Siberian children under her care suffer from immunological disorders caused by environmental pollution. Though she has absolutely no white blood cell data to prove the need, Nikiforova has ordered her staff to care for ailing children differently in 1997 from how their counterparts in 1987 were treated. Antibiotics are shunned in favor of Siberian herbs made from reindeer horns and rhododendron plants. Animal thymuses are mashed up and injected into the children. And in some cases vaccinations are avoided because, she says, the Siberian children are too weak to tolerate preparations made for stronger Western youngsters. Though there is little scientific evidence to support these beliefs, the notion is so widespread that doctors and parents living more than four thousand miles apart spout nearly identical claims. The only thing that varies from place to place is the culprit charged with the crime of generational devastation: in Belarus and Ukraine the finger is pointed at the Chernobyl nuclear power plant accident in 1986; in Siberia the horrendous industrial pollution is blamed; in Eastern Europe the old Communist mining and manufacturing centers are credited; and in Moscow they accuse the air and water of violating their children's vitality.

The pollution was undeniable. It assaulted the senses, both physically and aesthetically. Seen through Western eyes the Soviet style of industry was reminiscent of a Hollywood science fiction version of a postapocalyptic society replete with pollution-darkened skies, grayness, and hulking concrete-and-steel structures. Perhaps with more relevance it brought to mind America's Pittsburgh in the 1880s, London during the Industrial Revolution, or Germany's Ruhr Valley during World War II military production—all periods of capitalist development during which human health, aesthetics, and the environment were sacrificed in favor of enormous scales of productivity and profit. Soviet planners clearly believed in two principles: Bigness and Utilitarianism. The niceties of human health and aesthetics were ignored. Having grown up amid industrial filth dissident Russian poet Irina Ratushinskaya wrote: "Do we have to know why/the river turns black?"[42]

There was no denying that the environmental devastation was an affront to the senses. But was it killing people? What chemical and radioactive threat was actually present, and was it at least partly to blame for the observed deterioration of the health of the people of the former USSR and Eastern Bloc?

"At issue is not only the scope and coverage but also the quality of environmental and health information," wrote Feshbach.[43] "Many experts concluded that available statistics on air pollution, for example, are 30 to 50 percent lower than the real figures. . . . Communism may be dead, but Lenin's dictum that 'statistics are not scholarly but practical' lives on. The normal bureaucratic response to requests for information is often to conceal what might be embarrassing or costly."

Had Chernobyl radiation exposure caused widespread illness in people who lived more than twenty miles away from the nuclear power plant in 1986? Could it be blamed for perceived health deficiencies of the children living a decade later in the western parts of the former Soviet Union?

Cancer is genuinely a problem. Though national cancer rates are generally below those seen in the West, cancer hot spots exist all over the former Eastern Bloc and Soviet Union. In the industrial regions of Siberia, for example, the incidence of adult leukemia is nearly twice that seen in Western Europe (15 cases per 100,000 Siberians annually versus 8 per 100,000 Europeans).[44] Hodgkin's disease incidence is about double that seen in Europe.[45]

"We see oncological hematological problems—leukemias and lymphomas. There is a real upward trend among children, especially," Dr. Tatyana Boyko, deputy president of the Public Health Committee of Irkutsk, said. Diagnoses of cancer in adults increased 130 percent between 1992 and 1996, she said. And for children under fourteen years of age cancer was diagnosed 145 percent more frequently in 1996 versus 1992.[46] In 1996 the diagnosed child cancer rate in Irkutsk was 247.5 per 100,000 children—nearly fifteen times the U.S. pediatric cancer rate.

As far as Boyko was concerned the culprit was clearly "the ecological disaster—after all, the real concentrations [of pollutants] exceed allowed ones by many-fold in this region."

Official Ministry of Health data[47] indicated there has been a slow but steady increase over the last two decades of the twentieth century in the numbers of Russian children and adults diagnosed with cancer. The child incidence rose 14 percent from 1993 to 1995; adult cancer incidence rose 6 percent.

Overall adult and child cancer rates also rose in Ukraine, jumping from 300 per 100,000 in 1988 to 410 per 100,000 in 1994, according to physicist Valery Kukhar.

"But the problem is that since 1990 the health status—*all* markers of health—have shown a worsening situation in Ukraine," Kukhar said. Infectious diseases were increasing, as were heart disease, traumas, poisoning, accidents . . . everything.

"All these figures—including the rise in cancer—may be the result of the deterioration of the environment, but also of psychological stress, economics, political instability—all of it," Kukhar insisted. And he gave the example of an ulcer to illustrate his point. If a man developed a peptic ulcer in Kyiv in 1999 was it because of the stress of his unemployment, a lowering in the quality of his diet, a newly acquired bacterial infection, or ingestion of radioactive food grown in the Chernobyl zone?

"One thing we can be absolutely sure of is that the thyroid cancer is the result of Chernobyl," Kukhar said.

Even the most conservative officials in Moscow, and the current operators of Chernobyl, agreed that there had been a striking radiation-induced increase in thyroid cancer, particularly in children, since the accident. In Ukraine the incidence of thyroid cancer in children was by 1998 52 times higher than it was before the accident; the incidence in Belarus, which bore the brunt of the fallout, was 113 times above its 1986 level.[48] And as the century closed, the Chernobyl district led the world in thyroid cancer, with a rate of one diagnosed case in every 3,700 local residents, or 500 times the pre-1986 rate.[49] And the incidence of thyroid diseases of all kinds in children was far above normal. By the end of 1997 fifteen thousand pediatric thyroid disease cases had been diagnosed in Belarus and fifty thousand in Ukraine. And eight years after the accident 19.5 percent of Belarusan children who were exposed to the fallout were making antibodies against their own thyroids—only 3.8 percent of children in Belarus who lived in unradiated areas made such antibodies.[50]

The Ukrainian authorities estimated that 700,000 children who were under fourteen years of age at the time of the accident were exposed to Chernobyl radiation and that 336,107 children lived in 1998 in radiation-contaminated areas. Dr. Daniel Gluzman—brother of psychiatrist Semyon—and his team of molecular biologists at the R. E. Kavetsky Institute of Experimental Pathology in Kyiv used sophisticated immunological methods to study some of these children, looking for signs of developing leukemias, lymphomas, and other types of blood cancers that were seen in victims of the Hiroshima nuclear bomb. In one such study Gluzman's group found a variety of blood disorders—such as leukopenia and thrombocytopenia—in 1,275 of 7,250 Chernobyl-exposed children. And in half of those children there were clear changes in their white blood cells, particularly T cell lymphocytes.[51] The sorts of alterations Gluzman saw in the T cells of these children were not found in any of the cells of control children from other parts of Ukraine that weren't affected by the accident. But they did correspond to some of the lymphocyte changes seen in cancer patients.

Perhaps more disturbing were Gluzman's studies of children who were born within nine months after the accident to mothers who were definitely exposed to Chernobyl radiation. More than half of these children had abnormal lymphocytes.

"We have also seen forty cases of leukemia in cleanup workers" who entered Chernobyl shortly after the meltdown, the white-haired elderly Gluzman explained, chatting in his chilly Kyiv laboratory. "So probably we will expect to see an increase in breast cancer, lung cancer, central nervous system neoplasms," over coming years.

But in 1996 the Ukraine Institute of Biophysics convened a meeting of so-called radiobiologists, most of whom were from Moscow. The forum released a statement concluding that beyond the observed thyroid cancer cases, there was no long-term deleterious effect from Chernobyl at all, which, they argued, wasn't surprising given human beings could tolerate 70 rems of radiation. Based on average U.S. annual radiation exposure, however, it would take 19,000 years for a typical American to receive that dose of radiation.

A large-scale study done by researchers at Harvard University concluded that the incidence of childhood leukemias in the radiated areas was 50 percent higher than that seen in parts of Ukraine not exposed to Chernobyl fallout: 37.7 cases per 100,000 in the radiated zones versus 25.4 cases per 100,000 in control areas.[52]

Perhaps remarkably there was no evidence of birth defects, other types of cancer, elevated numbers of miscarriages, or heightened sterility among residents of the radiated area. Nor was there evidence of widespread damage to human immune systems.

But there was plenty of fear. Surveys showed that ten years after the accident up to half of the adults who had lived in radiated areas were still taking sedatives.[53] They were caught between information extremes, between polarizing views of their futures. At one extreme was the Ukrainian government, telling them that 125,000 citizens had already died in the first decade following the near meltdown, victims of unspecified forms of radiation damage. And at the other extreme were researchers who argued that only a handful of verified deaths had, or would, occur, all of them among the men who died in the accident itself, or children downwind who developed thyroid cancers.[54]

The Chernobyl radiation debate was mirrored all across the region as residents of the former Soviet states learned that nuclear waste had simply been dumped in local lakes, seas, and garbage heaps; ugly "factories" were actually secret nuclear facilities; nuclear submarines lay decommissioned upon the floor of the Baltic Sea; and within dense cities Soviet engineers had conducted dangerous radioactive experiments, leaving residue behind that would still emit radiation for thousands of years.

All of these sites, charged physicist Alesey Yablokov, contributed to an overwhelming burden of radioactive contamination across the region, especially in his beloved Russia. Having served as President Yeltsin's environmental advisor, Yablokov was privy to long-secret documents that delineated the horrors. In 1992 Yablokov lost a tooth and, out of curiosity, ran radiation tests on it. He was astonished to discover that it was highly radioactive, containing traces of several different isotopes. Determined to learn where the radiation had come from, Yablokov urged his colleagues in a Moscow laboratory to be tested: all returned with similarly disturbing results. Eventually, Yablokov found documents, he said, that proved his lab building, and many other Moscow structures, were built of concrete made in part from waste products produced by Soviet nuclear facilities.

He resigned after three years in Yeltsin's service, despairing of the obstacles against change. After 1995 the bombastic Yablokov worked from outside the government, acting as chair of the independent Centre for Russian Environmental Policy: "Your society wants to be protected," he said, "but ours is not mature. . . . My government has no money to combat pollution. And every new fact showing disaster demands more money. So the government doesn't want to have good information."

The Russian government created a "dirty cities" program—a rough equivalent of the U.S. Superfund for toxic waste cleanup. About thirty cities were officially designated "dirtiest" in Russia, giving them highest priority for the paltry reserve of funds Moscow could muster for ecological research and cleanup. In addition the Russian government during the 1990s designated two hundred cities as ones that posed "ecological danger to human health" due to toxic pollution of the air and/or water.

Dr. Boris Revich, of the Center for Demography and Human Ecology in Moscow, sits on the panel that decided which cities should receive the dubious "dirty" accolade, and what sorts of scientific interventions should be executed. As documents were declassified and data mounted the extent of Soviet pollution proved so overwhelming that Revich and his fellow scientists couldn't begin to decipher the impact it was all having on human health.

"So the first task we want to solve is to make a short list of the most dangerous contaminants for Russia. Where are the pollution/environment problems most acute? What are the problems? We have no sense of priorities," Revich lamented.

Efforts were hampered not only by money, Revich said, but also by horrible Soviet-era statistics and a dearth of skilled epidemiologists. The old database on such things as birth defects, child asthma rates, child deformities, and even child cancers was, Revich insisted, "almost useless."

"When they try to link [anything] to the environment they say, 'The level of unborn deformities has gone up.' We say, 'You didn't have any statistics before! They weren't calculated properly ten years ago,' " Revich said. And because all aspects of the study of environmental damage to health stepped on the toes of Soviet military and industrial planners scientists weren't foolish enough to wade into such research waters prior to 1991.

The Lake Baikal region of Siberia offered a perfect illustration of the problem. The lake itself is a national treasure of rare size and beauty. More than a mile deep and 636 kilometers long, Lake Baikal is the crystal clear source of one-fifth of the world's fresh water supply. During the winter the lake—which is larger than the nation of Belgium—freezes on top with an ice crust more than a meter thick. So solid is this winter ice mass that the Japanese Army drove over it and into Siberia during World War II, surprising

Soviet forces. Called the Pearl of Siberia, Lake Baikal holds a special, precious position in Russian culture.

In 1988 Soviet leader Mikhail Gorbachev gave his startling address to the USSR nation, disclosing for the first time the extent of the great Soviet pollution cover-up. He deliberately opened by referring to Russia's natural treasure, Lake Baikal. But he went on to tell the stunned Soviet masses that damage to their beloved lake was minimal compared to what had been done elsewhere in the nation, including in seven industrial cities located along the Angara River, the only body of water that flows out of Lake Baikal. Angara meanders first to the metropolis of Irkutsk and then northwest past the industrial cities of Angarsk, Usol'ye Sibirskoye, Cheremukhovo, Zima, and several smaller cities. As the Angara flowed farther from Lake Baikal its pollution levels increased significantly, particularly with dioxins, lead, and PCBs—all substances closely regulated in Western Europe and the United States.

At the Federal Medical University in Irkutsk Larisa Ignatyeva used mass spectrometers and gas chromatographs to measure dioxins in the region. Such dioxin compounds as 2,4-D, 2,4,5-T, and TCDD were used as pesticides and produced as waste by-products of pulp and paper processing. They were considered highly carcinogenic, teratogenic, and mutagenic, making these chemicals prime suspects for any observed increases in cancer or birth defects.

Ignatyeva found dioxins everywhere she looked: in local food, water, soil, sewage. The highest levels were in locally produced butter, milk, riverbank soil, and sewage water pouring into the Angara and Irkutsk drinking water.[55]

The TCDD levels Ignatyeva found were low—in some cases within safe U.S. standards. But Ignatyeva, who had been nicknamed the Dioxin Lady by her colleagues, was convinced that dioxins were causing a marked "effect on the human body, the immune systems," she said.

Toxicologist Nina Ivanova Motorova of the Siberian Academy of Science's research station in Angarsk wasn't convinced. While she was quite sure that the health of people living in the Angara River industrial cities had been severely damaged she did not think exotic compounds like dioxins were the key problem. It was the overall burden of pollution, compounded by social stress, that was killing people, she said.

The Taiga forests around Angarsk were denuded by acid rain. No floor of scrub and greenery formed a protective bed for dying trees, their trunks encrusted with black filth. Nearing the city the amount of blackness on struggling trees increased, covering not only their trunks but their limbs and leaf buds as well. Weighed down by their pollution burden trees leaned at sad angles, eventually collapsing.

The sky, too, changed as one neared the city, its blueness fading. In place of azure appeared grayness, haze, and, at sunset, a vermillion glow.

The city was ringed with oil refineries and energy production plants. The landscape was crisscrossed with enormous rusting steel ducts that carried petroleum products from one plant to another.

The city center of Angarsk, population 280,000, was bisected by streets that, as was the case in every city in the Soviet Union, were named after Karl Marx and Vladimir Lenin. Next to the requisite stern statue of Lenin was a sign: "Angarsk City—Born by Victory!" From behind the sign American disco music blared. Rows of concrete apartment buildings, each exactly the same as the last, lined the streets of Angarsk, creating a visually numbing landscape. It was hard to fathom in the 1990s, but thirty years earlier when Komsomol volunteers built the apartments and factories of Angarsk it was considered a great Soviet honor to live and work in the city.

All around the city stood gargantuan steel factories and plants, most built during or soon after World War II. Everywhere the ground literally smoked, smoldered, and flamed as some buried pipes leaked, their contents spontaneously combusting in the chilly Siberian air. The area was densely littered with abandoned hunks of machinery, oil drums, chemical containers, and trash. The air routinely exceeded all Russian air pollution standards, Motorova said, and the soil was severely contaminated with heavy metals and lead.

Everyone in the city was in some way connected to the chemical or oil industries. And all of the factories and plants dumped their wastes into the ice-cold swift Angara River, carrying the pollutants all over Siberia, Motorova explained.

When Nina Motorova moved to Angarsk in 1973 she found the city horribly polluted and was kept busy scurrying among factories and sites of contamination in her capacity as an environmental health scientist.

"I got enough of a pollution dose in the seventies to influence my body," Motorova says. Though only in her forties, blue-eyed Motorova maneuvers with difficulty, leaning heavily on a cane and any fellow pedestrian willing to assist. "I have a rare disease because I have visited so many polluted sites. So I have a disease of my central nervous system."

Motorova has reticulohistiocytosis, a profound, rare immune system disorder that is always crippling and may prove fatal. The cause of the syndrome, which is usually found in older women, isn't known. But she insists, "I got this syndrome from all the bad places I've visited."

As Motorova guides her visitors about the unsightly Angarsk mess, she nervously avoids eye contact with passing pedestrians and car passengers. Unemployment in all the old Soviet industrial cities was rising as these outmoded old plants went bankrupt. The people were angry, and they resented any outside inquiry that might further worsen their economic situation—even if it was intended to improve the health of the populace.

Once the stars of the proletariat state, Angarsk and dozens of other industrial cities in Siberia were, by the late 1990s, foci of mass public health fear. At the top of the phobia list, garnering the popular distinction of "most polluted place on Earth," was Noril'sk.

From the air, northern Siberia's mountainous, white frozen landscape, spotted with pockets of heavy pine forests, offers a breathtaking panorama. Until the plane nears Noril'sk.

A plume of chocolate brown air hovers over the city and a diameter area about fifty miles surrounding it. The white landscape takes on a dark, grayish-green tone from the air, though there are places where the snow is jet black. It is a devastated region—its chimneys belching out 2,041,000 metric tons of "atmospheric particulate" each year.

On landing, three alarming sensations took hold: a metallic taste in the mouth reminiscent of sucking on a nickel; a painful burning in the back of the throat that caused a reflexive tightening of the larynx and esophagus; and an almost constant tearing from eyes unused to the grit that quickly collected on eyelashes, crusting on the lids.

Welcome to the most polluted place on Earth, Noril'sk. Located 200 kilometers above the Arctic Circle. No sunlight four months out of the year. Population 280,000.

Once the cash cow for the Soviet Union, Noril'sk sits on more than a third of the planet's nickel reserves, a fifth of the platinum, half the palladium, and 10 percent each of copper and cobalt. It is rich in high-grade coal, is the world's second largest producer of diamonds behind South Africa, and contains significant quantities of gold and amethyst.[56]

But along with the sweet cream of these natural riches came curd: in addition to the airborne particulates, the area's mining and processing operation produced 28 million tons of solid waste, at least 10 million of which was toxic by Russian government standards. Every year some 5,500 tons of black particulate crud fell on each square kilometer of Noril'sk, giving each inch of surface a charcoal veneer. It was estimated that Noril'sk's industrial effluent routinely blanketed more than two thousand hectares of the Arctic.

And the pollution didn't stop there. Noril'sk annually pumped an astonishing burden of filth into the earth's atmosphere, including: 2.1 million metric tons of sulfur dioxide, 1.8 million tons of copper oxides, 1.2 thousand tons of nickel, 10.1 million metric tons of carbon monoxide, 19 million tons of nitrogen oxides, 43.7 million tons of lead, 30 million tons of hydrogen sulfide, a tenth of a million tons of sulfuric acid, and 0.3 million tons of chlorinated hydrocarbons.[57]

The wind blew toxic dust filled with heavy metals—30 percent of it iron oxide—swirling down in visible clouds off the black slag mountains dotted around the city. And when the wind didn't blow, in midwinter for instance, the pollutants hung heavily over the sunless city like a dirty, wet wool coat.[58]

Along Leninski Prospect, the city's main boulevard, the populace is taking its Sunday evening stroll. Dressed in mink and sable coats and hats the people parade down the boulevard, walking its seventeen-block length and then turning around. They wear their finest clothing on this popular promenade and many women stroll behind baby prams, taking care in their high-heeled boots lest they fall on the icy sidewalks. The men tug thoroughbred dogs by their leashes. Children toss soccer balls to one another as they play in parallel progress to their slowly meandering parents. Clusters of friends greet one another, remarking on the weather, their children's grades, one another's attire, maybe sports.

Remarkably—perhaps astonishingly—these Noril'sk paraders seem unaware that with each step they are pushing their feet into several inches of black metallic filth. The marching masses produce a *crunch crunch crunch* cacophony, treading upon industrial waste. Their fur coats and pets blacken as they go, accruing layers of carbon, iron, copper, lead, nickel, and other pollutants. To either side of the sidewalks, also seemingly unnoticed by the citizens of Noril'sk, stand banks of black snow. The only thing that appears to irritate those out for their constitutionals are the metal kiosks that have recently sprung up along the sidewalks, forcing occasional detours and bottlenecks. The kiosks, from which all manner of goods are vended, indicated that capitalism has come to Noril'sk.

And there was no mistaking the imprint of the old Soviet *nomenklatura* upon Noril'sk, which they dubbed "The Pearl Set in Snow." Though hints of Noril'sk's astonishing mineral wealth were known to Czar Peter the Great in the 1750s, the city was not built until 1935, when Stalin ordered its construction. Prior to that time the region was inhabited by nomadic Shamanistic tribes—the Evenkis, Tungus, Nganasan, Dolgan, and Nenets—who herded reindeer and hunted fish and animals along the Taimyr Peninsula. Stalin ordered them shoved into gulags, outlawed their languages, and did his best to obliterate their cultures.

Between 1939 and 1953 slave laborers, most of whom were interned for alleged acts or thoughts contrary to Communist ideology, toiled in the Arctic wasteland, building the "Pearl" of which the Moscow *nomenklatura* dreamed.[59] It is estimated that at the gulag's peak 100,000 political slaves toiled in Noril'sk, a quarter of them dying every year, quickly replaced by new shipments of dissident poets, intellectuals, nationalists, and labor organizers.

To lure otherwise rational, highly skilled human beings to lives of darkness, deadly freeze, and dismal pollution the Moscow *nomenklatura* created a second class within the "classless society," composed of privileged scientists, engineers, miners, and industrial personnel who enjoyed certain opportunities not afforded to the rest of the proletariat. Certain cities, such as Noril'sk, were designated "A

Class," meaning that their stores had top priority for all goods. Residents of Noril'sk took satisfaction in being able to fly—at state expense—all over the USSR on holidays, and see barren shelves in markets elsewhere, bereft of the same toys, tomatoes, and television sets that they could readily obtain back home. Workers in "A Class" cities were among the highest paid Soviet citizens.

No matter how bad things got in the icy darkness of a Noril'sk January the workers could always be consoled in knowing that they were superior to the slaves who toiled, and died, all around them. Russian poet Galich neatly summarized the caste system of Noril'sk, and other gulag/cities:

> We dug and we toiled,
> And we bit the iron,
> We offered our chests
> To the muzzles of submachine guns.
> And you, driving past
> On your Victory motorcars,
> Shouted to us:
> "Achieve your norm."
> And we forgot
> about sleep and food,
> And you led us
> From victory to victory.
> Meanwhile you
> Exchanged your Victories for Volgas,
> And later
> You exchanged your Volgas for Zims,
> And later
> You exchanged your Zims for chaikas,
> And later
> You exchanged your chaikas for ZILs.
> And we wore ourselves to the bone,
> We dug and we loaded,
> And you led us
> From victory to victory
> And shouted toasts
> To victory.[60]

By the 1990s the ugly history of Noril'sk, including the enormity of the Schmidt Mountain gulag cemetery, was known.[61] Nearly every resident was desperately trying to get off of what they called their "island," a place escapable only by air. But they were trapped. Pay was down—if it arrived at all. The airlines were no longer state enterprises that provided free tickets to Noril'sk's workers. To decamp Noril'sk in the late 1990s one needed money—more of it than anyone was now earning.

"It's an economic gulag now," Komsomolsky Mine director Hamby Kozhijev said.

Paranoia forced denial: fear of job loss, of freezing in an unheated Arctic hovel, helped keep complaints unsaid.

But denial was getting harder every day, as the populace learned long-secret public health truths.

Though precise, analyzed statistics were hard to come by; it was clear that the pervasive pollution was linked to internationally high rates of miscarriage, lung cancers, various forms of chronic respiratory diseases, cardiovascular disease, allergies, and skin disease. At one hospital in neighboring Talnakh, for example, 90 percent of patients admitted from 1993 to 1998 suffered from lung diseases and "practically 100 percent of the children hospitalized in the area have allergies and skin problems," said Vladimir Koshubarov, deputy chairman of Noril'sk's Committee on Environmental Protection.

"Lung cancer is the number one killer in Noril'sk. Cardiovascular disease is number two. Without any doubt we know Noril'sk has the lowest life expectancy in all of Russia," Koshubarov continued.

An average infant in Noril'sk suffered 1.7 bouts of respiratory illness per year. Mothers in Noril'sk were three times more likely to give birth to a child with congenital birth defects than were women living elsewhere on Taimyr Peninsula, and ten times more likely than was the average Russian mother.[62]

Outside Noril'sk, along the roadsides that connected the city to neighboring mines, smelters, foundries, and workers' settlements, the permafrost was disappearing under the heat of mile upon mile of leaking pipelines of pollution. In places hundred-foot-tall geysers of steam spewed from leaking conduits. Slag heaps, discarded automobiles and steel machinery, and sacks of mysterious garbage covered the imperiled permafrost. In places the permafrost had completely disappeared, all of its ice having long since melted and been replaced by lakes of red, putrid liquid that, like some organic mass, spontaneously belched, burped, and spewed forth fountains of nausea-inducing, putrid steam.

St. Petersburg–born Boris started life in Noril'sk as foreman of a metal furnace, rising through the ranks to reach one of the Kombinat's top positions. As a Jew Boris couldn't hope to attain such stature without having become a devout Communist Party member during Soviet times. With the KGB long gone, USSR dead, and the old *nomenklatura* vanished, Boris was still frightened—perhaps more so. He was afraid of the Kombinat.

In 1992–94 the Yeltsin government sold off most of the old state-run industries. A consortium of banking and investment firms, working with Russia's second largest bank, Oneximbank, bought 51 percent of the Kombinat Noril'sk Nikel and in its first year shared an estimated $2.4 billion worth of mined metals sales with the Russian government, which retained 49 percent ownership of the Kombinat. But at the end of 1994 Noril'sk's largest turbine engine blew up, killing several workers and plunging most of the citizenry into a long, horrible, heatless winter.[63]

Among the citizens of Noril'sk rumors spread of gangsters who had bought out several original partners and sent thugs to force greater productivity. For men like Boris this meant that where once they feared KGB spies in their midst, now it was the company thugs, famed for their brutality, who gave them daily cause for concern.

No wonder, then, that Noril'sk had become an island of paranoia. Parents pulled their children away from strangers, passengers on buses hastily moved to the far end of the vehicle when foreigners boarded, workers and the mayor declined to speak of their situation. . . .

Though Noril'sk is often cited for a dramatically lower than normal life expectancy for the region, it was difficult to confirm because of the Kombinat's retirement policy. Life in the mines and plants was so hard that men could retire at forty-five, women at forty, receiving full life pensions.

"A man works his shift, spends some time at home. He does this for years. Then he goes to the 'Continent' and dies. Who cares? Who blames Noril'sk?" Koshubarov says with a shrug.

"So data are hard to come by because usually when workers retire they leave Noril'sk and die elsewhere," Komsomolsky Mine chief engineer Alexander Borodai said. That could explain why there were few graves in Noril'sk's cemetery belonging to people who died after age forty-five. And why he was considered "elderly" in Noril'sk, fifty-five-year-old Borodai said.

"For us Noril'sk is an information black hole," said Russian government scientist Boris Revich. Moscow had repeatedly offered to designate Noril'sk a "dirty city," which would qualify the region for special cleanup and scientific research funds. But the Kombinat refused both the designation and Moscow's offer of scientific inquiry.

Or it may be true that *average* life expectancy for men was below forty. That wouldn't surprise Dr. Nikolai Pavlov, chief physician of Medical Sanitary Unit No. 2, located thirty-five kilometers from Noril'sk in the satellite city of Talnakh. Two of the Noril'sk Kombinat mines and seventy thousand people reside in Talnakh.

The incidence of lung disease in Talnakh adults is, Pavlov says, "Three times the average in Russia." His 310-bed hospital over the last six years admitted 1,207 lung disease patients, accounting for 90 percent of its inpatient clientele.

Malignant lung cancer killed 231 of them. Emphysema, tuberculosis, pneumonia, chronic bronchitis, and acute asthma claimed the rest.

The six-foot six-inch white-haired Pavlov strolled the noisy, crowded hallways of his hospital inured to the sounds of harsh coughs and raspy breathing. No longer subsidized by the state and ignored by the Kombinat, the hospital's unpaid staff survives by directly billing patients for each procedure and compelling the ill to purchase their own drugs, meals, linens, syringes—"the whole lot," Pavlov says.

Pavlov had recently logged a stupendous increase in drug-resistant tuberculosis cases, more than doubling in number in just two years. He had no resources to support scientific research, but he had a hypothesis: the pollution had so devastasted the lungs of the seventy thousand residents of Talnakh that any cases of TB brought by visitors from outside the area swiftly spread. Nearly 2 percent of the population had active pulmonary tuberculosis in 1997, Pavlov said. And his hospital "had no TB drugs."

"In the winter there is a waiting list here when we see outbreaks of upper respiratory infections," Pavlov points out. "And it keeps our surgeons busy, breaking up lung cavities of tuberculosis, removing cancerous lungs, cutting [tracheal] bypasses," so patients can breathe.

The future of Talnakh, Pavlov opines, could be one of "slow, slow death."

One thing was certain. Working conditions in the mines and plants were incredibly dangerous.

Down the road from Noril'sk is the huge Nadezhda ore processing plant, where 10-story-tall furnaces heat copper, nickel, and cobalt to temperatures of 1,100 to 1,400 degrees centigrade. Thousands of workers toil with the vermillion, molten ore in front of them radiating searing heat, and winter's minus 40 degree centigrade chill at their backs.

"You'll never know what that feels like," manager Boris says, noting that it "confuses your heart," because half the worker's body is exposed to frigid, subzero air, signaling a need for fast-pumping blood. And the other half is boiling hot, telling the heart to slow down.

A suppressed study by the Medical School of Sverdlovsk, provided to a visitor, showed that workers in the mines were far more likely to suffer cardiovascular disease and lung cancer, even when compared to other residents of Noril'sk. Measurements of their work space air revealed that they were inhaling 19.2 micrograms per meter squared of nickel and up to 134 micrograms of cobalt—levels 20 and 135 times more, respectively, than considered normal by Russian standards.

The study, which was completed in 1990, was never published, by order of the Kombinat. Nor were the results of a recent Kombinat-financed environmental survey of a 53,000 square kilometer Arctic area around Noril'sk. Geologists Yuri Melnikov and Sergei Snisar, both aged thirty, led a seven-man team that collected ten thousand samples in the vast region, braving all Arctic weather conditions. By pulling core samples out of the permafrost, drawn from appropriate depths, Snisar and Melnikov could compare contemporary pollution levels to those two hundred years ago.

In the areas farthest from Noril'sk, Melnikov said, "contemporary snow samples contain 18 times the amount of cobalt, 6 times the copper, 11 times the nickel, 14.5 times the barium, and 3.2 times the zinc," that was present two hundred years ago. Acid rain from the Kombinat's smokestacks has destroyed up to 90 percent of the original tree population.

Moss and lichen had become saturated with heavy metals at levels up to twelve times what they were before the Russian Revolution of 1917, killing off half the plants.

And, "we see a dangerous potential for avalanches due to degradation of surface plant life that protects the permafrost," Melnikov concluded.

Three days after Melnikov and Snisar shared their unpublished findings with their visitor, the Kombinat cut off all their funds and ordered the young scientists not to speak. The Kombinat representatives declined to discuss any health or environment-related matters.

According to the Russian Ministry of Health the relative hazard of dying prematurely in Noril'sk in 1994 was 85. In Angarsk, which ranked fourth worst, it was 15. No city ranked above a 22—except Noril'sk.

Noril'sk was at the extreme end of a Soviet ecological legacy that could be felt from East Berlin all the way to the Pacific Ocean. In Bohemia, the Czech Republic, fifty years of strip mining and coal smelting had devastated what once was the preferred vacation site of the Hapsburgs and aristocracy all over Central Europe. The fall of the Berlin Wall gave West Germans a shocking look at the industrial filth and putrid air of their eastern countrymen. The Central Asian nations of Uzbekistan and Kazakhstan were suffering from an insane irrigation scheme begun by Lenin, draining the vast, landlocked Aral Sea to provide water for cotton fields, resulting in elevated throat cancer due to environmental dust.[64] The visual and physical filth was pervasive. It assaulted the senses.

But was it the cause of the region's radical demographic shift?

On that experts stridently disagreed.

Former Yeltsin advisor Yablokov became visibly agitated when the question was posed. The gray-haired, bearded Russian dismissively said that despite reliable data the illnesses and deaths seen in Noril'sk "are obviously due to pollution."

"Look," he says, stabbing his points home with pokes in the air. "Fourteen percent of our young children in Russia meet primary school healthy child standards. Why?

"I have personally had a high level of radiation exposure—why? No one knows how. It may be possible that a pipe somewhere comes free, releasing radiation. All over Moscow every year an average of seventy places are discovered with dangerous levels of radiation. It's amazing," Yablokov, a physicist, says, gesticulating wildly. "Nobody can feel safety even inside Moscow."

Zoologist Maria Cherkasova shares Yablokov's views. As head of the Moscow-based Center for Independent Ecological Programs Cherkasova cites the same figures as Yablokov. Her chief concerns are rocket and missile launches, and the d-methylhydrazine fuel used as a propellant.

"The whole world should work on safe fuel for rockets," Cherkasova says, insisting that children all over Russia and Central Asia were dying due to exposure to missile fuel. Other key contributors to the region's rising death rates, the fifty-five-year-old ornithologist says, are dioxins, lead, DDT, and a generalized dampening of people's immune systems prompted by environmental assaults.

The key problems with the environmental argument were that the epidemiology, if it existed at all, was poorly done. And pollution had actually declined dramatically after 1991 all across the region due to the economic collapse of local industries. Thus, during the very time in which the region experienced its most dramatic increase in deaths and health crises the amount of pollution in people's environments decreased.

Boris Revich had no doubt that the ecological tragedy was playing a role in human illness, and he had personally documented pollution-induced asthma,[65] lead-associated child health problems,[66] and dioxin impacts[67] in Russia. But he found most assertions that the pollution was directly responsible for the region's demographic shift "nonsense—complete crap!"

Beldrich Moldan was the first minister of the environment in the Czech Republic following the fall of communism. His country underwent the same debate, perhaps starting three years earlier than did the nations to his east. The focus of the Czech public's fears was industrial Bohemia.

"In 1990 when I was minister I went there. And to my amazement there was a slogan: 'The first three words our children learn are *Mommy, Daddy,* and *inversion,'* " a reference to air inversions that held smog and pollution inside the Bohemian valleys. When just two months after the Czech revolution the populace was accusing Moldan of not doing enough to clean up their environment, he realized the depth of their collective panic. After decades of lies and cover-ups by the former Soviet-aligned government the Bohemians suddenly realized what was in their air, water, and food.

He pored over all available data, Moldan recalled, and found it was "mostly shit! Really! So bad you cannot believe it."

In the end blue-eyed, silver-haired Moldan concluded that "life expectancy in Bohemia is about five years behind the Czech average," for a number of reasons, including—but not limited to—the environment.

Six years after the Czech revolution that country's demographics shifted back, even in Bohemia, in favor of longer life expectancies and better public health,[68] "and nobody can say our environment has improved that much."

Moldan, dressed casually but seated in a meticulous office lined from floor to ceiling with books and scientific journals, saw the issue philosophically. After decades of communism, he explained, people had no sense of personal responsibility. Because they had little control over their personal fates during totalitarianism the new societies found individuals unable to imagine that their own behaviors—drinking, smoking, driving while inebriated—were key to their health.

"I told those people in Bohemia, 'Look, you have done nothing to clean this up. You just wait for the government to do everything. But if you don't take some responsibility, too, this place will look like Russia.'

"And I remembered that in 1987—maybe it was 1988—I met a young Russian colleague. We discussed political evolution, a favorite topic of mine. He said, 'I see you have hope—forty years of Communist rule is bad, but you can recover. But seventy years of Communists—we will never recover!' And that man's remarks will always live with me."

IV

What are the present Russian authorities offering the people? "Support Yeltsin and you'll live the way people do in America!" . . . How is it possible not to see that everything in Russia is being done not "like in America" (or in France or Sweden), but the way things were done in Uganda under President Idi Amin?

—Andrei Sinyavsky, 1997[69]

From the point of view of the United Nations Children's Fund the public health crisis of the nations of the former Soviet Union and Eastern Bloc boiled down to one thing: history.

"Hopes that, with the elimination of authoritarianism and the introduction of a demand-led market economy, the needs of children would be better met in the short-term have been largely betrayed," read UNICEF's 1997 report.[70] "Systematic changes have for the most part been too large and sudden, with negative effects to the economy; and the bursting out of national pride and ethnic intolerance has led to heightened tensions and, in a few cases, warfare. Child welfare has once again become the victim of dramatic historic changes.

"The transition has been accompanied by a severe region-wide economic crisis, the effects of which have hit even the most successful countries. Moreover, the transition is also based on market forces, which can free powerful human energies, but which also need support from societal values and social institutions for a balanced development. As social norms and institutions collapsed, values eroded—it will take time for new values to take root, which will also require support from laws, law enforcement and the recognition of a common interest."

As the demographic nightmare unfolded in the region UNICEF, viewing matters through the prism of children, felt that public health had collapsed because the societies themselves had lost their social fabrics. It was more than just economic peril that drove individuals to the brink, UNICEF argued, it was economic peril coupled with the cessation of all social cohesion.

In other words, change was killing people.

The World Bank, on the other hand, argued in its 1996 World Development Report that the problem wasn't too much change: it was that not enough change had occurred. Those societies that made the transition to market economies most rapidly, such as the Czech Republic and Poland, suffered the briefest demographic disaster. Public health catastrophes persisted, according to the Bank, where governments kept one foot in the old Soviet system and another in capitalism.

"What has happened to health during transition?" the Bank's analysts asked. "Two conclusions emerge: rapid reform is not necessarily detrimental to health indicators, but slow reform or the absence of reform does little to impede a long-run deterioration."

In 1993 the entire region appeared to be in public health hell. But by 1996 demographic disasters in Poland, the Czech Republic, Slovakia, and Hungary appeared to have reached their nadir and were heading toward recovery. This, the Bank's analysts felt, offered proof that populations could, indeed, tolerate "shock therapy" economic reform and, in the long run, benefited from such drastic measures.

From its inception the Soviet Union's economy was dictated by Communist Party planners in Moscow who seemingly cavalierly moved entire ethnic populations from one place to another, started industries in the middle of unpopulated tundra, demanded corn be grown in icy climes, and placed the means of production for different segments of the same industry thousands of grueling, wintry miles apart. Inefficiency was the rule of the game.

When the USSR collapsed, industries fell with it, as the various segments of its typically long outmoded production were now located in different countries. Overnight millions of workers lost their jobs, and the majority of the people residing in the Eastern Bloc and former Soviet Union fell into poverty—perhaps 25 percent of them were, according to UNICEF, living in acute poverty within eighteen months of the breakup of the Soviet Union.

In Russia 45 million people, or a third of the population, had incomes *below* subsistence level in 1995, meaning they were surviving off their wits and dacha gardens—or weren't surviving at all. Those who actually had paying jobs were earning a paltry average wage in 1996 of $153 a month, which was 10 percent less than they earned in 1992.[71] The World Bank and International Monetary Fund broke all historic lending records in a scramble to save Russia, and, of course, bring it into the capitalist fold. By 1996 the IMF had loaned the Russian Federation more than $12 billion, a good deal of which the Yeltsin government used to cover the cost of its war in Chechnya and, it would later be revealed, to line the pockets of the Yeltsin family and cronies.[72]

In 1997, however, there was talk of economic recovery. For a few financial moments Russia looked promising, as its trade balance and industrial production levels were both firmly in the asset columns at the dawn of 1997.

Yet these positive indicators glossed over a distressing picture that would have profound regional implications for public health: the concentration of wealth in the hands of an elite oligarchy. Rising out of the post-1991 chaos came the phoenixes of the supposedly free markets. The "New Rockefellers," as they were dubbed, snapped up de-nationalized industries, built regional banking systems, created vast energy and telecommunications monopolies, and without a second's concern for the once-dominant proletariat, shut down inefficient industries and created economic ghost towns that dotted the lands across twelve time zones. In some cases their cozy relations with government regulators and mobsters were so obvious as to recall Al Capone and Chicago in the 1920s. Indeed, many may have aspired to be John D. Rockefeller, but in practice appeared more reminiscent of the Familia Corleone.[73]

For ordinary Ukrainians, Georgians, and Siberians, this concentration of wealth in corrupt hands spelled disaster. As the greedy took over industries, they not only laid off upward of a third of the workforce, but also stopped paying those who theoretically still had jobs. Tens of millions of workers continued for years on end to tromp to work every day, toiling in increasingly unsafe, antiquated factories, in hopes that one day a miracle would occur and months of back wages would be paid. That occasionally this occurred supplied the necessary carrot that kept the old proletariat trudging its way to the means of production throughout the dismal 1990s.

Despair and gloom set in on a mass basis as the people came to appreciate that their futures were in the hands of gangsters. In Russia, for example, the Ministry of the Interior estimated that by mid-1997 forty thousand former state enterprises and five hundred banks were controlled by mobsters, and the gap between rich and poor had reached levels not seen since the days of the czars.

One by one government services collapsed as these gangster businesses became tax scofflaws, denying Moscow, Kyiv, Baku, and Tblisi billions of dollars' worth of revenue that might—ought—to have been used to run hospitals, pay schoolteachers, repair highways, and take care of the public health needs of the regional populace.

As the plight of the majority worsened, average, normally sane people in the region resorted to acts of madness. On a spring day in 1997 Muscovite Irina Smirnova threw her six-year-old daughter, Dina, out of a fourth-floor apartment window and then followed, plunging to her death. *Komsomolskaya Pravda* noted on May 23 that Smirnova was the third Moscow mother that week to commit suicide, taking her starving children with her. Weeks later Colonel Aleksandr Terekhov sat down in a Moscow subway station and set himself on fire. The same week, three thousand miles away, Private Sergei Polyansky stuck a pistol in his mouth and blew his brains out while on duty.[74] Everywhere groups of unpaid workers staged hunger strikes, hoping—in vain—that protests would promote government action.

Reactions took many forms, including the region's ancient bottom line, anti-Semitism. Average citizens and politicians blamed "the Jews" for the region's nightmares, sure, as they were, that behind every corrupt gangster and banker stood a vast Zionist conspiracy.[75]

Bad as all of this was, it soon grew far, far worse. After months of haggling amid concerns about corruption the IMF on April 13, 1998, finally approved a $22.6 billion loan package for Russia, offering $4.8 billion of it immediately to bolster the precarious ruble.

But by August 1, 1998, the Russian Central Bank was putting out half a billion dollars a day in a scramble to keep the ruble from collapsing. Though the government claimed that these efforts were keeping the currency stable, black market trade in rubles went wild, with the number of rubles needed to purchase one U.S. dollar inflating by more than 30 percent a week. Anticipating disaster, smart players moved their capital out of the country—at a rate of more than $2 billion a month. For several tense days the Yeltsin government continued the bailout until Western billionaire currency speculator George Soros said on August 13 that the ruble wasn't worth a fig.

The Russian stock market collapsed,[76] and the value of the ruble plummeted. An instant inflation backlash resulted, pushing the prices of food to levels never before seen in Russia. Beef soared in cost by 85 percent in a single day, milk by 60 percent. An already desperate populace fell into a mad scramble for the basics: food.

By the end of 1998 Russia's political and economic situations were in a tailspin, the nation owed $17 billion but only had $12.3 billion in its Central Bank, hyper-inflation set in at local food markets, the Moscow stock market had lost more than 100 percent of its value compared to the dollar, and capital hemorrhaged out of the country at an estimated rate of $3 billion each month.

"Each day without a government is a day closer to the abyss," a member of the Duma said.[77] Briefly in early 1997 it had looked like Russia might follow Poland and the Czech Republic down the road toward stability and free market success. Now it was clear that, instead, she was on a highway to hell. And she was dragging her neighbors down with her.

No nation owed the world's investors and IMF as much money in 1999 as did Russia, and the government wanted still more. The Russian bear was panhandling, offering the prospect of political instability in the nuclear weapons nations of Russia, Ukraine, and Belarus as ample incentive for continued Western spare change.

By 1999 many leading Western economists and politicians openly argued that it would be in the best interests of the Russians, Ukrainians, Moldovans, Belarusans, and others in the region if the flow of loans from the West simply stopped, cold.[78]

The threat of instability, however, seemed all too real, as terrorist bombings killed some three hundred Muscovites in the summer of '99, prompting a resurrection of warfare in the province of Chechnya. Billions of foreign aid dollars were drained, blood was shed, yet the war proved immensely popular among Russians, who favored strong, patriotic action to prevent further erosion in the nation's geographic and military influence. Riding the crest of that newfound national pride was Yeltsin's designated heir, former KGB operative Vladimir Putin, who was elected president of Russia in March 2000.

By then Russia's economy, along with that of its allied neighbors Ukraine and Belarus, was generating only 1 percent of global merchandise trade, and domestic inflation was running ahead of the nation's GDP growth rate. One man, Boris Berezovsky, controlled the bulk of the region's wealth and assets. And the once-feared Russian superpower was ranked by the influential Swiss International Institute for Management Development in 2000 as the least competitive large economy in the world, well behind such troubled economies as the Czech Republic, South Africa, Slovenia, Mexico, and India.[79]

Possibilities for the near future regionally included civil war, widespread anarchy, painfully slow stabilization of market economies, the splintering of Russia into as many as ten different nations, military coups, a regionwide return of Stalin-style Sovietism, and a sort of endless period of "muddling through."[80]

What all of this boded for public health was, of course, agony. By the end of 1998 at least forty-four million Russians were living on *less* than $32 a month:

that's one out of every three Russians. In Ukraine matters were so bad that the government couldn't even provide such statistics. In Belarus the Communist government may have had the grim numbers but refused to provide them.

Russian children bore the brunt of it all, turning into a massive, orphaned subpopulation that lived by its wits on the streets of the snowy nation. The Russian Association of Child Psychologists and Psychiatrists estimated in November 1998 that the number of abandoned and orphaned children suddenly doubled, to two million children—up from essentially zero in 1990. And the annual suicide rate among these cast-off youngsters was an astonishing 10 percent.[81] UNICEF estimated that since 1989 the region had experienced a 33 percent increase in the rate of child abandonment, suicide rates in under-nineteen-year-olds had more than doubled, and child school enrollment had fallen by more than 10 percent.[82]

In late 1998 the University of North Carolina conducted a survey that revealed that *all*—100 percent—of Russian children suffered iron deficiencies, most having only 3 to 4 percent of minimum daily requirement needs met in their terrible diets.[83] As Russians prepared for the bleak winter of 1998, a Moscow-based polling service queried them, asking how they expected to survive. Forty-four percent said that they hoped to live off the vegetables they had grown over the summer in their dacha gardens; 12 percent intended to live on game they planned to hunt in the Siberian tundra and taiga.[84] By 1999, the fastest-growing occupation in Russia was "dacha thievery," or stealing vegetables from strangers' gardens.[85]

Starvation was not common in the region's pregnant women and children, but malnutrition was. According to UNICEF, in Georgia, the average mother and child daily calorie consumption fell from 2,790 calories in 1980 to 1,940 in 1995: a 30 percent decrease. Russians were consuming an average of 21 percent fewer calories in 1996; Ukrainians 23 percent. Following the 1998 crash of the ruble caloric consumption fell still further.

Nothing weakens an immune system and overall health as efficiently as malnutrition, especially if families are, for economic reasons, substituting cheap fat and starch for more expensive proteins and fresh vegetables.

Georgian families in 1997 consumed only a third as much dairy products and almost four times less meat, poultry, and fish as they did in 1980, UNICEF figures showed. And Ukrainian, Russian, Estonian, and Armenian protein consumption declined by nearly as much.

The U.S. Centers for Disease Control and Prevention and World Health Organization considered the shocking deficiencies in micronutrients, such as iodine, potassium, calcium, and iron, to be so severe in much of the former Soviet Union that the agencies were blaming it for declining IQs, anemia, stunted

growth, and other developmental deficiencies seen on a mass scale in the region.[86] And some of these micronutrient deficiencies could also have rendered
the children more vulnerable to pollution and radiation.

A joint 1996 U.S.-Russian health study conducted by top government scientists from each country concluded that 60 percent of Russia's territory was
deficient in fluoride, accounting for the 85 percent tooth cavity rate in the nation's children.

When these nations were all part of the USSR and Soviet Bloc such things
as iodine and iron supplements were universally available, shipped from one
part of the vast region to another. After 1991, however, impoverished Georgia
struggled to find cash reserves with which to purchase iodized salt, and the
Ukrainian people had to do without fluoride entirely.

In the end, Russian analyst Revich said, it was clear that the children of
modern Russia and the rest of the former USSR were, indeed, less healthy than
their counterparts a decade previously. But the causes of their infirmities were
certainly more complex than the public believed. Pollution and radiation played
roles. But so did stress, economics, and diet.

"Any epidemiological research that uses immune system measurements
sees changes in the status of Russian children," Revich concluded.

"But as far as the quality and quantity of analysis and the reasons it has
happened—all of that we must say is unclear."

It might never be possible to empirically state how much regionwide malnutrition contributed to the 1990s demographic and public health catastrophe.
It certainly didn't help. During Soviet days the masses had money, but grocery
store shelves were empty.

But after the collapse of the Soviet Union the situation flipped 180 degrees.
Suddenly fruit, vegetable, and meat markets sprung up in even the remotest
parts of Siberia, where such exotica as Nicaraguan bananas, Dutch tomatoes,
and Florida oranges could be seen. But that was all most people could afford to
do: look. Food markets became something like museums through which the
masses strolled, their pockets bereft of *hryvnyas, laris,* or rubles.

And evidence of deprivation of even basic foodstuffs was starkly outlined
by visits to the marketplaces of the region.

In Zhitniy Market in Kyiv, Ukraine, gold-toothed peasant Galina sold an
average of two hundred kilos of potatoes a day in 1992—now she feels lucky if
she sells ninety. Tatyana says she can still afford to buy chicken once a week for
her five-year-old son, Dima, "because I deny it for myself."

The elderly babushkas who for years have made cheese in their village
homes and sold it in Zhitniy Market tell a visitor that the current sales are
"tragic."

"No customers! You stay here all day and then you take all the cheese home because you cannot sell it," toothless, elderly Katya cries.

Gori was Joseph Stalin's birthplace: a mountainous city of 160,000 residents, dominated by a three-story-tall, imperious statue of the "Father," as he was called, and a marble enshrined cabin in which Stalin was said to have been born.

About a mile from the Stalin shrine is a complex of rundown buildings, strafed with bullet holes during the mid-1990s civil war, that serves as the region's key hospital.

Pediatrician Tamriko Iluridze fights back tears as she speaks. "In comparison to ten to fifteen years ago we see that the quality of children's health is decreasing. We can't do neurological exams, but we see involuntary shivering, inabilities to hold their heads. The children's neurological status is impaired."

Behind her ten newborn babies, swaddled tightly in wool against the icy room temperature, lay two to a bassinet.

All too often Iluridze's boss, Dr. Nori Jorhadze, says babies here are born "hypoxic, the central nervous system is ill-prepared for external conditions. . . . The mothers say they are okay, but really they are not okay because the food isn't good enough for them. Nine out of ten women say they are eating, but what are they eating? Fat and bread."

Inside the central hospital's unheated corridors, lit dimly by clouded sunlight, the hospital director wrings his hands in despair, saying, "God save us from such conditions here! We are witnessing the ecological genocide of the nation."

V

The word progress *was always one of the key words in political speeches of my youth: look what progress we have made for a poor, peasant country; how many asphalt roads we have built, how many factories! Look how your life has improved! You're not starving any longer, your children go to school and have proper shoes, and everyone has electricity nowadays. No more tuberculosis or epidemics of other terrible diseases! Isn't that progress? And communism has brought you all that.*

—Slavenka Drakulić, 1997[87]

When the ancient scourge of diphtheria swept across the former Soviet Union beginning in 1990 the international health officials were stunned by its speed and frightened by its makeup. After all, diphtheria was a fully vaccine-preventable disease the occurrence of which in North America, Western Europe, and Japan was limited in the 1990s to one or two isolated cases per year.

When the *Corynebacterium diphtheriae* infected a human being the course of illness depended crucially on two factors: the site of bacterial colonization and which genetic subtype of bacteriophage was lodged inside the larger bacteria. The former determined the likelihood that an individual's immune system might bring the disease swiftly under control, with or without treatment. The latter was the key to diphtheria's virulence, as it was the viral corynebacteriophage lurking inside diphtheria bacteria that emitted lethal poisons. If the most toxic of bacteriophage were in an epidemic's bacteria, antibiotics would not prove effective in treatment and acute diphtheria cases would require antitoxin therapy.

In most cases *Corynebacterium diphtheriae* infected the mucous linings of the nose, mouth, and throat, forming a classic white membrane mass across the back of the victim's throat that prompted gagging and labored swallowing and breathing. In more severe cases the bacteria made their way into the victim's heart, brain, or nervous system, killing 10 percent of those so infected.

In 1994 diphtheria rates in the former Soviet region ranged from one case per 100,000 people to Tajikistan's abysmal 31.8 per 100,000—the highest seen anywhere in the world since the 1950s. Russia's was the second highest rate at 26.6 per 100,000, which was nearly thirty times the U.S. diphtheria rate and tolled to more than forty thousand cases in a single year. Cases were reported in every former Soviet and Eastern Bloc state, as well as Finland and Germany.

"This is the biggest public health threat in Europe since World War II," declared WHO's Dr. Jo Asvall. And it was one that "presents a danger and a risk for the population of a good many parts of the world that might have thought they were safe from such a disease as diphtheria," UNICEF's Richard Reid added.[88]

World Health Organization researchers, working with colleagues in Moscow, traced the epidemic backward, concluding that it was rooted in the long Soviet/Afghanistan war. During the 1980s Afghanistan had experienced a diphtheria epidemic involving nearly 14,000 cases of the disease. Beginning in 1988 some 100,000 Soviet soldiers left Afghanistan, returning to their respective homes or regimental bases. Unconfirmed anecdotes placed the first adult diphtheria cases in Russia in an army barracks located in Moscow, sometime in early 1990.

Most cases, they found, involved previously vaccinated adults, sparking fear that the epidemic that infected 200,000 people in the former Soviet Union, killing 5,000, could infect immunized adults worldwide. The last time that the USSR had experienced such a profound diphtheria epidemic was 1955, when

104,000 cases occurred. That was three years *before* the USSR began mass immunization. Was the world facing a new, resistant form of the disease, or was something else at play?[89]

In fact, experts discovered, something else was at play.

A 1995 study by the American Centers for Disease Control and Prevention found that nearly all of these cases occurred in a narrow group of people immunized either by natural exposure or with Soviet-made vaccines from the 1950s that didn't have enough diphtheria toxoid. The report went on to say that even though this group wasn't properly protected, they probably wouldn't have contracted diphtheria unless the level of disease in unvaccinated children during the late 1980s and 1990s was high enough to pose a threat.

Even though mistakes were made in the 1950s, it was the collapse of immunization in the 1980s and 1990s that put these adults at risk.

This collapse was fueled by two key factors: first, a surprising lack of expertise among immunologists trained during a Soviet era dominated by ideology, when access to Western medical journals—indeed, to any Western-based science—was banned; second, a mystifying theory of immunology that evolved in the region, suggesting that there were hundreds of good reasons *not* to vaccinate.

The theory—which ran counter to all Western scientific experience—held that vaccines sparked reactions that could be dangerous to "weak" children. Thus, any child who was ill for any reason (including a simple cold), who had a white blood cell count 5 percent below normal, or who had a family history of illness, would be harmed rather than helped.

"Vaccine coverage was very low in the 1980s. In Moscow in 1983, for example, only 40 percent of the children were fully immunized," Dr. Alexi Savinykh of the Russian Ministry of Health's MEDSOCECONOMINFORM, the government's major health think tank, said. And by 1992 the Moscow vaccination rate had dropped to an abysmal 34 percent, according to Dr. Eugene Tikhomirov of the emerging diseases division in the World Health Organization in Geneva. "It makes no sense to say Russian [or former Soviet] children are immunosuppressed and can't tolerate vaccines—none! But there it was."

While the diphtheria epidemic appeared by 1997 to have been brought largely under control in Russia, at least, with the help of health agencies from the United States and Europe, the attitudes and conditions that spawned it remained in place, driving other formidable diseases.

And vaccine expert Robert Steinglass, who was technical officer of the U.S. Agency for International Development–funded campaign to control the diphtheria epidemic, warned that "it's only a matter of time" before pertussis—or whooping cough—swept the region. This was because, he said, Soviets did not combine pertussis and diphtheria vaccines into DPT, as was done in the West.

Rather, pertussis was done separately and rates of successful immunization varied wildly across the region.

When Steinglass and his American colleagues first assessed the vaccination situation in 1992 they were stunned. In some areas, they found childhood immunization rates had fallen during the 1980s below levels seen in many sub-Saharan African countries. And basic requirements of vaccine delivery, such as consistent refrigeration of supplies—or maintaining a cold chain—were routinely ignored.

"They don't know how to manage stocks and inventories of vaccines," Steinglass explained. "They don't know how to manage a cold chain, which by now every African country understands."

It wasn't always so. Not at the height of the Soviet Sanitation and Epidemiology Service's (SanEp) power when upward of 280 million citizens could be lined up and immunized in a single month.

"It was a point of ideology," Steinglass explained. "People were pretty much told, 'You will report to this station on this date for a shot.' Period."

"Russian pediatricians were kind enough to try to save the Soviet children from vaccines," Dr. V. K. Tatochenko, chief pediatrician for the Russian Ministry of Health, said sarcastically. In 1978 and 1979, he said, Soviet officials introduced a long list of "contraindications" that told doctors to avoid vaccinating children with *any* condition—real or imagined—that could cause a child's white blood count to fall marginally. This, despite the fact that pediatricians in Western Europe and the United States found no need for such precautions.

Part of the problem, Tatochenko and others said, was that Western medical journals were banned in the Soviet Union for more than fifty years. So the "science" of immunology, as well as principles of pediatric practice, evolved despite controlled studies or serious data.

By the mid-1980s pediatricians all over the Soviet Union had been trained to believe, Tatochenko said, "that Russian children are weak, perishable. It doesn't mean [the child] has a pathology, but he's just not what he should be." And this belief eventually led to the "weak child" theory of immunology that at the dawn of the twenty-first century remained a major contributor to rates of death and disease that rivaled the third world.

Furthermore, in the absence of a sound, scientifically based concept of vaccination theory and practice during the 1980s doors opened for crackpots and pseudo-scientists, such as eighty-two-year-old Boris Nikitin, a bearded, bespectacled engineer and self-declared expert on child rearing who was often referred to as the Russian equivalent of America's Dr. Benjamin Spock. However, there was a key difference between the two highly read and influential authors: Nikitin lacked medical training and was proudly antiscience.

In the Moscow suburb of Bolshevo Nikitin lived in a three-story blue wooden home with his wife, seven adult children, and fifteen grandchildren. All of them went barefoot, even during the notorious Russian winter, and the grandchildren scampered about on a chilly, cloudy day in little more than their underwear.

This was all part of the Nikitin Doctrine, which held that most clothing, food, or water treatment and medical interventions weakened children.

"Nature," he tells visitors one spring afternoon, "has designed a certain stage in child development when natural immunity is formed. This natural mechanism is called children's infections.

"So this immunization of society is a great medical mistake."

As he plays with his naked granddaughter outdoors during the dusk chill, Nikitin explains his rationale: "Animals go barefoot. They don't have influenza or respiratory diseases."

Actually animals do have flu and respiratory diseases. But facts don't seem to stand in the way of Nikitin's philosophy: "You can decrease immunity," he says. "I don't know how, but I see the relationship. We must train our muscles. . . . Even medical people see that! But they don't see that you can train your immune system, as well."

Training, under the Nikitin Doctrine, is illness or exposure to pathogens. Indeed, Nikitin says he is thrilled that SanEp has lost its legal power to force immunization since 1991, allowing him to "save" two of his grandchildren from "the clutches of the vaccinologists."

But asked repeatedly about the diphtheria epidemic, he declines comment, changing the subject.

Journalist Boris Umnov—another key figure in the history of this sad doctrine—also refused to discuss the diphtheria epidemic. In 1988[90] Umnov wrote a much-cited article in *Komsomolskaya Pravda* declaring adamant opposition to vaccinations, based on a claim by a single Russian scientist—Dr. Galena Petrovna Chervonskaya, then a virologist in the Tereseeva State Research Institution of Medical Preparation in Moscow—that existing Russian-made diphtheria and pertussis vaccines contained dangerous poisons.

Since his publication[91] was read by young adults throughout the USSR, the impact was profound: parents began avoiding vaccinations for their children whenever possible, and pediatricians, fearing Chervonskaya could be right, did not aggressively push the vaccine on fretful parents.

Chervonskaya claimed the levels of Merthiolate (which she referred to as a pesticide, though it is not) and mercury salts found in the vaccine were toxic. And despite a study by the World Health Organization that disputed this, she and the influential Umnov continued a campaign into the mid-1990s—in most of Russia's leading newspapers and magazines—that suggested that use of the vaccine be ended.

Similar voices were heard in other former Soviet countries.

In Kazakhstan, for example, Dr. Raisa Sadykovna Amandzholova was in 1996 given the nation's highest meritorious award for her medical efforts. During the award ceremony, she argued that vaccination programs were killing children with "AIDS, tumors or blood cancer. The whole of children's oncology is over-filled. And that is the consequence of vaccination."

Amandzholova, who was seventy-six years old in 1996, said on the occasion of receipt of the "Honorary Degree for the honorary title of Peace and Culture" that vaccines were responsible for disintegration of the human gene pool.

"I want to pose a question as a scientist: what goal is harder? To protect children against infectious diseases but creating for them the risk of getting diseases and the plague of the XX century [AIDS and cancer]? As a result children are delivered unhealthy and this is passed from one generation to another. But it is time to think that perhaps natural selection is better than to spoil the genome of our people and cause mutations, the consequences of which are unpredictable."[92]

While voices such as Nikitin's, Chervonskaya's, and Amandzholova's got widespread play in the post-Communist media, vaccination supporters such as Tatochenko got virtually none. Tatochenko insisted that he argued constantly with Russian reporters, but realized they were looking for sensational angles. Steinglass and Tatochenko teamed up to spread a counterinformation campaign to the region's pediatricians and medical schools.[93] But it was tough going. Old ideas died hard.

For example, in the former Soviet state of Estonia, Dr. Toomas Trei explained, "The reason why the immunization rate in children is low is simple: 95 percent of the nation's doctors got their training at Tartu University. And the [Soviet] professor in charge of pediatrics taught that vaccines are dangerous. He said babies needed to grow without vaccines."

By 1991, according to the World Health Organization, only 60 percent of Russia's children under five years of age had received the three doses of diphtheria, pertussis, and tetanus vaccines necessary to ensure immunity—even though WHO experts contended a 95 percent rate was needed to prevent epidemics. The antivaccine sentiment had even reached Germany, on both sides of the Berlin Wall, where diphtheria vaccination was incomplete or absent altogether for nearly a quarter of the adult population in 1997.[94]

And that was only one part of the story, statistics showed. Russian measles vaccine coverage was only 78 percent in 1991; its polio coverage a mere 71 percent; and virtually *no* girls were vaccinated against rubella.[95]

The diphtheria epidemic first surfaced in the USSR in 1987, when the number of confirmed cases reached 2,000. Then in 1990 soldiers returning from Afghanistan apparently introduced the particular strain of the bacteria that would spread. That diphtheria toll then grew to more than 12,000 in 1991, when Moscow asked for help from the World Health Organization and the United States. The Bush administration agreed to provide assistance, sending scientific teams to Russia, Ukraine, Georgia, and other former Soviet states throughout 1992 and '93.[96]

What the Western researchers found was shocking. First, their own stocks of vaccine—indeed, global supplies—were desperately low.

And in the former Soviet nations, the Westerners learned, millions of children had received inappropriate adult-dosed shots, and these children had five times the diphtheria rate seen in children immunized with appropriate doses. And they found that, as Steinglass had noted, their Soviet counterparts knew nothing of one of the most essential principles of vaccinology, the so-called Cold Chain or necessity to maintain refrigeration of vaccines throughout transport and storage.[97]

Even more astounding were the regional death rates. By 1994 diphtheria had made its way into every single one of the former Soviet states, prompting an only marginally above-normal death rate in Russia of 2.8 percent of all active cases. But in Lithuania and Turkmenistan an astonishing 23 percent of all diphtheria cases proved fatal.[98]

After two years of intense effort and distribution of more than 30 million vaccine doses the international team had, by mid-1996, vaccinated 70 percent of all Ukrainians, pushing diphtheria incidence down by 30 percent. But as nearly a third of all children and adults in the country remain unvaccinated, the situation was still critical.

Dr. Alla Shcherbynska of the L. V. Gromashevski Epidemiology and Infectious Diseases Research Institute in Kyiv said that during the 1970s, before all of the antivaccine sentiment arose among Soviet pediatricians, Ukraine's fifty-two million people experienced an average of seven diphtheria cases a year. By 1990, she said, that number had risen to two hundred and in 1992 one out of every 100,000 Ukrainians (or nearly 50,000 people) suffered a case of diphtheria—a level of disease not witnessed since Czarist days.

The incentive to "smash" the antivaccine movement suprisingly might not be diphtheria but polio, which also resurged in the region. The paralytic effect of the polio virus upon children and the microbe's highly contagious nature rendered this disease especially worrisome. Further, the World Health Organization, backed strongly by the USSR, had long ago set a goal of complete global eradication of polio by 2000. Any return of polio to the former Soviet Socialist Republics was, then, a genuine slap in the faces of SanEp and its antecedents.

Between 1959 and 1991 all supplies of polio vaccine used in the Eastern Bloc and Soviet Union were manufactured by the Institute of Poliomyelitis and Viral Encephalitis, located in Moscow. Like the iodine to prevent goiters, chlorine for water purification, and fluoride for dental care, supplies of polio vaccines suddenly disappeared with the collapse of the Soviet Union. By mid-1992 every single one of the former Soviet republics—except the Russian Federation—was using up the last of their polio vaccine inventories.

In late 1991 a strain of the most virulent form of polio—poliovirus type 1—surfaced in Tajikistan. And it continued for four years, as Tajik public health leaders proved incapable of mounting an effective national polio vaccine campaign until late 1995.[99]

The Tajik polio strain spread to Ukraine in 1992, infecting thousands more people and causing a small number of paralytic cases.

The following year a different, thankfully less virulent, type 3 strain of poliovirus emerged in Uzbekistan, where all supplies of vaccine had long since dried up and thousands of youngsters were unimmunized. An estimated 146,000 children were infected between 1993 and 1994, equaling more than a third of the affected area's under-four-year-old children.[100]

These polio outbreaks, like the larger diphtheria epidemic, were brought under control through massive vaccination campaigns, underwritten by European and North American governments.

In war-torn Chechnya, however, all child immunization efforts ground to a complete halt in 1992. And in 1995 the Tajik type 3 virus found its way into Chechnya, resulting in an epidemic that infected by far the majority of all under-five-year-olds in the breakaway area, causing paralytic disease in 154 of them.

Fearing that the Chechnyan polio epidemic could quickly spread across Russia, Dr. Gennady Onyschenko, the Ministry of Health's top infectious disease official, loaded up vaccine supplies and flew to the Chechnyan capital, Grozny. A tall, charismatic man with piercing blue eyes, Onyschenko was accustomed to holding sway during Soviet health crises. In post-Soviet Russia, however, he said he had a "revelation—a rather unpleasant shot to us—to discover even the medical specialists were not aware how important immunization is."

Having spent considerable time arguing with Russian doctors in order to raise diphtheria immunization rates and halt that bacterial epidemic, Onyschenko was in no mood for debate about polio. Despite a bloody civil war, he planned to simply march into Grozny and start vaccinating every single young child he saw.

But the Chechnyan leaders had other ideas. One of the several gangs vying for control of Chechnya kidnaped Onyschenko and held him—and the precious polio vaccines—hostage for several months. Eventually freed, Onyschenko was physically and mentally exhausted by his captivity, and the polio vaccines he'd brought had long since deteriorated into useless glop.

At the war's end Chechnyan vaccination resumed, bringing an end to the polio outbreak during the final weeks of 1996.

A key set of lessons for public health were revealed. First, immunization levels could not be permitted to fall below the 95 percent level in any corner of the world without creating pockets of vulnerability into which lurking microbes rapidly emerged. Vaccine supply shortages, local wars, and cash flow problems could not be considered adequate excuses, as microbial surges were spectacularly swift and, ultimately, far more costly than continued immunization campaigns. Happily, the diphtheria and polio events also demonstrated that mass scale immunization works, halting outbreaks and swiftly slowing epidemics to manageable proportions. In short, vaccines remained marvelously effective elements in the public health toolbox.

Sadly, the same could not be said for antibiotics.

It came as a sad shock to anyone who meets him to learn that Irakli Sherodzle was fifteen years old. Frail and tiny, Sherodzle looks like an elementary school child of ten or eleven years.

Sherodzle and his mother, Rovena, are civil war refugees who live in a one-room apartment with no light, because they can't afford a light bulb. Their tiny apartment is inside an enormous hotel converted by the Georgian government to emergency shelter for civil war refugees. Ice-cold, lacking light bulbs in its halls, and with staircases ringing with sounds of arguments and political debates, it is a grim setting. On a day made colder by bone-chilling rain, mother and son huddle around an orange hot steel electronic coil on the floor—their only source of heat—and talk in gentle voices that whisper out of the room's darkness.

Weakened by illness, Irakli speaks with effort and deliberation. His mother, an unemployed widow, talks quickly. Irakli is dying from streptococcus, a type of microbe an American might pause to consider only for about as long as it takes to say the word *penicillin.*

"He has no father," Rovena tells a visitor. "Maybe America can help him."

Similar cries for help echoed all across the former Soviet Union where rampant misuse of antibiotics and archaic hospital hygiene practices were promoting the emergence of more and more deadly, drug-resistant strains of common bacteria.

Though the ingredients for antibiotic disaster were in place before the 1991 collapse of communism, the ensuing economic chaos dramatically worsened matters. As the pace of bacterial mutation and spread quickened in this region, neighboring nations in Western Europe and immigration destinations such as the United States and Canada were becoming concerned about the spread of bacterial superbugs.

In Georgia, Irakli pulls up his pant legs and with great difficulty stands, supported by Rovena's firm grip. Both legs have a large gash up the front, revealing fetid flesh-eating infection and the boy's shin bones. Irakli can only stand long enough to give visitors a quick glimpse of his osteomyelitis—a condition in which the streptococci eat both flesh and bone. Since January, when Irakli developed a high fever, heart flutters, and severe weakness, strep has invaded his heart, blood, flesh, and bones.

Back in January mother and child had gone to Republican Hospital—a huge, deteriorating medical complex in downtown Tblisi—where Irakli was hospitalized for what was then a routine infection: he was given penicillin. After several days of treatment, however, the boy's situation nose-dived.

"That's because every microbe in the nation of Georgia is now resistant to penicillin," said pediatric surgeon Irakli Gogorishvili, who did not treat the young patient. "People took it for everything—even for a bad mood. So for sepsis [blood poisoning], meningitis, and so on we now assume penicillin won't work. So we start with cephalosporins."

Expensive and more complicated to use properly, cephalosporins are a class of newer antibiotics. In February, the doctors told Rovena she would have to supply Irakli with cephalosporins, which in Georgia cost ten times more than penicillin. To buy the drugs—even at bargained down black-market prices—Rovena sold all but two outfits of her clothing, leaving her one set for winter, one for summer. She sold the emergency relief food she received as a refugee, and every memento except her dead husband's portrait. She even sold the wedding ring she had removed from his finger before he was buried.

After a week, though, Irakli's fever rose again. And doctors said Irakli's streptococcus was probably resistant to that treatment as well—though they weren't sure, since the hospital had no way to test the bacteria.

Laboratory capacity was largely absent throughout the former Soviet Union, both for fiscal reasons and because physicians in the former Communist regime were never trained to work with their microbiology counterparts. Laboratories existed in hospitals not so much to help with diagnosis and treatment, but to police SanEp hygienic practices that, in the end, contributed little to patient well-being.

Because no lab work was done, no one will know whether the bacteria that originally made Irakli mildly ill was the same strain that, after three weeks of hospitalization, is threatening his life. But given conditions in Soviet-era hospitals, it is quite possible that Irakli's deadly strep was a microbe acquired in the very place he sought refuge from infection: Republican Hospital.

In Georgia's hospitals, Gogorishvili said, "Ciprofloxacin you can forget about. People use it like tea in the morning. Doxycycline—people buy it on the black market and use it for STDs [sexually transmitted diseases], so it's useless now." Amoxicillin is following the same route, he said, though tetracycline remains effective.

The doctors treating Irakli told Rovena to find more money, to buy third-generation cephalosporins. When she discovered that a week's worth of those drugs, plus syringes to inject them and vitamins to help rebuild his body, would cost more than $300, Rovena was horrified.

Many stepped forward to help. "The head of the committee of refugees . . . here raised the money for his antibiotics," Rovena said; the surgeon who dressed Irakli's infection wounds waived his fees; the hospital charged nothing for three weeks' stay; friends brought donated meals to the bedside.

But it was not enough. Though the boy improved briefly from the initial treatment, returning home in March, Rovena couldn't afford to keep the treatment up indefinitely and, in April, mother and son huddled together in their icy room, without options, watching the streptococcus resurge.[101]

In the Deserters Bazaar—so named because hundreds of Georgian draft dodgers congregated there during the Soviet war in Afghanistan—Goga sells antibiotics to customers like Rovena. An economics student with no medical training, Goga advises customers on how to use the drugs and which to take for their ailments—which he is also happy to diagnose, if asked. Goga's stand offers everything from Ukrainian transfusion kits, Turkish syringes and IV saline, and Indian-manufactured condoms, to Bulgarian-made kanomycin and expired antituberculosis drugs bearing insignias of Western humanitarian organizations.

"The official pharmacies have to pay taxes, rent, and so on," Goga explains. "So their prices are two times higher. I also have a much greater supply of drugs here and no drug lies on a table for more than two days. We have a huge turnover."

The Deserters Bazaar, and hundreds of markets like it all over the former Soviet Union, was full of such impromptu, illegal drugstores. At a similar stand in Kyiv, Ukraine, a former schoolteacher diagnosed an elderly woman's arthritis and sold her ampules of steroids that the bewildered woman was told to self-inject. In the Siberian city of Irkutsk, a woman who described herself as a housewife diagnosed ailments in an open market and freely prescribed antibiotics.

While quacks and marketeers dispensed admonishments against vaccination and bolstered the widespread misuse of antibiotics, infectious disease tolls rose dramatically.[102]

Rheumatic fever raged across western Ukraine, for example, in the rural Lviv area. Caused by type A streptococcus bacterial infection, rheumatic fever was an infection of the heart that commonly led to growth stunting and severe, lifelong cardiac disease.

"The problem is very severe," elderly Dr. Miraslava Strouck, chief statistician for the Lviv Institute, explained in an insistent, throaty voice. "About 19 percent of the patients become invalids."

In 1994 Strouck began to realize that doctors were filing too many heart disease reports on teenagers. When she added up the numbers it looked like nearly one out of every one hundred youngsters aged fifteen to seventeen years were suffering major cardiac disease, which on the face of it made no sense. Then, in 1995, she received reports on 710 "heart defects" in teenagers—a figure far too high to be due to any normal event.

Working backward with her painstaking attention to detail Strouck realized that western Ukraine was in the midst of a largely unrecognized strep A epidemic, prompting astonishing rheumatic fever rates. In 1996, she found, the teenage rheumatic fever rate was 7.1 per 1,000 and the adult rate was 9.3 per 1,000.

The U.S. rheumatic fever rate in 1995 was about one case in every 2.6 million Americans, for a total nationwide of 112 cases.

"By the end of 1996 we had about 20,000 cases in Lviv Oblast," Strouck said. "There were 1,500 pediatric, 800 teenager, and 18,000 adults."

Donated American antibiotics proved far more effective in treating the strep A infections compared to locally available drugs, Strouck said, causing her to conclude that the Lviv strain was resistant to first-line, affordable drugs. But she didn't know for sure.

"In the former USSR there was only one laboratory, in St. Petersburg, which could identify strep A. That's why there are no labs in all of Ukraine which could identify this streptococcus and give us data about its virulence. . . . To start such a lab we need supplies, reagents, and, unfortunately, the economic conditions right now prevent us."

So rheumatic fever continued its spread in rural Lviv Oblast.

At the World Health Organization's Geneva headquarters Dr. Maria Neira was wringing her hands over an even more basic public health crisis in the East: water. Everywhere that she cast her surveillance net Neira found more outbreaks in the formerly Communist world of cholera, typhoid fever, shigella—all diseases that were entirely preventable with proper water and sewage treatment facilities. There need not be epidemics in the modern world of any of these diseases, Neira argued, as treatment was cheap and highly effective.

So Neira was stunned, she said, by the East's inability to control such outbreaks. Beginning in 1992 she and other WHO technical experts made frequent trips eastward, hoping to decipher the causes of both the outbreaks and treatment failures.

"We did a seminar in Kyiv, Ukraine [in 1995], and it was *very* hard to convince the old [public health] leadership," Neira recalled. "They wanted to call the army in, encircle the entire place where cholera broke out, go out to the frontiers and round people up, forcing them into hospitals. And then they wanted to keep them in those hospitals until they had three successive stools negative for cholera vibrio," after, typically, fifteen to eighteen days of hospitalization.

That was the old Soviet, SanEp, model: bring in the military and police, compel obedience from the masses, and enforce a treatment protocol that was both phenomenally expensive to the state and personally offensive to the affected population.

Meanwhile, simpler, cheaper solutions were ignored. For example, when a cholera epidemic exploded in Romania in 1994, lasting two years and felling thousands of Romanians with severe diarrheal disease, Neira's office was dumbfounded by the country's public health response:

"In Romania they injected all sorts of high-dose antibiotics to treat cholera. They don't understand that cholera vibrio do not respond to antibiotics," Neira said, her face expressing frank astonishment. "They want electrophoresis and amyloid analyzing equipment," all expensive and entirely unnecessary. When Neira's team carefully explained that worldwide cholera was best treated simply with oral rehydration therapy—a mixture of clean water and salts that stop the deadly dehydration induced by cholera—the Romanian public health officials snapped at WHO experts: "Don't come here with your guidelines for African poor people—cholera guidelines are for Africans. We are Europeans!"

But WHO concluded that some former Soviet-dominated countries—particularly Ukraine—had "sanitation that is worse than in Africa," Neira said.

WHO water engineers discovered that all over the region Soviet urban planners had bundled drinking water and sewage pipes, burying them one atop the other under the region's densely populated cities. The pipes, which typically were of iron or steel, had been subjected to decades of freezing winters during which they were encased in ice, followed by summer thaws when rust claimed the conduits. There had been little attention to maintenance over the years, and by the 1990s sewer pipes commonly leaked directly into drinking water carriers.

The result was that the populaces of such places as St. Petersburg, Tblisi, Bucharest, Dushanbe, Kyiv, and Moscow were—literally—drinking and washing in their own waste. That obvious disaster was compounded by acute chlorine shortages that were the result of the same production and distribution problems that rendered the region deficient in micronutrients, such as iron and iodine.

A long litany of diarrheal epidemics ensued, and due to leaking stagnant water supplies, so did mosquito-carried diseases such as malaria and encephalitis.[103]

At the close of 1995 the Russian Environment Ministry concluded that half of the nation's drinking water supply was unsafe, either due to severe industrial pollution or biological contamination. Without funds to improve the situation the water remains at the close of the twentieth century only marginally better in most of Russia than it was at the century's beginning.[104]

"How can a nation feel safe if her air and water are polluted . . . and half of the population drinks water that doesn't meet basic standards?" asked the Russian Academy of Medical Science's Gerasimenko in 1997.[105]

The typhoid fever epidemic was a particularly critical example of the water crisis. Spread through contaminated water supplies, the *Salmonella typhi* bacterium readily exploited any disaster situation that led to reduced water safety. In January 1996 in Tajikistan's capital city of Dushanbe a handful of typhoid fever cases were diagnosed. By mid-1997 hospitals in the capital were diagnosing 200 new cases *per day*, 10 percent of the city's 600,000 residents had active cases of the disease, and no one could even count the typhoid rates outside the city—in part because of the nation's ongoing civil war.

In addition to eroded water and sewer systems, massively scaled, badly conceived Soviet water projects also ended up increasing the incidences of human waterborne diseases.

Taking a visitor to stand before a map-covered wall in his small office Ivan Rusiev, ecosystems expert for the Soviet Plague Laboratory in Odessa, pointed to the Dnieper River: "The main idea in the Soviet Union was that they planned to transfer fresh water from north rivers—here—to the south—down here. They planned to pump the Danube River into the Dnieper. And the first stage of the master plan was here—Saslyk Lake."

All of southern Ukraine was, Rusiev explained, a swampy delta estuary, right up to the Black Sea. The Soviets wanted to bring fresh river water down to the delta region for irrigation. The fresh water was dumped into salty Saslyk Lake, which actually was a Black Sea estuary.

The plan was a disaster. Misguided Soviet engineers ended up miscalculating the ratios of salty and fresh water in Saslyk Lake, flooding the delta fields with overly salty water that left sixty thousand devastated hectares upon which no crops would grow. And they turned Saslyk into a gigantic blue/green algae pond in which all sorts of mosquitoes and disease-causing microbes thrived. For two decades—well into the Brezhnev era—Soviet planners ignored the rising diseases incidence, refusing to acknowledge their profound environmental plumbing fiasco. Finally in 1985 they erected a dam across the Dniester River, hoping to improve matters. But this completely eliminated fresh water supplies to the delta, turning the area into a salted moonscape.

Meanwhile, Saslyk and other similarly altered lakes in Ukraine bred cholera vibrio, which thrived in the new algae colonies. And the dams slowed waterflow rates so badly that there was little mixing. The lakes became bacterial stew pots, especially in the summer, when the water was sixteen degrees centigrade, emitting classic organic stenches. They also bred mosquitoes that carried malaria, West Nile Virus, and Sindbis virus. And the slowed rivers no longer flushed out the tons of unprocessed human waste dumped into them by upstream municipalities.

By the time all of this water reached Odessa and the Crimean Sea ports it was so microbially contaminated that local water, if consumed unboiled, was guaranteed to cause dysentery.

"Our authorities do their best, but everything stumbles over finances," Rusiev says with a shrug. But then he amends his statement: "But I tell them we have not only problems with finances, but also problems with our brains. When problems arise you need to think of the river. It's the source of water for ten million people!"

What could be more basic an element of public health than water? Or immunization? Or safe and adequate food supplies? Or elimination of antibiotic-resistant microbes?

Yet in each of these cases the Soviet leadership failed, blundering its way through one poorly designed and executed scheme after another. What happened in these arenas after 1991 constituted collapse of houses of Communist cards, not decimation of once-solid systems of public health.

VI

When a prolonged, stubborn, and heated struggle is in progress, there usually begins to emerge after a time the central and fundamental points at issue, upon the decision of which the ultimate outcome of the campaign depends, and in comparison with which all the minor and petty episodes of the struggle recede more and more into the background.

—V. I. Lenin, "One step forward, two steps back," 1904

Konstantin, an emaciated, bedridden thirty-nine-year-old former Soviet soldier, lies dying at the Moscow Tuberculosis Research Center. Drug-resistant TB has invaded his lungs, liver, kidneys, and heart.

Still, he says with a smirk that he appreciates the irony of the situation. "It's like a joke," he notes, his soft, ruined voice interrupted frequently by fits of coughing, "a particularly Russian joke."

It's hard to see the humor in Konstantin's situation. An IV drip pumps cocktails of antibiotics into his body twenty-four hours a day. Despite a bath of warm sunlight spread across his hospital bed Konstantin wears a wool knit cap and two sweaters, lies under layers of blankets, and still shivers. His colorless face and sunken eyes betray Konstantin's peril, and a doctor whispers that there is little hope for the man, as every vital organ of Konstantin's body is overwhelmed with tuberculosis bacteria.

Still, Konstantin sees irony in his plight, he says between bouts of coughs that seem to shake his lungs right out of their protective rib cage. And for a Russian, he continues, irony equals a joke. A Russian joke.

"I did it all," Konstantin begins. "Komsomol, Communist Party, fighting in Afghanistan . . ."

A decorated intelligence officer in the Afghanistan War, Konstantin returned to Moscow suffering from post-traumatic stress and was discharged in 1991, just before the Soviet dissolution. When Moscow radio announced in 1993 that fellow-Communists and a hodgepodge of other anti-Yeltsin forces had seized the Russian White House, Konstantin grabbed the Afghani rifle he had brought home with him and dutifully reinforced the barricades.

"In 1993 I took an active part in the political turmoil. I supported the coup," Konstantin recalled.

But the rebellion failed, and a year later Konstantin was arrested for high treason. He was sent to Butirka prison without a trial, or formal sentencing, where, he recalls, "I got TB in 1995."

For months after that, his health deteriorated as he was transferred from one prison facility to another, his medications constantly interrupted and changed. Finally, in January 1997, a judge reviewed his case for the first time, ruling that since he wasn't in the army when the coup occurred, he couldn't have committed high treason. And for the first time in nearly three years, Konstantin was free.

But the exoneration was cold comfort. "In principle," Konstantin says with Russian stoicism, "I was given a death sentence. The paradox is that most people are in there like me, waiting for court action, not even sentenced. I remember several people in prison who died of TB and never had a day in court."

Mirian wanders the halls of the Moscow TB sanatorium, bored but exhausted. The skinny, pale Georgian also caught tuberculosis in jail—in his case at the notorious Matrosskaya Tishina prison—in 1993 and four years later is still struggling with the now multidrug-resistant microbes that have overrun his lungs. Arrested for robbery, Mirian served three years in a thirty-square-meter jail cell inhabited by more than a hundred prisoners, he softly says. Each prisoner, then, had less than a half a square meter of space, or about a chunk of personal turf measuring one foot by one foot. To sit or sleep the men rotated, Mirian said, taking turns alternately packing like sardines to stand for eight hours while other men lay down and slept.

The crowding in Russian jails and prisons was a post-1991 crisis born of the new nation's need to create a judicial system. Where once a mere KGB whisper backed by no evidence had been enough to land someone in a lifetime of imprisonment now judges were required to impartially oversee trials in which prosecutors and defense attorneys argued over the merits of available evidence. But few such judges and attorneys existed in Russia, as the very concept of legal defense in the face of prosecution had long been anathema. While the nation struggled to invent a system of jurisprudence men piled up in the nation's jails, most having never formally been indicted. As Russia's crime rate escalated after 1991, so did the size of her unindicted prison population, reaching 500,000 in 1996.[106] And Russia was hardly alone: the entire region was struggling to create judicial systems while untried prisoner populations piled up.

Released in October 1996 Mirian transferred to the Moscow sanatorium. And there he remained nearly a year later, held captive by tubercular microbes.

Asked why his TB has proven incurable, twenty-five-year-old Mirian shrugs: "I can remember that at Butirka there were different tablets we got once a day. Different ones, changing all of the time."

According to TB experts, staying just three years in the Russian jail system—home to an amazing 1 in 148 Russian residents in 1997—was tantamount to a death sentence from tuberculosis. And world health experts argued that unless Russia stopped the rampant spread of TB there, it hadn't a prayer of controlling it in the society at large.

"The easiest way to bring the Russian TB epidemic under control is with a focus on prisoners," said Belgian physician Tine Demeulenaere of Médecins Sans Frontières (MSF). "Cure them. Stop the recycling of TB."

With up to one million people jamming the jails, overcrowding had become acute. At Moscow's Matrosskaya Tishina pre-trial detention center, for example, there were 140 prisoners per 35-bed cell, with a per-prisoner "space" rate of 0.1 square meters, according to photo documentation provided by the independent Center for Prison Reform. By the summer of 1995 people were actually dying of lack of oxygen, as there were simply too many men packed in each cell.[107]

"We now know that some 50 percent of [Russian] prisoners are estimated to have TB," says Murray Feshbach. "And we also are now told that some 850,000 to one million persons are in prison."

So it seems logical, he said, to conclude that there were up to 500,000 Russian prisoners with TB—a rate forty times higher than in the general population. Indeed, an unpublished Ministry memo supported that claim, noting that prisoners in Siberian jails, alone, were contracting more than 6,500 new cases per year per 100,000 prisoners—the highest infection rate recorded in the latter half of the twentieth century in any risk group in the world, according to the World Health Organization.

Nestled in the Caucasus Mountains in the southern region of the former Soviet Union, the little nation of Georgia was in the late 1990s trying to tackle its tuberculosis epidemic with a strategy that met Western approval. And key to stopping its TB epidemic was elimination of the disease in Georgian prisons.

Dr. George Nashievili, director of the nation's TB services, was waging a two-pronged attack on the problem, focusing on Georgia's urban centers. Following a World Health Organization approach called DOTS (Directly Observed Therapy System), Nashievili was trying to rebuild Georgia's demolished network of TB outpatient clinics and from them dispense appropriate antibiotics to identified tuberculosis cases and carriers. But he knew that it would be impossible to stop the spread of TB in the general population unless it was first eliminated from the nation's jails and prisons.

Though the numbers of prisoners dying each year of TB in Georgia paled when compared to neighboring Russia, tuberculosis was the leading cause of death in prison, surpassing violence and heart disease, according to Givi Kvarelashvili, head of the National Committee of Incarceration.

To conquer the TB problem in prisons, Kvarelashvili's medical staff regularly scours the prison population in search of visibly ill men, who are then given chest X rays. Those who are confirmed TB cases are separated: acute cases go to one special holding area, chronic tuberculosis sufferers to another. All patients are given DOTS antibiotic therapy, involving four drugs, daily. In addition, TB prisoners are put on special, highly nutritious diets and issued wool blankets.

As a result of this program TB death rates have fallen by 50 percent over the two years of the new prison program, Nashievili said.

Normally that would be cause for joy, but Nashievili was cautious about interpreting TB trends either in the jails or on the outside—due to unreliable Sovet-era records and nonexistent records during the post-1991 chaos and civil war. Still he was convinced that Georgia's TB situation had begun to improve.

Dr. Maya Sharashidze wasn't so sure. Her privately funded Georgia Foundation surveyed and treated TB in the remote Sagarejo region of the country. In every village the medical team had found hidden cases—individuals who for one reason or another never sought medical attention for the TB that they knew was responsible for their weakness and coughing.

"Georgians feel ashamed of TB," Sharashidze explained over tea and khachapuri cheese bread in her Tblisi home. "They try to keep it confidential. They do not tell neighbors, and do not go to doctors."

Though no one in Georgia had the necessary laboratory equipment to conduct drug resistance tests, Sharashidze said, it was also clear that most TB in the country was resistant to at least one of the five antibiotics used in the primary treatment cocktail.

So even if Georgia one day managed to get its prison outbreaks and Tblisi epidemics under control, Sharashidze said, the rural epidemic would persist and increase in drug resistance. Furthermore, in the wake of the civil war Georgia faced newer TB problems among refugees and civilians living in the contested areas.

In Southern Ossetia, for example, four tuberculosis patients huddle in a bombed-out hospital, trying to absorb heat from a log that smoldered on the concrete floor. They are the only patients in what had been the City Hospital of Tskhinvali, population 42,000. Volunteers from Médecins Sans Frontières built a toilet at the site, and puttied glass into the windows of the TB ward. But the patients use the former operating room to chop wood and furniture for their tiny fires. They are, in essence, camping out inside the rubble hull left by war.

MSF nurse Jean-Luc Seugy says the people of devastated Ossetia approach TB with "aggressive denial," taking whatever antibiotics they can buy on the black market until their money runs out. And never seeking medical attention. In the process they are breeding drug-resistant strains of tuberculosis. Even when family members die of TB the relatives refuse to be tested.

Amid the chaos that had become the norm in Ukraine's health system, children were suffering the highest levels of TB seen in that country since the 1950s, when antibiotic-based public health approaches to the disease were initiated.

"The situation is just dreadful. It is dreadful," exclaimed Dr. Victoria Kostromira, director of pediatric services for the Kyiv Institute of Pulmonology. "There are not only many more children with TB than we've seen in the past, they are getting forms of the disease we've never seen before."

The number of diagnosed tuberculosis cases in Ukrainian children under age fifteen doubled between 1990 and 1996, Kostromira said, and with diagnostic capacity down to near-zero levels for mild cases, it had become almost impossible to estimate the disease's true rate.

And more of the Ukrainian pediatric tuberculosis cases were proving fatal. Prior to 1992, for instance, Ukraine had no TB-related meningitis cases. In 1996 there were thirty such cases, and twenty-four children died.

Kostromira's institute had a supply of just four first-line antibiotics, she said, and every day their usefulness diminished. That was because the front line TB dispensaries in the former Soviet state of 52 million people had run out of money.

When the Soviet Union was intact, Moscow created single production centers for specific items and shipped the products all over the vast nation: chlorine, vaccines, iodine. In the past, raw materials for antibiotics were made in one area, and packaged as useful drugs in another. Almost immediately after the 1991 breakup of the Soviet Union the chain of production collapsed. The result, in terms of TB treatment, was that Ukraine had to import all of its antibiotics; nothing was manufactured inside the country. And that meant that the essential drugs were anywhere from ten to one hundred times more expensive for Kostromira and her patients in 1997 than they were in 1987.

Once the frail tubercular children reached the institute their care—including meals—was free. The trick for anxious families spread out over the large nation was getting diagnosed at a local TB clinic and finding the resources to travel to Kyiv.

"We used to be full," Kostromira said of her institute, built under the Soviet regime to serve patients diagnosed at local TB clinics throughout the large republic. "Now patients can't afford to get here." Galina managed to bring her grandson, Janya, to the institute in August 1996. They lived only fifteen kilometers outside Kyiv, so it wasn't a difficult journey, Galina says.

On a cold, overcast day, she and her grandson lie quietly on his hospital bed in a room that is also home to three other children. The lights are turned off to save hospital electricity costs, and there is no heat. In the late afternoon shadows, Galina reads slowly to the tiny five-year-old boy, whose growth has been visibly stunted by his bout with tuberculosis. She hesitates while he coughs, which is frequently, since he suffers from a bronchial infection.

But it was Russia's out-of-control tuberculosis epidemic that most worried WHO and Western public health experts. By the close of the 1990s, the multidrug-resistant tuberculosis epidemic, spawned in packed prison populations, spanned the entire nation, often at incidence rates unseen anywhere else in the world at that time.

Prison treatment options were limited. While the Russian Interior Ministry made TB treatment available to prisoners at its own medical facilities, health officials throughout Russia complained that the treatment could do more harm than good. That was because it remained standard practice to give prisoners only one or two antibiotics at a time, rather than the four or five recommended by the World Health Organization. And the drugs were often catch-as-catch-can, since ministry officials allocated little money to the effort. Further, prisoners were subject to frequent transfers among jails, which meant they often underwent the type of treatment changes that promote the emergence of drug resistance. And once released, 95 percent fell out of the public health system entirely.

The result: Dr. Alexey Priymak, then director of TB services for the Ministry of Health, said that about 80 percent of all infected ex-prisoners in Russia carried drug-resistant strains of bacteria, and half would die of TB-related symptoms within twelve months of their release from prison.

In Soviet times TB care was simple and straightforward. Every single man, woman, and child in the USSR was required by law to undergo an annual chest X ray. Any suspicious X-ray films were sent to SanEp, which rounded up the possible TB carriers and compelled sputum tests. If proven infected, the individual was placed in a sanatorium for months, often years, isolated from contact with friends or family until several repeated sputum tests came up negative for TB. This was policy for infants, as well as older children and adults. During their sanatorium stay the Soviet TB patients received, typically, one or two antibiotics in high doses.

But with the collapse of the Communist state no one had the power to impose TB incarceration upon Russian or Georgian citizens. As a result all public health TB control measures had fallen to pieces because they rested during Soviet days upon the power of the state to impose screening and treatment upon its citizens.

So by 1997, officials said, Russia's primary drug resistance rate was 23.4 percent; 21 percent to two drugs; 19.4 percent to three drugs; 6.4 percent to more than four antibiotics.

In the jails incidence of TB, and resistant tuberculosis, continued to rise. At the Tomsk central prison, for example, the TB incidence was 7,000 per 100,000—ten times the general Siberian TB rate.[108] Estimated rates in other Russian prisons ranged from 2,481 per 100,000 to more than 7,000 per 100,000.

And the prison system was every day feeding costly, multidrug-resistant, TB-infected patients into the beleaguered state public health network. A 1997 Ministry of Interior memo leaked to a visiting foreigner contained these disturbing lines:

"By the year 2000 the incidence [of tuberculosis] will increase fifty times compared with now; mortality will increase seventyfold; and deaths in children are expected to rise ninetyfold."

Murray Feshbach interpreted that statement as follows: "In 2000, according to these numbers, tuberculosis deaths in Russia will reach approximately 1.75 million, whereas I estimate that heart disease and cancer deaths will number about 1.5 million. This says something extraordinary about the state of public health."[109]

Meanwhile, Russia's prisons only worsened with time.[110] With the 1998 collapse of the ruble came a government services crunch that, among other things, signaled food shortages and reported starvation in some Russian prisons.[111] By late 1998 the Yeltsin government, realizing that imprisonment, even in the absence of indictment, had become a death sentence, enacted waves of amnesties, releasing inmates who hadn't been convicted of major violent crimes. Tens of thousands of TB-ailing former inmates were released into the arms of a grossly overwhelmed health care system.

Every TB hospital and sanatorium in Russia was full: some had waiting lists. The staffs were going unpaid or, if they were lucky, underpaid. Less than half of the public health system's TB-related equipment, such as laproscopes and X-ray devices, worked. The number of doctors and nurses willing to endanger their own health, working without protective gear in such facilities, steadily declined: by 1997 nearly half nationwide had quit. Who could blame them: mortality rates among health care workers employed by the tuberculosis system was ten times higher than that of the general population.[112]

Of greatest concern was Russia's eastern Siberian region, where TB traditionally ran at rates higher than were seen in Moscow and west of the Ural mountains.

When nature calls for Dr. Galina Dugarova, the sixty-two-year-old head of tuberculosis control for Russia's Southern Buryatia state has to hike down a flight of dilapidated wooden stairs and step outside to an outhouse. The chief TB dispensary, which contains all the administrative offices and laboratories for the state of 1,150,000 people, has no running water, no sewage system, no heat, no laboratory supplies, scarce supplies of antibiotics, no modern chest X-ray devices, no protective masks and gloves for the staff and physicians, and no money to pay said staff. It resides inside a 150-year-old wooden building that leans sharply to one side, has gaping holes in its roof, and is sinking.

The semiautonomous Buryatia Republic, located in Siberia just 150 miles north of the Mongolian border, hasn't a spare ruble to deal with tuberculosis. But it has plenty of TB.

"It's like a genocide," declares Dugarova. "A holocaust. We're dying."

Though she was until recently a prominent member of the Soviet Communist Party, Dugarova concedes that the dramatic tuberculosis epidemic sweeping over her people began during the USSR days and has steadily worsened since 1991.

She is one of 260,000 ethnic Buryatis living in the mountainous republic—high cheekboned Buddhists (or in the case of devout Communists, atheists) who proudly declare their heritage to include Genghis Khan. Probably for genetic reasons, though no one was sure, ethnic Buryatis and other indigenous peoples of Siberia are especially vulnerable to the tuberculosis mycobacteria. In 1996 some 211 of every 100,000 Buryatis suffered active, symptomatic tuberculosis. That's twice the TB rate seen in their ethnic Russian neighbors.

For Buryati Minister of Health Blair Balzhirov the particular susceptibility of his Mongolian people to TB was a focus of great sorrow. He hoped that a blend of seventeenth-century-old Tibetan medical practices and Soviet-style TB control approaches would soon obliterate the tuberculosis crisis. But he had few health care workers at his disposal trained in either tradition—who could travel the 354,000-square-kilometer republic in search of TB cases.

It's Patriot Day in Ulan Ude—May Day in the West—and the city's population is pouring into Ploshehad Sovietov, a central square accessed via Ulitsa Lenina, a broad, tree-lined boulevard. Though it is still chilly, the sun bathes the celebrants as they parade past the two-story-tall, black head of Lenin, which nestles atop a marble pedestal like the decapitated, neckless face of John the Baptist setting upon Salome's platter. Russian Army soldiers and sailors stand at attention in dress uniforms while units of protofacist Cossacks, red flag–waving Communist Party members, and World War II medal-bedecked veterans march past.

So it comes as no surprise to discover Buryati's TB officer, Dugarova, and her political leaders favor a return to the old Soviet methods in their search for a way to staunch the area's rapidly expanding tuberculosis catastrophe.[113] Every individual found to have tuberculosis in Ulan Ude is, by Dugarova's command, brought to the log cabins that currently constitute her TB sanatorium. One is entirely pediatric, housing children—forcibly separated from their parents— aged twelve months to fourteen years. Tiny Misha, fifteen months old, has languished on the ward for three months, separated from his loving parents during key weeks of infant development. He has pulmonary TB.

Pretty, blond Tatyana, her hair wound in tight braids, plays with her "doll," a baby named Dulma. For more than a year Tatyana has lived in this tiny cabin, alongside a horde of other children, playing with the babies that at an increasing rate are dying in Dugarova's sanatorium.

Dugarova has no resistance laboratory test kits, no medical microbiology capacity, and—worse yet—no drug options. She just keeps giving the patients what antibiotics she can find, generally one or two drugs daily, and hopes the babies and adults muddle through. It's less than satisfactory, she admits.

But things will be better, Dugarova insists, when the giant 200-bed concrete sanatorium that has been under construction for six years is completed. The TB director takes her visitors to the edifice, which must be guarded twenty-four hours a day by armed men who shoot at would-be thieves. The nine-square-meter, six-story building is Dugarova's pride, though all its windows are broken, its stair banisters are rusted, and the entire structure seems about to collapse.

Yet, Dugarova insisted repeatedly, this shell will one day be a sanatorium. And a sanatorium will stop the Buryatian epidemic.

Though the Buryatia Republic's situation may have ranked as the worst in the world—especially for ethnic Buryatis—there were hot spots within the former Soviet Union that, remarkably, had even higher incidences of tuberculosis in specific risk groups. Officials at WHO described the situation as "eighteenth century," and were doing all they could to pressure the governments in the region not only to pour more money on the problem but to change the way they tackle tuberculosis control.

Some of the governments, particularly those of Georgia, Armenia, Azerbaijan, and the Kyrgyz Republic, were listening and had radically altered their TB control efforts to follow WHO guidelines. But the huge nations of Ukraine, Belarus, and Russia, as well as much of the Baltics and Central Asia, remained stubbornly locked into old Soviet approaches to TB.

New York City learned its lesson in 1991 when TB erupted in the city, driven by neglectful therapy, inappropriate antibiotic use, emergence of multi-drug-resistant strains of the bacteria, and the presence of a uniquely vulnerable population—hospitalized AIDS patients who lacked immunological capacity to fight off infection. After a few months of bumbling and fumbling the city adopted the Stiblo Model, instituting a Directly Observed Therapy System—DOTS—to monitor medicine compliance every day in the city's identified TB patients. It worked.

WHO had promoted the DOTS approach vigorously worldwide. And wherever it had been properly implemented, officials said, TB rates fell dramatically.[114]

But the approach adhered to—stubbornly and rigidly—in Russia, Ukraine, Belarus, and most of the rest of the former USSR was diametrically opposite. Tuberculosis was handled in the 1990s as it was in the 1950s when Nikita Khrushchev ran the far-flung nation with a Communist iron hand.

A massive system of sanatoriums staffed by doctors, nurses, and phthisiologists (a TB specialty that no longer existed in the West), coupled with an even more sizeable network of outpatient screening clinics, monitored the population, testing every citizen annually with chest X rays. Anyone who came up positive was given skin and culture tests—laboratory assays. If either of those also proved positive, the individual was removed from employment for two years, placed in mandatory sanatorium confinement for a minimum of one year, and treated with huge injections of one or two types of antibiotics. All of the patient's family members and coworkers were also tested, ensuring that the patient's TB was publicly known. If any of them proved positive, they, too, were pulled out of school or stripped of employment for two years. If therapy after one year appeared successful, the patient would be given a temporary job involving no contact with food products or the public. If therapy hadn't proven successful, infected parts of the patient's body were surgically removed. Twenty to 25 percent of all TB patients underwent lung surgeries in which some or all of the lung was removed.

To the degree that dwindling finances permitted this highly labor-intensive, repressive approach to TB control, it was still practiced. But few TB officials could afford routine X rays, tracing to find all of the familial and social contacts of every infected patient, or appropriate drug treatment.

And those in charge, such as Dr. Alexey Priymak of the Russian Ministry of Health, said that the rising TB death toll stemmed not from a failed approach to tuberculosis control but from inadequate financing of that old model.

"Underlying it all is a struggle for the survival of these huge, hulking old hospitals and institutions," Richard Bumgarner, deputy director of WHO's Global Tuberculosis Program, insisted. "They charge patients now for things that were free, and discharge them when the money runs out. Therein lies the reason for the resurgence of TB. The Russian health minister doesn't see this. TB is Ebola with wings, and she is busy creating it."

At Priymak's urging the Ministry of Health lobbied successfully in 1996 for

Duma passage of a tuberculosis five-year plan. Three billion dollars (eighteen trillion rubles) were allocated for expenditures starting in 1997 on upgrading the existing TB infrastructure. Even if the government only actually came up with 30 percent of the allocation it would more than double spending on the disease. And if Yeltsin's people didn't come up with the funds, Priymak warned, "By year 2002 the annual new caseload officially in Russia will be 200,000, and the incidence in children will increase 100 percent."

In fact, Priymak's system had already failed to cure at least 249,000 TB cases by 1996. It was an idle threat. But it worked, politically.

And it infuriated Western Europeans, who felt certain that Russia's drug-resistant bacteria were crossing their borders. By 1998 the Copenhagen office of WHO had documented that 25 percent of all Russian TB cases involved multidrug-resistant forms of the bacteria.

"Tuberculosis is at our [European] doorstep, and it is uglier and more frightening than ever," Dr. Arata Kochi, WHO Tuberculosis Programme director, concluded.

In fact, it had already crossed Europe's threshold, and forms of tuberculosis found in Russian and Baltic states were cropping up all over Scandinavia. More than half of all TB cases documented in Sweden, Denmark, and Norway in 1996 to 1999 were seen among emigrés from the Baltics and Russia, Dr. Nils Pederson, of the Statens Serum Institut in Copenhagen, said. By 2000 Russian-originated drug-resistant strains of TB bacteria were turning up all over northern Europe, according to WHO.

Yet Priymak and the Russian government refused to yield. Open public health warfare ensued, pitting Western and Communist policies against one another in a battle that could cost tens of thousands of lives and spread untreatable forms of tuberculosis across all of Europe.

There were dissident voices within the old Soviet tuberculosis system. The loudest and most influential was that of Priymak's former teacher, director of Russia's largest TB clinical research center, in Moscow. Operated by the Russian Academy of Sciences, Dr. Alexander Khomenko's huge TB facility was independent from the Ministry of Health—and from Priymak's influence. The former teacher and student locked horns in a battle over the future of Russia's tuberculosis epidemic, and there could be little doubt that the winner would influence not only Moscow's approach to TB but also the attitudes of counterpart health agencies in Kyiv, Minsk, Alma-Ata, and capitals of other former Soviet states. Khomenko, who served as the USSR's representative to WHO in Geneva from 1965 to 1970, favored the DOTS approach.

Khomenko had watched the incidence of TB rise throughout the former Soviet Union by 10 to 15 percent a year every year since 1990. He had seen budgets crumble to the point where he, earning $400 a month, was one of the

most highly paid TB doctors in the nation. And even more worrisome, he asserted, was the phenomenal increase in drug resistance.

Under his direction, the Ivanovo Oblast, a region northeast of Moscow,
was trying the DOTS approach, and it had already reduced its TB rate by 8
percent since 1995. As part of the ongoing experiment the laboratory capacities
of Ivanovo's TB hospital were vastly improved, and drug sensitivity tests were
performed on sputum samples from the region's patients. More than half—58.1
percent—of all samples contained mycobacteria that was partially resistant to
one or more antibiotics. One out of every eight patients in Ivanovo carried a
multidrug-resistant strain of TB.

At Khomenko's Moscow facility most patients had drug-resistant TB—that
was one of the reasons they made their way from as far as Vladivostok, searching
for last-ditch treatments that might save their lives.

In 1996, for example, Paulina Mahachela brought her twenty-one-year-old
son, Khoubanov, all the way from Dagestan, a mountainous Russian state on
the Caspian Sea. A champion weight lifter with Olympic dreams, Khoubanov felt
fatigued and weak in March 1996—doctors in his hometown of Makhachkala
diagnosed tuberculosis. By then the young Muslim man already had enough TB
bacteria in both lungs that X rays revealed bilateral damage.

"For one and a half months he stayed at home, and he seemed all right,"
Paulina, a short, middle-aged brunette, recalled. Because she is a physician—
though not a TB specialist—Paulina was confident that home treatment with
four antibiotics would be sufficient.

But she didn't know Khoubanov was infected with drug-resistant TB. Nobody did because none of the Dagestan hospitals had equipment to conduct
drug sensitivity tests on his sputum samples. Worse yet, the young, dark-eyed
man developed a toxic liver reaction to the only one of the drugs that was effective against his TB.

Hospitalized in Dagestan, Khoubanov's condition by August 1996 was dire.
When doctors switched him from the four drugs he had been taking to expensive
cephalosporin antibiotics Khoubanov had a severe allergic reaction to the medicine. That's when Paulina decided it was time to pool the family's financial
resources and bring her son to Moscow—to the famous Dr. Khomenko.

"By then he was resistant to all available drugs," Paulina said. And X rays
revealed that both his lungs were completely infected. Khomenko's staff felt
there was no option—in November the patient was rolled into the OR.

When the surgeons opened up Khoubanov's lungs, they were stunned.
Inside his left lung was a "giant cavity," one of the surgeons recalled—hard as a
rock, the formation was full of tuberculosis bacteria. And all but the lower lobe
of his right lung was similarly infected. The surgeons removed the cavity and
half of the man's right lung.

For 130 days, Khoubanov's remaining lung musculature refused to function and the man's life hung on little more than his mechanical ventilator and Paulina's prayers. His weight fell precariously from 84 to 53 kilos, and Khomenko's staff feared every day that the young man would die.

But during the worst of Moscow's 1996 winter, Khoubanov's lungs spontaneously started working again. When some of his strength was restored doctors noticed that it was his right lung—which had been surgically reduced by half—that was doing all the work. X rays revealed that TB had once again claimed his left lung.

So on May 14, Khoubanov's entire left lung was surgically removed, leaving the man with only 25 percent lung capacity.

In the spring of 1997 Khoubanov lay lethargically in an isolated room in the intensive care unit, breathing through a one-inch-diameter hole cut in his trachea. Painted daily with emerald disinfectant the hole gapes at horrified visitors. When he can gulp enough air through his mouth, Khoubanov covers the disturbing hole with a piece of gauze bandaging. If breathing becomes particularly difficult doctors insert a ventilator tube directly into the aperture.

Khoubanov tries to speak, but cannot muster enough air across his voice box to make clear noises. Paulina knowingly leans over, placing her ear directly over his tracheal hole, her mouth inhaling what her son exhales. She—and the staff—do this many times a day. And no one wears masks. The protective gear is in such short supply that it can only be used during invasive and surgical procedures.

"The doctors are very enthusiastic but they don't have enough money or drugs," Paulina says.

"It's true," one of the physicians adds. "It's only due to the relatives that he survives."

Since Khoubanov was diagnosed in March 1996 the Mahachela family has spent 80 million rubles on drugs (about $14,000) and 55 million on surgery (some $4,000). Paulina could not recall how much she has spent on hospitalization and housing for herself in Moscow—perhaps another $4,000. Even an American family would be hard pressed to come up with $20,000 in cash—for Dagestanis it's almost unimaginable. The typical Dagestani family with employed heads of households survives on about $2,400 a year. Khoubanov's tuberculosis has not only destroyed one and a half of his lungs and bankrupted the Mahachela family but also left his entire clan in debt back home in Dagestan.

Such severe measures—and patient expenditures—weren't even possible for most of the region's TB patients. The majority, said Dugarova, in Buryatia, were "jobless, homeless, and poor." And it was precisely because of the poverty of both the patients and TB treatment system that Dugarova sided with Priymak, not Khomenko, and opposed DOTS.

"Okay, it's cheaper, it's cost-effective. And maybe other areas have fruit and vegetables all the time, but not here," Dugarova said dismissively. "If these drugs are available, okay, but they aren't. We haven't even got vitamins, so come on!"

What did Dugarova have for TB treatment? Sacks full of isoniazid powder intended for injection but given orally in capsules. Old supplies, Soviet made, that Stiblo had analyzed and said "is just like sand." She also had two other basic antibiotics and, occasionally, a third. Supplies varied, so patients rarely got a steady, consistent course of therapy. And consistency, experts said, was the key to avoiding development of resistant strains.

"We don't interrupt therapy, but we may get down to just one drug," Dugarova admitted.

At the Buryatia "sanatorium"—the three log cabins, packed wall-to-wall with patients—Dugarova declares that "at least there is running water," though the rooms are ice-cold in the winter. Between the children's cabin and one of the adult log hospitals long clotheslines are stretched; the children's hand-washed bed linens flap in the crisp mountain wind.

In the adult wards patient beds are stacked so closely together that plump Dugarova cannot make her way between them. The hospitals have no pajamas or linens—these, the adult patients must provide for themselves. The dining hall consists of three hot plates and a few tables. "I want to go home," cries sixty-three-year-old patient Yekatarina Chernykh when she spies Dugarova.

In the intensive care ward—so designated not by virtue of any better technology, but because the patients are sicker—four men lay inert, their tableside meals untouched. Three have advanced pulmonary TB, the fourth has tuberculosis meningitis.

"They are all going to die," Dugarova whispers. "These forms of TB—I never saw them, even in the fifties. They are, of course, sentenced to death. We cannot treat them. No way. We would like to give them four drugs and some protein but we have no money, and they have no money. They are sentenced."

One of the attending nurses had been eavesdropping on Dugarova's conversation. On hearing the chief physician's somber pronouncement she silently bows her head, ties a wad of gauze bandaging around her mouth and nose, and tiptoes to the bedside of a twenty-one-year-old man. Dugarova looks on impassively as the nurse gently strokes the bony body outlined by a red blanket.

Thousands of miles away in Tartu, Estonia, Heinart Sillaustu, president of the Estonian Society of Respiratory Medicine, denounces such practices as "old-fashioned, inflexible and overstaffed. The Soviet TB system was one in which the Party dominated everywhere."

Sillaustu warmly greets visitors into his comfortable home, serving tea and offering data via a home slide show. Retired, Sillaustu devoted decades of his life to challenging the Soviet view of tuberculosis. When he began in 1953 Estonians suffered tuberculosis at a rate of 417 primary cases per 100,000 citizens. Through a combination of Soviet methods and his own uniquely Estonian brand of Stiblo's DOTS approach Sillaustu managed to push TB rates down to their nadir of 21 cases per 100,000 in 1992. But since then TB had been climbing back up, reaching 44.5 primary cases per 100,000.

"In Russia they didn't give the real data," Sillaustu says, "but these numbers are real," illustrating that although public health lost some ground after the fall of communism in Estonia, no tragedy on the scale of the Russian debacle occurred.

Still, Sillaustu continues, nearly 20 percent of all Estonian TB cases are drug resistant and the average age of tuberculosis patients has shifted down, from fifty-five to sixty years in 1981 to, in 1996, an average of thirty, "the productive workforce," he notes. Regrettably Sillaustu wasn't making much headway with Estonian politicians because the officials would always point to Byelorussian and Russian TB data and say, "See, we're not so bad off."

"But I say to them, 'Let's not compare ourselves to Russia—we are rid of Russia! Let's compare to our neighbors, Finland,' " Sillaustu said, noting that Finland had one-fifth Estonia's TB rate.[115]

"Our politicians just don't understand," Sillaustu says, shaking his balding head. "We must have money to build facilities to carry out DOTS. If we don't, we will be unable to control TB."

So much in the region hinged on Russia. If that behemoth country didn't change its TB public health policies, few politicians in other former Soviet countries were likely to support DOTS and WHO policies.

Realizing that, Viktor Aphanasiev was in 1997 preparing to do battle with Moscow. It was a high-stakes game the St. Petersburg physician was playing, but he said lives were on the line. Lots of lives.

As director of tuberculosis services for Leningrad Oblast (or state), Aphanasiev had grown weary of following the Ministry of Health rules and watching the death toll from TB rise. He was going out on a limb—defying national TB director Alexey Priymak's orders and siding with the World Health Organization and Western Europeans. He was going to treat his patients with DOTS.

"Without a doubt we will have this DOTS, with the support of our governor," the forty-something robust Aphanasiev declared. "Whatever it takes!"

Since the fall of the Soviet Union in 1991 the TB rate in Leningrad Oblast had doubled, antibiotic resistance had developed in the microbes, the death rate had soared, and all the money for TB services had run out. It had been so long since the staff received full paychecks that much of the patient care was handled by retired health workers who lived off their meager pensions.

In 1996 Aphanasiev ordered drug-resistance tests on sputum samples from

1,160 St. Petersburg patients—nearly every one contained microbes that could completely resist treatment with one or more of the quintet of drugs available in the city.[116]

"Drug resistance is our greatest fear. If you face this problem in America, well, what about here," Aphanasiev exclaimed. "It's one more reason to try DOTS."

Aphanasiev and his assistant Dr. Tatiana Dolubava succeeded in gaining financial and political support from the Leningrad Oblast's newly elected governor, and hoped to get further funds from nearby, worried Sweden.

With adequate funding Aphanasiev hoped to purchase enough antibiotics to be able to put nearly all TB patients on outpatient therapy taking five drugs a day, confirmed by an observing nurse or TB official every day. The dynamic Dolubava/Aphanasiev duo wanted to get away from following the old Soviet approach of mass X-ray screening, forced sanatorium incarceration of those who have TB, and long rounds of treatment with injections of two or three drugs a day.

"I'm not happy—we administer three drugs now. And we still have active TB," Aphanasiev said. "Yes, we see a decrease in mortality, but we get an increased morbidity [illness] rate . . . from the point of view of epidemiology it's terrible because it increases the chances of spreading TB."

But switching from the Soviet model that was favored by powerful Priymak carried huge risks. It could result in even further constraints on St. Petersburg's already all-but-nonexistent budget.

"We are in a very difficult position," Dolubava explained. "We have to have courage to deviate. . . . As the philosophers say, you cannot enter the same water twice. We cannot keep working as we did in the 1930s. Conditions have changed."

In the fall of 1996, billionaire American financier George Soros set up a $12.3 million grant with the Manhattan-based Public Health Research Institute (PHRI), aimed at offering technical assistance and advice to stem Russia's TB crisis. PHRI, in collaboration with Médecins Sans Frontières and the London-based MERLIN group, set up a pilot DOTS project in Tomsk Prison in Siberia, demonstrating that appropriate antibiotic therapy had a cure rate more than double that of traditional Soviet approaches at a cost savings of $2 million for the prison in a single year.

PHRI also conducted training workshops throughout Russia, showing their counterpart microbiologists how to do drug-resistance assays on tuberculosis samples.

But the Tomsk Prison success still wasn't enough to persuade Priymak and the Russian TB establishment, PHRI's Dr. Alex Goldfarb said in 1998. "It's a vicious circle. . . . It's not just resistance to DOTS, it's something that is combined with the severe economic crisis. All of the people are primarily concerned with saving their jobs. We said in Tomsk they could decrease costs by about 50 percent, and use the money to pay [unpaid] salaries," Goldfarb continued.

But the Tomsk doctors still resisted, "because all they think when you say, 'restructuring of TB services' is that it means nonpayment of salaries."

Cracks in Russia's anti-DOTS resolve began to show, however, as other tuberculosis control officials followed the examples of Khomenko and Aphanasiev, openly defying Priymak's policies. With the August 1998 economic crisis came still more fissures in the old system, pried wider by Western pressure placed directly upon President Yeltsin.[117]

Later in 1998 the same organizations initiated a $100 million campaign to tackle Russian drug-resistant TB. And on October 28, 1998, the White House convened a meeting attended by some of the most powerful leaders of the capitalist world,[118] focused on Russia's tuberculosis situation.

The gathering's paramount concern was that Russia adopt DOTS strategies, install drug-resistance laboratories, and remedy its prison problem. Despite such international pressure, money, and expertise, Russia's epidemic continued to expand. In early 1999 the International Red Cross issued a bulletin: "a serious tuberculosis outbreak is killing one person every twenty-five minutes in Belarus, Moldova, Russia and Ukraine."

As the twenty-first century dawned tuberculosis was raging out of control all across the former Soviet states, and drug-resistant superstrains had emerged regionwide. Even in Ivanovo, where WHO had executed its pilot DOTS project, drug-resistant TB rates had more than tripled since 1996, topping 10 percent of all diagnosed tuberculosis cases.[119] And in Kemerovo, where Europeans tried DOTS in Siberian prisons, drug resistance rates in 1999 exceeded 20 percent.

Once considered a triumph of global public health, tuberculosis had become the world's great shame. All systems of control had failed. As Harvard University TB expert Dr. Paul Farmer put it, the globalized economy had brought "into relief the flabby relativism of the public health *realpolitik* that leaves us with a double standard of therapy": immediate multidrug treatment for the infected affluent, and inadequate treatment of the poor. The latter was leading to the emergence of drug-resistant microbes which, in turn, imperiled the whole world, rich and poor alike.

VII

Oh no,
They've gone and named my home
St. Petersburg.

What's going on?
Where are all the friends I had?
It's all wrong, I'm feeling lost like
I just don't belong.
Gimme back,
Gimme back my Leningrad.

—Leningrad Cowboys[120]

I like Edgar Allan Poe. His poems are about death. Live fast, die young.

—Aruslan Kurcenko, age twenty-seven, after injecting heroin in Odessa

Tuberculosis, diphtheria, typhoid fever, cholera, alcoholism, malnutrition—all are diseases that worsened after 1991 but whose rises predated the demise of communism. The Soviet Union's public health infrastructure had rules and regulations for each of these illnesses, but whether these structures were working to contain them was another matter. In any case, though, the ailments were familiar, as were methods of preventing and treating them.

Not so with the new public health catastrophes of the post-Soviet era.

The first of the new scourges surfaced during the Gorbachev years but did not reach catastrophic proportions until well into the Yeltsin era.

His slides were amateurish, handmade. His voice quivered. The notes he clutched made loud fluttering noises over the conference amplification system as his trembling hands struggled to hold the papers still. Dr. Viktor Zhdanov wasn't an officially invited speaker to the Second International Conference on AIDS, held in Paris in 1986. But he clearly was the bombshell speaker.

The elderly Russian scientist, dressed as he was in a frumpy suit and well-worn shoes, stood out in the fashionable Paris crowd even before he spoke. After his brief speech the hall of some five thousand AIDS experts buzzed with amazement, for Zhdanov had openly defied Soviet authorities by revealing that Moscow's claims that it had virtually no incidences of HIV or AIDS cases were untrue, and small outbreaks of the virus were appearing in various parts of the vast nation.

Though the audience at the time understood that Zhdanov's action was a courageous one, few realized exactly who the scientist was. Even fewer had any idea what happened to the venerable old researcher after he returned to Moscow.

When seventy-two-year-old Viktor Mikhailovich Zhdanov returned from Paris in 1986 the Soviet secret police force, the KGB, "hounded him relentlessly," one source said. His stature as one of the Soviet Union's most prominent virologists didn't protect him. Despite membership in the prestigious Soviet Academy of Sciences, his position as head of the Ivanovski Virology Laboratory in Moscow, his receipt of four orders of Soviet honor, his discovery and development of the first live measles vaccine—despite all these accomplishments Zhdanov was targeted for "destruction."

"He was denounced as a CIA spy," Dr. Eduoard Karamov of the Ivanovski Laboratory recalled bitterly. "He died less than a year after he returned from Paris, and I have no doubt that, despite his age, the witch hunt gave him that stroke."

Soon after the Paris meeting the KGB and top Communists in the Soviet scientific establishment mounted a campaign that was a textbook example of how intellectual voices were silenced under the old regime. It began with a series of unsigned articles in Soviet scientific journals questioning Zhdanov's credibility as a scientist, and his loyalty as a Soviet citizen. Many of those articles, Karamov said, were written by men who Zhdanov considered his best friends.

Zhdanov's most dangerous enemy would prove to be the affable leader of the Soviet Academy of Medical Sciences—and post-1991 head of the Russian equivalent agency—Dr. Valentin Pokrovsky. A seemingly jolly man who enjoys his vodka and readily hugs visitors, Pokrovsky was, several sources insisted, very close to the KGB.

Pokrovsky set up a commission within the Academy to investigate claims made against Zhdanov, most of which were filed in the form of unsigned letters. The commission summoned Zhdanov to appear on a Tuesday morning to defend himself—an order the senior scientist found so astounding that he appealed to his friend, Pokrovsky, for an explanation. Pokrovsky ordered him to go.

Monday night Zhdanov suffered a stroke after, Karamov insists, "five phone calls hounding him to go" before the commission. Despite his stroke Zhdanov appeared before the commission, "where they were tearing him to pieces," Karamov said.

Just days later Zhdanov, age seventy-three, died.

And a few weeks following that it was announced that Valentin Pokrovsky's son, Vadim, was the head of a new HIV/AIDS laboratory and clinical center in Moscow. In the 1990s that facility was called the Russia AIDS Centre, still headed by Vadim Pokrovsky.

After several rounds of vodka at a reception in the Russian Academy of Medical Sciences Valentin decried the social changes that seemed to be spawning Russia's AIDS epidemic as "this wild dance of unharnessed democracy."

His son, Vadim, told a visitor that nothing short of a resurrection of socialist rule could prevent an HIV cataclysm.

At the Leningrad Republican Infectious Disease Hospital, located in the Russian countryside near St. Petersburg, a city of 4.5 million, the sorry history of the Soviet HIV explosion in Russia could be seen at once at a Salvation Army prayer meeting.

A ten-year-old girl demurely bows her head, a large pink bow in her hair, as she prays. Beside her a nine-year-old girl, her hair filled with carefully entwined artificial flowers, shifts impatiently in her seat. Across from them two tough-looking men in their midtwenties nibble on the free meal, only half-listening to an ongoing Bible reading.

In all, nearly thirty people sit around a large lunch table. Ranging in age from six to fifty, they represent a cross section of Russian society. And they're all infected with the human immunodeficiency virus.

"See little Misha over there? The twelve-year-old boy?" whispers Svetlana, a thirty-two-year-old Salvation Army volunteer who is also HIV positive. "He says, 'It's okay, I'll get married when I grow up and my HIV will go away.' "

Some of the adults in the room, like Svetlana, got HIV through heterosexual intercourse. Others—probably the majority—were infected through contaminated needles they shared with fellow opiate users. And one, Nikolai, got the virus through homosexual sex.

But the children were all infected in Russian hospitals in a series of transmissions known within the health care system as the "Elista incident."

The Elista tragedy signified for many a substantial rip in the fabric of basic health care. In conversations over several months in Russia, Georgia, and Ukraine, many people spoke vehemently of avoiding minor surgery and dental visits because they feared getting AIDS via reused or contaminated instruments. They also feared repressive measures—including military quarantines—that were routinely imposed upon HIV sufferers during Soviet times.[121] Physicians told of the dangers they faced caring for their high-risk patients.

The chain of tragic events known as the Elista incident began around 1982, when a sailor who had worked in Africa unwittingly acquired HIV. He passed it on to his wife, and she, in turn, infected her fetus.

In May 1988, the child was admitted to Elista's pediatric hospital with a variety of intractable infections, all without apparent causes. The baby died soon afterward, still undiagnosed. Meanwhile, the baby's mother, by now twenty-three, began to develop the same type of unusual infections.

The mother went to Moscow for treatment, where she ran into a woman with similar symptoms, who had also lost a child at Elista. When the two mothers compared notes, they determined that their children had been in the neonatal ward at the same time, and had suffered the same type of infections. At the mothers' insistence, doctors finally added up the coincidences and gave both HIV tests, determining that the country's first AIDS outbreak was under way. A joint Russian/UN probe later found that by the time the last mother and child in the chain were infected, in 1994, about 250 cases had occurred through hospital injections with recycled syringes and catheters, the mothers via bites from breast-feeding babies.[122]

In the Soviet health system, healthy babies, or those suffering minor ailments, routinely received up to three hundred injections yearly of vitamins and antibiotics that were given with needles used on one patient after another all day long. And babies who were very sick typically received implants of recycled, poorly sterilized catheters.

"There was just one case to begin with," said Dr. Saladin Osmanov, of UNAIDS. "But the terrible medical practices were enough to create an outbreak."

And the outbreak didn't end at Elista. Some of the HIV-positive babies were shipped to other hospitals in the Russian cities of Rostov-on-Don, Volgograd, and Stavropol before their diagnoses were clear. And doctors in those facilities, repeating the same health care practices, passed the virus around their pediatric facilities as well.[123]

After Elista, Soviet authorities panicked, stepping up mandatory HIV testing to levels unheard of elsewhere, and allowing doctors to screen their patients without consent.

They could, indeed, use the testing to isolate individual infections. But since the rate of infection remained tiny, the Soviets felt no pressure to follow with infection control efforts that would have ensured adequate supplies of sterile syringes and protective equipment, not to mention extensive retraining of caregivers.

Instead, Soviet leaders created centers for the quarantine and study of HIV-infected citizens who—like those gathered in prayer in St. Petersburg—faced futures of near imprisonment and boredom. The job of tracking down Soviet HIV cases fell, as did most public health responsibilities, to SanEp, which executed the task in classic Soviet fashion. No one had a right to refuse HIV tests, and no nation conducted as many involuntary screenings as did the USSR. From the moment the first HIV case was identified in Moscow, and with even greater vigor following the 1989 Elista incident, HIV testing was executed at a phenomenal pace. Between 1987 and 1995 some 165,470,049 Russians alone were subjected to state-mandated tests. Records on the numbers of non-Russian Soviets who were tested are not available but surely would substantially increase that toll of 165 million.[124] Testing in Russia peaked in 1992, when 24.4 million people, or one out of every 6.8 citizens, were screened by the state.

But, like so many SanEp approaches to public health, it was an extraordinarily inefficient strategy. Between 1987 and 1991 some seventy-two million HIV tests were executed in Russia, netting 522 cases of infection; more than half of them stemmed from the Elista incident. In order to conduct all of those tests—138,000 for every single Russian case identified—the Soviet Union had to maintain an enormous central laboratory in Moscow dedicated to manufacturing test kits and analyzing millions of blood samples every year. Further, SanEp field workers had to round up all of those blood samples and ship them to Moscow. Most of the tests were conducted on blood donors, pregnant women, prisoners, and Soviets who traveled outside the country—tests were mandatory upon re-entry.

In 1996 Russia spent about $1.75 million on testing. But 1997 opened with a smaller HIV/AIDS budget, unpaid doctors and nurses countrywide, and hospitals with empty pharmaceutical shelves. Far from being able to afford $10,000 to $40,000 a year to treat HIV patients in ways that met U.S. standards, or to continue a nearly $2 million testing program, Russia couldn't even find the wherewithal to buy television advertising time on national television to promote AIDS education.

The same policies, including extensive, expensive involuntary testing, were the rule throughout the former USSR.

Svetlana was nineteen years old when the Chernobyl nuclear accident occurred. A Ukrainian, Svetlana lived near the power plant and was exposed to enough fallout that she suffered immediate radiation sickness. For four years Ukrainian physicians gave Svetlana blood transfusions, hoping to replenish her vital red and white blood cell populations that were killed by radiation.

In 1993 Svetlana, then living in Kyiv, tested positive for HIV, sparking a panic among the apparatchiks responsible for Soviet blood supplies. Tens of thousands of donors thought to have given blood during the post-Chernobyl years were retested in a frantic search for the source of Svetlana's HIV.

But she knew that it hadn't come from the blood.

"I know who I got it from," Svetlana, a tall, robust, blue-eyed blond adult recalled. "And he has passed away. He was from Italy. His sister wrote to me from Italy and told me that he died of AIDS. I realized that I was in danger and sought medical assistance."

Nevertheless, Soviet public health officials insisted on retesting the Ukrainian blood supply. And Svetlana, who had already suffered years of hardship resulting from Chernobyl, was shipped off to the Republican Infectious Diseases Hospital outside St. Petersburg, where she lived throughout the rest of the 1990s. Her Ukrainian family was permitted to visit, but the long journey from Kyiv proved an expensive one in the post-Soviet period, and Svetlana soon realized that the Elista incident survivors and a handful of adults who contracted HIV infection from other sources were to be her only comrades. She watched the tiny Elista children grow up—and, in eighty cases, die—acting as their surrogate aunt and occasional nurse.

"The children are charming," Svetlana tells visitors. "Their mothers are making matches between the little boys and girls, so someday the HIV-positive children can grow up and marry."

Svetlana lowers her voice to a whisper: "Most of the children don't know about their diagnosis."

Since 1989 the youngsters, most of whom arrived as newborns, have known no other world save the ramshackle hospital, its personnel, and the views of distant dacha fields and a river that they can see from their windows. Life perked up a bit for the youngsters in 1993 to 1995 when diphtheria cases—thousands of them—filled the hospital. But since that epidemic's end the hallways of Republican Hospital have grown silent, and the only additions to their sad quarantine colony have been drug addicts and their babies, most of whom have come from Kaliningrad. All of them are HIV-positive.

Nikolai Nedezelski, a handsome twenty-seven-year-old, was diagnosed HIV positive in 1991 in Moscow.

"I got it from my Russian partner," says Nikolai, who is gay. Eloquent and schooled in the ways of European AIDS activitists Nedezelski spent his days visiting quarantine centers, such as the one in St. Petersburg, and lobbying for humane policies. He also was one of the only HIV patients in all of Russia in 1997 who was receiving state-of-the-art combination drug therapy—the result of frequent trips he managed to make to Los Angeles and Paris. He wanted all of his fellow HIV patients in Russia to get the life-extending drugs, but due to an arcane set of Soviet laws still on Russian books, only infected residents of Moscow could obtain even one such drug. Outside of Moscow and St. Petersburg no one received the full cocktails commonly used in Western Europe.

In 1995 Nikolai was selected by his HIV-positive peers to plead their case to the international community at the Paris Summit on HIV. He pulled no punches, telling the conference that "in Russia it's still a political disease. Everything related to treatment and prophylaxis is political. Society says, 'Why spend money on prostitutes, homosexuals and drug users? . . . Why should we provide combination therapy . . . the people will die sooner if we don't. Good.' "

Nikolai's speech was aired on Russian television.

"When my mother watched my speech on TV she said, 'I'm so glad you were born in these times rather than earlier. In the old days the gulag would be crying for you,' " Nikolai recalled.

In a sense, however, the gulag did still call to Russia's HIV patients, as the laws of the post-Communist state forbade most of their sexual activity, condemned infected drug users to the tuberculosis-infested prison system, and greatly limited their access to treatments.[125]

Mikhail Ivanovich Narkevich, chief of AIDS Control for the Russian Ministry of Health, says that in retrospect Elista and the tragedy of the St. Petersburg colony "taught us a lot. If not for that tragedy I don't know how many more people would have been infected in Soviet hospitals."

After the breakup of the Soviet Union each of the new, independent countries muddled through for a while, largely ignoring HIV in favor of more immediate public health crises, such as diphtheria and tuberculosis. If not for the Elista and Romanian pediatric cases the region's HIV rates would have, in the global scheme of things, been negligible. Even including those roughly 2,300 cases didn't put Russia, Georgia, Lithuania, Poland, or any of the other former Communist nations in apparent HIV jeopardy.

Until 1996.

"That was the year the situation got worse," Narkevich insisted. Actually, it was sometime in May 1995.

"It's clear it came from Ukraine to Russia," Vadim Pokrovsky added. "The question is how it got from the Ukraine to Belarus, and from Belarus to Russia. It is an A clade virus—not the B clade that we saw before—so we know it was new. But where did it come from?"

The "where" might never be clear, Narkevich countered, but the "how" was horribly obvious. It rested with *narkomania*, or drug abuse: between May 1995 and 1996 the number of Russian IV drug users found infected with HIV increased nearly a hundredfold. And Russia's *narkomania* crisis was running a few laps behind the drug-use explosion in Eastern Europe, Belarus, and—most importantly—Ukraine.

It's Monday night at 7 P.M. and Artur is ready to "walk the thread" through Odessa's prime narcotics neighborhood, Palermo. The plan is for him and pal Oleg to score enough opium poppy straw and the necessary solvents to be able to cook up a batch of *chorny* sufficient to get two people high.

The energetic—perhaps hyper—Artur zips his coat up high against the cold wind and fog and heads first to a block of large concrete apartment buildings near the Ukrainian city's railroad tracks. After two years of shooting opium into his veins, the twenty-one-year-old knows exactly where to go.

He moves swiftly, cutting his way through the thick, bone-chilling fog, into one of the many look-alike Soviet communal housing buildings, and bounds up ten flights of urine-soaked stairs. Artur knows that the elevator doesn't work—few do in this city of post-Communist decay. As he catches his breath on the top floor Artur unzips his jacket, removing an empty plastic water bottle and eight *hryvnya*—about $5.50. He approaches a specially constructed steel chamber that securely seals the apartment behind it off from the rest of the world. There are two cutout holes along the side of the steel fortress: through a two-inch by two-inch hole, Artur passes his money; into the other, slightly taller slot, he places the empty bottle. Artur presses a loud buzzer and waits.

A hand appears, withdrawing the money and bottle. Five minutes later a door opens in the steel, revealing an inner steel cage behind which lies still another door—the one originally built for apartment 10A. An elderly gypsy woman, dressed in a long-flowing multicolored skirt and equally colorful but clashing silk blouse, silently returns the bottle to Artur, passing the now-filled object through the cage bars, along with a syringe filled with acetic anhydride. As the steel barriers slam shut in successive loud clanks, Artur sniffs the contents of the bottle, verifying it is the paint remover solvent he expected.

Ten minutes later Artur climbs into the backseat of an old Lada, nods to Oleg, and the pair drive the unpaved, pot-holed road into the neighborhood dubbed Palermo. The Gypsies keep the road rough, Artur explains, so that the police cannot make any surprise raids. About halfway into the Palermo neighborhood, where there are some ten thousand Gypsies and their "slaves"—drug-addicted Ukrainian adolescents who work for nothing more than daily hits of narcotics—the road becomes impassable.

"Now we walk," Oleg announces, getting out of the car and disappearing into the dense, ice-cold fog. Artur follows, and the pair "walk the thread," as the local addicts put it, winding their way rapidly along the alleyways that zigzag between large, cinder block gypsy fortresses. Each fortified home has high, thick walls around it with small, ground-level, hand-size holes designed for passage of drugs and cash.

It's dinnertime, dark, and moonless. Few people are outdoors. A pair of colorfully dressed Gypsy girls look Artur and Oleg disdainfully in the eyes as they pass. A fashionably dressed Gypsy man polishes his 1996 BMW sedan. A middle-aged woman pops her scarfed head out of a gate and shouts a command to her German shepherd. The dog runs in the opposite direction, its tail between its legs.

Oleg and Artur pause in front of one of the fortress-houses from which blasts loud rave music, its techno-pop beat reverberating off the neighbors' walls. The men whisper to each other, and it is decided that Oleg should hold back, letting Artur approach their preferred dealer alone.

Across the muddy road from the pulsating house, Artur walks up to an eight-foot-high steel gate and shouts, "Luba! Luba!" Middle-aged Luba, her shiny clothes of many colors billowing in the night air, comes out of the house and peers at Artur. They exchange words, but she turns him away. Artur is stumped.

From the opposite direction a new 1997 Ford Taurus arrives, the driver steps out, and he, too, calls to Luba. As the driver passes cash to the Gypsy, Artur again presses her for poppy straw. Luba tells him no—she doesn't recognize his close-cropped hair and dark jeans. Artur looks like a cop.

Suddenly the aggravating music stops in the house across the dirt road. A fourteen-year-old boy wearing a Sony Walkman steps out of his house, recognizes Oleg, and calls out to Luba in Russian: "They're okay, I know this guy."

Luba nods, disappears into her house, and returns with two packages. She sells one to Artur, but as she passes the other to the Taurus driver the wily German shepherd appears, leaps at Luba's outstretched hand, and steals the poppy straw. In an instant the sneaky dog disappears into a neighbor's house.

Artur and Oleg, anxious now that they are in possession of the rough opium stems and dried bulbs, race back to the car.

At 8 P.M. they arrive at the apartment of Oleg's grandmother, whom he calls simply, Babushka.

"Don't worry, Babushka," Oleg says, "nothing bad will happen." The grandmother, seeing she has no choice, lets the young men enter her tiny apartment but immediately telephones Oleg's mother, Svetlana.

Artur sets to work in the kitchen, removing his shirt because "it's going to get hot in here. You'll see." While Oleg calms his grandmother and almost instantly present aunt and mother, Artur scrubs a set of cooking pots and a meat grinder with steel wool.

"The first step," he explains, "is to remove all the fat from the poppy straw. We must get it out because it will induce human allergies. We have to scrub all the fat off these things."

Artur toils in Babushka's hundred-square-foot kitchen, with its peeling white ceiling and walls, warped lime green linoleum flooring, four-burner gas stove, sink, one-man eating table, and minifridge. And in the living room Oleg comforts his pretty blond mother, whose transparent blue eyes are brimming with tears. He promises Svetlana that he will not inject the drugs Artur is making in the kitchen—"if I slip down again I want to die," he tells his mother. The widow, who lost both her father and husband last year to heart attacks, acknowledges that Oleg has tried to stop. But she is unconvinced.

"I learned two years ago that he was addicted for three years already," Svetlana explains, nervously tugging at her dress and fingers. "It wasn't noticeable. He managed to keep himself together and I couldn't see it. He graduated from university and had a prestigious position."

Oleg nods: "It's true, I had a good job—five hundred dollars a month. More than twice the average wage in Odessa for men much older than me. I was married, optimistic."

Oleg avoids his mother's reddened eyes. Silently, she slips into the kitchen and watches Artur, who is now dripping with sweat despite the chilly night air, grinding up the hard dried poppy pieces into a coarse powder that spills over yesterday's Ukrainian newspaper. "If you have an intelligent son, you really grieve when he becomes an addict," Svetlana whispers, her voice breaking on the word *narkoman*.

By eight-thirty all the poppy straw has been ground to a powder and Artur dumps it into a small tin cooking pot, along with some baking soda and about three tablespoons of Odessa's notoriously contaminated tap water.

"This will infuse into the poppy straw under heat, breaking it up," Artur explains, displaying skills that under different circumstances might have made him a good organic chemist. It must be steadily stirred, he says, as he wipes sweat off his brow and the high gas flames heat up the kitchen, turning the poppy straw into a paste.

Ten minutes later danger begins.

Now Artur and Oleg will perform the extraction steps, which involve highly flammable solvents. Both men have seen plenty of friends be severely burned by accidents at this stage; some have even died as their kitchens were engulfed in flames. Artur decides to proceed in a slower, but safer manner, using a frying pan full of boiling water as a barrier between gas flames and the opiate concoction that now cooks with three cups of paint thinner and acetone. He must stand over the high heat stirring constantly, or the mixture could explode in flames.

Within minutes the kitchen fills with a powerful stench and the chemical fumes make everyone in the room gasp for air, their eyes watering. Oleg opens the windows, hangs a blanket over the kitchen entry to prevent the fumes from escaping into the rest of the minuscule apartment, and sends Svetlana to the living room.

The three distraught women sob in the spartan living room. Stripped of all valuables long ago—sold by Oleg for drug money—the room has the feel of a prison cell. Babushka cries out between sobs that all the neighbors will smell the acrid stench and know that drugs are being made in her apartment. Svetlana and her older sister murmur that Oleg claimed he stopped taking drugs two months ago—how can they believe him now?

At 9:05 Artur removes a stinky, hot brown liquid from the stove and pours it through a cloth into a tin bowl. The stench nearly overwhelms him, and Artur comes dangerously close to spilling the boiled opiate extract on himself. As it passes through the cloth the liquid takes on a greenish hue.

Artur puts the tin bowl into the jury-rigged double boiler and cooks it another twenty minutes until nothing remains but a thin dark green film reminiscent of pond algal scum. He grabs the syringe full of acetic anhydride and carefully injects it into the pot, producing yet another vile vinegarish odor. He stirs slowly, his tattooed wrist rotating round and round, bearing the Russian phrase, GOD BE WITH US.

By 9:46 the process is complete, and a dark brown/green puddle of about five cubic millimeters beckons from the tin bowl. From 250 grams of poppy straw, three cups of water, about a liter of solvent, and a few drops of acetic anhydride, this is it—enough opiate extract, called *chorny*, to get two addicts high. The cost: about $10 and three hours of dangerous labor.

At the urging of his family, having sworn that he was only making the concoction to demonstrate to his visitor how *chorny* is made, Oleg "proves" he is no longer an addict and dumps the final drug into the kitchen sink. Artur watches silently, no expression on his tense face. A cold wind blows into the kitchen, dispersing the sickening fumes. Oleg's eyes fill with tears, and it is unclear whether he is regretting dumping the opiates, or merely reacting to the gaseous stench.

A few days later, the air still damp with Odessa's early April chill, a visitor crosses the train tracks and lingers for a while on a knoll overlooking a vast open meadow and, beyond, Palermo. A steady stream of adolescents pours past, their pace quickening as they eye Palermo and descend into the open field. It's easy to tell which of the youngsters have been using *chorny* the longest, as they no longer possess clothing and shoes adequate against the early spring chill and shiver uncontrollably. Those more recently inducted into the opiate world haven't yet sold their winter coats and boots for a few *hryvnya*; enough, perhaps, for another hit of *chorny*.

The opium concoction he's been shooting into his veins for two years no longer satisfies Sasha, a pale, wiry, twenty-year-old laborer. "Even so," he says, "I can't quit. Something keeps drawing me back here."

He pauses a moment to watch a cluster of other adolescent drug addicts scurry past into Palermo. "It doesn't matter anyway," he adds. "I'm HIV positive. Whether it's from drugs or AIDS, soon I will die."

Many of the friends Sasha grew up with have already died—of overdoses, alcohol, and drug-related violence, tuberculosis, AIDS, suicide. Now he is awaiting his turn.

When the Soviets fell in 1991, experts say, men like Ukraine drug lord Karabas began to rise throughout the region—gangsters who took advantage of the turmoil inherent in the historic change to target a generation of alienated young men and women, people like Sasha. Drugs were suddenly cheap and readily available, prostitution became a huge regional industry, and the stage was set for the birth of a regional AIDS epidemic of third world proportions.

"This isn't just an explosion," suggested Dr. Alla Soloviova, a Ukrainian working for UNICEF in Kyiv. "This is an A-bomb."

In 1996 some 7,000 new HIV cases were registered in Ukraine. And one international agency projected that by 2001 they would have 20,000 AIDS cases, perhaps a quarter million accumulated HIV infections, and 4,000 new AIDS cases a year erupting after that. These were startling numbers for a country that recorded only 214 cumulative HIV cases prior to 1994.

"Imagine the impact on the health care system then," said epidemiologist Luiz Loures of UNAIDS, which made the turn-of-the-century prediction.

It wasn't until mid-1996 that health experts in Odessa began to understand why the HIV "A-bomb" was exploding so dramatically in that city, as well as the rest of Ukraine. At that point, volunteers such as Odessa attorney Sergei Minov opened a discreet needle exchange center in Odessa and began questioning young people about their habits. What they found, Minov explained, "was a nightmare." Nearly all drug users said that they frequently shared needles and syringes, and that they typically pulled some of their own blood into the syringe after the initial injection in order to flush any remaining narcotics out.

It also became clear that the Gypsies of Palermo and organized drug gangsters elsewhere in the region were selling their poppy straw in forms already contaminated, Minov said. This was because the drugs were mass-produced, then checked for potency by young addicts who took free narcotics in trade for these life-threatening tests. To test the samples, the slaves, as these addicts were called, repeatedly dipped their personal syringes into large pots, and often pulled the plunger in and out several times.

Finally, Minov said, local addicts reported that Gypsy children were ordered by the drug suppliers to collect used syringes: the supplier would "fill them with narcotics and put them back in circulation."

This practice ended, Minov said, when he and other volunteers put the word out among the addicts that he wanted to talk to the "Gypsy Baron," who led the poppy straw trade in Odessa. Weeks passed.

Then one winter morning in 1996, he said, two large limousines came to Minov's apartment building, bodyguards leapt out, and the lavishly dressed drug lord knocked on Minov's door. Minov told him that selling contaminated opiate and syringes was "bad business" since it would quickly kill off his clientele.

The drug lord, whose identity Minov had sworn to keep secret, saw the wisdom of the lawyer's comments and forbade the children from collecting used syringes.

One small victory in an "A-bomb" war.

But the shooting field in front of Palermo was covered with used syringes, and desperate teen addicts often plucked an unbroken one off the ground for a quick *chorny* injection, if need be.

Down on the shooting field young people huddle in small groups, trying to find uncollapsed veins into which to inject one another. Pain writ upon their grimacing faces the teenagers poked and prodded one another, desperate to get the drug into their bloodstreams. So viscous is the opiate compote that the users needed 10 and even 20 cc needles—volumes far in excess of the 1 cc syringes used to inject heroin in North America or Western Europe.

Minov and the staff of a small drug addiction clinic called Trusting Spot collected thousands of syringes found in the Odessa shooting field in January 1997: fully a third of them tested positive for HIV.

"It's an explosive outbreak," Grigory Baavsky, a UNAIDS epidemiologist working in Odessa, says. "Every month we find six hundred new HIV cases. . . . In Odessa we have three thousand registered drug addicts. The real number is ten times that—"

Minov interrupts: "That's in a city of 1.1 million people. Think of that— thirty thousand for sure, out of 1.1 million."

Baavsky drew a chart, plotting the mounting Odessa HIV toll since the first cases appeared in 1995. He draws dotted lines, extending to 2012: "Within fifteen years the whole Odessa society could be up to 70 percent infected," he says.

UNICEF's Soloviova, a pretty, intense blonde, says that blood tests performed in the spring of 1995 revealed that nearly three-quarters of Odessa's IV drug-using population was HIV positive. Even she has a hard time believing the data, realizing that the virus overwhelmed the community in less than six months. Surveys of the drug users indicate that nearly all of them are under thirty years of age, have completed high school, and are unemployed.

Back in 1995 Soloviova attended a regional UNICEF meeting, where she pleaded with her fellow United Nations employees to commit resources to what she foresaw as an AIDS crisis.

"The policy makers said, 'Oh, only three hundred cases in all of Ukraine? We have so much more cardiovascular disease, cancer . . . this HIV isn't a problem.' "

The next year Soloviova pled her case again, directly to UNICEF chief Carol Bellamy. By then Soloviova had numbers that revealed a sudden surge of cases in Kyiv and Odessa, "and it was like a bomb went off. They said, 'My God, is it really so?' " Soloviova recalled.

Soloviova set to work, discovering that none of the governments in the area had any public health strategy for dealing with HIV. And, she said, "The speed of this epidemic is the fastest in all of Europe."

Even at the Plague Laboratory, once the bastion of SanEp efforts in Ukraine, Drs. Lev Mogilevsky and Elena Yugorova believed the numbers of HIV cases in teens and young adults were huge.

"Our main task is to save the younger generation," Mogilevsky sternly says. "If we manage to pull them out of the reach of the Mafia structures, we will win this battle."

Stopping the Mafia, Gypsy gangs, and other narcotraffickers in the region would be tough—perhaps impossible, psychiatrist Pavel Bem said. Handsome, long-haired, thirty-four-year-old Bem was one of Eastern Europe's leading experts on drug abuse, and chair of the Czech Government Anti-Drug Commission. Bem insisted that regardless of what factors were driving the region's young adults toward lives of drug addiction—and he felt a rather complex array of issues was involved—the real crisis for governments in the region was how readily, and cheaply, the killer products were available.

Almost without exception, narcotics and amphetamines could be purchased easily and openly, even in rural areas of Siberia or the frozen Arctic Circle. And sophisticated networks of gangsters and Gypsies, working with traditional drug traffickers from Nigeria, Afghanistan, Pakistan, and the Asian Golden Triangle, were moving across the newly porous borders behind the once-Iron Curtain.

"If you look at stable economies [such as the United States] there has been little increase in drug use in recent years," Bem said. "But these new economies are great opportunities for organized crime. And they are holding their prices way down at introductory levels."

Following universal rules of marketing, drug traffickers were creating clienteles in the region by selling everything from raw opium to heroin at rock-bottom prices, more than tenfold lower than equivalent drug sales in New York City.

The cheapest high was *vint*, an extract of ephedrine allergy pills that were chemically oxidized to ephedrone, a powerful hallucinogen. In Moscow *vint* sold for three dollars.

And the *vint* sellers were elderly babushkas who supplemented their meager Russian pensions by gaining free pharmaceutical ephedrine, as was their right as senior citizens who allegedly suffered allergies or hay fever. The women did the chemical extractions in their kitchens, loaded the *vint* either on sugar cubes or inside syringes, and sold the addictive concoction to teenagers—at a 200 percent profit above the babushka's total costs.

The primary selling spot for *vint* was Lubyanka Square, directly across the street from the headquarters of the Russian police force formerly known as the KGB.

The low cost and ready availability of these drugs explained why unemployed youngsters could afford to be high all of the time—even on top-grade heroin.

And youngsters desire to inject the deadly drugs, Bem said in fluent English. "It has something to do with the information overload and increasing demands on certain values and abilities. If you look at young teens today, to build a career and to be valuable to society it means you have to fulfill a lot of very difficult tasks . . . to be effective. And a lot of young people say, 'We cannot do it! We cannot fulfill this demand. We are not counted. It's senseless.' The technoculture emerging has no sense of grounding—you are flying somewhere in space. It's not a way to understand, it's only a way to feel. As a psychiatrist I would call it a separation from authentic feelings. It's something the older generation—the parent—is not able to understand."

The upsurge in drug use was most pronounced in the industrial areas that were erected, for the most part, during or immediately after World War II, as the

USSR built itself into a superpower. Millions moved to such cities during the 1960s and 1970s, mostly voluntarily; the pay was good, and Moscow gave its top industrial centers highest priority for shipments of fresh food, new clothing, televisions, and consumer products. In times of great scarcity for the rest of the USSR, workers of Novosibirsk, Noril'sk, Kemerovo, or Narva had tropical fruit in February.

But with the collapse of the USSR came a tough transitional economy in which the antiquated, inefficient industries of the past closed down. And that new openness allowed television images and magazines that showed the startled residents just how horribly sharp the contrast was between their bleak existences and that which was available to those in Moscow who could afford to buy the dreams of the West. Once elite, the ugly, dirty cities became little more than filthy centers of disappointment, envy, unemployment, alcoholism, and drugs.

In Estonia, for example, the Russians built a heavy-industry complex in the old medieval village of Narva, located a literal stone's throw from Russia's northwestern border. Prior to 1991, Narva averaged a population of 81,000 people, most of them Russians who were given priority job status over the native Estonians. It was a prosperous city.

But by 1998 only 75,000 people remained in Narva, nearly all the cement, textile, and metal factories were closed, and officially 39 percent of the population was unemployed. Located at the same latitude as Helsinki, Finland, the city saw no sunlight for three months out of the year, and then was entombed in snow.

"Democracy is good, but it's better when you have something for young people to do," moans Narva's Deputy Mayor Viktor Veevo. The burly Estonian-born Russian estimates that three thousand young people in Narva are drug addicts—about one out of every five residents aged fourteen to twenty-five years.

In Narva the incidence of hepatitis B and C increased 400 percent between 1992 and 1996, according to Dr. Olev Silland, director of Narva's hospital. And he is skeptical of Veevo's estimate of the number of IV drug users in the city—it's far more, he says, than three thousand. Perhaps more like ten thousand, or one out of every 7.5 residents of the beleaguered city.

HIV numbers were still low in Estonia, but Dr. Lea Tammai, the elderly epidemiologist of Merimetsa Hospital of Infectious Diseases in Tallinn, couldn't believe what was happening with hepatitis. In 1990, she said, the incidence of hepatitis B in Estonia was 6.9 per 100,000 people; hepatitis C was 2.6 per 100,000. By 1996 that was up to 24.5 per 100,000 incidence for hepatitis B and hepatitis C incidence had doubled.

Two floors of the hospital were full of hepatitis cases, all of them IV drug users.

At Narcology Hospital No. 17 in Moscow deputy director Tatiana Lysenko sees addicted boys every day. They come now in droves, their young bodies sickened by the drugs—and by hepatitis. Her Moscow 3,300-bed facility is full, and she, like her counterparts from Odessa to Vladivostock, has no idea what to do about it. Since 1982, when Narcology Hospital No. 17 opened, Lysenko has been the SanEp representative inside the massive facility, and during Soviet times her job was fairly straightforward. Narcology, or the medical discipline that dealt with *narkomania*, had extraordinary powers then to seek out drug users and incarcerate them in hospitals like No. 17—sometimes for years. Lysenko never had to resort to persuasion, methadone—which was, and remained after 1991, illegal across most of the region—behavior modification, or any of a long list of tactics Western physicians working with narcotics and amphetamine addicts utilized. Until 1991 Lysenko, and hundreds of health care workers like her, simply called in the police and locked up the users. And the patients cold-turkeyed, repented, underwent political re-education, and either learned the error of their ways or were sent to prison. It was simple.

But after 1991 and the collapse of Communist rule narcologists had no idea what to do.

"Drug use estimates from the [Russian] Ministry of Interior say there are about two million IV drug users, 300,000 long-term users," UNAIDS Moscow representative Zdeněk Ježek said. "Ten to 15 percent of the Russian population has some experience with IV drug use."

Ježek, a white-haired Czech scientist who had worked all over the world for the United Nations, was flabbergasted. He found public health officials regionally were mired in old Soviet ways of thinking, completely unable to grasp how to stem the tide of hepatitis and HIV in new, democratic social systems.

Ježek grabs a stack of charts and tables, telling a visitor that these very tables had been shown to one government official after another, usually with no effect. One chart shows, for example, that in 1995 only 0.3 percent of Russia's known HIV cases were IV drug users. But by December 1996, Ježek said, "61.2 percent of all HIV was in IV drug users. To plot the rate of growth in this population we have to use a log scale."

In May, Dr. N. F. Gerasimenko, of the Russian Academy of Medical Sciences, announced that new HIV cases there rose eightfold between 1995 and 1996 to around 1,500, and the Ministry of Health said it expected 800,000 people to be infected by the turn of the century, or about 5 percent of the country's projected population. By comparison, only 0.3 to 0.5 percent of the U.S. population is thought to have contracted HIV or AIDS between 1979 and 1999.

Like Ukraine, this rapid HIV expansion was occurring in a country that just a few years before was labeled an "AIDS-free zone" by Russian health officials citing exhaustive state-mandated HIV testing, which failed for years to turn up significant signs of the pandemic.

"We are now experiencing a true explosion of HIV in this region," UNAIDS director Dr. Peter Piot insisted. "We see the same potential as we saw in North America sixteen years ago, which makes us worry that we're really not learning from our mistakes."

Belarus state epidemiologist Vladimir Yeremin offered this chilling example: the economically depressed industrial city of Svetlogorsk, population 72,000, had zero detectable HIV cases until January 1997. Then, suddenly, there were eight hundred, all among young drug users, and Yeremin estimated that one out of every nine residents of the squalid city were infected.[126]

Worse yet, scientists at UNAIDS in Geneva identified eight of the ten known HIV subtypes circulating in a region stretching from Belarus to Vladivostock, from the Baltic states in the north to the Eastern European nations along the Danube and Dneiper Rivers. And this, in turn, prompted concerns that it would be here, in this well-traveled region, that the disease would recombine genetically, taking on new forms.

HIV was one of the world's most rapidly mutating viruses, and it responded quickly to changes in its target human population. For example, most infected drug users and gay men in the world carried the B subtype of HIV, while female prostitutes in Africa and Asia predominantly had the C, D, A, and E subtypes.

But only a tiny minority of the world's AIDS population moved in social circles that allowed them exposure to widely divergent HIV subtypes, so few people in the 1990s carried two or more subtypes in their bodies at the same time. When such superinfections occurred, HIV had a golden opportunity: it could trade genetic chunks of its RNA from one subtype to another, creating new genetic forms that could include the ability to infect a wider range of cell types, outwit certain drugs, or cause more rapid illness.

And, true to forecast, a new form of HIV did emerge in Russia's Kaliningrad during 1997. The new strain represented a blend of B and A clade viruses. The A clade was identical to a strain previously seen among IV drug users in Odessa; the origins of the B clade were unknown. The new virus contained the genetic capabilities of both clades.[127]

"It's unbelievable," virologist Saladin Osmanov of the UNAIDS Programme in Geneva said. "It now seems that the East will be the mixing pot for all of the elements of the last fifteen years of HIV worldwide: subtypes, sex, intravenous drug users, nosocomial [hospital spread]. This is it."

All this viral diversity implied that HIV had entered the region several times, from different parts of the world. Osmanov said that there were at least five epidemics in the region—reflecting five separate times and places in which particular strains were introduced.

It was questionable whether all five would continue to develop; experts said it was clear that beyond the narcotics-driven dominant epidemic lay a bur-

geoning heterosexual epidemic that could be more explosive than seen anywhere—including Thailand, which went from a handful of cases in 1989 to a 70
percent infection rate in prostitutes in 1991.

"You really need to understand the nature of sex networks in Eastern Europe" to understand the potential in the region, explained Dr. Luiz Loures of the
UNAIDS Programme. "Clearly the rates of multiple partner sex are higher than
in Western Europe. And though no one knows the size of the sex worker population, it's large and growing.

"It's all very dynamic," he added, "and the situation is hard to forecast
right now."[128]

Despite such grim information, Ježek said government officials still declined to take appropriate steps to slow the spread of HIV among IV drug users.

"The government sees drug users as criminals," Ježek explained. "During
the Soviet period drug use officially did not exist. So all of these people were
underground. And if people are underground you cannot reach them, cannot
educate them."

The strongest anti-AIDS program in the region was in Prague, the Czech
Republic. There, Dr. Marie Bručkova ran a national AIDS laboratory that collected and analyzed blood from individuals who voluntarily gave samples in
confidential or anonymous settings. Those infected got free treatment, counseling, and safe sex education.

Meanwhile, on-the-street AIDS education was done through needle
exchange centers with support from the nation's president, Vaclav Havel, and
safe sex education had been introduced into school curricula.

Since mid-1997 the Czech Republic had identified only 318 citizens with
HIV, 95 of whom had developed AIDS, and Bručkova described the national
mood in terms of AIDS as "alert, but not in panic mode."

The Georgian government, which was deeply cash poor as a result of post–
civil war economic despair, couldn't match the Czech campaign in size but followed a similar approach, at least in intent, said Dr. Tengiv Tsertsvadze, who
headed up the Caucasus nation's anti-AIDS efforts, coordinated through a small
laboratory in Tblisi, the capital city.

The education and voluntary testing program was done in collaboration
with Dr. Jack Dehovitz of Downstate Medical Center in Brooklyn, Tsertsvadze
proudly said, noting, "It's a very civilized program."

But there were other problems in this war-torn country that doctors like
Tsertsvadze had to contend with—including a highly questionable public blood
supply. In Tblisi, for instance, fewer than half of all blood transfusions involved
sera or plasma that had been screened for HIV or hepatitis contamination.

According to Tsertsvadze's staff only seventeen thousand of fifty thousand
blood bank donors were tested in 1996, and at least half of the nation's emer-

gency blood donations weren't tested at all—for HIV, or any other virus. Only 3 percent of the nation's blood donations were screened for hepatitis B or C.

"In old times we had blood banks," Tsertsvadze said. "But not anymore."

Blood banks in Georgia were, in fact, rather sorry affairs: Tsertsvadze said that about 5 percent of the donations were hepatitis B positive, and an equal percentage carried hepatitis C. But he admitted that C testing was rare and "nobody knows the real number of cases."

Sources in Western embassies warned visitors that Georgia's blood supply was absolutely unsafe and urged them to undergo even emergency procedures that might require transfusions outside the country.

It was not hard to see why. The central blood bank system of Georgia fell apart from 1992 to 1995 during its civil war. In its place emerged a chaotic hodgepodge of hospital banks and blood donation clinics, all of which paid donors, thus attracting alcoholics and drug users in need of quick cash. One such clinic in Tblisi had only sporadic electricity to ensure safe storage of its three refrigerators full of whole blood and two small freezers of plasma. The majority of its blood was "donated" by professional donors who came as frequently as doctors allowed them, to give a few pints in exchange for 12 *laris* (about $9.60)—which they in turn used to purchase a pint of booze or hit of opium extract, blood bank director Bella Kvachantivadze conceded.

Two such donors, Yuri Nevandovski and Viktor Yakovlev, reeked of alcohol as they stuck their arms through a portal in a glass wall. On the other side of the barrier a nurse drained their blood. After which the men pocketed their *laris* and staggered off in search of strong Georgian wine.

While some other countries in the region had better blood banking systems, only a handful had resources for universal screening of donors for hepatitis B and C, HIV, or any other dangerous viruses. Given the extraordinary explosion of these viruses occurring in the IV drug-using population, and the local practice of paying donors for providing blood or plasma, this seemed an extraordinary regional public health time bomb.

Nowhere was that possibility as scary as in Russia. Across the entire eleven-time-zone length of the vast nation, hepatitis, in particular, was emerging from obscurity into a full-fledged epidemic. In the short run, treatment costs were minimal, as there was not much Russian hospitals could do for viral hepatitis cases short of nutritional support and gamma globulin shots to boost patients' immune systems. Ten years down the road, however, Russia, and the other Eastern countries, will face tough economic choices as the advanced cirrhosis and liver cancer cases appear.

In the United States, advanced hepatitis-associated disease could make an individual a candidate for antiviral and cancer chemotherapy or liver transplantation—if the local board overseeing priorities in organ donations was willing to give a precious transplant to a virally infected recipient. But such procedures were extremely costly and required advanced medical technology. A six-month course of antiviral chemotherapy for hepatitis C cost $200,000 and was fully effective in less than 20 percent of all cases.[129]

If Russia's medical system advances far enough by 2007 to be able to handle such cases, it still is unlikely to find treatment affordable for any but the richest patients who can pay their own piper.

Officially Russia had a combined hepatitis incidence in 1996 of 26.7 cases per 100,000 adults and 5.9 cases per 100,000 children, according to the Ministry of Health. This represented a doubling in officially recorded hepatitis cases since 1992.

But in a report filed at the close of 1996 by the Russian Academy of Medical Sciences to President Boris Yeltsin, the toll of hepatitis appeared far graver and was described as "unfavorable."[130] In 1995, it stated, more than 52,000 Russians were hospitalized for viral hepatitis, primarily types B and C. The incidence of type B, alone, topped 36 per 100,000 Russians. Combined viral type hepatitis was said to be far higher, but no reliable estimate of numbers could be given because so few tests were performed for types C through G.

When the Soviet Union fell apart in 1991, fewer than 6 percent of all hepatitis cases in Russia were among intravenous drug users. By 1995, however, 21 percent of all Moscow hepatitis hospitalizations were drug users, as were 40 percent of those in St. Petersburg.

The underreporting of hepatitis infections was a serious problem, aggravated by two factors: the lack of appropriate laboratory test kits to allow diagnosis and patient failure to seek medical assistance before their infections had reached acute phases. Often the young drug users, oblivious to their health needs, were canary yellow from jaundice and suffered full-fledged cirrhosis by the time they sought treatment. Since most non-A hepatitis infections were asymptomatic for weeks, even years, the number of reported hospitalizations represented only a fraction of actual viral infections. In no part of Russia had scientists done systematic surveys of drug-using adults and teenagers to determine the genuine, asymptomatic infection rates.

In the southern Siberian city of Novosibirsk, officially registered numbers of hepatitis B and C cases did soar, approaching 180 cases per 100,000 in 1997, according to Dr. Tatyana Boyko, deputy president of the Public Health Commission. And Novosibirsk Oblast Hospital infectious diseases expert Dr. Evgeny Bocharov said that whenever he tested hospitalized *narkomani* for the viruses, "It's everywhere. It's a common cold already. We've seen a fivefold increase just since 1995."

Once these viruses found their way into a hospital—via a drug-using cirrhosis patient, for example—they could spread to the general population with terrifying efficiency if appropriate precautions were ignored. That was why Bocharov shouted when asked about the hepatitis risk in his Novosibirsk hospital: "Shortages, shortages, and more shortages! We have no latex gloves, syringes, anything!"

At the large Oblast Hospital in Odessa, Dr. Vasiliy Gogulenko was similarly distressed about contamination, particularly because, he said, "To be infected we [health care workers] need to have less than a drop of blood exposure. It takes only 10^{-9} viruses per milliliter of blood to cause hepatitis C infections."

Senior nurse Lila Brynchuk said that nurses on the hospital's surgical staff openly complained because it was illegal for health care workers to go on strike in Ukraine. They wanted the state to pay for protective hepatitis B vaccines, which cost twenty *hryvnya*, or about 15 percent of a nurse's monthly wages—when she got paid at all.

Fear of treating drug-addicted patients had nearly paralyzed the staff of Odessa's infectious disease hospital, chief Dr. Konstantin Servetskiy said, "Because we have no financial possibility to purchase gloves for our staff."

The health care providers also feared for their patients, because they could not afford to routinely test blood for hepatitis contamination. At the Institute of Oncology and Radiology, Dr. Grigory Klinenyouk would do anything necessary to protect the forty children who were under his treatment for cancer—including giving pints of his own hepatitis-free blood on a regular basis to the leukemia and lymphoma patients. He had to bleed himself and his nurses dry, the dedicated young doctor said, "Because unfortunately for the recent months the institution cannot find funds for hepatitis testing. Even HIV tests can only be done if indicated" by donor symptoms.[131]

At a clinic in Kyiv, Alexander, a television repairman by trade, sits in the converted seventeenth-century Ukrainian monastery that serves as that country's primary AIDS hospital. The forty-six-year-old father of three speaks of his room as his "cage" but says he appreciates the kindness of the staff.

One of the nurses—a woman who has treated HIV patients for more than two years—rolls up Alexander's sleeve and takes a blood sample. Although she's not wearing protective latex gloves, she uses her forefinger to apply pressure on the site of injection after she removes the needle. Then, still bare-handed, she injects the blood into a test tube, manually removing the needle from the syringe.

When her supervisor, Dr. Alla Vouk, is questioned about the incident later, she flatly denies that any of her staff ever performs blood-related procedures without appropriate precautions. Her denial is unaltered by a visitor's insistence that these events were eyewitnessed, and photographed.

Throughout areas of the former Soviet Union witnessing an upsurge in HIV, health providers seemed woefully behind the times. While concerned about their own safety, many were seen routinely without protective attire performing procedures that put them in direct contact with patient blood.

Meanwhile, some continued to demand the right to decrease their personal risks by performing HIV tests without patient approval, and refusing care to those who were infected. It was a discussion painfully familiar to American nurses, physicians, and dentists, who collectively confronted the same issues and debates more than a decade earlier.

One crisp June morning in St. Petersburg Dr. Aza Rakhmanova, chief infectionist for the city, rushed between the numerous buildings of Botkin Infectious Diseases Hospital, heading for the Neurosurgery Institute. The month before, the short, plump woman recalled breathlessly, "Surgeons did brain surgery and afterward realized the patient was an HIV-positive drug user from Kaliningrad. And the surgeons weren't wearing gloves! They claim that the brain is a fine structure and gloves impede their work. I told them it's a crime!"

Rakhmanova disappeared into the Neurosurgery building, where she would deliver the sorry message that first-round testing had turned up some tentative HIV-positive results in six of the surgeons and nurses who were in that operating room. The tests will have to be repeated, probably several times over coming months.

Ironically Rakhmanova has just come from her AIDS ward, where she dispensed therapy that would be sophisticated even in New York City, epicenter of the North American epidemic. To twenty-eight-year-old Costa she suggested adding anabolic steroids to his protease inhibitor combination therapy to enhance the man's metabolism.

"It makes sense," she said brusquely. The patient was left wondering how to pay for still more drugs, as Rakhmanova strolled next door to the room of a long-haired bearded man who was sitting on the edge of his bed and slowly, tentatively spooning food into his mouth.

"How is the invirase?" Rakhmanova asks. Timour Novikov looks up, his eyes fixing on a spot a few inches shy of the doctor's position. As he carefully slides his borscht soup aside, Novikov smiles and says, "I can swallow the pills— it's not too difficult."

Novikov, an artist, lost his eyesight recently when an opportunistic viral infection invaded his brain, causing encephalitis. Now he sells his paintings to pay for the protease inhibitors that have restored some of his weight and his ability to walk.

As Rakhmanova and her staff move from room to room making patient rounds they know when it is necessary to wear gloves—and when it is not.

But outside the rarefied world of a handful of such AIDS-specialized sophisticated hospital settings, ignorance reigns. At the Kyiv AIDS Clinic, for example, thirty-eight-year-old postal worker Viktor has had AIDS for three years.

He won't take AZT—the only treatment available in Ukraine. Instead he sees a popular Kyiv healer, "who has invented an apparatus to measure biocurrents from my body. She charges the currents with a piece of tin, which we call a bullet. And the bullet counters my negative biocurrents."

Viktor opens his shirt to reveal a bullet-shaped piece of tin taped to his chest.

And in Odessa, where abortions are the preferred form of birth control, doctors make extra cash by performing the procedures outside the hospitals. "In that case the physician doesn't know that [the patients] are HIV positive," prominent obstetrician Igor Boychenko said. "And she may be treated with the same tools and instruments as the next woman."

As the HIV toll mounted at a frightening pace in the former Soviet Union, Eastern Bloc governments found themselves in the unique position of having a small window of time to take public health actions that might forestall medical disaster. But despite nearly two decades of vivid AIDS history and experience from around the world the authorities were unable to agree upon courses of action, lacked funds to support the few steps they are willing to take, and had no experience—with any medical problem—in modern approaches to public health.

In some places, such as the Baltic nation of Estonia, freedom and candid discussion were considered the ideal approaches to stemming an HIV tide. But in many other parts of the former Communist world top AIDS doctors and politicians claimed that only a return to totalitarian control of society could stop the virus.

"From my point of view it's necessary to bring back socialism," Vadim Pokrovsky told a visitor to his HIV research and clinical care facility in Moscow. "This psychology of socialism is more acceptable for Russians—the so-called democratic way is not realistic at the moment. The sense of working for society is very important for young people. In the present moment they don't understand, and the result is drug addiction, prostitution, and so on."

Extreme as that may sound Pokrovsky was reflecting a sentiment popular among members of the Russian and Ukrainian public health elite—most of whom gained entry to the top circles of science and medicine during the Soviet period when such stature could only be obtained with membership in the Communist Party. These leaders looked at their countries in the post-Communist world and saw lawlessness—an anarchy that microbes easily exploited. And they said they saw a state of disorder that needed to be arrested by classic Communist means: secret police, Young Pioneers and other rigid youth groups, large prisons, and harsh penalties.

Noting that the "world community forced us to comply" with its notions of human rights, Russian Ministry of Health official Belaeyev said his country was compelled to abandon methods that had kept HIV in check for a decade. Now, he insisted, it was hard to believe Russia was supposed to follow AIDS control measures promoted by American human rights advocates.

"It's more than 500,000 AIDS cases in the U.S.A. That's not a good example for us!" Belaeyev insisted.

By the end of 1998 the Russian Ministry of Health had to acknowledge two things: nearly all new HIV cases were among youthful IV drug users, and the ranks of said narcotics and amphetamine injectors had swelled dramatically. The Ministry's Onyschenko said that 90 percent of all new HIV cases—those diagnosed since January 1996—were IV drug users. And, he noted, there were officially one million IV drug users in Russia in early 1998. Where spot checks were performed around Russia, from 20 to 70 percent of the nation's IV drug users were HIV positive in 1998, which would indicate, assuming all of the above numbers were reasonably accurate, that between 200,000 to 700,000 IV drug users in Russia carried the virus. Given that Russia's infection rates were, until 1996, among the lowest in the world, such numbers, if accurate, pointed to one of the pandemic's most rapidly evolving epidemics. And expensive: nearly all of those cases were young adults who would, had they been healthy, have formed the backbone of Russian economic development in the early twenty-first century.

At the close of 1998 UNAIDS estimated that 270,000 people in Eastern Europe and Central Asia were HIV positive. This was certainly a conservative guess, probably a gross underestimate. Given apparent infection rates in the IV drug users regionally it was hard to imagine that HIV numbers were of such moderate size. As of the end of December 1997, 7 percent of the Russian military tested positive for HIV infection. That was roughly 105,000 men, or more than a third of the UNAIDS estimate.[132] As the twenty-first century dawned, the pattern of drug behavior and spread of HIV seen in Odessa and Kaliningrad in the mid-1990s was repeating in hot spots across the region. The results were HIV wildfires, fueled by shared narcotics needles, in Moscow, St. Petersburg, Irkutsk, Krasnoyarsk, and scattered outposts in the Baltic nations of Estonia and Lithuania, as well as Siberia. Addiction rates as high as 50 percent were common among teens and young adults in these hot spots, and statisticians were hard pressed to calibrate the explosive spread of HIV by 2000.[133]

In most respects the region's HIV epidemic appeared in the late 1990s to be following the tragic model set by Thailand a decade earlier. In 1988 HIV rates in all population groups in that Southeast Asian nation were quite low, with fewer than 3 percent of any group testing positive for infection. In early 1989, however, surveys of Bangkok IV drug users jumped ominously, with just over a third testing positive: eleven months later half of them were infected. And by the end of 1991 IV drug users all over the country were infected: less than 15 percent had escaped HIV.

Lagging just a few months behind that IV drug epidemic was an upsurge in HIV seen in prostitutes and their male clients. Nationwide in mid-1989 less than 4 percent tested positive. Twelve months later the infection rate in prostitutes was 10 percent. And six months after that a whopping 70 percent of the prostitutes in tourist mecca Chiang Mai were infected. By the end of 1991 upward of 90 percent of the lowest-class prostitutes—those who served more than five customers every day out of hellish brothels—were infected nationwide. And by 1992 HIV had so thoroughly spread into the general population that life expectancy for the year 2000 was expected to plummet by an average thirty years and the population was predicted to see shrinkage, with twenty-five million fewer Thais than would have existed in the absence of HIV.

All of that in a time span of just two and a half years.[134]

For Eastern Europe's HIV epidemic to follow that tragic pattern either a high degree of promiscuity in the adolescent populations across the region or substantial prostitution need exist.

While the end of communism may not have in most countries in the region signaled a rise of genuine democracy, it did generally usher in a freer atmosphere among young adults. With that came a rise in adolescent and post-adolescent promiscuity. In the absence of readily available condoms, or male willingness to use the protective devices, this 1960s-style free love atmosphere was woefully cavalier in the face of a 1990s HIV pandemic.

But in every country in the region the sexually transmitted diseases data tracked wrong: the genders were out of synch. Females had far higher disease rates than the males in their age groups. And that was because more and more of the girls weren't having sex with boyfriends but with older adult men who had money. And it was paid sex.

Dr. Jaromir Jirašek, for example, was at the end of his rope. He had done everything he could to stop the prostitutes, pimps, and their German customers from taking over his little Czech town. But under the new post-Communist Czech constitution any attempts to ban prostitution represented illegal violations of human rights.

So Jirašek and his fellow citizens of the small Bohemian village of Dubi were forced to turn a blind eye to the Ukrainian, Slovakian, Russian, Bulgarian, Romanian, and Gypsy girls who stood half naked in glass booths along the E-55 highway, wiggling to an unheard rhythm, presenting their "goods" to the drivers of passing BMWs, Audis, and Mercedes.

Dubi is just twelve kilometers from the German border, not far from Dresden. The tiny town is one of many strung along E-55 that during the 1990s had become little more than brothels, strip joints, roads full of streetwalkers, parklands littered with discarded underwear, and school playgrounds strewn with sex leaflets written in East German dialect.

But the forty-something Jirašek was no prude. His office was adorned with naked pinup girls and, he said with a wink, the doctor knew how to have a good time. A middle-aged man with a sharply receding hairline and wire-rimmed bifocals, Jirašek spoke sitting in front of a large calendar depicting Miss June— a naked blonde sporting bandolier crisscrossed shell casings and holding an AK-47 rifle. His objections to the new, yet already titanic, prostitution industry were those, he said, of a physician.

"We're seeing syphilis, gonorrhea, soon HIV," Jirašek explained. "Since 1989 it started with pimps here with two, maybe three, girls in a car. And later they bought houses right on the highway . . . and by a year ago the situation was one of girls lined all along the side of the highway—in a huge line [several kilometers long]. And Germans drove by and chose which one. And they had sex in these houses, in the forest, in the cars—anywhere.

"Sometimes local people are involved, but the business is run by foreigners. And they don't provide health care to their prostitutes. They're all over the Czech Republic, all over Eastern Europe, in fact, and when one [prostitute] gets ill they just replace her. That's it."

Since the 1989 Velvet Revolution of Czechoslovakia, the 1990 fall of the Berlin Wall, and then the 1991 collapse of the Soviet Union prostitution had transformed in the vast region from a tightly controlled cottage industry into a multibillion-dollar, multinational enterprise controlled by sophisticated organized crime rackets that transported tens of thousands of women—and in all too many cases girls and boys—from the poorest formerly Communist countries to pockets of plenty along the borders of wealthy Western Europe and the Middle East. The scale of these operations was staggering. It was globalized sex—and globalized sexually transmitted diseases.

The International Organization of Migration had struggled since 1991 to keep track for the United Nations of the woman-smuggling operations out of Eastern Europe. The trafficking of women, the IOM's Marco Gramegña said, was so massive and so rapidly expanding that the agency could provide only ballpark estimates.

"These [ex-USSR] women are the new merchandise," Gramegña explained. "And it is a new form of slavery. I would say it is following exactly the model we see in India. These women are given a contract—a phony contract—for legitimate jobs in Western Europe. The trafficker charges her bank account or debits her future earnings for her plane tickets and lodging. When she reaches the destination the trafficker seizes her passport, plane ticket home, documents, and tells her she must work as a prostitute until she earns back her debt. And of course she never does."

In this manner about a half million women from Eastern Europe and the former Soviet Union had been smuggled into Western Europe and forced into prostitution by 1995, Gramegña said. And thereafter the scale of the operation escalated, with up to 300,000 more women trafficked into Western Europe annually, most of them from Russia and Ukraine. By early 1998 the "slave prostitute" trade was netting at least $20 billion a year in Western Europe and untold additional amounts in the Middle East and Asia. No one knew how many more women from the region were being smuggled into China and Japan, or southwest into the Middle East. But it was possible that the combined scales of those operations nearly matched that of the Western European smuggling enterprise.[135]

At the international level, Gramegña noted, the crime syndicates involved in the trafficking of women and girls were also key players in narcotics and weapons smuggling. Some of the business was handled by decades-old Mafia gangs, but there were "new Russian ones. And they are investing financially in [legitimate] Western European businesses—they are Europe's new nouveau riche."

"A Mafia man told us that the girls are bought as slaves and every mark or dollar they earn is taken away from them," Jirašek said. "They are beaten. Their identity papers are taken away from them. And they can't go anywhere without a guard who keeps them from running away." Every Bohemian official and physician in the area confirmed that more than 95 percent of Bohemia's prostitutes were non-Czech women lured to the area under false pretenses, such as alleged disco dancing jobs, by organized crime figures. The women came from Ukraine, Russia, Belarus, Slovakia, Bulgaria, and Romania and were, in the word most commonly used to describe their plight, "slaves."

The prostitution syndicates appeared to be beyond regulation, out of police control. In little Dubi, for example, two of the more than twenty brothels were situated along either side of a police station. Gypsy and Russian women dressed in hot pants and spiked heels called out to cars twenty-four hours a day in plain view of the police. Prostitutes also worked in front of local schools and parks, angering helpless parents.

"Since 1985 we have seen a thousandfold increase in syphilis," Dr. Alesander Moroc of the Central Hospital in Ustí Nad Labem said. Ustí, also a Bohemian town, is about a twenty-minute drive from Dubi. Moroc is the city's clinical expert on sexually transmitted diseases (STDs).

"Sixty-eight percent of the syphilis is among fifteen- to twenty-four-year-old females. And often we see syphilis in late pregnancy women. They come in during the second half of pregnancy when nothing can be done. Before 1995 we never had any, but now we do see congenital syphilis here," Moroc said. "In one case the baby died right away, but normally the child is healthy looking, but serologically positive. . . . Often these kids are lost to follow-up" and go untreated.

The other major STD, gonorrhea, was also on the rise, but "we see a paradox that gonorrhea rates appear to be decreasing as syphilis rises," Moroc explained. "This is because general practitioners treat the gonorrhea and don't report the cases."

Syphilis was harder to diagnose and treat—it required more extensive antibiotic therapy—so patients typically sought clinic or hospital assistance and ended up as registered cases. Gonorrhea, in contrast, could be treated with a single penicillin injection. So privacy-conscious people sought discreet care for their gonorrhea, leaving the disease woefully underreported.[136]

Worse, widespread self-medication or physician misuse of antibiotics resulted in mutant strains of gonorrhea that are drug resistant.

"Resistance to penicillin is actually the norm now," Moroc said, noting that there was no drug-resistant gonorrhea in Bohemia prior to 1991. In Dubi, Jirašek said that only three physicians were licensed, and none of them would treat the prostitutes. So, he concluded, the pimps were obtaining penicillin and other antibiotics through black market suppliers.

A 1992 Czech government survey of Ustí prostitutes showed that 30 percent carried either syphilis or gonorrhea. Rates were believed to have doubled since then, Moroc said, but the pimps forbade the women from participating in such studies.

A plump, middle-aged man with sparse black hair, Moroc has a face filled with warmth and sincerity. It emits genuine pain when he reveals that 68 percent of all female syphilis cases reported in the Czech Republic in 1996 came from his hometown district of Ustí.

Moroc shakes his head.

"There were surveys done among the prostitutes and it showed that the women are forced NOT to use condoms by their pimps because they make more money," Moroc said.

It was impossible to interview prostitutes in Bohemia: none would talk. Even taking photographs drew protests and threats. Jirašek said a German photographer who made photographs in 1996 on E-55 was shot at but escaped unharmed.

Gynecologist Pavla Vitagfásková worked with Prague-based Pleasure Without Risk, a nongovernmental outreach group that tested for HIV and STDs

among Czech prostitutes. Rates of infection weren't as high in Prague as in Bohemia, she said, but they were climbing steadily. Worse yet, even her group
couldn't get past the pimps and Mafia to educate and test the prostitutes.

"From time to time the girls get beaten," Vitagfásková said. "The pimps
don't want us talking to them. And some of them are only sixteen. There's an
area around the main railroad station where there are many homeless women.
They come often from Slovakia looking for jobs and can't find any. The girls are
sick, homeless. They have sex in toilets. Sometimes merely for a bowl of soup.
We found there a Slovakian woman with secondary syphilis."

In Ustí chief epidemiologist Dr. Josef Trmal, of the Regional Institute of
Public Health, found evidence in 1997 that the Bohemian STD epidemic "seems
to have gone well beyond the prostitution circle to all sexually active young
adults. We've seen an increase in the numbers of people seeking STD counseling
and treatment and most of them are teenagers and very young adults."

"We do see a connection between drug abusers and prostitutes," Trmal
said. "With girls it is a strong problem—dual drug use and prostitution. Some
girls said they were prostitutes only when under the influence of drugs.

"For five hundred deutsche marks you can buy a [slave] girl from Turkish
dealers," Trmal continued. "The pimps are buying the girls and then forcing
them to be prostitutes forever. The girls are on drugs, they don't have documents."

Nationwide the Czech syphilis rate jumped from 50 cases per 100,000 in
1986 to 320 per 100,000 in 1996, according to Dr. Bohumir Kriz, head of the
National Center of Epidemiology and Microbiology—the Czech equivalent of
the Centers for Disease Control and Prevention. In 1995, Kriz said, the Czech
Republic saw its first congenital syphilis case ever entered into public health
records: "Terrible," he exclaimed.

In every sizeable Russian city prostitution strips or neighborhoods
emerged in which complex networks of young prostitutes, female pimps, and
male gangsters serviced both local and traveling business clienteles.

On an ice-cold night in front of Moscow's Red Square pretty Ula lures
customers with her teenaged charms. Dressed in a Dolce & Gabbana black
jacket, tight black patent leather pants, high-heeled boots, and a fluorescent pink
mohair skin-tight sweater Ula looks like a teen queen from suburban Americana.
She says she is eighteen, but blushes, betraying a poor ability to lie. She doesn't
look a day over fifteen. She left her family home in frigid Syktyvkar, about five
hundred miles northeast of Moscow, during the summer of 1996 to better herself, Ula says.

Now she stands in front of the Intourist Hotel, greeting men who drive up
beside her. The moment they arrive Ula's stern thirty-five-year-old *mamochka*—
her pimp—rushes up and negotiates a place, a price—the details of Ula's next

hour's work. If the men meet the right price Ula gets 50 percent of the take, which for one hour of sex in the hotel or back of a Moscow disco comes to $150 to $200. Her female pimp, who insists the girls call her by the affectionate Russian term for "mommy," takes the other half of the income. A typical Moscow *mamochka* works ten to twenty girls a night, earning on exceptional nights more than $5,000. On a dreary winter night like this, however, even the *mamochka* has to hustle hard to get enough customers to cover her overhead: bribes to the hotel and payoffs to local thugs who sit in a warm Mercedes ready to beat up any overtly kinky customers or men who try to stiff the girls with inadequate payments.

A few blocks away Marina pimps her six girls in front of Russia's legislative building, the Duma. The blue-eyed brunette is well bundled-up against the cold—after all, she's not selling her body. She ran into "some financial troubles" last year, Marina says, so at age twenty-four during the winter of 1997 she took on the title of *mamochka*. A dozen other competing pimps race Marina to cars as the men pull over. Duma security guards dressed in combat fatigues watch but do nothing.

"That's the Duma across the street. If they can't do anything how can we," asks the tall guard, who says his name is Sasha. "It's been like this since 1980 when the Olympics happened. Now it's more open. People used to be afraid, but now we have democracy."

His short partner—also named Sasha—laughs, adding, "That's democracy for you!"

Prostitution in Moscow was far from subtle. The girls, their *mamochkas*, and the protective thugs could be seen day and night along highways, in train stations, in front of the state's sacred Red Square and Duma, inside discos and casinos, and in hotel bars. In Moscow's most exclusive nightclubs high-class hookers charged $1,500 for a night's "entertainment." At the extreme opposite end of the economic scale were women along Moscow's Ring Road who demanded $50 a night—or, lower still, illegal immigrant girls, homeless, who serviced their customers for a train station $2 kiosk meal.[137]

In the daytime abandoned or runaway children dashed among cars in Moscow's heavily congested streets, hawking prostitute pamphlets and "hot sex" tip sheets. Tiny ten-year-old Natasha, who clearly hadn't bathed in days and said she lived on the streets, darted among cars around Pushkin Square hawking a book that was a guide to Moscow prostitutes.[138]

"Gimme fifty thousand rubles [about $8]," Natasha demanded. "It tells you addresses, prices, and so on."

A Fagin-type figure skulked along the sidewalk shouting out to Natasha and several other apparently homeless little girls. "Hurry up! Sell more! Watch for the police!"

Natasha shot a frightened look at the man, said she was afraid of the police, and dashed off down the stairs of Chekov Metro station.

Little Natasha apparently could not read. Had she been able to she would have known that the book, authored by Edvard Maksimovsky, was subtitled *An Anti-Brothel Guidebook.* In page after depressing page Maksimovsky detailed the horrors of the lives of Moscow's sex workers, underscoring the coercion and fear that both brought the women into the trade and compelled them to remain—despite the obvious risks to their health and well-being. For example, Maksimovsky wrote, "In 1993 when the spring Moscow River ice melted there were six women's bodies found. That was a warning to all the girls: this is the fate of those who try to quit."[139]

The police often sat among the *mamochkas*, enforcing traffic regulations and parking laws—only rarely arresting the prostitutes, and never busting their clients. Because September 1997 marked the 850th birthday of Moscow the mayor moved the most blatant Red Square–area prostitution out of the city center. While that temporarily decreased the visual assault of Moscow's trade in flesh, it did not affect the industry's health impact. And, of course, the prostitutes were displaced for only a few weeks.

In 1988 Russia had a total of 5,704 registered syphilis cases, according to the Ministry of Health. In 1996 a staggering 386,935 cases were registered—a sixty-eight-fold increase in eight years.[140] And this whopping figure was most certainly an underreported total, according to a study conducted in 1996 by Dr. Adrian Renton of Westminster Medical School in London.[141] Joint British-Russian analysis revealed that the old Soviet system of tracking down and forcibly registering all the sex partners of identified syphilis cases virtually collapsed, along with the rest of the health care system. Further, in many parts of Russia the Dermatovenereology Service, as it was called, ran out of funds for drugs and now charged patients up to $300 for a twenty-eight-day course of syphilis treatment.

Wishing to avoid having their names on lists and lacking funds to pay the state doctors, more and more syphilitic individuals were either going underground for treatment or not getting treated at all. Even under the best of conditions syphilis could be hard to diagnose in women because the infection hides far inside their reproductive tracts and may lurk there—contagious to her fetuses and sex partners—for years before causing obvious hard-to-treat symptoms in the female. As the old system of syphilis screening deteriorated in Russia the risk to both women's health and to general public health rose.

But even the officially registered—grossly underreported—numbers were chilling.

In 1995 the national syphilis rate in eighteen- to nineteen-year-old boys was 359 per 100,000; girls in that age group had an astonishing 922 syphilis cases per 100,000.[142] (By way of comparison the combined male/female syphilis rate for that age group in the United States was 13.7 per 100,000.)

For 1996 the overall national syphilis rate was 221.9 cases per 100,000—thirty-seven times the U.S. rate. And in the city of Moscow, with a population roughly the same size as New York City, twenty thousand cases of syphilis were officially reported. The entire United States of America, with a population of over 260 million, had fewer than seventeen thousand syphilis cases that year.

What most troubled demographers when they looked at the syphilis numbers was how sharply the slope of the climbing curve of cases veered upward—almost at a ninety-degree angle. In 1994 the incidence nationally was 81.7 per 100,000—by 1995 it was 172 per 100,000. In 1996 it reached 221.9, and syphilis topped 330 cases per 100,000 in 1997, making Russia's syphilis rate one of the top ten worldwide. Even far outside Moscow rates were soaring. For example, in the medium-size Siberian city of Irkutsk syphilis reports jumped 78 percent from 1995 to 1996, reaching a rate of 422 cases per 100,000 people of all ages in the city, according to Irkutsk Oblast official data.

Watching this nervously from their offices in Geneva, Switzerland, officials with the UNAIDS Programme were convinced the official Russian figures understated the true syphilis rate by 10 to 20 percent. By 1998 UNAIDS was regrettably reporting that one out of every four hundred Russians had syphilis, rates of the disease were five hundred times greater than those seen in Western Europe, and since 1991 congenital syphilis rates had risen thirtyfold.[143] And they saw the same deeply disturbing STD trends in other former Soviet states, particularly Ukraine.[144]

In Ukraine the STD epidemic was being driven by the activities of young people aged thirteen to twenty-one years. While the Ukrainians who were over thirty had seen a steadily soaring syphilis rate since 1990, it was still below 180 cases per 100,000. Among adolescents, however, rates weren't soaring, they were rocketing to the moon—especially in girls.

According to the Ukrainian Ministry of Health girls fourteen years old and younger had about 600 syphilis cases per 100,000. And fifteen- to sixteen-year-old girls had syphilis rates since 1993 that fluctuated between 1,550 and 2,000 cases per 100,000. That meant one out of every fifty sweet-sixteen girls in Ukraine not only was sexually active, but also had seen enough male partners to have acquired syphilis. Estimated combined syphilis and gonorrhea rates in teenaged boys and girls in 1995 were 4,500 cases per 100,000. But by far the majority of those teen syphilis cases were girls.

"I always make my customers use condoms," claimed a fourteen-year-old girl dressed in hot pants, knee-high boots, and a fur bolero jacket. She laughed and gave a knowing wink to another teenaged prostitute working in front of Odessa's Philharmonic Hall. The girls all claimed to use condoms, but the truth was they merely charged more for customers who refused to use the protective latex devices.

The girl in hot pants, who declined to give her name, was part of a well-organized contingent of fifty prostitutes who solicited customers in front of the stately Philharmonic Hall, charging $50 for a "quickie" or $100 for an all-night dalliance. On the complex hierarchical scale of Odessa's vibrant sex industry the Philharmonic girls were middle class, according to psychologist Valeri Kiunov, who mapped out the sex trade for the UNAIDS Programme and Odessa State University. During Odessa's cold winter months about two thousand girls worked as prostitutes. But in the summer when the beachside city was a popular Ukrainian vacation spot the prostitute population more than doubled.

Kiunov has found six distinct social strata of prostitutes. Most of the youngest girls—ages eleven to seventeen years—worked as what he called "chaotic prostitutes," flagging down customers on the streets after school two or three times a week. They typically earned $39 to $50 a week and used condoms.

A second group, averaging twenty-six years of age, worked through female pimps and tended to have steady customers. Kiunov said two-thirds of these women had at least one STD during his three-year study (1994 to 1997).

The most promiscuous groups, called "the Pacifiers," tended to congregate around factories and large workplaces where they serviced twenty to forty clients a week. The mean age of the group was nineteen years, and nearly all of them had an STD during any given year.

Lucky girls worked their ways up to the Philharmonic crowd or the top rung—call girls toiling for gangsters who ran high-class operations inside all of Odessa's Londonskaya and other elite hotels.

But the most vulnerable group, Kiunov said, was also the largest, accounting for more than half of Odessa's sex workers. They worked particular streets, averaged eighteen years of age, and, he said, "agree on everything. And they are the most likely to get beaten, raped, have sick stuff done to them. They can't afford condoms [which cost twenty-five cents each], and when you talk to them about 'safe sex' they think it means avoiding beatings. They have no idea you're talking about STDs and AIDS."

Half of that group injected local opiate concoctions, and in recent years the average age of these prostitutes had been dropping.

"Last summer I saw nine- and ten-year-olds working in this group," Kiunov said. Some seven- and eight-year-olds even worked during school recesses doing what they called "hot sex"—quickies performed with adult men behind food kiosks for about two dollars.

The regional STD explosion was staggering,[145] and no government or United Nations agency possessed a public health strategy for tackling the problem.

"The situation in Moscow is grim," epidemiologist Nikolay Briko of the Moscow Medical Academy said in 1998. "Syphilis rates in the Russian Federation have increased fiftyfold over the last seven years. Special anxiety is caused by a fortyfold rise in syphilis cases among children and teenagers and a thirtyfold rise in congenital syphilis."

The highest levels of syphilis—in some cases more than two thousand times the U.S. rates—were in 1998 seen among girls aged sixteen to twenty.

"We consider assistance from the international community essential," Dr. Leonid Barabanov of the Belarus Ministry of Health said. "Unfortunately our government does not have adequate financial, technical or human resources to fight the STD epidemic on its own."

At the Geneva headquarters of UNAIDS public health experts were scrambling at the close of the 1990s to come up with strategies that could prevent the seemingly inevitable marriage of the prostitute-driven STD epidemic and burgeoning HIV/hepatitis crisis in IV drug users. With syphilis levels astronomically high, predominantly in girls aged fourteen to twenty years, and HIV/hepatitis rates soaring in boys and girls of the same ages, an AIDS catastrophe seemed tragically inevitable.

German scientist Karl Dehne tried out of his tiny UNAIDS office to coordinate prevention efforts across twelve time zones. Dehne's bleary eyes and jerky body movements betrayed lack of sleep, and the urgency in his voice showed genuine anxiety.

"They don't know anything [in former Soviet countries] about outreach, behavioral change, counseling. They say, 'Information! Information!' When I say, 'Information isn't enough to change behavior,' they say back, 'Well what else is?' Imagine—they have no methodology at all for outreach."

And why should they? During the heyday of SanEp, "outreach" consisted of forcibly rounding up the public and submitting everybody to whatever intervention was deemed worthwhile. The narcologists were only trained to imprison patients. The venereologists were taught how to maximize shame in order to limit spread of disease. Nowhere in the region's public health toolbox were the skills of peer education, persuasion, and nonjudgmental behavioral intervention.

"They tell me to find the people there, but it's just not there," Dehne exclaimed. "There are several million prostitutes there and not one prostitute outreach program."

Having done such work for years in Africa Dehne was stunned by the Eastern European dilemma: in no African country had he ever encountered such severe public health skills limitations and social obstacles to averting drug and sexual diseases crises.

"I think we have a window of opportunity here and I'm still hoping we can prevent an epidemic calamity. It's very new," Dehne said. Then his shoulders slumped and he concluded, "But I'm afraid I'm not really winning." A few months later Dehne, distraught over the situation, left UNAIDS, forming a private organization dedicated to training Russians and other former Soviets in public health outreach skills.

Brazilian researcher Luiz Loures had an office down the hall from Dehne, and although he had faced tough obstacles to AIDS prevention in Latin America he, like Dehne, was finding the former Soviet nations a dismal challenge.

"First of all," Loures said, pointing to charts and tables strewn across his data-cluttered desk, "look at the economics. Ukraine, for example. In 1992 it ranked sixty in the Human Development Index," a United Nations Development Program Scale in which higher numbers indicate greater progress in all facets of social and economic advancement and infrastructure. "By 1993, a year later, it was down to nineteen. By 1994—seventeen."

Now, Loures continued, add an overlay of a quarter million IV drug users and millions of teenaged prostitutes and it was obvious that Ukraine would have twenty thousand full-blown AIDS cases by 2001.

UNAIDS director Dr. Peter Piot, a Belgian, had been battling HIV since the virus first surfaced in the early 1980s. He had witnessed the evolution of epidemics in one nation after another. And he knew from experience that only one thing could avert disaster in the former Soviet region: "political leadership.

"Fundamentally the problem everywhere is public health leadership. Without leadership and political commitment [AIDS prevention] is not going to happen," Piot concluded. So in late 1997 Piot traveled the region, meeting with Yeltsin and other heads of former Soviet states. He went to the Davos economic summit, and the powerful G-8 meeting in 1998. He pleaded with the world's most powerful political leaders, asking that they draw a line in the sand along the former Iron Curtain, saying, "No more HIV."

At the G-8, Yeltsin, multinational corporate leaders, World Bank, and all of the leaders of the Newly Independent States nodded in agreement, issued bold resolutions, and lent written support to Piot's UNAIDS efforts.

But in concrete terms, they did nothing.

VIII

It is characteristic of Russia that the majority of people were reconciled to the fact that the guaranteed salary was wretched and the guaranteed medicine was awful. People who are not used to living in conditions of freedom are now feeling nostalgic for what they have lost.

—Andrei Sinyavsky[146]

G iven all the infectious disease scourges that physicians suddenly faced in the 1990s hospitals could no longer view themselves as cavalierly as they had during the previous decade. Under the Soviet construct medical care was farmed out to unique, specialized centers: alcoholics and drug users to narcology clinics; tuberculosis patients to the sanatoriums; infectious diseases patients to contagion clinics located in rural areas where the patients' germs couldn't cause urban epidemics. Even common colds and minor flu cases landed in isolated facilities where workers were spared having to toil while ill, but removed from their families until well. In this way the Soviet public health planners believed risk was segregated, and thereby limited: the society at large need not fear syphilis, TB, or diphtheria because all of the carriers were routinely rounded up and placed in sequestered facilities.

It was a system with much in common with Soviet political control. Possessors of deviant ideas were similarly rounded up and sequestered in gulags lest they might contaminate the masses with their subversive notions. For nearly seven decades it worked.

But by the 1980s, well before the USSR fell apart, hospitals were facing new threats about which the physicians and doctors knew very little: antibiotic-resistant bacteria; untreatable multidrug-resistant tuberculosis; hepatitis B and C. And after 1991 the trend accelerated, adding a host of once-controlled ancient infectious diseases and the new scourge of humanity—AIDS—to the mix. The microbes did not respect the hospital segregation system: infectious diseases would not oblige physicians' demands that they turn up only in designated facilities. And the patients were increasingly reluctant to abide by the sequestration system, preferring to stay at home among loved ones rather than bide months, even years, of time in isolated medical gulags—particularly as funds for the facilities diminished and hospitalization often involved stays in boring, ice-cold rooms with little to do, and even less to eat.

Thus, the 1990s signaled the region's need for a sort of public health shock therapy in which SanEp either disappeared or transformed into a seriously beneficial epidemiology and surveillance service. And one in which the notion of sequestered patients and diseases was abandoned in favor of strict, across-the-board infection control standards in all health care facilities, wherein it was assumed that *every* patient might be a microbe carrier, therefore precautions need be standardized and universal. No emergency room physician, for example, could confidently treat *any* patient in 1999 without wearing protective gloves, gown, and goggles or glasses—not when the region was in the grips of so many profound epidemics caused by organisms that could be contagious in the absence of obvious symptoms.

The new era also signaled an urgent need to decrease the amount of time patients were hospitalized, both to decrease costs and lower risks. Patients ultimately lived longer if they spent less time in medical facilities, where they were exposed to other patients' bacteria and viruses.

Outside in the community public health's image needed to change overnight, from its old Soviet authoritarian and paternalistic structure into one that recognized the individual's right to refuse vaccines, found funds for repair of water supplies, adhered to appropriate antibiotic use, offered IV drug rehabilitation services, promoted safer sex through use of condoms, and other preventive interventions that could protect the society at large. The individual right of refusal could no longer be overcome with the power of the state: only the powers of persuasion, peer education, health marketing, and common sense would do.

But it was no easy matter to transform an entire, gigantic infrastructure. Though the Soviet Union no longer existed, its public health apparati and apparatchiks still did.

The system—most of which was executed in 1999 as originally designed in 1937—worked like this: medical students and future epidemiologists were trained from age eighteen onward in different institutions, and rarely interacted. Once the epidemiologists were professionals, they joined SanEp, where they were trained to "basically function as policemen who came to hospitals and brought grief," said Russian-trained Dr. Elena Bourganskaia of American International Health Alliance in Washington, D.C. "So physicians learned to see epidemiologists as threats."

"The surveillance of infections is not lab-based at all," Bourganskaia said. "And it's passive. They [SanEp] wait for physicians to report [hospital-acquired] nosocomial cases. But in the old system physicians were punished if they were related in any way to an infection. So you basically have to be out of your mind as a physician to report cases."

Under Communist dictator Josef Stalin's rules, every system in the Soviet Union had to be monitored by a parallel, Communist Party–controlled apparatus. For the medical system, that apparatus was SanEp. And survival as a hospital administrator was absolutely contingent upon supplying SanEp with rosy reports, not word of an outbreak of antibiotic-resistant staphylococcus in your cardiac postop ward.

Worse yet, SanEp's entire procedural structure was based on false biology. Its concept of infection was an environmental one not terribly dissimilar from the ancient Greek concept of "miasma," meaning "bad air." Germs flew about in the air, and illness arose as a result of filthy environments. Soviet hospitals were required to expend enormous amounts of manpower scraping off samples of whatever film or muck might be on the walls, ceilings, and floors. And hospital microbiology laboratories devoted 70 to 90 percent of their resources to scrutinizing these samples for bacterial contamination.

If contaminants were found, SanEp marched in and someone took the fall.

If diseases spread within a hospital then a mad scramble was initiated, in search of the dirty wall or floor responsible for the spread of the microbes.

If patients failed to respond to first-line therapy then treatment typically followed an empirical course: Plan A didn't work, switch to Plan B. Rarely were patient samples sent down to the laboratory with instructions to find out why Plan A had failed.

"Virtually no one in [the former Soviet Union] is a clinical expert in diagnosis, management, and prevention of nosocomial [hospital-acquired] infections," said Dr. Ed O'Rourke, an infectious diseases expert at Boston's Children's Hospital, who, during the 1990s, shuttled around Russia and other former Soviet countries trying to spread the gospel of Western-style infection control.

"We talk about the abuse of antibiotics here, but here it's usually using overpotent drugs for simple infections," said O'Rourke, who was also on the faculty of the Harvard Medical School. "There they simply add one on top of another without any particular rationale. . . . And when the patient worsens they just add another drug to the regimen."

O'Rourke's main message was that more patients would survive simple bacterial illnesses, fewer such illnesses would be acquired inside hospitals, and everyone would save both lives and money if they stopped using antibiotics and conducting hospital hygiene in the manner they were taught under the Soviet regime.

There was no way to quantify the extent of nosocomial infections and antibiotic resistance in Russia or any other ex-Soviet country. The first—hospital-spread disease—couldn't be quantified because the old Stalin-era infrastructure of infection control was so punitive that doctors rarely reported cases. The second—drug resistance—couldn't be quantified because few clinical laboratories had adequate supplies or skills to perform drug sensitivity tests.

Nevertheless, it was obvious that the spread of drug-resistant microbes was proceeding at an alarming pace, and the sorry saga of Irakli Sherodzle—the strep-infected Georgian teenager—was becoming more commonplace every day.

At the Russian Ministry of Health's Central Microbiology Laboratory in Moscow, Drs. Nina Semina and Viktor Maleyev screened bacterial samples drawn from patients all over Russia. Their approach allowed them to determine what sorts of mutant microbes were out there, but not how frequently they were causing human disease. Despite the drawback, they had already found unnerving evidence of rapidly expanding antibiotic resistance.

Since 1993 the Moscow scientists found new drug-resistant strains of staphylococcus, klebsiella, pneumococcus, salmonella typhi (the cause of typhoid fever), shigella (dysentery), and cholera. By 1994, more than 10 percent of all staph samples sent to their lab were methicillin-resistant and 3 percent of all pneumococci were penicillin-resistant.

"It's becoming a real crisis now," Maleyev said.

In Ukraine the picture was similar, Dr. Anatoly Shapiro, of the L. V. Gromashevski Epidemiology and Infectious Diseases Research Institute in Kyiv, said. "Our physicians, maybe this is a drawback in their education, but their first thought isn't to go to the laboratory. They'll just prescribe and see what happens. . . . And now Ukraine is flooded with new Western antibiotics; the physicians don't understand them—cephalosporins and such."

Streptococcus and pseudomonas bacteria developed widespread multidrug resistance throughout Ukraine, Shapiro said. And ampicillin no longer was effective against enterococci. With each additional layer of antibiotic resistance the bugs got harder—and far more expensive—to treat. As physicians escalated their weaponry from simple penicillins to powerful broad-spectrum antibiotics, it was a little like starting out with an expert sniper and ending up using an all-out aerial strategic bombing campaign. The collateral damage, in the form of ravaged stomach, intestines, liver, kidneys, and other organs increased and had to be managed by physicians, often with other drugs. In a country like Ukraine, physicians were unfamiliar with such antibiotic collateral damage and didn't know how to treat it. And while all sorts of alternative antibiotics were after 1991 readily available, patients had to buy them, with cash—cash few possessed. As a result, many bacterial infections were economically incurable.

Microbiologist Vera Ilyina of the Novosibirsk Oblast Hospital tracked antibiotic resistance in Siberia since 1994. At that time so many untreatable infections suddenly turned up in the region's children that, she said, "It was a real problem. We were begging for humanitarian aid."

The American Merck, Sharp and Dohme pharmaceutical company donated laboratory supplies for bacterial sensitivity assays, and Ilyina discovered that staphylococcus all over the hospital—indeed, all over Siberia—was acquiring resistance to methicillin, a crucial antibiotic. She also found evidence that streptococci were resistant not only to the third-generation cephalosporin drugs—the kinds Rovena searched for in Georgia for poor Irakli—but also to the even more expensive new fourth-generation cephalosporins, drugs that weren't even available in Siberia until 1993.

At that point, she began hunting around the massive Novosibirsk Oblast Hospital, trying to find sources for these new, lethal microbes. She looked for connections among the infected patients and noticed that those with drug-resistant strains tended to have spent a long time on a mechanical ventilator in the burn ward, or were babies in the neonatal intensive care unit.

But in the spring of 1997, her inquiry ground to a halt when she ran out of money to buy the culture medium to complete her study.

That was a perfect example, Dr. Mikhail Yan said, of the degree to which the medical community of the former USSR suffered in the 1990s for having been isolated from the rest of the scientific world for seven previous decades. After all, it was very well known everywhere else that burn units, neonatal ICUs, and mechanical ventilators were key sources of nosocomial infection. But it was not because something was "growing" there; it was because the patients and equipment in all three sites were subject to a lot of contact with the ungloved hands of doctors, nurses, orderlies, and family.

"We have been very cut off from international experience," Yan, a Buryatia Republic state epidemiologist in Ulan Ude, explained. "WHO bulletins, medical journals, scientific books—we haven't seen them, ever. And we don't know what has been working elsewhere. Information is simply not available."

How bad was the information gap? Think of hand washing.

From the poorest to wealthiest of hospitals in most of the rest of the world, doctors and nurses understood that they must scrub their hands and forearms thoroughly with disinfectant soap before touching any patient or device that will come in contact with a patient. In lieu of hundreds of scrubbings a day health providers ideally wore latex disposable gloves, donning a different pair for each patient or procedure.

The reason for all this gloving and scrubbing was that human hands were the primary vector of person-to-person bacterial transmission. Lack of attention to hand cleanliness guaranteed that, for example, the staphylococcus on Mrs. Jones's arm would get to Miss Smith's mouth by hitchhiking on the unwashed hands of Dr. Brown when he examined the Jones wound and then put a thermometer under Smith's tongue.

It seemed terribly obvious. Yet it was revolutionary thinking to doctors and nurses trained under the old Communist regime.

"I can't tell you how surprised I was by their lack of infection control," Howard Cohen, former executive director of Coney Island Hospital in Brooklyn, said, referring to hospitals in Odessa, Moscow, and Kyiv. "In the operating room they had commonly used soap bars, commonly used towels. Surgeons were going from one patient to another without washing. . . . They thought airborne infection by bacterial spores was the key. They really didn't appreciate that the key was dirty hands."

In some operating rooms in Russia and Ukraine devices that looked like upside-down umbrellas hung from the ceiling. Inside were ultraviolet lights. The contraptions were designed to zap "flying" bacterial spores, doctors explained, which then "fell dead" into the umbrella, sparing the patient any risk of infection.

"Three years ago when I first went there my initial impression was—my god!—they sacrificed their entire population for the sake of satellites in space and their military. For seventy years they sacrificed public health," said Regina Napolitano, Coney Island Hospital's infection control chief.

For example, the cash-strapped Children's Hospital No. 17 in St. Petersburg had stopped purchasing both paper towels and rubber gloves. The staff, oblivious to the crucial need for clean hands, either stopped scrubbing or did wash (especially after using toilet facilities), but shared cloth towels with dozens of coworkers a day.

In the Siberian Oblast of Irkutsk, infection control was hampered in all the hospitals by "shortages, shortages and more shortages," cried Dr. Tatyana Boyko, deputy president of the Committee on Public Health. The lack of latex gloves, paper towels, disinfectant soap, and disposable devices such as catheters has, she said, sparked a 30 percent increase in sepsis among newborns since 1995—with the majority of cases being fatal.

In Ossetia, an autonomous region inside Georgia, a hernial resection surgical procedure was underway. Some of the staff in the operating room wore no masks or gloves—including the scrub nurse. And midway during the operation she collected bloodied instruments, carried them to a wash tub filled with water that had been in place, uncovered, for hours. She dunked the instruments in the water, gave them a quick shake, and returned the surgical equipment to the surgeon's table. Within seconds one of the hemostats the nurse had rinsed was inside the patient's intestines, holding tissue aside while the surgeon probed the hernia.

Napolitano said that in every hospital she visited in the region, "There were no [infection] barriers that we would consider acceptable for preventing blood-borne infection. They were reusing needles, gloves were scarce."

Dr. Gennady Onyschenko, who was in charge of all infectious diseases issues for the Russia Ministry of Health, was dismissive of the problem. He was well aware, Onyschenko said, that some Russian hospitals were diverting scarce resources from purchase of such things as latex gloves to doctors' salaries and fancy high-tech equipment purchases. But the Russian nation "has everything: reagents, test kits, gloves, enough for our patients. We are not importing anything. In principle, we are self-sufficient."

Furthermore, Onyschenko insisted, antibiotic resistance was a trivial issue in Russia, noting, "There are much more important ones to think of here."

Onyschenko to the contrary, the nosocomial and drug-resistance problem in the region was massive, but went largely unseen because of the very nature of the Soviet system of SanEp.

In addition to resistant bacteria, the enormous, antiquated medical facilities were spreading—rather than halting—hepatitis B and C, HIV, and other blood-borne diseases. Though comparisons with conditions in Africa always drew rage from health providers in the formerly Soviet region, it was hard to avoid reflecting on Kikwit's Ebola virus outbreak or other epidemics that were propelled on that continent by the medicinal reuse of syringes and poor hospital infection control. There was a difference, however: most trained African physicians knew what decent infection control entailed but lamented the poverty of their facilities and paucity of appropriate supplies. In Russia, Turkmenistan, Moldova, and the rest of that region, however, even where supplies were plentiful they were not properly used, and standards of infection control were not maintained.

While the majority of hospitals and physicians remained after 1991 entrenched in old SanEp thinking, a few were beginning to step away from it.

Coney Island Hospital's Napolitano spent a lot of time in Odessa Oblast Hospital in Ukraine during the 1990s teaching New York standards of hospital infection control to her counterparts in Odessa. And staff from the Ukrainian facility rotated through Coney Island, where they felt right at home because 45 percent of the patients spoke Russian. After four years of such an exchange, sponsored by American International Health Alliance (AIHA), chief Odessa physician Vasily Gogulenko was proud to say he had reduced the average length of patient hospitalization from fifteen to eleven days and decreased the death rate by a whopping 29 percent.[147]

AIHA hoped that the Odessa hospital experience would serve as a lightning rod, sparking reform across the region.

But O'Rourke said change "doesn't just spring up like wildflowers [because] the whole concept of infection control has been so punitive. . . . The system here is still find the scapegoat and punish them. The focus is always to get the bad guy and throw him in the slammer. . . . So infection control is a bunch of rules, it's not a thought process."

Bourganskaia said it all boiled down to thinking about biology. Doctors prescribed combinations of antibiotics in Russia, for example, that made no sense because they all targeted the same aspect of the bacteria rather than hitting a microbe at two or three different vulnerable points. But they didn't actually understand how antibiotics worked, she insisted, so the precious drugs were almost universally misused.

"We calculated that they could save millions of dollars if they just changed that practice," Bourganskaia said. "Similarly, if hospital administrations realize that infection control improves quality of care and saves money, then maybe they can change. If they can just change the way they think about what they do, and how they do it."

The former Soviet states need not view Bourganskaia's critique as some sellout to the West. They need only look slightly westward, to the Czechs, for a clear illustration of this principle.

The Czech Republic not only performed the job of infection control well—it did it better than the United States and nearly all Western European countries.

The Czech Republic had the lowest antibiotic-resistance rates in disease-causing pathogens in the former Communist world and was rivaled by few nations in the world for the number one slot, overall. Many antibiotics that had been rendered useless in the United States and former Soviet Union because of widespread drug resistance still worked as well in Prague and the rest of the Czech Republic in 1998 as they had twenty years earlier. And some of the most worrisome forms of antibiotic resistance, such as enterococcal resistance to vancomycin, never emerged in Czech hospitals.

"We are an island, you could say, in terms of resistance," said Dr. Anna Jedličková. "Slovakia and Hungary—all our neighbors—are much worse off. So we are in very good shape."

Though the Czechs were governed by many of the same SanEp-type health policies that were the law in the Soviet Union, the country's microbiologists and physicians strived to be more scientific and, as best they could, follow Western European trends.

The nation's microbiologists, caught up in the spirit of resistance that permeated Czech life in '68, broke with Soviet policies and set up their own system. They didn't know what the West was doing to control new bacterial infections, but they realized that the Soviet model was a disaster.

Cut off from the West, the Czechs invented their own unique system. By law all uses of antibiotics had to be cleared by a control microbiology lab, such as the enormous one that Jedličková ran in Prague. Physicians could not prescribe the drugs willy-nilly, prompting emergence of resistance bacteria. Instead, they had to submit sputum, blood, or infected tissue samples to the laboratory for analysis, where the precise nature of the infection would be determined.

If, for example, the lab diagnosed streptococcus, the physician was told, "Okay, it's strep. Here is a list of three antibiotics we recommend you use."

The "recommendation" was actually a command, and the central laboratory in Prague periodically modified drug-use guidelines according to observed trends in bacterial mutations and resistance. Policies often varied regionally in the country, reflecting differences in the local bacterial ecologies.

Hospitals were also told which disinfectants they could use, and what equipment needed sterilization. This, too, reflected constant vigilance on the part of the microbiology laboratories, searching for trends in microbial resistance to chlorine bleach and other antiseptics.

"And we introduced a specialized laboratory of sterile controls," Jedličková said. "It is unique. It will detect the sterility of the environment and of autoclaves and disinfecting machines."

Ironically, the entire system nearly toppled following the successful 1989 Velvet Revolution that overthrew the Czech Communist dictatorship.

"Some doctors thought that antibiotic use policies were undemocratic," Jedličková said. "These people wanted to abolish the [microbiology] centers. But fortunately common sense won. Even the opponents to antibiotic centers started to understand that bacteria don't recognize democracy."

Soon a new challenge faced Jedličková and her fellow microbiologists— free market medicine. The Czech government was easing its way out of nationalized medicine into a mixed economy of health care similar to what existed in the United States. This meant private practices, managed care, health maintenance organizations, and personal health insurance were all swiftly replacing five decades of Soviet-modeled socialized medicine. For the microbiologists this signaled loss of control.

Jedličková was still able to dictate antibiotic and infection control practices for the prestigious three-thousand-bed University Teaching Hospital in Prague, but her wide influence over the private prescribing practices of individual physicians was quickly evaporating.

The impact was felt most sharply in treatment of syphilis, gonorrhea, and other sexually transmitted diseases, according to Czech Deputy Minister of Health Dr. Miroslav Čerbák. Fueled by both the desire to protect patients' sexual privacy and the enormous amount of money that could be made in off-the-books treatment of prostitutes and their customers, Czech doctors were risking their licenses and prescribing drugs without seeking microbiology lab testing and approval.

In Russia the lessons of modern science had yet to permeate most medical and public health facilities—except, of course, at the Kremlin. That was why you'd never be able to convince Texan J. T. Peoples that Russia had a medical system in chaos.

"Hell no!" Peoples declared in his Beaumont, Texas, twang. The sixty-year-old American Embassy electrical engineer said his major symptom on May 9, 1997, was "Death!"

"I figured I only had a few hours," he recalled. Diverticulitis and a perforated abdomen had Peoples doubled over in agony. But he was lucky. As an American Embassy employee Peoples qualified for admission to the most advanced facility in all Russia, the Kremlin Hospital, otherwise known as Moscow Central Clinical Hospital.

It's no wonder Peoples felt right at home in the Kremlin Hospital—he practically was. The fully renovated luxury floor on which Peoples recuperated from surgery had wall-to-wall American pile carpeting, walls papered in American synthetic fabrics, lovely American sofas on which patients rested while watching American television, American nurse Marianne Hess on staff to provide that down home touch, American magazines to read. And in case all of this is too subtle there was an American Stars and Stripes standing right next to the Russian tricolor in the front lobby.

A plaque on the wall read: "Training for the unit has been provided by the following health care members of Premier Health Alliance, Chicago, Illinois, with the support of the United States Agency for International Development and American International Health Alliance."

This was where Russian President Boris Yeltsin got his heart treatments and checkups. Seventy percent of the patients were deputies in the Duma, senators, or members of Yeltsin's cabinet and top staff. The remaining 30 percent of the patients were either Western embassy personnel like J. T. Peoples, or wealthy executives from the newly privatized major corporations and banks of Russia, cardiology unit director Dr. Marina Ugryumova said.

"We have some rich people that can be treated here," Ugryumova said. "But we do not want robbers and killers treated here because we have serious security concerns."

In other words, if you had enough money you could be treated where the American flag flew—unless your money was blatantly ill-gotten.

The Kremlin Hospital had always offered a better class of care. But it wasn't easy to get into the facility—and never had been. The elite central Moscow compound, with its well-manicured grounds and expansive buildings, was surrounded by a perimeter of walled security. Entry was closely monitored by armed guards, video cameras, and gated driveways.[148]

As would be expected, considering the clientele. It was here that President Leonid Brezhnev was treated for his strokes during the 1970s and final cardiac death in 1982. And his successor Yuri Andropov died in the Kremlin Hospital two years later of kidney failure; his successor, Konstantin Chernenko, was treated here for heart failure, hepatitis, and multiple other health problems the following year, dying in 1985.

But by the 1980s the hospital had become little more than a high-security, fancy geriatric care center, catering to the Soviet Central Committee and Politburo dinosaurs. It stopped advancing, Ugryumova said, because treatment of the septuagenarian elder statesmen of Russia was too predictable, and easy.

Then in 1996 the world learned that president Boris Yeltsin was suffering life-threatening heart disease. No facility in Moscow was up to Western standards for the quadruple bypass cardiac surgery Yeltsin desperately needed. But it was unthinkable that the president of the Russian Federation would disgrace his nation's bruised, but proud, health care system by seeking treatment overseas. So the U.S. government hastily renovated not only the Kremlin Hospital's physical appearance and equipment but the structure and skills of its staff as well.

The result was a facility so many cuts above what was generally available in Russia as to seem from another planet.

The region's hospitals and medical clinics outside the hallowed Kremlin walls ranged from appalling to astonishingly horrible.[149] Most were staffed by personnel who rarely—if ever—were paid. Supplies of all kinds were scarce. Physical maintenance had long since been abandoned, and many health structures were poorly built in the first place. So everywhere hospital administrators had for more than a decade patched and painted peeling walls, cracked floors, caving ceilings, and shattered windows.

And, remarkably, little thought was given to patient mobility. Central planners in Moscow dictated that the region's hospitals have elevators of one size but gurneys of another—incompatible—length. In many hospitals patients had to be carried up and down stairs by relatives in order to reach X-ray machines or other diagnostic and treatment equipment. Virtually no hospital was wheelchair accessible. Beds were rarely more than basic, nonadjustable affairs. For some procedures—notably, abortions and childbirth—anesthesia and painkillers were used minimally, if at all. And in general pain management was not a priority.

The situation only worsened after 1991, as elevators broke down, compelling ailing individuals to scale stairs in order to get from test sites to their hospital beds. Food fell into short supply, with most hospitals stating frankly that families needed to provide rations for their ailing relatives, much as they would in India or Zaire.

The old Soviet medical system was titanic in size but utterly lacking in efficiency or cost-effective management. Like the polluting, inefficient industries that shut down after 1991 all across the region, the Soviet model of health care simply could not function in the New Reality. In Russia, for example, there were 10,280 hospitals, 1,601 clinics, 6,107 outpatient centers, and 450 university teaching hospitals. For a population of 147 million people in 1995 Russia had nearly two million hospital beds, for a patient-to-bed ratio of 1:118. The average hospital stay in Russia in 1995 was *seventeen days.*

A fee-for-services form of medicine had emerged in which patients' ability to pay (or barter) determined the extent and quality of their care. To a certain degree this had always existed. During the Soviet period—particularly during the Brezhnev years—patients were expected to provide their surgeons and physicians with under-the-table cash or services, such as free auto repairs or caviar and vodka.[150] But the situation spun into marketplace chaos after 1991, with doctors and nurses demanding arbitrarily set payments for everything from cardiac surgery to changes of bedpans.

Dr. Yuri Komarov of MEDSOCECONOMINFORM noted that by the late 1990s nearly 100 percent of all health care in the Caucasus nations (Georgia, Armenia, Azerbaijan) was paid for directly by the patients: cash up-front for every single service.

"We are still living in lawless countries," Komarov said. "We are still at the mason's stage, building we don't-know-what," as a health care system. More than 80 percent of the annual 1997 Russian state health care spending, for example, went to hospitals, which used it largely to maintain their inefficient, overly large staffs.

"We need to change that around," Komarov insisted.

In Turkmenistan the 1990s witnessed radical changes in health care as reformers like Annageldy Gaipov, of the Ministry of Health, pushed successfully for complete elimination of Soviet-era priorities. Average inpatient hospitalization was reduced by 4 percent from 1994 to 1997, Gaipov said. The number of physicians on the national payroll was slowly reduced, first by making medical school admission far more difficult and licensing fewer new physicians, and then by eliminating duplicative medical departments. The number of inpatient beds was cut by a third. And all priorities for state-funded medical care shifted from lengthy, tertiary care in hospitals to public health.

The result? From 1990 to 1997 Turkmenistan decreased its maternal mortality rate by 10 percent, Gaipov said, its measles rate by a third, its anthrax rate by 60 percent, and eliminated all cases of polio by 1996.

"We're pretty confident that we're on the right path," Gaipov said, grinning.

But it was a comparatively easy path for little Turkmenistan, population 4.5 million, to follow. The challenge of health care reform was greater in nations with more difficult geographic or population obstacles. In Kazakhstan, for example, the population was so spread out that human density averaged just 1.5 people per square kilometer, Dr. Bakhyt Tumenova, social affairs director for the city of Semipalatinsk, said. Amid rising economic chaos many of the rural clinics had turned into lawless entities in which health providers extorted patients for huge sums of money, or refused care. To counter this trend, Tumenova said, the state created a competitive bidding system, privatizing the small clinics and forcing them to compete.

In Georgia health reform ran smack in the face of resistance from the medical community, as providers realized that many of them would be unemployed by the time reform was completed. Georgia had about thirty-seven thousand physicians and fifty-five thousand nurses on the state's payroll in 1990—enough, experts say, to adequately meet the public health and medical needs of a nation of sixty-five million people. But Georgia had only five million citizens. Like all Soviet states, Georgians overdiagnosed illnesses and hospitalized far too many people.

For decades Georgia's health care system was based on enormous facilities like Republican State Hospital, located in downtown Tblisi. The twelve-story, two-thousand-bed concrete facility was so full during the 1980s, doctors said, that patients often lay upon gurneys lining the hallways.

By 1997, however, a visitor found all of the hospital's elevators broken, and scaled ten stories of concrete stairs, littered with bloody bandages and medical detritus, before finding any patients. Around them was evidence of little more than decay: swaths of linoleum flooring curled up and bubbled in waves of self-destruction, holes gaped in the plaster walls, and stretches of assorted types of tapes covered cracks and holes in most of the windows, proving inadequate in the face of gusts of icy winds. The thirty-year-old hospital was disintegrating.

As the Soviet state issued dictums from Moscow, local government workers had no choice but to follow—or, at least, appear to obey. In the case of health planning Moscow's orders always focused on two things: goals for percentage reductions in various infectious disease rates and construction of hospitals.

"In old times with these five-year plans they would write, '1957: must build one thousand new beds.' And two thousand the next. This was the nature of planning. All of this was *not* improving health in the country," Minister of Health Avtandil Jorbenadze, a forty-something, dashing brunet, said. With policies that were driven by pursuit of gigantism—always assuming that bigger meant better—the Soviets set their health system on an upward spiral they could not afford.[151] Building more hospital beds meant staffing the ever-larger hospitals and polyclinics with more trained personnel to tend to those beds. By the 1960s it was obvious to everyone in the medical system that supply far exceeded demand, so the Soviets simply expanded the list of medical conditions that required hospitalization and lengthened the recommended durations of hospital stays.

"In the old days we lived in a country with a strange system of health care," Jorbenadze said, chuckling. "And not all of it was bad. But we had an excess of technical and capital investment. After 1991 we had to imagine the main role of the state, health care, and people in our new society. And we had to evaluate our resources and needs. And, most of all, we had to change this vertical system into a horizontal one, with partnerships among the state, managers, and employees."

Critical to any reform, Jorbenadze said, was elimination of SanEp. In its place he hoped to create a system of public health and disease control that was clearly rooted in sound science. He dreamed of the U.S. Centers for Disease Control and Prevention, which—at least in Jorbenadze's fantasies—used epidemiology as a scientific tool for providing a data-driven basis for health policy. It was Jorbenadze's ambitious goal for Georgia.

And it would be a tough one to meet.

IX

In order to renovate our state apparatus we must at all costs set out first, to learn, secondly, to learn, and thirdly, to learn, and then to see to it that learning shall not remain a dead letter, or a fashionable catch-phrase (and we should admit in all frankness that this happens very often with us), that learning shall really become part of our very being, that it shall actually and fully become a constituent element of our social life.

—V. I. Lenin, "Better fewer, but better," March 2, 1923

When hard-line Communists staged their failed coup against Soviet President Mikhail Gorbachev in 1991 the job with the highest prestige in the land was Scientist. The twenty-story, white marble Russian Academy of Sciences was built just four years before the coup out of anodized gold aluminum and titanium and featuring cut-crystal light fixtures: it was meant as a paean to scientific discovery. The giant white edifice cast an impressive shadow over the Moskva River. Atop the building was an odd five-story-tall golden aluminum and titanium construct that glistened in the noon sun.

But the strange, massive pseudosculpture atop the Academy headquarters was a poor cover for an unbelievable mistake. Convinced Soviet science would one day rule the world the Communist Party architects planned a building of more than fifty stories in height, and spent a fortune on Georgian marble and fantastically expensive titanium to adequately proclaim its glory. But less than halfway up the engineers noticed that the building was sinking. Laden with marble, the construct was heavier than the Moskva River landfill site could bear. To cover their abominable oversight in failing to conduct a geological assessment before designing the gigantic mess the architects simply halted construction and created the strange aluminum/titanium "sculpture" to cover the partially built twenty-first through twenty-fifth floors.

Years after the collapse of the USSR the Academy headquarters had a sad look to it, reminiscent of an abandoned American shopping mall circa 1975. Footsteps echoed across the emptiness of the meeting halls and reception areas, unreplaced light bulbs left dark cavernous shadows, and behind the leather-padded doors lay hundreds of empty offices.

The scale of the Soviet scientific enterprise was staggering before 1991.

What it may have lacked in quality was certainly offset by quantity. In Russia alone there were 250 civilian scientific institutes employing sixty thousand scientists. In some institutes—particularly outside Novosibirsk—scientists often functioned with a sort of privileged sense of freedom, able to indulge intellectually in ideas that would land any other Soviets in gulags.[152]

That was then.

After 1991 everything changed.

The average Russian scientist in the late 1990s earned 500,000 rubles a month, or about $88—if he or she was paid at all. Once the best paid members of the Soviet society, Russian scientists had fallen dramatically in prestige and earned only 80 percent of the median national income, according to Boris Saltykov of the Russian House for International Scientific and Technological Corporation.[153] In Russia the number of employed research scientists and technicians had dropped to just 1,300,000—down from 3,400,000 in 1985. During the 1980s scientists were bedecked with Orders of Lenin and praised as socialist heroes. But as the twenty-first century approached, according to the Centre of Science Research and Statistics in Moscow, scientists ranked among the lowest professions in public esteem, just 1 percent above the military.[154]

At least fifteen thousand Ph.D. scientists left Russia between 1991 and 1996, forming the largest peacetime brain drain in world history.

The Russian scientific collapse was mirrored in most of the other nations of the former Soviet Union and Eastern Bloc—with the striking exception of the tiny Baltic States. Even before the USSR collapsed East German scientists got sobering glimpses of the price they were going to pay for decades of isolation from their more advanced West German peers. In 1989, months before the fall of the Berlin Wall, the Iron Curtain weakened enough to allow some 400,000 Germans from the East to visit the West, and 1 percent of her scientists relocated westward. Those scientists who went west told colleagues back home that they found their skills woefully backward. In particular, the almost complete lack of computer skills and knowledge of computer-driven research tools put the Easterners twenty years behind.[155] And after the fall of the Berlin Wall the West German scientists were shocked to see how completely the Communist Party controlled Eastern science, allowing dogma to carry greater weight than such seemingly irrefutable foundations as the law of physics.[156]

Czechoslovakia awoke from its 1990 Velvet Revolution to the realization that most of its fifteen thousand scientists had been cowed or jailed after the Soviet invasion of 1968. Only the Communist ideologues in the ranks of Czech and Slovak scientists had, for twenty-two years, received lavish research funding and prestigious academic positions.[157]

Georgia's ten-thousand-strong Academy of Science was in a state of utter chaos after the country's civil war, from 1991 to 1994. Virtually all of its research institutes went without electricity, resulting in destruction of all frozen laboratory samples and what little computer-stored information had existed. So desperate had economic conditions become that by 1996 laboratories were stripped by thieves of equipment, copper wiring, electric transformers, even light bulbs.[158]

Hungary's scientific establishment shrank swiftly, as federal funding all but disappeared and the National Academy of Sciences was forced to reorganize. Between 1985 and 1996 Hungary lost 27 percent of her biologists and chemists: some moved west, some simply had no choice but to find new ways to earn a living. Poland, Bulgaria, Romania, Latvia, and Lithuania followed similar courses.[159]

Ukraine particularly suffered, as more than 70 percent of the country's scientists were, prior to 1991, employed by the Soviet military.[160]

Sadly, the sinking of the titanic Soviet science came at the time when the health and survival of the region's populace hinged on innovation, research, and course corrections in the directions of medical thinking. Though money was horribly absent, solutions rested less with cash infusions than with fundamental changes in the ways policy makers, hospital administrators, physicians, nurses, epidemiologists, and biomedical researchers thought about what they did.

"Basic research science has fallen apart. And even before [the collapse of the USSR] the quality of research was very low," Elena Bourganskaia said in 1997. "You can't trust the results. There are no case-controlled studies. There is very little appropriate statistical methodology. And the research need is huge! They have to change what they're doing, but they can't just base practices on American or French data. Their practices must be appropriate to the setting."

Bourganskaia, at age twenty-seven, embodied the tragedy of Russia's loss. Trained as an M.D. in Moscow, the pretty, energetic Bourganskaia spoke fluent English, was earning two Ph.D.'s at major American universities, and was curious about her world, energetic in her work, sophisticated in her views of the role of modern science in public health, ambitious, and personable. She worked, however, not in Russia but in the United States and won't return anytime soon for anything more than a visit, she said. She was Russia's loss, and America's gain.

"The concept that you need data to determine the efficiencies and efficacies of your practices—it's not a concept that's in use. Medical school training does *not* include the scientific method: hypothesis, study, data-driven solution. You never see denominators in reports. . . . Everything was a 'science' in the Soviet view—history was a science, politics was a science, philosophy was a science. Any academician can be called a scientist. And the stuff that gets published is horrifying!"

Bourganskaia's wish list for Russian scientific research included establish ment of key labs that could determine the extent of antibiotic resistance in disease-causing bacteria and develop appropriate treatment strategies. And she wanted to see tests done to determine if many medical techniques in general use across the region actually worked—or worse, caused harm.

At Children's Hospital No. 5 in Moscow microbiologist Valery Stroganov would have loved to tackle some of Bourganskaia's questions. But the thirty-four-year-old scientist had a more basic problem: he couldn't get a decent culture media to grow bacteria in, and he couldn't get appropriate biological supplies even to conduct simple screenings for antibiotic resistance.

"That's why Russian microbiologists don't have the possibility of clearly interpreting the results of their work," Stroganov said. "We don't have any tools."

In Ukraine, Russia, Belarus, and Estonia physicians concerned about HIV and hepatitis were desperate for information about drug abuse: were the bizarre concoctions used in the region—which could include such hellish chemicals as acetone—more addictive than the counterpart narcotics popular in the West? And how do you prevent and cure such addictions?

"The drug users come to us and ask for help. They are injecting heroin and opium dissolved in acetone and paint thinner," Dr. Svetlana Danks of the AIDS Information and Support Center in Tartu, Estonia, said. "The answer is we just don't know. Like with everything else, we just don't know."

Danks wanted to see more carefully controlled scientific testing done on several methods suggested within the region, but this hadn't been a priority with regional governments. And money was not available.

In the old days, the Soviet Union's Gamaleya Institute was the nation's top medical science facility. After 1991, however, Gamaleya rented out most of its land and office space to small-time entrepreneurs, a beer brewery, and a parking garage in order to pay its taxes, heat, and electrical bills, said its director Sergei Pozorovskii.

"In the old days we were guaranteed funding. Okay," said Gamaleya scientist Henry Dolgov. "But some of the work may not have been the best. Today we must compete for funds. Well, we have to learn the grants process. We have to learn to compete. That's the way it is."

In Moscow physicist Michael Alfimov was doing his best to create a competitive grants process for Russia modeled after the way the National Science Foundation in the United States dispensed funds that it received from Congress. Since 1994, Alfimov—who spoke fluent English—had led the Russian Science Federation, modeling it closely after the NSF in Washington, D.C.

The main problem for Alfimov was that the Russian legislature kept reneging on its promised funds for science. In 1996, for example, the Russian Science Foundation received fifteen thousand grant proposals, of which three thousand were judged by panels of experts to be worthy of funding. The Duma promised nearly one trillion rubles ($200 million), but by December 1996 the RSF had only received 170 million rubles ($340,000).

By 1998 Russian spending on science had fallen from a 1991 level of $11.6 billion to $1.5 billion, prompting Science Minister Michael Kirpichnikov to say that "today's situation is the worst it's ever been for Russian science. And the most difficult times are in the future."[161] And, true to prediction, funding for scientific research fell further still, in 1999 sinking to just a half billion dollars. The average research grant was a mere $5,000.[162]

Many outside organizations, including George Soros's Open Society, the Howard Hughes Medical Institute, U.S. National Institutes of Health, and the European Union, sank substantial funds into the region's scientific enterprises, picking out the most promising researchers and awarding reasonably sized grants. But the scientists still had to toil within the political economic realities of their countries, which often proved impossible.

Russia's 1996 minister of science, Boris Saltykov, said that at the core of all the flaws in the region's scientific enterprise lay one key point: until 1991 more than 75 percent of all Soviet scientific research—in all subject areas—was controlled by the Soviet military.[163] The military closed science off from the rest of the world, rewarded those ventures that had potential strategic applications, and created a vast scientific bureaucracy in which, Saltykov said, "Obedience and tolerance for bosses' views were valued higher than freedom of creative works."

The dominance of the military also explained why Soviet leaders rarely funded research done in universities, a key component of scientific progress seen in Western society.

Which may not have been altogether bad, given the quality of some of that science. For example, the man in charge of all psychiatry and psychology research in post-Soviet Ukraine, Dr. A. P. Chuprikov, published numerous studies claiming that color-tinted glasses, laser surgery of the brain, and insulin-induced comas all could cure schizophrenia. An independent panel of Dutch and Canadian psychiatrists judged the work "reminiscent of the KGB/psychiatric circuit" and "a direct violation of Human Rights," not to mention shoddy science.[164]

Such shoddy psychiatry had immediate implications for public health. As drug abuse, alcoholism, and suicides skyrocketed regionally the legacy of absurdist approaches to psychology rendered the profession ill-equipped for the challenge.

In Georgia, for example, psychiatrist George Nanieshvili, head of the nation's largest psychiatric service, sadly watched the suicide toll mount among Georgian men, particularly forty- to sixty-year-olds.

"Why? Of course, the social situation," Nanieshvili exclaimed during a discussion in his dark, ice-cold, unheated, and unelectrified office. "Because traditionally the father takes care of the family. With the [post-Soviet] change the man has to bring food to his family but he cannot. And the man's reaction is . . . to commit suicide."

In Nanieshvili's institute a middle-aged woman who declined to give her name was recovering from a complete nervous breakdown. It wasn't having her home seized by rebels in Georgia's breakaway district of Ossetia that made her crack. Nor did four years of living in a squalid refugee encampment inside a former hotel in Tblisi. Even the kidney stones diagnosed in one of her three children and the heart and lung problems in another didn't put the woman over the edge. Or the complete bankruptcy of her family of six, all of whom lived in one 400-square-foot room.

What did it was the fire, she said. It started when refugees in the apartment below made a mistake while cooking dinner on a hot plate and the flames soon devoured her apartment. She jumped from a second-story window, breaking her leg. And as she watched the fire eat up all that remained of her former life in Ossetia—her family photographs, embroidered clothes, bits of hand-me-down jewelry—the woman suffered an absolutely complete nervous breakdown.

The stress caused by the former Soviet Union's transition from communism to capitalism was producing such pronounced psychiatric difficulties, Nanieshvili said, that it could be likened to Leningrad Syndrome—the sociopsychiatric state experienced by the population of St. Petersburg during World War II when German troops surrounded the city for more than a year in a siege that left millions starving or dead.

And this psychological burden had to be borne by societies that, in many cases, almost completely lacked any tradition of psychotherapy or modern psychopharmacopoeia. Indeed, during the height of Soviet totalitarian control over the vast region psychiatrists worked hand-in-hand with the KGB and police, certifying that individuals who held dissident views were insane and should spend the rest of their days in Siberian gulags and asylums.

Dr. Semyon Gluzman of Kyiv, Ukraine, spent ten years in a Siberian gulag. His crime? He found that noted Ukrainian General Petro Grigorenko, who opposed the use of nuclear weapons, was "sane and the doctors committed an act of injustice," Gluzman recalled. Grigorenko spent the 1970s in an asylum for challenging the concept of a "winnable" thermonuclear war.

"The KGB used psychiatry for political purposes," Gluzman said in his Kyiv office. "And that was doable because psychiatrists were inadequately trained. The majority of psychiatrists just aren't ready for modern practice. It was very important in Ukraine [during Soviet days] to explain everything very simply, without ambiguity and forever. That's why it was impossible for a psychiatrist to say, for example, 'we don't know what schizophrenia is.' We had to say, 'It is X disease and it was discovered by the Soviets and it will exist forever.' In the mid-twentieth century Western doctors realized it's better not to treat an unknown disease, but to help the patient lead a normal life. In the Soviet system it was forbidden to use the term *psychologist*. And psychologists were forbidden to participate in treatment."

During the seventy years of Soviet rule of Ukraine no Western psychology or psychiatry books, articles, or journals were allowed in the country. The pioneering works of Freud and his followers were ignored, as was the striking 1970–1980s revolution in the understanding of the chemistry of the brain and the development of drugs that could adjust specific chemical imbalances. Most psychiatric disorders were simply classified in one of five boxes: psychoses, senile dementia, schizophrenia, neuroses, and mental retardation. Notably absent was the world's most common psychiatric disorder, depression. It was assumed that the only individuals who could be depressed under communism must be anti-Communists, not depressed.

Throughout the former USSR and Eastern Europe psychiatry and psychology suffered similar fates in the past and were proving woefully inadequate to meet the tasks of the post-Soviet era.[165]

Dr. Toma Tomov of the Medical University in Sofia, Bulgaria, said that the real question was, "How does the Self gain esteem if the social organism is sick? That requires facilitation—it means coming to terms with reality." A reality that included the knowledge that everything you were taught to believe about the world, and your place in it, was wrong. It was, many psychiatrists argued, a situation that induced regional mass paranoid psychosis.

Even in the Baltic States, which were only occupied by the Soviets for forty-six years and retained strong Western traditions, the psychiatric profession was controlled by Soviet ideology and was struggling to cope with what Dr. Lembit Mehilane called "a nation suffering a broken heart."

Mehilane, who was on the faculty of Estonia's prestigious University of Tartu, catalogued the tragedy: a doubling in suicide rates between 1988 and 1994 with six thousand suicide attempts in the tiny nation during 1994, alone. In 1996, he said, there were more than sixty thousand cases of clinical depression diagnosed in Estonia, or one case in every twenty-five people. Only 53 psychiatrists had private practices in the country, 170 were inside hospitals, and nationwide there were only 40 clinical psychologists.[166]

Classic psychiatric disorders such as psychoses and schizophrenia did not increase in frequency after 1991—and would not be expected to, experts insisted, as they were usually genetic in origin. The increase was primarily in depression. After all, millions of workers in all imaginable professions were toiling in expectation that someday they would be paid. No one had a count of these people. The Russian government conceded only that "trillions of rubles are owed" in back pay; the Ukrainians and Byelorussians gave even fewer clues.[167] Laid-off workers, who comprised anywhere from 28 to 50 percent of the region's potential workforce depending on where you looked, wouldn't be collecting welfare or getting unemployment checks.

The smart ones were getting by, working in the massive unofficial economy of trading and hustling, smuggling and small-time entrepreneurship. The World Bank estimated, for example, that the Ukrainian unofficial economy in 1996 topped $10 billion, which, given that its official net private capital flows were only $247 million, may have far exceeded the size of the official economy.[168]

Increasingly, then, survival depended on skills most people raised under communism didn't have: individual initiative, monetary smarts, and competitive instincts. Those who couldn't cope were suffering nervous breakdowns, depression, alcoholism, drug addiction, and suicide.

"I think that's the main reason for this psychological crisis," Gluzman said. "For us, having grown up with a Soviet mentality, we don't realize we have to pay a price for freedom. Secondly, the average Soviet person sees it as freedom for *oneself,* not freedom for the whole society, *for everybody.* And third, not everyone realizes that a better life can come as a result only of very hard work."

Totalitarianism was obviously a terrible, repressive force. But it also offered predictability and stability. No surprises. Steady checks, repeated habits. "In old socialist times we weren't comfortable but we were in a cage—and this cage protected us," Georgia's Nanieshvili said. "Don't think I am a Communist, but a totalitarian system offered stability."

There might not have been much on the shelves of the USSR but everyone had money—just in case some moldy beets turned up at the market. Now the reverse was true: in even the most remote Siberian outposts Pepsi and Coke vied for consumer loyalty and Norwegian salmon competed on the shelves with local sturgeon.

But most of the population could only look. They hadn't enough cash to buy.

Genuine psychiatry disappeared as a profession prior to World War II.[169] During the 1960s and 1970s Soviet psychiatrists were obsessed with psychic research: extrasensory perception, evidence of UFOs, telepathy, telekinesis, astrological birth control, psychotronic generating devices, pyramid power, and unusual uses of acupuncture. Joseph Stalin was an admirer of psychics, as was Nikita Khrushchev. The Soviet Navy spent enormous sums of money training sailors to psychically communicate with submarine captains, thus allowing Moscow to issue orders to its fleet without using radio signals that might be intercepted by NATO or U.S. eavesdroppers. The line between vaudeville-style magicians and Soviet Academy of Sciences members was fine in this area, perhaps undetectable.[170]

By the 1980s the parapsychology of the previous decade, coupled with the extraordinary KGB-granted power psychiatrists had over the lives of Soviet citizens, pushed many members of the profession to extraordinary heights of grandiosity. Some psychiatrists, particularly in Ukraine, Siberia, and Belarus, came to see themselves as religious figures. Around them grew cults, featuring everything from medieval black magic and doomsayers to faith healers and a colorful variety of pseudo-Christians.[171]

Even at the once-prestigious Russian Academy of Sciences' Institute of Clinical Immunology in Novosibirsk scientists were absolutely convinced that stress, combined with pollution, had wiped out the Siberian people's immune systems. But they were curiously unable to offer a shred of laboratory evidence for this assertion—no T cell measurements, lymphocyte counts, allergy test results, or other standard tools used in the West. Pseudoscience was hardly unique to Soviet psychiatry: all biomedical fields suffered from a fair amount of hocus-pocus.

The Immunology institute, which had suffered devastating budget cuts over the post-Soviet years, survived in large part off treating the public's perceived immune deficiencies, on a fee-for-service basis. Thirty-year-old Sivieta, for example, suffered chronic bronchitis and headaches for three years. The institute treated her with injections of pig spleen extracts that were intended to boost her antibody production.

Former gulag judge Leonid was, at age sixty-eight, having trouble breathing. So he was living in the institute and undergoing immune system treatments that included consumption of *Topim ambur* Siberian herbal bread— patented by the institute—and foam made from an oxygenated form of a green liquid, the contents of which clinical director Dr. Valery Shirinsky declined to name.

"But it will lift you," Shirinsky declared. "It will raise you—lift your immune system. You must feel high! Your spirit must be light."

And every patient spent time in a device ubiquitous in Soviet-era medical facilities: hyperbaric chambers. The patients were sealed, prone, into contraptions that created a sensation of pressure akin to that achieved in deep-sea diving. There were chambers designed for people of all ages and sizes—even newborns. And though no controlled, valid scientific studies were ever presented to an inquiring visitor, physicians all across the region affirmed that these chambers boosted immune responses, through unknown biological means.

Dr. Yvan Hutin was part of the enormous Russian scientific diaspora.

Working with the CDC in Atlanta Hutin documented a pattern in Eastern Europe of overuse of medicinal injections, and resultant spread of hepatitis B and C. In Romania and Moldova Hutin found that people had four to six therapeutic injections annually, typically given as treatment for such vague diagnoses as simple fever, the blues, mild diarrhea, and stomach aches. Vitamin supplements and antibiotics were, typically, the injected substances given with little or no basis in science.

And given with nonsterile needles.[172]

Many of these injections were part of the theory of "weak children" so popular among pediatricians from Budapest to Sakhalin. Overall, the theory held that living creatures—plants and humans alike—"reacted" to their environments, eventually, if all went well, "adapting." But adaptation was hampered, according to the view, if the living being was weak, and *all* of the region's children were, by the 1990s, as per popular belief, severely weakened; therefore, they were unable to "adapt" after "reacting" to such things as pollution, vaccines, common colds, and allergies.

This adaptation concept originated with the work of an obscure Ukrainian agronomist, Trofim Denisovich Lysenko. Born to an impoverished peasant family in 1889, Lysenko rose after the Bolshevik Revolution because of a series of experiments he conducted in 1925 in Azerbaijan. The effort boiled down to one tantalizing assertion: under appropriate conditions plants could be forced to adapt to frigid surroundings, providing ample yields of vegetables. In subsequent years Lysenko claimed to have experimentally "adapted" strains of peas, barley, wheat, rice, and oats—all of which could thrive in Siberia.

The peasant agronomist was catapulted to the most vaunted levels of Soviet scientific power overnight because he fulfilled two of the Communist Party's needs: he promised he could increase food production and he represented a heroic peasant figure at a time when Stalin needed to coax Soviets to turn their backs on traditional intellectuals in favor of the new proletariat leaders of thought and science.[173] The Marxist thesis of human malleability through social change was threatened by Mendelism, bolstered through Lysenkoism.[174] In 1927 his ascendancy to dominance over all Soviet biology and medicine began with a well-placed article singing Lysenko's praise in *Pravda*.

By 1929 Lysenko had enough power to be able to hold sway at all major genetics gatherings in the USSR, where he adamantly pushed his concept of "vernalization," in which crops could be coaxed to grow in climates and during seasons in which they did not usually thrive.

Lysenko unabashedly extended his vernalization theories to human beings. Chromosomes, and the DNA they held, had no relevance to the nature of offspring. Indeed, Lysenko argued, they were mere artifacts:

When a nuclear dye such as gentian violet is used, the whole preparation is heavily stained. Chromosomes become visible at a certain point in the removal of the dye. But when this process is continued, the chromosomes simply disappear. Hence the chromosomes are just temporary pictures observed during the removal of the stain.

When Lysenko was reshaping Russian genetics, based on "vernalization" and "adaptation," every college student in Europe and North America was imbued with the writings of Darwin and Mendel.[175] The West's geneticists were thoroughly convinced; the Soviets were not.

By 1945 Lysenko was Stalin's darling, so powerful that he had received eight Order of Lenin medals, the highest honor in the Soviet Union, was a deputy in the Supreme Soviet, became director of the Genetics Institute of the Soviet Academy of Sciences, and in 1945 got the ultimate honorific: "Hero of Socialist Labor."[176]

And as Lysenko's power grew, terror rose among the Soviet Union's legitimate scientists. The purges began in 1932. One by one the nation's leading geneticists were packed off to gulags or summarily executed, as Lysenko purged from the halls of Soviet science all "Morganist-Mendelists." His power extended to Poland and much of Eastern Europe, where scientists who believed in chromosomes—literally, simply believed in the existence of chromosomes—were obliterated.[177] In their places Lysenko promoted quacks and sycophants who decried every single aspect of what were then the frontiers of biological sciences in the West.

It is impossible to overstate the impact Lysenkoism had on Soviet medicine, science, and public health. Not only did this ideologue set Soviet biology on a course backward into the eighteenth century, but the belief system also created a legacy of death that would continue to affect public health policies regionally well into the 1990s and early twenty-first century.

Consider this: if one asserted that chromosomes, and modern genetics, were irrelevant it would be impossible to comprehend such things as viruses, antibiotic resistance, immunology, and inherited disease. Thus, Lysenko's coterie insisted that viruses formed spontaneously out of organic matter. And clusters of viruses spontaneously became bacteria. And, conversely, by placing the antibiotic crystals of penicillin in a slurry one could spontaneously grow *Penicillium* fungi.

By the time Lysenko finally fell from grace in the USSR in the 1960s scientists outside the Soviet Union had delineated most of the elegant biochemistry and molecular biology of DNA, inheritance, cell function, mutations, antibiotic resistance, viral structure, cellular infection by viruses, the existence of promiscuous DNA plasmids, protein chemistry, hormone interactions with cells, and—

fundamentally—the "central dogma," elucidated by Francis Crick in 1956. Its simplicity belied the dogma's import: life boils down to DNA, which is transcribed into RNA, then translated into a chain of amino acids, forming a protein.

In 1965 every college biology student in the non-Soviet world knew these simple truths.

Yet not one word of *any* of it appeared in a medical school or graduate biology text in the USSR or most of Eastern Europe until the late 1970s, and Lysenkoists still held prominent positions in regional science in the 1980s.[178]

With Lysenkoism as a framework it is suddenly easier to comprehend the public health policies of SanEp, Soviet hospital administrators, and physicians. If, for example, bacteria could spontaneously arise from crud on a wall it made sense to create a SanEp police force tasked with penalizing doctors who failed to keep their hospital walls well scrubbed. If viruses spontaneously arose from organic matter there need not be concern about reused syringes. Why worry about inappropriate antibiotic use or radiation exposure if chromosomes are irrelevant artifacts?

The Lysenko legacy was crippling.[179] As American scientists geared up for the dawning "biotechnology century" in 2000 their former Soviet counterparts were struggling to catch up, begging for research funding, and devouring scientific literature for so long denied them.[180]

"Our biomedical science really is in not-bad shape, largely thanks to Lysenko," said leading Estonian scientist Endel Lippmaa sarcastically, "since it was forbidden to investigate the molecular basis of life, then, obviously, it was fashionable [in Estonia] *because* it was forbidden."

To see how science could be done right the former Soviet nations need in the 1990s look no further than to tiny Estonia. While molecular biology and genetics remained in the Dark Ages in most of the Soviet Union, the rebellious Estonians dove into genetic engineering and cellular studies with relish.

"We were able to establish quite serious research which percolated even to medicine," Lippmaa said proudly. "But why should you compare us to *them* [Russia]? After all, our country was an occupied country. It is their hard luck if they have rotten science, not ours."

This turn-your-back-fast-on-Russia attitude was pervasive in Estonia, and explained why the tiny nation salvaged its scientific enterprise so quickly. It looked in 1991 "like all the most senior thirty-five- to forty-year-olds were going to leave Estonia. And science here would collapse like in Moscow," Dr. Richard Villems, director of the Estonian Biocentre in Tartu, said.

As soon as Estonia's *kroon* stabilized against the deutsche mark in late 1993 Villems and his colleagues took decisive action to save science.[181] They used available funds to, as Villems put it, "buy back" scientists who had left, luring them with new lab equipment and guaranteed good salaries. And they asked the

Royal Swedish Academy of Sciences to conduct an impartial review of all of Estonia's science, grading the work and helping the tiny nation spot its weakest areas. Instead of bolstering the weak, Estonia sunk resources into enhancing its strongest areas, making them competitive with European and American science.

The key to Estonia's success was its willingness to not only build up strong departments but also eliminate those that produced the poorest science. In 1970 Estonia had seventy-two research institutes; in 1990 that was pared down to forty-seven. In 1970 anyone who gained membership in the Estonian Academy of Sciences was guaranteed funding, regardless of the quality of his or her research. But in July 1991 the government created a grant and peer-review system that dispensed funds based on research quality, much as was done in nearby Sweden.

The big winner was medical science, which included molecular biology. In 1990 medical science garnered 7.7 percent of all grant funds—by 1995 it had snagged 16.5 percent and was expected to grow further, largely at the expense of engineering and agricultural sciences.

With only 0.3 percent of the population of the former Soviet Union, in 1996 Estonia won 14 percent of all grants dispensed to the ex-USSR by the European Union, Villems said with no small amount of pride.

Toivo Maimets, the vice rector of the University of Tartu, said the trick then was to translate that new scientific vigor into changes in the way medicine and public health were practiced in Estonia.

"The fights are sometime quite active," Maimets laughed, "because physicians were quite conservative, wedded to old Soviet ways. The problems are deep. The medical community is quite closed. It doesn't let new ideas—troublemakers—in."

"I personally have problems when I take my children to doctors," Maimets continued. "They prescribe an antibiotic and I ask, 'How do you know this is the right one?' And they say, 'Well, that's what I usually prescribe.' They have no idea if it's the appropriate drug, biologically."

Maimets, who spoke fluent English and had studied tumor biology in Britain, was doing research on the p53 oncogene, looking at a relationship between expression of that gene and infection with human papilloma virus.

It was research that would have been unimaginable for a Soviet scientist.

By the end of 1999 it seemed that Estonia wasn't the only country that had created a nascent scientific renaissance. Billionaire George Soros sank hundreds of millions of dollars into supporting such science, in hopes of halting the brain drain from the region. Hungary, the Czech Republic, and Poland all saw science blossom out of painful pruning processes similar to that experienced by Estonia's research community. But the blossomings were few and isolated, still surrounded by the old, tired Soviet-era debates, inefficiencies, dogmas, and ideologies.[182]

X

What is to be done?

—V. I. Lenin, 1902

In the end public health—its failures and hopes for its future—was tightly bound with the social, political, and economic status of a nation. And in the once-Soviet and Eastern Bloc nations on the eve of the twenty-first century the precarious futures of each were tied, to varying degrees, to the most problematic among them: the Russian Federation.

Prognostications worked overtime at the turn of the century trying to envision Russia's future.[183] Most Western observers, in the end, concurred with Washington analysts Yergin's and Gustafson's perspective:

> Russia's path to capitalism in the twenty-first century does not . . . start from nowhere. Rather it marks Russia's return to a journey that it abandoned, under duress, in 1917. By 2010, the post-Soviet transition will be far from complete. Russia could well run off the road in the meantime, once or more than once. But a democratic Russia is possible; a non-imperial Russia is possible. A capitalist Russia seems almost certain.

Perhaps. But it also appeared likely that the Russian Federation would defederate, splintering into wayward provinces that followed the course of Chechnya: Dagestan, Samara, Novgorod, Krasnoyarsk, Vladivostock, Saratov. Russia's federal government was imploding under the weight of its own corruption, incompetence, and lawlessness. It had long since lost control of the farflung provinces. Vladivostock, for example, stopped passing tax rubles to Moscow in 1996, and its governor ran Russia's easternmost Pacific oblast as if it were his own private domain. Boris Yeltsin's longtime rival, Alexander Lebed, was similarly inclined as governor of Krasnoyarsk, which bisected the nation north-south through the center of Siberia.[184]

At the local level laws were passed that flouted contradictory federal legislation.

Public health law, what little there was at the federal level, was flagrantly ignored at the local tier. Lacking federal rubles to pay such basics as salaries and electricity few health policy and administration leaders felt much cause for allegiance to Moscow. And the forecast called for more pain.

Sadly, public health desperately needed centralization, as none of Russia's constituent parts had, by themselves, the essential tools of the trade: vaccines, pharmaceuticals, databases, sterile medical equipment, qualified scientists.

The rest of the region had its own problems, which generally were less severe as one progressed westward. But a collapse of the ruble, Russian hyperinflation, a civil war inside Russia—any of these events could have profound ripple effects across the length and breadth of the former Soviet world.

Any simplistic answer to the demographic puzzle was useless. The regional trend toward declining life expectancy and rising premature mortality was, in the end, due to a complex constellation of factors, both Soviet in origin and unique to the post-1991 transformation.

The Soviets under the despotic rule of Stalin created public health, from its outset, as an ideological tool. The practice of public health was executed in a manner that stressed, in every facet, the primacy of the collective over the individual. At times—even, perhaps, frequently—public health was a cruel mistress of the state. Certainly its leadership was devoutly Communist, its scientific underpinnings rested more on ideology than on any set of experimental facts.

The collapse of the Soviet Union foisted its former socialist states into the world community, which had three impacts. First, long-sealed exit doors were opened, allowing for a record-breaking brain drain that stripped the region of most of its brightest scientific and medical minds. Second, doors also opened inward, allowing both the aspirations and sins of the external world entry into the long-sequestered societies: the populations for the first time realized their comparative material poverty, experienced resentment and avarice, and discovered drugs and other ways to dull the pain of that awakening. Third, the legacy of Soviet-era science, psychology, public health, and human rights left the professionals, their infrastructures, and individual citizens without the tools to cope with the New Reality: narcology, TB sanatoriums, SanEp, venereology, KGB-affiliated psychiatry, and Lysenko-devastated biology could not protect the health of a free public.

The Soviet public health infrastructure, in short, required authoritarianism. In the absence of centralized despotism and the intrusive powers it extended to public health authorities, the fundamental flaws in the system were frightfully exposed.

The anguishing transformation, even anarchy, of the post-1991 years in the ex-Soviet region did not, of course, occur in a global vacuum. A New Reality greeted every nation on earth at the same time, spawned by the end of the fifty-one-year Cold War and rise of globalized capitalism, a key feature of which was shared excruciation. It was not an equitable participation in pain: Americans felt little, Europeans got off easy, but Asia, Africa, Latin America, Canada, and all of the former Soviet sphere of influence suffered economically and socially.

Globalization did involve shared risk, however, as escalating drug markets had ways of spilling over into other nations; prostitute slave markets became sources of exported sexually transmitted diseases; new mutant strains of bacteria that could defy modern medical options swiftly spread beyond country or regional borders; tuberculosis was an airborne transmitter; disease-ravaged regions often spurned mass human migrations to other regions of the planet; and instability in any strategic part of the planet could reverberate with geopolitical impact across the globe.

"In sum, those specializing in geopolitics, economics, and the military who ignore these issues or put them into a 'who cares?' pocket do so at the hazard of not understanding what is going on and its consequences," Murray Feshbach said.[185] "Perhaps the Russian population will be dead or so ill that there will be no solution to the economic, military, and political problems of the country. Neither the past system managers nor the current leaders should take any solace in blaming the others; both are or will be responsible."

While the region's old guard fought tooth and nail against change, the agents of the West pushed their agendas into the vacuum. It was not always a pretty picture. Private North American and European insurance, health management, and pharmaceutical companies swarmed over the region during the 1990s, hoping to snag lucrative deals that would commit the new societies to mixed economic structures of health. Government agencies marched in from the West to preach the gospels of health management organizations, managed care, global pharmaceutical patent protection, and social marketing. The World Bank and an assortment of United Nations agencies tried carrot-and-stick approaches, hoping to lure the region's governments toward Western models of reconstruction in exchange for substantial interest-free or low-interest financial aid.[186] They met with varying degrees of success, particularly in their overall push toward health insurance–based systems.

"In general, given the chaotic nature of the economic reform and democratization processes, Russia may simply not be ready for a market-based insurance scheme at this time," wrote a top team of American public health experts.[187] "Certainly, it must have seemed persuasive to Russia's health care decision makers, in light of the failure of socialized medicine to fulfill its mandate, to embrace 'insurance' as a kind of antimodel. Many Russians, however, are now realizing that at least some elements of the old system, with its 'assurance' of universal health care at state expense, may be worth preserving until 'insurance' can fulfill its promises."

"We don't know, actually, where we're going, or what is happening, especially in science," Dr. Alexi Savinykh of Moscow's MEDSOCECONOMINFORM think tank explained. "We now have a blanket made of pieces—a quilt. Each local government is free to do whatever they want. . . . And as to public health and health care, it's not an easy question. We have *no* standards for the current time."

In Georgia Minister of Health Avtandil Jorbenadze eagerly embraced American models of public health and health care. But he admitted that public health was getting short shrift, as most funds still went to the nation's overly large hospital system. Less than forty cents was spent per capita on public health during the 1990s, Jorbenadze acknowledged.

He leaned heartily on American advisors, Jorbenadze said, laughing. "It was part of building a new state with market economic relations and democracy."

Which echoed clearly the U.S. government's position on public health in the newly independent nation. "We're here to do democracy building," a top U.S. official working in the region said. "We are *not* focusing on health sector reform."

Smugly the official added that "the public health leadership of this country is not looking [to Russia] for ideas—it's looking West. That's what matters."

Perhaps.

But the moves were tenuous, at best. WHO advisor to Georgia, Dr. Archil Khomassuridze, acknowledged that his country, for example, had embarked on a distinctly American-style reform of public health and health care.

"The country is on a path of progress, but they are *only* at the beginning," Khomassuridze said. "It could still slip back. If war breaks out again. If there is a cataclysm in Russia. Remember: if Russia sneezes Georgia catches pneumonia."

Estonia's minister of social affairs, Jaan Ruutmann, drank his morning coffee from a U.S. government coffee cup emblazoned with Old Glory. In his spacious office, decorated in wood and pastels, the raffish, robust Ruutmann spoke sternly about changes in his Baltic country. Since 1991 he had imposed strict accounting and financial controls on the nation's hospitals—the first time most administrators had ever been required to tell the government how they spent their money.

Key to public health was assuring that those hospitals spent adequately on basic preventive services, such as immunization, STD screening, surveillance of diseases, and health education. Though Ruutmann felt that "it's obvious" that spending on prevention ended up saving money by avoiding severe diseases in the future he was uneasy. He could see profiteering emerging in the Estonian health system. As the insurance industry moved in, more and more doctors seemed to be after short-term, high-yield medicine, rather than the less profitable preventive health measures.

In the Czech Republic the pendulum had swung too far in the direction of managed health and private insurance, complained Dr. Victor Kayak, who had the largest private pulmonary medicine practice in the nation. The hallways of his Prague clinic reverberated with the sounds of tubercular coughing. Between 1995 and 1996 he saw a 35 percent increase in tuberculosis cases at a time when government public health authorities recorded only marginal elevations in TB levels.

"How would they know?" Kayak, visibly exhausted, asked. "In the Czech Republic it's a question of financing of health care. Our government and Ministry of Health didn't even consider TB. . . . The state should finance bringing TB under control. But it doesn't. We are now financed through insurance reimbursement and that's not enough for TB. . . . It's a horrible situation!"[188]

Terribly upset, the tall, lean doctor, dressed in his spotless lab coat, had eagerly embraced the new democracy, even the new health economy. But now, he nearly shouted, public health was pushed aside, "and the government is giving up all of its responsibilities."

The last thing we need, he mumbled, is your American system.

CHAPTER FOUR

PREFERRING ANARCHY

AND CLASS DISPARITY

The American public health infrastructure
in an age of antigovernmentalism.

*Public health is purchasable. Within natural limitations a community can de-
termine its own death-rate. . . . No duty of society, acting through its governmental agencies, is paramount to this obligation to attack the removable
causes of disease.*

—Dr. Hermann Biggs, New York State Commissioner of Health, 1913

Government is not the solution to our problem; government is the problem.

—Ronald Reagan, presidential inaugural speech, January 20, 1981

*As the scientific case for public health becomes stronger, politics and popular
support has not kept pace. Public health programs in the United States—and
the situation is similar in many other countries—are either not being improved
or, in many cases, are being allowed to wither. . . . Overt resistance to public
health is rare. On the contrary, public health has been subject to the death of a
thousand cuts, some of them noticed, others not.*

—Daniel Callahan, The Hastings Center, 1998[1]

The twenty-first century dawned with America's public health system in dire
disarray. Some might argue that there actually was no system per se, but a
hodgepodge of programs, bureaucracies, and failings.

As incredible as it might seem, given America's breathtaking prosperity at
the close of the 1990s, most of the problems and crises noted in the health
apparati of central Africa, the Indian subcontinent, and former Soviet Union
could also to one degree or another be found in the United States. American
public health leaders of the 1990s were struggling to ensure that the nation's

food and water were safe, that diseases like HIV and hepatitis C didn't over-whelm the populace, that the country's children were appropriately vaccinated: item by item the travails of the rest of the world were also America's. And America had its own additional bugbears, reflecting unique political and eco-nomic dimensions of the society.

If the former Soviet states suffered from an overemphasis on the public health needs of the collective, at the expense of the individual, America at the end of the twentieth century was reeling under the weight of its newfound lib-ertarianism: the collective be damned, all public health burdens and responsi-bilities fell to the individual. It was an odd paradigm and an about-face from the attitudes and sense of duty that had formed the foundation of American public health at the dawn of the twentieth century. While the 1991 end of the Cold War brought public health chaos and despair to the losing side, for the American victors it unleashed a national me-first sentiment that flourished during the country's most phenomenal and lengthiest period of economic prosperity.

Less than a decade after the fall of the Berlin Wall, the middle class of the United States had grown blasé about the word *millionaire*, the New York Stock Exchange scaled heights that would have been unimaginable in the 1980s, and few citizens of the United States seriously doubted that the New World Order hailed in 1991 by then-president George Bush meant anything less than Amer-ican dominance over the global marketplace.

It seemed, in short, a good time to be smug—if you were a fortunate Amer-ican.

The nineteenth-century and early-twentieth-century creators of America's public health systems would have found this emphasis on individualism amid such grand prosperity shocking. For them, the health of a community was the key measure of its success, and if pestilence and death stalked even one small segment of the population it was a stark indication of the community's political and social failure. They were zealous in their beliefs, imbued with a sense of mission and, in most parts of the country, empowered by law to execute their plans—even if such efforts entailed battles with governors, mayors, or legislative politicians: "The public press will approve, the people are prepared to support, and the courts sustain, any intelligent procedures which are evidently directed at the preservation of the public health," New York City health official Dr. Her-mann Biggs declared in 1900. "The most autocratic powers, capable of the broadest construction, are given to them under the law. Everything which is detrimental to health or dangerous to life, under the freest interpretation, is regarded as coming within the province of the Health Department. So broad is the construction of the law that everything which improperly or unnecessarily interferes with the comfort or enjoyment of life, as well as those things which are, strictly speaking, detrimental to health or dangerous to life, may become the subject of action on the part of the Board of Health."[2] If disease raged, the objective, in short, was to stamp it out by any means necessary.

These crusaders would find it amazing to witness the erosion of America's public health infrastructures during the later twentieth century, the low status ascribed to public health physicians and scientists, the legal limitations placed on their authority, and the disdain with which Americans viewed their civil servants. In the early 1890s America led the world in designing and executing the primary missions of public health; in the 1990s, the same nation turned its back on most of the key elements of the enterprise known as Public Health.

For example, American hospitals had once been death traps from which few patients emerged in better health than they had been in when they entered. Public health zealots of the late nineteenth century cleaned up the hospitals, ordered doctors and nurses to scrub up, and brought death rates way down.

But a hundred years later, while Zaire might have been the only nation with the dubious distinction of having twice spawned Ebola epidemics out of its hospitals, it was hardly alone in an apparent state of helplessness before wave after wave of nosocomial, or hospital-acquired, infections. Throughout the former Soviet Union infection control—or the lack thereof—was in a calamitous state. In the poor regions of the world resource scarcities could always be blamed when dangerous microbes passed from one patient to another via the hands of a physician, who, ironically, had sworn to the first maxim of medicine: do no harm.

But scarcity could hardly explain why nosocomial disease was, like a dark horseman of death, sweeping over American hospitals. Nor could lack of resources justify the apparent helplessness and impotence with which public health officials greeted the tidal wave of mutant, drug-resistant superbugs.

Even in wealthy America, hospitals had become places where many patients grew *sicker* than they had been when they checked in, catching diseases on the wards. By 1997, 10 percent of *all* patients who spent more than one night in the average U.S. hospital acquired a nonviral infection nosocomially, carried to their fragile, ailing bodies on contaminated instruments or the hands of medical personnel.[3] The more severely ill the patients, the greater their likelihood of being nosocomially infected. This was simply because individuals in an intensive care unit recuperating from, for example, open-heart surgery were subjected to far more potentially contaminated needles, shunts, devices, and manipulations than were, say, women recovering from childbirth. In intensive care units the odds that any given patient would be infected in this way approached fifty-fifty. And all too often those infections were fatal.[4]

A few hospitals in the United States cooperated with the CDC to form the National Nosocomial Infection Surveillance System. Their lab work showed steady increases in the percentage of drug-resistant organisms that could defy conventional treatments in every population of common hospital microbes during the 1990s.[5] A University of Iowa–run Sentry Antimicrobial Surveillance System in Europe, Canada, and Latin America spotted the same trend, as did a WHO global surveillance network that monitored the emergence of mobile rings of DNA that carried drug-resistance genes. These rings, called plasmids, were readily shared among bacteria, even across species.[6]

For reasons nobody could quite pin down, New York City had the highest rates of drug-resistant bacterial diseases and deaths in its hospitals.

"We seem to be leading the nation on this, which is a dubious number-one position, to say the least," the city's health commissioner, Dr. Margaret Hamburg, said with a sigh.[7] Hamburg's assistant commissioner, Dr. Marcelle Layton, said in 1997 that the city faced an unparalleled scale of public health challenges that might be contributing to the steady rise in drug resistance her staff had observed over ten years.

"There are fifty-three thousand people per square mile in New York City," Layton said, and "about two hundred thousand of them are HIV-positive. A quarter of the population lives below the poverty line. One point three million have no health insurance."

Layton stopped and shrugged her shoulders, her body language saying, "What can we do?" And, indeed, public health officials all over America were stymied, as they anxiously watched death tolls rise, the bugs mutate, vital drugs get rendered useless, but lacked any powers to stop what seemed an inevitability: the arrival of the postantibiotic era. And nowhere was that terrible prospect looming more precariously than in the nation's hospitals.

Unfortunately, hospitals had become physicians' sacred grounds, not to be trammeled by public health authorities. A century earlier Layton's counterparts could have marched in and shut down any hospital that, like Kikwit's Ebola-spreading General Hospital, created epidemics. Not so in the 1990s. Instead Layton and her counterparts nationwide counted death tolls and issued warnings.

The numbers were truly horrible. One of the key sources of nosocomial infection was contaminated intravascular catheters. Such devices were placed in nearly all postsurgical patients. If contaminated with pathogenic bacteria or fungi the result was blood poisoning, or septicemia. Twenty-five percent of the time such septicemia episodes during the 1990s proved fatal. For the 75 percent of such patients who survived, nosocomial infection added an average of $33,000 in medical costs. In 1996 there were an estimated four hundred thousand nosocomial septicemia survivors in the United States whose total additional treatment cost was $13.2 billion.[8]

The bottom line: by the close of the 1990s somewhere between one hundred thousand and one hundred fifty thousand Americans were dying each year, felled by infections they caught inside U.S. hospitals. And the deadliest of nosocomial microbes were newly emerging, mutant bacteria that could resist antibiotic treatment.

The crisis brewing in New York City during the nineties involved four ubiquitous pathogens: *Enterococcus faecium, Enterococcus faecalis, Streptococcus pneumoniae,* and *Staphylococcus aureus.* The enterococci were troublesome, but not usually lethal, intestinal bacteria that produced digestive problems, diarrhea, and bowel and colon pain and spasms. If an individual was highly stressed or immune deficient—as were the cases with most hospitalized individuals—these bacteria (particularly *faecium*) could be lethal.

Strep and staph were, of course, far more worrisome. Strep pneumonia bacteria were leading causes of ear infections, disease-associated deafness, pneumonia deaths, and what was commonly called strep throat. Severe strep infections could result in bacterial colonization of the meninges tissues, leading to meningitis and life-threatening infections of the central nervous system. In the preantibiotic era, 30 to 35 percent of all *S. pneumoniae* infections were fatal.[9]

In 1996 *S. pneumoniae* was the leading cause of pneumonia in the United States, producing four million adult cases annually. Outpatient treatment costs alone topped $1 billion a year. And for patients over sixty years of age such infections were, despite vigorous antibiotic treatment, fatal about 7 percent of the time.[10]

Staphylococcus aureus was the cause of wound infections, sepsis (blood poisoning), toxic shock syndrome, bedsores, osteomyelitis bone disease, endocarditis heart infections, boils, abscesses, and bacterially induced arthritis. Because some strains of the organism exuded powerful toxins, staph infections could be terrifying, escalating in a matter of hours from little more than a small, pus-producing contamination of a wound to life-threatening blood poisoning and cardiac arrest. It was primarily because of staph infections that tens of thousands of soldiers' limbs were amputated during the Civil War and World War I.

Staph bacteria tend to cluster in tight groups, like grapes on a vine. Under stress, the organisms can expel the water from their cytoplasm and go into a dormant state as hard, dry "beads." In that state they are virtually invulnerable and can survive in air, water, food, soap, soil—almost anywhere. Strep are also spherical, but rather than forming clusters, they tend to gather single file, forming long chains, like pearl necklaces. They, too, are capable of resisting environmental stress by expelling water and going into a dormant state.

New York's troubles with these organisms had been severe in the late nineteenth and early twentieth centuries, but had virtually disappeared with the arrival of the penicillin era. These were among the first microbes to acquire penicillin resistance, however, and all over the city by the early 1990s Dr. Hamburg's department was finding strep that was resistant, or completely impervious, to penicillin.[11]

A citywide survey of seventy-three hospitals found that penicillinase-resistant infections in all age groups of patients had soared from 8 percent in 1993 to more than 20 percent in 1995, said Layton in a speech to the 1996 American Public Health Association meeting in Manhattan. The incidence of resistant strep was highest in children under one year of age, with eleven cases per 100,000 New York City infants occurring in 1995.

That year, Hamburg noted, only one antibiotic was still universally effective against New York City strep *pneumoniae*: vancomycin. It was also the only treatment for drug-resistant staph—MRSA (methicillin-resistant *Staphylococcus aureus*)—which by 1993 represented fully a third of all staph cases in the United States.[12]

And there was the rub: three different species of common bacteria were acquiring powerful drug-resistance capacities simultaneously. And all three left medicine with the same last-resort drug:. vancomycin

The critical concern was that the vancomycin-resistant enterococci (VRE) would share their resistance genes with strep or staph. Test tube studies in the early 1990s showed that VRE resistance genes were carried on mobile transposons, or plasmids, and that the changes they mediated in the enterococci could also be carried out in strep or staph bacteria.[13]

Remarkably, some enterococci actually became "addicted to vancomycin," Rockefeller University microbiologist Alexander Tomasz said. The bugs not only could *resist* vancomycin, they actually evolved to *depend upon it*.[14]

Looming over New York City in the mid-1990s, then, was the prospect that, within a hospitalized patient who was infected with enterococci, some VRE would share its awesome genetic machinery with staph or strep, resulting in a terrifying, highly contagious superbug.

It was a nightmarish public health prospect.

"We're just waiting for the other shoe to drop," Dr. Hamburg said nervously. Hamburg's staff, together with Tomasz and scientists from the local Public Health Research Institute and area hospitals, formed the BARG—Bacterial Antibiotic Resistance Group—in 1993 to watchdog microbial trends in the area. And Hamburg warned the area's hospitals in the strongest possible terms that their infection-control standards needed to improve or they would soon see death rates soar due to drug-resistant microbes. The New York State Department of Health toughened infection control guidelines, too, and ordered that every single hospital employee in the state—from intake receptionist to brain surgeon—had to undergo state-certified infection-control training every year, beginning in 1994.

As part of that first year's training, infection-control nurse specialist Kathleen Jakob warned an audience of health providers at Columbia College of Surgeons and Physicians in Manhattan that lapses in infection control usually were the unintended results of becoming overly habituated to the hospital environment. "People outside the medical profession have a very hard time discussing rectal abscesses over dinner," Jakob said, drawing guffaws from the medical students. "We don't. We don't see our environment the way visitors do. We get so used to it that we don't see risks, the chaos, the filth."

But when it came to controlling the spread of tough bacteria inside hospitals, the time-honored Semmelweis technique for scrubbing hands before touching patients—an insight that had revolutionized medicine more than a century earlier—had more than met its match. Now microbes such as *Staphylococcus* were capable when dormant of living on tabletops, curtains, clothing, even in vats of disinfectant. Despite strict scrubbing, careful health workers could pick up such organisms when their uniforms brushed against a patient's wound or sheets, and then carry the bug to the next patient's bedside.

Of the more than fourteen thousand germicides registered in 1994 with the U.S. Environmental Protection Agency (EPA), few could kill such bacteria in their dormant states, and some required hours of soaking to guarantee disinfection. Indeed, some bacteria had acquired additional supercapabilities to resist disinfectants and soaps. They could, for example, shunt all chlorine-containing compounds out of their membranes, rendering all bleaches utterly useless.

The only cleansers guaranteed to kill dormant bacteria were quaternary ammonias and formaldehydes, Jakob told her Columbia audience. And those compounds were associated with cancer and birth defects, so the EPA discouraged their use on neonatal and pediatric wards.[15]

An alternative to cleansing was cooking the germs in autoclaves, flash sterilizers, gas chambers, and steamers. But there, too, hospitals were encountering problems because of the tenacity of the bacteria, the sloppiness of personnel, and new medical equipment that was extremely difficult to clean. Additionally, some bacteria mutated to tolerate high temperatures, forcing either longer or hotter sterilizations.

The only way hospitals could track lapses in infection control was to monitor the organisms found in their sicker patients and run laboratory analyses to determine which—if any—antibiotic could still kill those microbes. If highly resistant bacteria were uncovered, tests were done on patients bedded nearby. If they were infected with the same bacteria, a stern-faced Jakob told her anxious audience, "It's a sure sign that a break in infection control took place somewhere on the ward."

At that point, every piece of equipment on the ward, every millimeter of surface area, each television set, chair, bed—*everything*—had to be scrubbed thoroughly with effective disinfectants. Patients had to be placed under quarantines (ranging from total, air-lock isolations to merely being asked to remain in their rooms, away from other patients), all ward personnel had to be tested to determine whether any of them carried the mutant bacteria in their bloodstreams, and all staff operational procedures needed to be scrutinized to determine where lapses might have occurred.

Sometimes the microbes—particularly MRSA—proved so tenacious and resistant to disinfection that hospitals had no choice but to shut down the ward, strip it of all organic matter (rubber, cotton, wool, silicone, plastics), repaint all walls, retile all bathrooms, and apply new linoleum to all floors.

Only after that mammoth task was completed, and all equipment had been replaced, could the once-contaminated wards be reopened.

Such procedures were horribly costly and almost always led to patient lawsuits against hospitals. And all too often the carrier of resistant microbes turned out to be a nurse or doctor who unknowingly harbored the germs in his or her blood; harmless to the health care worker, but lethal to the susceptible patient. So it was in the hospitals' and health providers' interests, whether they recognized it or not, to take tedious steps to avoid such extreme contamination.

It sounded straightforward enough, but even at an elite institution like Columbia-Presbyterian—one of America's best hospitals—preventing spread of VRE and other drug-resistant organisms was all but impossible.

For example, at Columbia-Presbyterian Hospital, nurse Janise Schwadron was handling postsurgical intensive care patients. When word came that the patient in "contact isolation" had to be taken downstairs for a CT scan, Schwadron sighed, "What a pain."

In addition to recuperating from lung transplant surgery, the patient was infected with a mutant strain of enterococcal bacteria resistant to *every* antibiotic used for its treatment. To protect the rest of the hospital's patients, moving the patient to radiology was quite a job. Everything that touched the patient had to be disinfected before and after making the move. Schwadron ordered up three helpers. Then—dressed in head-to-toe protective gowns, latex gloves, and gauze masks—they began scouring every inch of each piece of equipment before changing the patient's bedding. Hours later, after the CT scan room had also been disinfected and the transplant patient was back, Schwadron relaxed. A simple diagnostic test that usually involved just two employees and an hour's time had taken up more than six hours' time for five employees, as well as a heap of expensive protective gear.

Hospital staff were only part of the problem. Schwadron was also responsible for watching others who entered the transplant patient's room, from family members to attending physicians—reminding them to follow proper precautions and, if they failed to do so, ordering them off the ward.

Some of the patients seemed to do everything they could to make matters worse. For example, Columbia-Presbyterian had a patient the nurses called the Wanderer. Normally, patients who insisted on walking the halls and popping their heads into other patients' rooms were nothing more than a nuisance. But the Wanderer was infected with VRE. If, in her travels, the Wanderer were to meet with another patient infected with a mutant version of either staph or pneumococcus, they could easily infect each other, their bugs could share genes, and both patients could end up carrying completely drug-resistant staph or pneumococcus infections.

In the late-nineteenth-century day of public health pioneer Hermann Biggs, recalcitrant, belligerent patients like the Wanderer would have been restrained, placed in quarantine, or locked up for the good of the community. But in 1994 such actions weren't legal. The only power nurses had over the Wanderer was the power of persuasion—and this patient wasn't heeding their pleas. Indeed, she had slapped a nurse who tried to push her away from nibbling food off another patient's tray.

Public health had lost so much power and authority by the 1990s that Commissioner Hamburg's options did *not* include the three steps that offered the greatest likelihood of slowing the spread of deadly drug-resistant bacteria. All evidence indicated that physician's overprescribing antibiotics was driving up drug resistance, but years of successful American Medical Association lobbying had stripped public health authorities of all powers to affect doctors' prescription practices. Ideally, Hamburg would like to have put vancomycin in some special legal category, requiring doctors to seek the Department of Health's permission before using the precious drug. That might preserve its utility a few years longer, but she and her colleagues nationwide were powerless to implement such a stopgap measure.

The second and third options were to order forced confinement of patients who carried highly drug-resistant strains of bacteria and mandatory testing of medical personnel on a routine basis to ensure that they weren't unknowingly infected with such bugs. But there, too, Hamburg's legal powers were minimal. Indeed, inside hospitals all over America there were modern "Typhoid Mary" doctors who flatly refused to undergo tests to see if they were carriers of drug-resistant bacteria.

One New York City burn ward—the largest burn treatment center east of the Rockies—had an outbreak of MRSA, which was *extremely* dangerous for burn patients because so much of their bodies were exposed, unprotected by skin. Every single person who worked on the ward, save its chief physician, was tested. All came up negative as MRSA carriers. The physician refused to be tested. When that physician transferred to another hospital, that hospital, too, experienced a MRSA outbreak. But Hamburg's department could do nothing legally to compel the physician to undergo testing or treatment to cleanse the lethal bugs from his body.

When the legal authorities of public health were stripped during the mid-twentieth century, nobody anticipated that hospitals would become centers not only for disease treatment but also for disease creation. VRE first appeared in the United States in 1988 when it was reported in three New York City hospitals. But a survey of twenty-four hospitals in New York City, neighboring Long Island, and Westchester County found it had surfaced in every single one by the beginning of 1994.

Nationally, cases of VRE increased twenty-fold between 1989 and 1993, and about 7.9 percent of all 1994 enterococcal infections involved the mutant bacteria, according to the CDC. That was up from less than 1 percent just four years previously.

Hospital by hospital, it was extremely difficult to obtain information on VRE rates—nobody wanted their institution labeled a center of drug-resistant bacteria, and public health authorities were powerless to order hospitals to be candid about their nosocomial infection rates. So Hamburg had to cut deals with the hospitals, promising to keep secret the details of their VRE rates in exchange for gaining access to their laboratory records. Publicly, she said, the department could never reveal that " 'Hospital X has this much VRE.' We will say, 'Overall, there's this much in hospitals in the city.' That's the only way we can do it."

All but three hospitals in the New York metropolitan area declined to provide an inquiring reporter with their VRE details. Those three hospitals all reported steadily climbing VRE rates.[16]

One institution that was very open about its VRE situation was Cabrini Hospital, a private facility in Manhattan that in 1993 published a detailed rundown of VRE cases detected on its wards between 1990 and 1992. Over a thirty-six-month period, Cabrini treated 2,812 enterococcus cases, 213 of which were vancomycin-resistant. More important was the trend over time. In 1990, 85 percent of all enterococcal infections were fully vulnerable to vancomycin. By the end of 1992 only 25.8 percent of all enterococcal infections treated in the hospital remained fully susceptible to the drug.

"We have been living in an era when if you got sick, there was always a pill to take," said Rockefeller University's Tomasz in later 1995. "We are approaching an era when that will no longer be true."

"Every bacterial species you can name has increased its level of drug resistance over the last twenty years. . . . It is probably the number-one public health issue in the United States," the CDC's expert, Dr. William Jarvis, declared in 1995. And, he insisted, if VRE ever shared its resistance genes with staph or strep, "it would be a catastrophe."

By 1997 the trend regarding MRSA and VRE was clear in New York City and nationwide, Dr. Louis Rice of Emory University said.[17] "If we want to control resistance in the community, we have to control it in the hospital first, because that's where it starts."

And the larger the hospital, the more MRSA and VRE lurked on its wards, Rice continued. In 1997 hospitals with fewer than two hundred beds had MRSA in 16 percent of their staph-infected patients, but hospitals with more than two hundred beds had a 27 percent incidence of MRSA. The implication was that infections spread more readily in the chaotic atmosphere of large, generally public hospitals.

Once these organisms surfaced in a hospital, "infection control is not going to be the answer," Rice insisted. "I'm not all that optimistic that we're going to be able to control this."

When resistant organisms emerged on a ward, drastic cleanup and escalated infection control could slow their spread, Rice said, but hospitals also needed to take radical steps to change their prescription practices; for example, completely stopping vancomycin use when VRE emerged. Still, he acknowledged, even that didn't always work. One hospital reacted to its first MRSA outbreak by ordering a full stop to the use of methicillin, telling doctors to instead use mupirocin on their staph patients. In a year, staph infections in that hospital went from involving 2 percent to 64 percent mupirocin-resistant organisms.

New York-Cornell Medical Center had a similar experience with drug resistant *Klebsiella* infections: switching all antibiotics simply led to emergence of multidrug-resistant *Klebsiella*.

On the other hand, changing drug-use practices had, indeed, lowered bacterial disease rates in some other settings, Rice said, indicating that when it came to controlling mutant bugs in hospital ecologies, "one size definitely doesn't fit all."

At Queens Hospital in New York City, Dr. James Rahal had discovered that the nature of the mechanism a resistant bug used to get around antibiotics was a key determinant of how tenacious that bug could be: were plasmid transposons the key to its resistance or was it actual mutations of the bacteria's DNA? The latter, Rahal argued, were the toughest to eradicate once they emerged.[18] After all, plasmids could pop *out* of microbes as readily as they popped *in*, making resistance a transient event. But if a germ mutated, if its *chromosomes* were altered, resistance was permanent not only in that individual microbe but also in all its progeny for generations to come.

For example, Rahal said, the percentage of *Klebsiella* infections in his hospital that were resistant to ceftazidime went from 6 percent in 1988 to 37 percent in 1995. Those were transposon forms of resistance and were moderately controllable through drug switching and standard infection-control measures. But in 1995 a new strain of chromosomally resistant *Klebsiella* emerged in the hospital—a form that had mutations in its primary DNA—and by Christmas of that year *every single Klebsiella* bacterium they found in the hospital was fully resistant not just to ceftazidime, but to the entire cephalosporin class of antibiotics.

At that point, the hospital ordered a full stop on the use of cephalosporins to treat *Klebsiella* infections. And then a strange thing started happening: resistance emerged in an entirely different microbe population. The hospital decreased its total cephalosporin use, for all purposes, by more than 80 percent during 1996, and increased use of the expensive alternative drug imipenem by 59 percent. That cut *Klebsiella* drug resistance down by nearly half. But it prompted emergence of imipenem-resistant *Pseudomonas aueriginosa*, a pneumonia-causing organism.

"So the problem just shifted from one microbe population to another," Rahal sadly concluded.

With cleanup so tough, and new superbugs emerging in the best hospitals in America, "I suppose that we're back in the preantibiotic era now," said Dr. Matthew Scharff of Albert Einstein Medical School in the Bronx. Speaking before a 1993 gathering of the Irvington Trust, an investment banking group that funded medical research, Scharff said patients who underwent cancer chemotherapy, transplant surgery, radiation, or who had AIDS commonly died of what, for other people, were fairly benign fungal or bacterial infections, even though they received high intravenous doses of antibiotics. *Staphylococcus, Meningococcus, Pneumococcus, Cryptosporidium*—all those germs could devastate such people.

"In the absence of our own immunity, even antibiotics cannot kill these agents," Scharff said, adding that even otherwise healthy individuals were at increasing risk for some diseases because the bugs had acquired drug resistance.

The evidence was clear on the cancer and AIDS wards of large hospitals in the greater New York area, Scharff insisted. Some 10 percent of all people with AIDS died from cryptococcus—a ubiquitous fungus found in bird droppings. Once it got into their brains, the microbe caused meningitis. Similarly, a variety of bacterial infections were essentially incurable in cancer lymphoma patients—former First Lady Jacqueline Kennedy Onassis died in New York as a result of such an infection.

Scharff thought that doctors in public health pioneer Hermann Biggs's day, before the invention of antibiotics, had had at least a partial solution to the problem: antisera. In the early twentieth century, physicians injected samples of the bacteria that were infecting their patients—say, pneumococci, which caused pneumonia—into a horse. The horse made antibodies against the pneumococci. The doctors withdrew blood from the horse, separated out and purified the antibodies, and injected the resulting antiserum into their dying patients.

"About thirty percent of the time it worked," Scharff said. But it was also often toxic because humans developed acute allergic reactions to horse proteins that were residual in the antisera.

At the close of the twentieth century, however, technology existed that would allow scientists to make pure human antisera in mice or in test tubes. So-called monoclonal antibodies were in use for other medical purposes, and Scharff's group had already made anticryptococcal monoclonal antibodies and proven that they worked in immunodeficient mice.

"I think we should look back at this," Scharff argued. "We have to. We have nothing else."[19]

Few New York physicians were willing to accept Scharff's dire view of the situation. Bad as antibiotic resistance problems were, *something* usually, eventually, worked—most of the time. Or so they argued in the late 1990s.

Not so, said the New York State Senate's Committee on Investigations in early 1999.[20] That committee issued a report concluding that hospital-spread infections in New York City alone in 1995 had caused 1,020 deaths and $230 million worth of extra patient hospitalization and treatments. Chaired by Senator Roy Goodman, a Manhattan Republican, the committee drew its conclusions from evidence presented by Nobel laureate Dr. Joshua Lederberg and Tomasz, both of Rockefeller University; Dr. Willa Appel of the New York City Partnership; and rheumatologist Sheldon Blau of the State University of New York Medical Center in Stony Brook.

Based on testimony and studies presented to the Senate committee, its report charged that between 1975 and 1995 the number of days patients were hospitalized nationwide rose 36 percent due to nosocomial infections. In 1995, the report continued, 1.7 million people in the United States acquired infections in the hospital that proved fatal to eighty-eight thousand of them and added $4.5 billion to the nation's health costs.

Further, the report charged, cost-containment measures under managed care were severely exacerbating the problem because nursing staffs were overworked and so tired that they made mistakes; and more hospitals were cutting costs by replacing skilled nurses with poorly trained nurses' aides. Within the New York City Health and Hospitals Corporation, for example, nursing staff was cut by 21 percent from 1994 to 1999.

Worse, 70 percent of all such hospital-acquired infections involved drug-resistant organisms. In metropolitan New York City alone, 7,800 patients acquired drug-resistant staph infections during hospital stays in 1995: 1,400 of them died as a result.

And about half of all hospital-acquired infections could be eliminated by simply imposing stricter hygiene regulation inside hospitals and reducing the rate at which doctors prescribed antibiotics.

"Some five years ago I entered a good, prestigious hospital," Blau said, "for a routine angioplasty. . . . I developed a hospital-acquired, drug-resistant staph infection, and I was so close to dying that last rites were said." Blau charged that his infection resulted from spread of staph within the hospital by doctors and nurses who failed to wash their hands and instruments between patients. And, he said ominously, "the next time you're in the hospital visiting a relative, you see how often the doctor washes his hands."

"This is a shocking thing," Goodman said. "It's almost unbelievable that something as basic as the washing of hands is being ignored by doctors." Incredible as it might seem American doctors were, apparently, almost as likely to shun essential infection-control procedures as were their counterparts in Siberia.

The Senate report scolded New York hospitals: "Health care workers seek to heal us and, first and foremost, must do no harm. Yet their failure to consistently follow even the simplest hygienic practices is a major reason for the contraction of bacterial infections in hospitals. Good long-term financial incentives exist for hospitals to insist on strict infection-control procedures; yet short-term financial considerations have militated against the consistent use of such procedures."[21]

Four decades earlier Lederberg had won a Nobel Prize for demonstrating how bacteria evolve, eluding antibiotics. In the 1950s he warned the scientific and medical communities that, unless carefully used, antibiotics would become less useful with time simply because the microbes were master mutators. By the close of the 1990s evidence supporting his prognostications was abundant, but public health actions aimed at preventing the otherwise inevitable end of the antibiotic era were nearly nonexistent. A dignified man, Lederberg rarely expressed public anger. But he was, nevertheless, enraged. He felt that the solutions were many and attainable, but lack of social, political, and economic will was blocking every rational path toward restoration of hospital safety and drug efficacy against resistant bacterial populations.

"We're running out of bullets for dealing with a number of these infections," Lederberg pronounced soberly, slowly shaking his white-bearded head. "Are we better off today than we were a century ago? In most respects, we're worse off," he pronounced.

Citing declining government support for public health, increasing globalization of humanity and its microbial hitchhikers, and the rise of managed care in America, Lederberg held out little hope for the future. "The world really is just one village. And our tolerance of disease in any place in the world is at our own peril," he insisted. "Patients are dying because we no longer have antibiotics that work. And there's no way we're going to eradicate all of these organisms. We have to learn to live with them, as moving targets."

It *was* possible to develop new antibacterial drugs, Lederberg insisted, if the pharmaceutical industry were so motivated. And it *was* possible to control the spread of resistant bacteria, if public health authorities were sufficiently funded and empowered to do so.

"But to say public health is going to be left out in the cold by Washington is an understatement," the visibly angry Lederberg continued. "It's already out in the cold. Public health—that system is very close to being in a shambles at this time."

It took centuries to build a public health system, and less than two decades to bring it down. Once the envy of the world, America's public health infrastructure was, at the end of the twentieth century, indeed in a shambles.

I

Hot, dry winds forever blowing,
Dead men to the grave-yards going:
Constant hearses,
Funeral verses;
Oh! what plagues—there is no knowing!

—Philip Freneau, written during the great yellow fever epidemic, Philadelphia, 1793

Public health—the discipline, the profession, the infrastructure that bears that moniker—was born at a time when hospitals were little more than warehouses for the dying, and the biggest enemy of humanity's healthy well-being was human behavior. In New York, political corruption, slavery and racism, urban squalor, and gross wealth disparities all gave microbes fantastic opportunities to spread, killing nearly half of all children before they reached their twelfth birthdays. In the Midwest, profound ignorance and medical corruption were key culprits. Out in the far West of America, where the climate limited microbial possibilities, religious and racial biases, coupled with boomtown growth that outstripped the pace of infrastructure development, left public health leaders bereft of popular support for their activities well into the twentieth century.

Yet the foundations of public health were built out of such travails, and the very tools of the trade that nurses on Columbia-Presbyterian's wards needed to apply in hopes of controlling the Wanderer and VRE had been developed more than a century previously. Indeed, as early as 1629 American colonists in Virginia realized that they couldn't protect their people's health unless they had numbers—hard facts, entered dutifully by quill into log books: births, deaths, illnesses, and marriages were, by law, recorded, chronicling the vital statistics of the colony.

Colonial leaders also recognized, despite their lack of any theory of contagion, that great epidemics followed the arrival of ships with ailing crews and passengers. While the Great Plague ravaged London in 1665, the port cities of the Americas held British ships offshore in strict quarantine. This set a striking precedent: thereafter each colony instituted increasingly strict quarantine regulations, detaining ships and even incarcerating their crews on islands offshore for periods of time deemed safe, for the sake of the public's health.[22]

Despite such early public health efforts, the colonial cities were visited periodically by epidemics of such magnitude as to seem terrifying in retrospect. For example, smallpox—which had arrived in 1679 aboard a slave ship—hit New York in wave after wave of deadly assaults beginning in 1689.[23]

In addition to smallpox, New Yorkers and other colonials suffered and died in enormous numbers from measles, scarlet fever, yellow fever, typhoid fever, malaria, and a host of other diseases, nearly all of them infectious. The waves of disease and death could not be rationally explained, though colonial leaders blamed satanic, anti-Christian forces of various kinds. That religious rationale yielded to the miasma theory, which saw malodorous and malevolent forces in the environs that, on occasion, enveloped humanity.

Despite the ravages of smallpox, the disease that sparked the greatest fear, claimed enormous numbers of lives, and ignited public health policies for decades to come was yellow fever. Depending on the strain of virus and the level of immunity in the local population as a consequence of prior yellow fever epidemics, death would claim anywhere from 5 percent to half of everyone infected.

Unbeknownst to the Americans of the seventeenth and eighteenth centuries, the yellow fever virus was passed from one person to another by *Aedes aegypti* mosquitoes. It wasn't actually a new disease, but it seemed so to the American Indians and white colonials, particularly because it appeared unique in claiming whole families, not just the children. Both the virus and its *Aedes aegypti* carrier were native to West Africa, and, like smallpox, they made their way to the Americas via slave ships.[24] Fear of yellow fever prompted passage of new, tougher quarantine laws and creation of offshore detention centers for ailing crew, passengers, and slaves.

During the 1743 yellow fever epidemic that claimed an estimated 5 percent of New York City's population,[25] an immigrant physician from Scotland began to see the light. Dr. Cadwallader Colden recognized a crucial connection between homes located around filthy standing water and higher incidences of disease, surmising that poor water supplies, inadequate diet among the city's poor children, and general filth caused yellow fever. In a series of striking essays,[26]

Colden drew the old miasma theory of disease toward a new concept—what would eventually be dubbed sanitarianism. With some subsequent refinements, sanitarianism would become the key framework for all American public health activities for more than 150 years.

In practical terms, Colden's yellow fever theory translated into a call for clean water and improved sanitation in New York. Both were tough goals for a city that, remarkably, lacked any source of fresh water save that drawn from wells, and had long failed to enforce its garbage and waste regulations. Physicians generally ignored Colden's "notions," as they were dubbed, as well as those of other medical thinkers of the day.

Desperate to control the economically devastating scourges of smallpox and, in particular, yellow fever, the New York State Legislature in 1796 passed the nation's first comprehensive public health law. It created the office of a State Commissioner of Health, a New York City Health Office, pest houses for isolation of infected citizens, vigorous maritime quarantine regulations, and a system of fines for failure to comply with quarantine and sanitation ordinances.[27]

Yellow fever fear inspired a wave of similar organized public health activity elsewhere in the United States. In 1798 Congress ordered the creation of the United States Marine Health Service, conceived of as an agency that would monitor sailors and protect American ports from incoming disease. Two years later the nation's capitol was built upon a large swamp located between the strategic states of Maryland and Virginia. Immediately overrun by yellow fever, smallpox, viral encephalitis, and a host of other diseases, Washington, D.C., constituted a public health disaster from the moment of its conception. In 1802 the District of Columbia enacted a series of public health ordinances modeled after those in New York.

In 1805, facing yet another summer yellow fever onslaught, New York City created the nation's first Board of Health. Armed with a budget of the then-considerable sum of $8,500 and authority to do whatever it deemed necessary to stop yellow fever, the board set out to sanitize the city. The board worked in tandem with John Pintard, the country's first city inspector.

Both Pintard and the Board of Health were strongly supported by New York's powerful commerce class in 1805. But as the city's efforts paid off, and yellow fever diminished, the popularity of public health measures ebbed. By 1819 the Board of Health's budget had fallen to a mere $500, and the business community was lobbying for its elimination.

The clash between New York's wealthiest men of commerce and its civic authorities over public health was a classic conflict between pursuit of short-term profit and prevention of often longer-term threats to the populace. Men of commerce, most of whom depended directly or indirectly on foreign trade and shipping, recognized the need for strict health measures during epidemics, even where such steps as quarantines impeded their business operations. But in the absence of crisis the economic impacts of such activities far outweighed any perceived health benefits, and opposition arose from the commercial sector.

This theme—of tension between business and health sectors—would repeat itself so frequently in coming decades in America as to constitute a primary motif of the nation's struggle for population health.

By 1819 commercial sector pressure brought New York's Board of Health to its knees, curtailing not only its activities but even its meetings. And, predictably, the city suffered another yellow fever epidemic in 1822. By 1835 the power of the Democratic Party organization called Tammany Hall—a corrupt political machine that would manipulate New York and national politics for more than a century—was virtually synonymous with entrepreneurial interests in the city. Tammany seized control of the board, stacked it with cronies, and corruption set in.

In 1850 New York City death rates (driven predominantly by infectious diseases) would be a full 10 percent higher than those estimated for 1750.[28] Clearly, the public's health was failing. This was not progress.

Ironically, New York City's health laws and its Board of Health became models for the nation. If Tammany corruption rendered those laws unenforced in New York, and staffed Gotham's Board of Health with fools and cronies, the structures were still sound ideas. So much so that, propelled by the fear of yellow fever and cholera, cities all over America adopted New York's Board of Health laws: Washington, D.C., Boston, Chicago, New Orleans, and dozens of other cities all created boards of health between 1810 and 1840 that were nearly identical in structure and intent to that originally designed in New York City in 1805.

On the East Coast, the combination of waves of impoverished immigrants (primarily from Ireland)[29] and overall urban disorder was driving the public's health downward. Epidemics swept over the cities regularly, claiming huge tolls among the poor.[30] None of America's densely packed cities had appropriate infrastructures: safe water, decent housing, paved streets, sewer systems, ample safe (not rotten) food, and public health control of contagion. In 1850 the average U.S. male life expectancy was thirty-six years, female was thirty-eight years. Huge epidemics were part of the problem: in 1853, for example, 11,000 residents of New Orleans died in just two months of cholera. But the real factors holding down life expectancy were huge maternal and child mortality rates.

In 1857, twenty-four out of every fifty-four pregnancies in the United States resulted in postpartum puerperal fever, an infection physicians and midwives did not then understand. As a result of puerperal fever, nineteen of every fifty-four pregnancies proved lethal to the mother.[31] Given that most women at that time gave birth to more than six children, the risk of premature death over the course of their reproductive lives was enormous.

Child mortality was also astronomical. In 1850 children growing up in large American cities had about fifty-fifty odds of reaching the age of five years without succumbing to disease or malnutrition. Odds were even worse—three to one against them—for children of the poorest urbanites: immigrants and African-Americans.

What was missing from American urban society—but would soon appear—was a middle class. Prior to the Civil War, most of the country's cities were largely populated by the working poor, entrepreneurial poor, and desperately poor. A small, elite group of urbanites possessed enormous wealth and employed large numbers of servants. They and the poor lived parallel but rarely intersecting lives.

In the absence of a strong, civically invested middle class, the cities became centers of political corruption. And the public's health worsened.

This theme of public health—the need for support from a sizeable middle class—would resonate throughout the future history of America. In the absence of a middle class, the rich simply lived separate and unequal lives, maintaining spacious homes along clean, tree-lined boulevards and raising their families through private systems of health, education, and cultural training. That a city might starve, politically and economically, in the absence of the elite's interest and finances seemed of little but occasional Christian concern to them. And the poor lacked the education, money, and skills to choose and run an effective government.

American public health would improve in tandem with the rise of the urban middle class, which paid taxes, supported cleanliness and public education, recognized and abhorred corruption, and, as home owners, had an investment in their cities. This was the interest group that would put into practice public measures based on the notion that "cleanliness is next to Godliness." In 1820 such a social class was virtually nonexistent; by 1850, pockets of middle-class professionals and small businessmen were surfacing in most American eastern cities. And following the Civil War, the middle class would steadily expand in America, becoming by the mid-twentieth century the dominant force in municipal and regional political life.[32]

In 1842 two crucial documents were published that compelled urban leaders and physicians to consider health in the light of the social, particularly class, context of industrialization. In London, Dr. Edwin Chadwick published *Report on the Sanitary Condition of the Labouring Population of Great Britain*, a remarkable survey of that country's living standards right down to the numbers of people using any one privy and the odor of particular London neighborhoods.[33] Chadwick would, under twentieth-century labeling, be considered an epidemiologist and perhaps a demographer, and very good ones at that. But his contribution went well beyond dry, statistical accounts of English filth, poverty, and pestilence. Chadwick correlated the three.

Chadwick called for organized public health, and he defined its mission as one of sanitary cleanup. An old-fashioned miasma thinker, Chadwick believed that if one lived amid filth, disease would be one's constant companion. Thus, the way to rid England of pestilence and premature deaths was to give her a good scrubbing. It was in the 1840s an astonishingly revolutionary insight.

Chadwick's counterpart in the United States was New Yorker John Griscom, who published *The Sanitary Conditions of the Laboring Populace of New York* in 1842 and his battle cry, *Sanitary Reform*, in 1844.[34] Griscom's goal was slightly less ambitious than Chadwick's: he didn't hope to scrub clean an entire nation, just New York City.

By the 1840s New York and most other large American cities were horribly crowded, disgustingly dirty affairs. Horse manure formed a thick, redolent layer over all of the streets, dead animals were usually left for days wherever they fell, tenement garbage was piled high in every vacant space, and everyone, save the rich, had to walk through this filth daily.

By 1845 Griscom had followers in the form of a loosely organized civic group known as the sanitarians that advocated New York cleanliness. Their call soon spread all over the United States, with the ranks of sanitarians swelling swiftly to include Christian leaders, civic activists, politicians, some doctors, and the growing middle classes. Their target was filth, which generally was seen to be associated with immigrants. Like England's Chadwick, the American sanitarians weren't particularly interested in raising the standard of living of urban workers. In fact, many nativist[35] sanitarians blamed the poor for their own poverty; they labeled slum and tenement residents lazy, idle, and immoral.[36]

The early sanitarians in America were also reluctant to rely on government to fulfill their dreams of hygiene. Most Americans in the 1840s were staunchly antigovernment, as well as anti-intellectual.

Doctors themselves were hardly a sophisticated lot anywhere in America during the first four decades of the nineteenth century. The oldest American medical school, established by Benjamin Franklin in Philadelphia in 1765, graduated only a handful of doctors every year, and most American "physicians" hadn't undergone any training at all. In 1780, for example, there were about four thousand doctors practicing medicine in New York City, only four hundred of whom had ever obtained a medical degree.[37] Though medical schools had been established in New York and Boston before the American Revolution—institutions that would eventually be known as Columbia University College of Physicians and Surgeons and Harvard Medical School—few practitioners ever availed themselves of such academic training.[38] And, as the typical sojourn in medical school lasted a mere nine months, with the bulk of that time spent studying Latin and philosophy, even those who did have training were ill-prepared for handling epidemics. In 1869, the president of Harvard University would denounce his school's medical training as "not much better than a diploma mill."

It was widely believed in the early nineteenth century that the best physicians were French.[39] U.S. medical men tended to ignore European advances in their profession for years: the Semmelweis technique[40] of sterilizing the hands by thorough washing before touching patients was developed in 1840, but was not practiced in the U.S. until well into the 1890s. Neither did they jump on two other crucial European developments for decades. In 1848 they paid little heed when the British parliament passed the Public Health Act. This legislation compelled every city and town in the United Kingdom to construct water systems, sewers and proper drainage, and pave primary thoroughfares: a feat accomplished in just over twenty years.

American health leaders also failed to take note of Dr. John Snow's 1853 insight that by removing the pump handle (and thus the source of contaminated water) from the well in a London neighborhood with an especially high cholera rate, that neighborhood's cholera epidemic promptly slowed. Though Snow had no concept of the bacterial cause of cholera, he realized that filthy water carried the disease.

Despite the early sanitarians' best efforts, and perhaps in part because of antigovernment sentiment throughout America in the 1850s, truly awful epidemics continued and were just beginning to ignite action. In Providence, Rhode Island, Dr. Edwin Snow harangued the city government for months until, in 1850, he won passage of the nation's first compulsory vaccination law, mandating smallpox inoculation of school children. Many years and court challenges would pass before such laws would take hold elsewhere in the United States. And resistance to vaccination, despite its clear efficacy as a disease prevention strategy, would remain one of the themes of public health 150 years later.

Just as yellow fever had pushed the first public health measures in America, the terror of cholera was enormous, and it became the impetus for both change and inappropriate panic in the mid-nineteenth century. When rumors spread of cholera's arrival to a region, cities sought, and usually obtained, authority to forcibly detain the disease's victims in hospitals or pesthouses—facilities that functioned as little more than holding cells for ailing individuals, generally those from the poorest classes. Though such measures surely violated all concepts of personal liberty and usually proved lethal to the sufferers, quarantine enjoyed a fair amount of popular support, primarily because cholera was such a horrifying disease.

The sanitarians missed the message of John Snow's Broad Street pump.

Rather than accept the possibility that a contagious agent might lurk in unclean water, the sanitarians continued to insist that filth, in and of itself, was the cause of disease. Spurred by fear of cholera, however, their zeal for cleanup was boundless.

While civic leaders targeted hogs, dirt, and horse manure, more sophisticated notions of disease were percolating overseas: talk of Charles Darwin's *On the Origin of Species* was on everyone's lips. Rudolf Virchow in 1858 published *Die Cellularpathologie*, which drew from his extensive laboratory studies to demonstrate that human illness functioned at the cellular level. The following year in Paris, Dr. Claude Bernard published the first modern book of human physiology. And in 1862 Louis Pasteur had published in France his theory of the existence of "germs," which, he argued, were key to fermentation. But America was focused on the Civil War. By far the majority of the 535,000 deceased soldiers were victims of disease or the hideous health care practices that resulted in the amputation of most injured limbs and proved fatal to 62 percent of those with chest wounds and 87 percent with abdominal wounds.[41]

While public health improved in most other northeastern cities, save among soldiers, New York's stagnated. In New York City the war had heightened tensions between immigrants, African-Americans, nativists, and politicians. Under Tammany Hall's control both the city inspector's office and the Board of Health were inept, corrupt, and stacked with Tammany sycophants. In 1865, at war's end, Francis Boole was Tammany Hall's man in charge of the New York City Inspector's Office. In a matter of months Boole hired 928 public health "inspectors," all of them cronies who either did nothing for their wages or used their inspectorial authority to blackmail the owners of restaurants, bakeries, slaughterhouses, produce markets, and private hospitals. The Board of Health was similarly inept, corrupt, and controlled by Tammany.

In far off Minnesota, Dr. Charles Hewitt was fighting his own war on corruption. His targets were not, however, the likes of "Boss" Tweed and his Tammany thugs but the state's physicians. A native New Yorker, Hewitt knew what constituted quality medical care in the 1860s, and what most certainly did not. In 1858, shortly before it became a state, Hewitt set to work mapping the demography of the territory's population, health, and disease. In his travels he was astonished by what passed for medical care.

"There is so little fact and so much theory, that I am sometimes tempted to think a medical practice founded upon the honest experience of *one* practitioner of sterling common sense would be safer and more successful than a practice based on what is vauntingly called 'the united experience of centuries,' " Hewitt wrote in 1856.[42]

Convinced that many Minnesota physicians were unintentionally killing their patients with toxic tinctures, salves, and potions, and that the doctors were worsening public health catastrophes such as smallpox epidemics through inept handling of patients, Hewitt went on a professional rampage. In doing so he aroused the ire of most of the state's medical practitioners. Despite attempts by rival doctors to discredit him, Hewitt's words resonated with average Minnesotans who were sick to death of paying doctors for hocus-pocus, snake oil, and Christian homilies. Hewitt used his popularity to pressure the state's political leaders into creating a Board of Health and a rudimentary vital statistics system that tracked Minnesotans' births, deaths, and diseases.

Hewitt became Minnesota's first secretary of the State Board of Health and began behaving like a government official, ordering hand cleansing among health care workers, smallpox vaccination statewide, and quarantines of the sick. He told the state's politicians that if they gave his office legal support the legislators could, in return, trust in him: he would stop epidemics and slow disease. It was a trust Hewitt would never betray, though the politicians would often fail to keep their side of the bargain.

In 1877 Hewitt began a disease detective tradition that some one hundred years later would be one of the state's true claims to fame.[43] Smallpox had broken out and, not satisfied merely to issue pamphlets calling for immunization, Hewitt set out to find the source of the outbreak—the index case. In so doing, Hewitt demonstrated that well before the issue was settled in the East, he favored a contagion—rather than the sanitarian—theory of disease origin. While Hewitt certainly supported clean cities, such filth could hardly explain the spread of smallpox in his sparsely populated, largely rural state. No, Hewitt reasoned, smallpox was caused by *something* that was spread from person to person.

Though he didn't know what, exactly, that "something" was, he felt certain that only the existence of a communicable, deadly entity of some sort could explain why quarantine could effectively slow epidemics. Hewitt soon spotted a connection between the first 1877 case of smallpox in Minnesota and a recently constructed train line that connected St. Paul to neighboring Wisconsin. The first case in the state, he discovered, was a woman who caught the disease in Wisconsin, boarded the St. Paul and Sioux Railroad, and traveled to Mankato, Minnesota. She unwittingly spread the illness to fellow passengers on the train who, in turn, took smallpox to towns all over the state. At all train stations that were at the state's borders, Hewitt established checkpoints where physicians examined passengers and crew for signs of smallpox. He stopped the epidemic in a matter of days, leaving only seven dead Minnesotans in its wake. It was, by 1877 standards, a spectacular feat.

Hewitt used that smallpox victory to once again castigate the physicians, telling them it was high time they accepted his contagion theory of disease and commence some local detective work when measles, scarlet fever, or other microbial scourges surfaced among their clientele. In the post–Civil War nineteenth century, however, physicians—like Tammany Hall—typically held public health in open disdain, seeing it as little more than a combination of meddlesome government and sanitarian scrubbers. Hewitt had already alienated scores of doctors by exposing their medicinal frauds. Now he dared demand that they accept his belief system, seeing diseases as ailments caused by as-yet-undiscovered, mysterious, contagious elements, the spread of which was preventable. In Minnesota, and all across America, doctors balked at the notion. They felt their autonomous powers over patients were threatened. And they resisted the population-based activities of Hewitt and his compatriots. The healers, it seemed, opposed the would-be preventers of disease.[44]

Friction between healers and preventers, between would-be curers and sanitarian scrubbers, and, eventually, between independent doctors and government regulators would form another lasting theme of American public health. A century and a half later this tension would limit Dr. Margaret Hamburg's ability to control antibiotic-resistant diseases in New York, as she would be powerless to change physicians' prescription practices. In the 1860s Hewitt ran Minnesota public health services but was at odds with organized medicine. All over America men like Hewitt would for decades do battle with the American Medical Association and individual physicians.

The severity of such tension would vary across the nation because American public health grew up in a manner entirely different from its counterpart in Europe. There, public health policies were promulgated from the top down, birthed as an essentially federal (or royal) function: American public health, in a manner characteristic of its fervor for democracy, arose from the local level, and no two cities or states had precisely the same policies. In some regions, medical systems grew along with those of public health; in most, they followed separate, often oppositional, courses. Not only was there no genuine federal leadership in public health in nineteenth-century America, few states had laws and policies that extended to all of their counties and cities. In New York and Massachusetts, for example, New York City and Boston were the tails that wagged their state health dogs.

On the East Coast the large cities were getting still bigger and more crowded, so their public health needs revolved around essential urban services, such as sewers and paved roads. Out on the prairie, men like Hewitt were focused on quarantines and epidemic control. And in the far West health wasn't even on the political agenda. The climate was benign, Anglos were, generally, far healthier than they would be in the cities of the East, and nearly the *only* thing on the western agenda was land and the mad scramble to bump Indians and Spanish descendants off it, in favor of Anglo, or Yankee, control. By 1865, at the end of the distant Civil War, the destitute *Californios* were huddled into the state's first ghettos, located in neighborhoods of Los Angeles such as Chavez Ravine.[45]

Bad as these barrios were, they paled in public health significance when compared to the new ghettos of the East's cities. Waves of impoverished immigrants were flooding into New York, in particular, only to be warehoused in such states of squalor as would be unimaginable a century later. Indeed, the quality of drinking water, sewer conditions, the safety of local produce, and housing all worsened considerably for New York workers by 1866, compared to those in 1776. Any disease adapted for spread via human waste and contaminated water would find the ecology of 1866 Gotham spectacularly favorable. That year, fed-up citizens bypassed Tammany and created a new Metropolitan Board of Health. Spurring its creation was word of an enormous, terribly virulent cholera epidemic in Paris.

Having spotted cholera from Europe aboard a ship in New York City's harbor, the new board—ardent sanitarians all—ordered immediate cleaning of every street and sewer in Manhattan and Brooklyn, among other measures. Crucially, board member Dr. Elisha Harris made the bold contagionist assertion that cholera infected people as a result of contact with water that was contaminated with fecal matter from other cholera victims. He knew, of course, of John Snow's Broad Street pump experiment in London, but Harris went a critical step further, mixing the Snow observation with Semmelweis's handwashing insights.

Harris told New Yorkers to wash their darned hands with soap and clean water.

By summer's end, though cholera had ravaged Paris and London and would wreak havoc throughout the United States, New York came away with few deaths.[46]

Despite such successes, Tammany-controlled judges and attorneys plagued the Board of Health for decades with lawsuits and injunctions, blocking as many quarantines and other actions as possible. The goal was to eliminate board enforcement of violations committed by Tammany-allied businesses or by Irish owners of tenement buildings. To gain public support for their obviously self-interested efforts, the Tammany machine rallied Irish tenement residents, telling them—falsely, of course—that the rules and regulations were being used prejudicially against their neighborhoods and that quarantines bypassed "niggers"—the Irish immigrants' key enemies—in favor of targeting those who had recently arrived from Erin.

A similar tension between immigrants and blossoming public health departments surfaced in other American cities as the flow of poor European transplants hastened west. It was to highlight another perennial theme of public health, one that would haunt America well into the twenty-first century: tension between the health concerns of native-born Americans and the fears and suspicions of recent immigrants.

In the mid-nineteenth century the U.S.-born population often saw immigrants as little more than sources of disease and filth, readily blaming them for all epidemics and, indeed, supporting sanitarian interventions that prejudicially targeted the newly arrived poor. Even when prejudice was not behind health department actions, political leaders could readily tap immigrant apprehensions, guiding the newly arrived Americans to see discrimination where it did not exist. Throughout the nineteenth century public health leaders tended, on balance, to side with the needs and biases of the native-born population. During the twentieth century the imbalance would persist, prompting federal officials to, for example, designate Haitian immigrants a "risk group for AIDS." And the same public health agencies would underplay issues that did preferentially afflict immigrants, such as the impact of pesticides on the health of Mexican farm workers, the remarkably high infant mortality rates seen in Latinos living in Los Angeles, and a plague outbreak among Chinese immigrants in San Francisco. Throughout the twentieth century, public health leaders would, with considerable difficulty, walk a fine line between the exigencies and suspicions of the immigrant communities and those of the native born.

II

It is in health that cities grow: in sunshine that their monuments are builded. It is in disease that they are wrecked; in pestilence that effort ceases and hope dies.

—Annual Report of the Commissioner of Health, Milwaukee, 1911

In retrospect, the turn of the century now seems to have been a golden age for public health, when its achievements followed one another in dizzying succession and its future possibilities seemed limitless.

—Paul Starr[47]

The revolution was about to begin. Genuine public health was gestating and soon would be birthed by the likes of Minnesota's Hewitt and New York City's Hermann Biggs. The profundity of Biggs's insights, in particular, would prove so deep and powerful that a century later they would guide New York City leaders through the horror of an epidemic of drug-resistant tuberculosis.

The ideas were sparked in far-off Europe, but it was in America's atmosphere of middle-class democracy that genuine systems of population protection would be spawned.

In Europe during the late nineteenth century a great intellectual revolution was under way that would make disease definable and, with that, relegated to the status of problems humanity might solve.

The great debates of the past—spontaneous generation, miasma theory, sanitarianism versus contagion—would be resolved, or would take on new tones, as Science stepped into the picture. And if public health would suffer from any intellectual sins amid the pell-mell delineation of disease information they would be arrogance and hubris.

On the eve of this great revolution, however, a host of essentially nonscientific measures had, by the 1880s, already vastly improved the public's health. Sewer and privy construction, improved drinking water quality, quarantine policies, street cleaning, enforcement of safer food, meat and milk production standards, paved roads—each of these measures had had its impact. In addition, railroad and teamster transport networks developed in post–Civil War America radically improved people's diets as fresh crops made their way into urban centers in bulk and at prices most working families could afford. While many children still lacked protein-rich and adequately varied diets, there was no doubt that fewer of them were nutrient deficient and malnourished in 1875 than had been so two decades earlier. In addition, many cities—notably New York and Boston—set up distribution stations that doled out fresh milk to poor children. That alone had a profound impact on the strength and stature of urban youngsters.

Though housing in urban areas remained atrocious for many of America's poor, sanitarians were doing their utmost to improve the squalor surrounding tenements and slums.

Death rates from yellow fever, smallpox, and cholera, three chiefly adult diseases, fell as swamps were drained, window glass installed, sewers built, vaccination improved, and, perhaps, because nutrition was enhanced.[48] The impact of such measures was limited, however, before the advent of vaccines, and great sweeping plagues, like the 1878 yellow fever epidemic that killed at least twenty thousand people in the Mississippi Valley,[49] were yet to come.

Also still to come were ebbs and flows in the great scourges of childhood: measles, whooping cough, diphtheria, typhoid fever, and scarlet fever, each of which would, just forty years later, claim comparatively minor numbers of American lives.

With the devastating yellow fever epidemics at center stage in the 1870s, and the then-slow pace at which information traveled, it was initially hard for U.S. sanitarians and health leaders to take note of the staggering scientific advances that were occurring across the Atlantic. Further, the sanitarians, among whom Christian moralists predominated, were slow to note advances in science. But advances there were indeed.

Antiseptics were discovered in 1870 by England's Dr. Joseph Lister, who found that by pouring carbolic acid on a wound or a suture site, infection would never take hold there. Beginning in 1876 Drs. Robert Koch in Berlin and Louis Pasteur in Paris were racing to identify the individual germs that caused disease.[50]

In 1880 Pasteur published his landmark *Germ Theory of Disease*, in which he argued that all contagious diseases were caused by microscopic organisms that damaged the human victim at the cellular level—as Rudolf Virchow had argued—and spread from person to person.

In Berlin, Paul Erlich went a step further, discovering that animals that survived an infection had substances in their blood that could successfully fight off the disease in other affected animals. He called the agents of ailment toxins and his newly discovered substances antitoxins. So enthusiastic was Erlich about the miraculous powers of antitoxins that he dubbed them "magic bullets."

At a dizzying pace between 1880 and 1889 the rival Berlin and Paris laboratories discovered the bacteria responsible for tuberculosis,[51] cholera, and diphtheria. They developed a vaccine against rabies. And they named the mosquito responsible for spreading yellow fever.

Among the most progressive public health leaders in America it was understood that if the identity of each great microbial killer was established, diagnostic tests, vaccines, and cures couldn't be far behind. Suddenly there was a rationale for vaccination, which they had long urged but never could explain to skeptics.

Even more profound was the shift in perspective from outward, mysterious miasmic origins of disease to microscopic. In Minnesota Hewitt lobbied the state legislature in 1888, raising funds for purchase of the region's first microscope. Similarly, New York City's health leaders realized that the age of laboratory-informed decision making had arrived and constructed the nation's first public health laboratory.

To really grasp the revolution then under way, however, men like Hewitt and his New York counterparts sailed off to Europe to sit at the feet of the great Koch and Pasteur.

All over America there were individuals inside local health departments who wholeheartedly embraced Pasteur's germ theory of disease, reveled in the newfound possibilities of their laboratories, and, practically overnight, changed the methods, strategies, and tactics of government public health. Past measures of disease prevention and epidemic control may have been effective—at least in some cases—but they lacked scientific explanation. Without a clear rationale for draining swamps or vaccinating children, health advocates had little choice but to await an epidemic and, capitalizing on the public's hysteria, twist the arms of politicians and men of commerce in order to obtain the desired laws and funds.

The germ theory changed that. While funding would continue to ebb and flow with the tide of politics and the level of public concern about contagion, support for prevention efforts became more sustainable. Advocates could now use their new laboratories to provide scientific evidence of a specific contamination or infection. In addition, they could prove to skeptics that a particular intervention was, indeed, responsible for lowering germ levels in the social milieu where it had been applied.

In short, public health suddenly had an empirical basis that rested upon demonstrable facts.

Nowhere was the impact of germ theory more powerfully felt than in New York City, which, in a few short years, would metamorphose from one of America's sorriest, most cesspoollike excuses for a metropolis into the world's paragon of government action on behalf of the public's health. Chief among the architects of this change were Drs. T. Mitchell Prudden and Hermann Biggs, both of them firm adherents to the germ theory of disease.

Biggs and Prudden had been appointed to the city's new bacteriology laboratory in 1885 by none other than President Grover Cleveland. The nation's leaders feared that escalating waves of "filthy, dirty foreigners" arriving daily in New York harbor would import further epidemics. As most immigrants passed through New York harbor, President Cleveland reasoned that he ought to place a pair of top scientists inside that city's laboratory.

Theophil Mitchell Prudden was, at the time of his federal appointment in 1885, a thirty-six-year-old graduate of Yale Medical School. The son of an immensely wealthy New York family, Prudden was one of the rare members of his social class who dedicated his life to science. Educated at the best of America's schools, Prudden was well-versed in Europe's bumper crop of scientific discovery and imbued with a youthful zeal over Pasteur's germ theory. During the early 1880s he studied in the best laboratories of Germany and Austria and even toiled beside the great Robert Koch.

Hermann Michael Biggs was ten years Prudden's junior but already an awesome presence on New York's medical landscape. A native of that city, Biggs had trained for medicine at Bellevue Hospital. Though his scholastic experience paled in comparison to that of Prudden, his uncanny political skills more than compensated. More than any other individual in America in his day, Biggs understood the intimate relationship between politics and public health and could successfully maneuver around corruption, complacency, and cronyism. In less than twenty years, backed by the power of the germ theory, Biggs would move public health from near the bottom of New York's ladder of political clout and public esteem to the top.

Although the nation's first bacteriology laboratories were actually established elsewhere (in Laurence, Massachusetts; Ann Arbor, Michigan; and Providence, Rhode Island), it would be the New York City bacteriologists who would reshape both their usefulness and their authority. Prudden would prove to be the intellectual giant, Biggs the street-savvy political force.[52]

In 1888 the city's Board of Health named Biggs and Prudden "consulting pathologists," appointing them as city employees. The pair immediately set to work to formulate, and back up, public health measures based on laboratory science.

In swift order the duo dispensed with tubercular cow's milk, built up both the size and clout of their laboratory, and began confronting the child killer diphtheria. They invented a screening test for cholera—the first that could identify human carriers of the deadly bacteria. And when the disease arose in Hamburg in 1892[53] and spread across Europe with terrifying ferocity, claiming upward of three thousand lives a day, Biggs and Prudden used their test and powers of quarantine to identify the first carriers that arrived in New York that summer on ships from Europe. The handful that escaped their grasp were tracked down by an army of health department staff and volunteers who hunted through every housing unit in search of diarrhea victims and filled privies and toilets with disinfectants.

Thanks to these actions, in 1892 only nine people died of cholera in New York City, while tens of thousands perished from Vladivostock to Lisbon to London.

It was a phenomenally successful demonstration of the strength and dynamism of germ theory-based public action. The forces of sanitarianism worked in tandem with the laboratory-based scientific efforts of Biggs and Prudden. The impeccably dressed Dr. Biggs, in particular, became an overnight sensation and, at barely thirty years of age, the hero of New York.

The Gay Nineties, as the 1890s were called, were times of social change that benefited public health. Some such changes arose from a growing civic pride—parks, paved roads, public transit. Some were the result of mass activism on behalf of labor and the poor. The antitenement movement focused scrutiny on the lives of slum dwellers, lives made unbearably grim by the appalling conditions of their crowded, pestilent, unmaintained dwellings, workplaces, and schools. In addition, union agitators, anarchists, socialists, and Communists were all gaining strong followings. Social movements were arising across the industrialized Northeast and Midwest. Even in the Pacific states of the far West, socialists and anarchists were finding favor among poorly paid laborers.

Chief among the demands shared by all these geographically and ideolog-ically disparate movements were the calls for greater occupational safety and improved housing.

The most influential social activist of the day was Danish-born photogra-pher and writer Jacob August Riis. In 1890 Riis published his masterpiece of text and photographs, *How the Other Half Lives*. It gave his appalled readers both a visual image of tenement hellholes and a vivid description of their odors, sounds, and claustrophobia. In the worst of them, located on what was called "Lung Block," could be found the city's densest concentrations of infant mortality, tuberculosis, and pneumonia.[54] Lung Block was inhabited by four thousand peo-ple, ten-fold more than lived on any average New York block. Crammed five or six to the room, its inhabitants witnessed 265 cases of tuberculosis during the 1880s for a case rate of 6.6 per 1,000 people—possibly the highest in the world at that time. Riis estimated that there were 1.5 million people living in such New York City tenements in 1890, or about 60 percent of the population of metro-politan New York.[55]

On an entirely different front, a variety of organizations were demanding improvement in the lots of women and children—the right to vote, to birth control, to abortion. Margaret Sanger, for example, published and distributed pamphlets on birth control, decrying the extraordinary death toll among women who, despite the continuing risks of puerperal fever and other pregnancy-associated ailments, were expected to give birth to six or more children.[56]

All of this social unrest and discontent would grow, further polarizing ur-ban America over coming decades. For the expanding middle classes and the old, native-born elite of eastern cities, these movements were cause for consid-erable consternation and evoked two key responses: anti-immigrant sentiments and capitulation to nominal reform sparked by fear of all-out social unrest and disease contagion. These responses would continue to cast a shadow on the public's health into the twenty-first century.

For the middle class had embraced to an extreme the idea of a germ theory of disease, becoming germ-phobic. While the wealthiest urbanites may have abhorred germs, they could avoid the riffraff or escape to distant estates. The middle class, however, felt trapped. For them, everything from public library books to dust could harbor lethal germs. Germicide sales boomed, as did the installation of indoor plumbing, flush toilets, and modern kitchens that included iceboxes to keep food fresh.[57]

This germ phobia and resolute commitment to stomping out the bugs ultimately fueled support for grand public health schemes. Because the middle and upper classes were convinced that the poor—particularly immigrants—were the source of all truly terrible microbial scourges, they were willing to pay the price in higher taxes for *biological*, as opposed to *class*, warfare. The sanitarians supported provision of some health hygienic services to the working people in America's cities. By 1890 in New York City, for example, nearly a quarter of all health care was provided free by tax-supported municipal dispensaries, and in 1887 the Board of Aldermen had agreed to spend funds to install toilets in all of the city's public schools. But the sanitarians also imposed a moralistic judgmentalism that openly expressed disdain for the religious, family, and cultural lives of the poor.

Harper's Weekly put the matter of class tensions starkly in 1881 with a cartoon depicting a conversation between the goddess Hygeia and a top-hatted man of wealth. Pointing to streets of filth and poverty, Hygeia berated the man, saying, "You doubtless think that as all this filth is lying out in the back streets, it is of no concern of yours. But you are mistaken. You will see it stealing into your house very soon, if you don't take care."[58] By 1890 the message was hitting home. The public health revolution began.

Projects of enormous scale, particularly water and sewer works, that would profoundly improve communities' health, were undertaken at the behest of the wealthy and middle classes.[59]

With so many social forces swirling about his public health world in Gotham, Biggs and his colleagues set the immodest goals of completely eliminating diphtheria and tuberculosis. Though Biggs declared a "War on Consumption" in 1893, he first set his sights upon diphtheria and, like Minnesota's Hewitt, made the journey to Europe to learn from the masters of microbiology. The New Yorker settled into the laboratory of Louis Pasteur, working beside Émile Roux.

Upon his return to New York in 1894, Biggs immediately set to work with his staff building a diphtheria antitoxin production facility and lobbying for funds. The Hospital for Sick Children in Paris had just begun using diphtheria antitoxin with remarkable results—an immediate 50 percent reduction in pediatric death rates. Seizing upon that evidence, Biggs did something almost unheard of in 1894: he held a press conference. And for weeks he systematically and deftly maneuvered several of New York's many newspapers into supporting his diphtheria antitoxin laboratory. By early 1895 Biggs's charitably funded laboratory was the world's largest diphtheria antitoxin producer and was also mass-manufacturing smallpox and anthrax vaccines and a host of other "magic bullets."

Soon, distraught immigrant mothers from the tenements were turning up in dispensaries demanding "magic bullets" for their ailing children. And diphtheria death rates in New York City plummeted, going from an 1875 high of 296 per 100,000 people to 105 per 100,000 in 1895 to 66 per 100,000 five years later.

By 1912 New York's diphtheria death rate would have fallen to just 2.2 per 100,000 residents per year.[60] Soon every city in America was buying antitoxin from the Biggs laboratory.

With such diphtheria success at his back, Biggs set full sail into the seas of tuberculosis, which was then overwhelming New York's tenements. In an 1897 speech before the British Medical Association[61] Biggs enumerated his War on Consumption strategies, tactics, and biases and received worldwide press attention for delivering the first clearly delineated strategy for attacking the disease. Many of his comments, delivered before a hall full of openly skeptical physicians, became the often-quoted battle cries of TB fighters worldwide and would remain so a century later. Then just thirty-six years old, Hermann Biggs was already the undisputed leader of the new public health movement:

> The government of the United States is democratic, but the sanitary mea-
> sures adopted are sometimes autocratic, and the functions performed by
> sanitary authorities paternal in character. We are prepared, when neces-
> sary, to introduce and enforce, and the people are ready to accept, mea-
> sures which might seem radical and arbitrary, if they were not plainly
> designed for the public good, and evidently beneficent in their effects. Even
> among the most ignorant of our foreign-born population, few or no indi-
> cations of resentment are exhibited to the exercise of arbitrary powers in
> sanitary matters. The public press will approve, the people will support,
> and the courts sustain, any intelligent procedures which are evidently di-
> rected to preservation of the public health.
>
> The most autocratic powers, capable of the broadest construction,
> are given to them under the law. Everything which is detrimental to health
> or dangerous to life, under the freest interpretation, is regarded as coming
> within the province of the Health Department. So broad is the construction
> of the law that everything which improperly or unnecessarily interferes
> with the comfort or enjoyment of life, as well as those things which are,
> strictly speaking, detrimental to health or dangerous to life, may become
> the subject of action on the part of the Board of Health.

It was a declaration of war, not just against tuberculosis but against any group or individual who stood in the way of Public Health or the sanitarians' Hygeia.

But while easterner Biggs was exercising his "autocratic powers" on behalf of public health, residents of the far western states were sneering at, or ignoring, Hygeia. In Los Angeles County, poor J. L. Pomeroy, first to hold the title of health officer, tried hard to impress upon the leaders of his county's many towns that "it must be clearly recognized that diseases recognize no boundary lines, and that the health and social problems of the rural areas . . . are closely associated with those of urban areas."[62] Pomeroy (a practical, though uninspiring physician) conducted health surveys in 1915 that indicated that his county's equivalent of New York's tenement population was its nonwhite population. Among the Mexicans and Mexican-Americans, for example, infant death rates routinely exceeded 200 per 1,000 births (compared to 80 for whites), and in 1916 would top 285 per 1,000—that is, nearly one-third of their babies perished in infancy.

From its quite late inception in 1915,[63] organized public health in Los Angeles was more a county than a city function, and, also from the beginning, took on the role not of Biggs's antidisease crusades but of a service provider. Rather than ruffle feathers with great Biggs-style campaigns, Pomeroy's county team concentrated on racing to give the ever-burgeoning towns and cities of Los Angeles the basics: food and water inspection, vaccines, and medical care. It made sense at the time, as the basics were desperately needed and the epidemics that ravaged the East were less severe in the mild climate of the West. Besides, Pomeroy won little support from apathetic Angelenos for much else.[64]

The still-sparse population and favorable climate were Pomeroy's only allies, holding Los Angeles death rates well below those of most of the United States: 7.9 per 1,000 residents per year. In contrast to New York City[65] and similarly dense eastern metropolises, the majority of Los Angeles's annual deaths were among people over fifty years of age. Children under ten years of age accounted for just 14.5 percent of the total. Most of them succumbed to diphtheria, measles, or whooping cough—and to smallpox.

Pomeroy found that delivering vaccines often ran into a wall of resistance. The nation's strongest antivaccination movement arose in his county and consistently blocked all attempts to impose both compulsory immunization of schoolchildren and some uses of diphtheria antitoxin. Though more than two million people resided in Los Angeles County by the end of the Roaring Twenties, fewer than a hundred thousand took advantage of free vaccination programs; most of the population actively opposed immunization.

Antivaccine organizations sprouted up all over California during the early twentieth century, driven by Christian Scientists,[66] opponents of the germ theory of disease, and groups generally opposed to government interference in personal affairs. As a result, smallpox rates rose steadily at a time when most of the country saw the disease disappear.

Elsewhere in America, vaccine opposition hit its peak in the 1890s, but in the far West it was still an effective obstacle to public health in the 1930s. Despite a 1905 Supreme Court ruling that the rights of individuals to opt for or against a medical procedure were far outweighed by the powerful need to protect the community as a whole,[67] as each new vaccine was developed and health authorities pushed to add it to the list of compulsory child immunizations, a nationwide pattern of opposition was repeated. It surfaced, for example, when New

York City passed a compulsory diphtheria vaccination law in 1920, when typhoid fever immunizations were introduced during the same period, following initial rounds of polio immunization in the early 1950s, and later with measles, rubella, whooping cough, chicken pox, and hepatitis vaccines.

As early as 1905, then, another critical and lasting theme of public health was emerging, largely from the far West: the needs of the community versus the rights of individuals. In the twentieth century, public health leaders and courts would tend to interpret—and reinterpret—appropriate balances between those often opposing needs, usually falling into positions that reflected the cultural and political moods of the nation at that time. Because during the early part of the century, bacteriology-based public health was perceived as extraordinarily powerful and the background of disease was obviously grim and urgent, both public health leaders and the courts tended to tip the balance far in the direction of community needs. By the end of the twentieth century, the scales would have swung to the opposite extreme, favoring individual rights.

Between 1901 and 1930 New York City officials routinely deployed police officers and zealous nurses or physicians to the homes of those suspected of carrying disease, and force, or the threat thereof, was commonly used to overcome vaccine refusers. In some cases, police officers pinned the arm of those who refused while a city nurse jabbed it with a vaccination needle.

Biggs often spoke of the "absolute preventability" of disease, proudly noting that nowhere else in the world had "sanitary authorities granted to them such extraordinary and even arbitrary powers as rest in the hands of the Board of Health of New York City."[68] He used that power to search out TB sufferers and (forcibly if necessary) place them in sanitariums. He also used it to find and destroy contaminated food and drugs.[69] No hearing, no appeals. The payoff was in steadily declining death rates.[70]

The most notorious example of Biggs's willingness to push the legal and ethical envelope in order to protect the collective health of New Yorkers was the case of Irish immigrant cook Mary Mallon. In 1902 Germany's Koch proved that healthy people could, for years on end, be contagious carriers of *Salmonella typhi*, the bacterial cause of typhoid fever.[71] Biggs and an army of disease detectives sleuthed their ways through a series of typhoid illnesses and deaths, finding Mallon to be the common link, and a laboratory-proven carrier.[72] They incarcerated her on an island in New York's East River until she pledged to quit working as a professional cook, for that was fostering her spreading the disease. But after her release Mallon illegally returned to that profession under a pseudonym. When Biggs's staff tracked the belligerent and thoroughly uncooperative woman down, they exiled her to that island again, this time for the rest of her days. She would forever be remembered as Typhoid Mary.[73]

Moving westward, however, there was a gradient of discontent with such forceful public health measures, with Los Angelenos in extreme opposition. Remarkably, such adversity for public health came during a time of spectacular scientific and social success for the profession.

In 1900 the American Public Health Association began to professionalize the calling by giving advanced degrees. By the time the Panama Canal was finished in 1913, the U.S. military effort to drain that country's swamps had virtually eradicated malaria and yellow fever from the Canal Zone, and similar drainage campaigns were under way all over North and South America.

Their imaginations fired by the bacteriology revolution that was in full swing, U.S. philanthropists endowed other bold campaigns. John D. Rockefeller created a scientific foundation bearing his name that in 1906 declared war on hookworm.[74] Ten years later Rockefeller's foundation put up millions of dollars to create the Johns Hopkins School of Public Health in Baltimore. It opened just seven years after other philanthropists funded the creation of the Harvard School of Public Health.[75]

And a foundation set up by steel tycoon Andrew Carnegie aimed to improve the quality of education in the 160 medical schools of the time. Abraham Flexner, who was put in charge of the effort, in 1910 wrote arguably the single most influential indictment of medical education ever published in the English language.[76] The Flexner Report, as it was called, not only revealed in truly gruesome detail the abominations of medical training at the time, but recommended detailed steps for repair, with the ultimate goal of transforming American medical schools into rigorous centers of science.[77]

The primary benefit of this for public health care came from the far higher level of belief in germ theory and vaccinology among graduates of the improved medical schools. And hospitals were transformed from nineteenth-century warehouses that merely isolated the diseased from the community into genuine treatment centers.[78]

But as physician skills and hospital quality improved, medical costs rose. And with that came debate over what, if any, role government should play in the provision not only of essential public health services, but of medical treatment. New York City already had public hospitals, funded by tax dollars. Out west, Los Angeles County was well on its way toward being the *sole* provider of medical care in its region. But no state, and certainly not the U.S. Congress, had yet addressed the question of where responsibility for paying for medicine lay. Debates over government provision of universal health coverage began in 1912 and would continue—unresolved—into the twenty-first century.

Over time, the nexus of basic research science was shifting continents. In the 1820s France had led the Western world's race of medical discovery. By the 1840s, it was Germany that dominated medical sciences and, with the exception of the Pasteur laboratory, produced most of the key discoveries of the latter half of the nineteenth century. By 1910, however, the American output was, by far, dominant, with most of the discoveries emerging from laboratories in New York City.[79] By the First World War's end, U.S. science, which had escaped war on its own territory, was in a position of dominance and would, in most fields of research, remain there throughout the twentieth century.

Everything, it seemed, was working in favor of public health. The germ theory crusaders were at the zenith of both their power and respect in America. It seemed no disease could go unvanquished by the scythe of their science.

Until 1916. And polio.

The microbe responsible for polio would not be successfully isolated and grown in laboratories for more than forty years. Until then, it shared with smallpox, rabies, and yellow fever—like polio, all viral diseases—the dubious honor of being an infectious disease whose microbial agents could be indirectly demonstrated to exist but not seen or understood. Science, and with it public health, had hit a major roadblock.

It would be decades before experts would understand that it was the triumph of turn-of-the-century public health that caused polio: the microbe was ancient, but the disease was not. Before sanitarians set to work cleaning up the water, infants were exposed to minute, immunizing doses of the virus from the moment they were weaned. Disease-free water meant such childhood exposure to the polio virus was much rarer. The generation born after 1900 in cities like New York, Boston, Chicago, Paris, and London had little, if any, immunizing exposure to the microbe.

All it took to spark an epidemic, then, were a few days during which water supplies were inadequately filtered—a common occurrence during the hot summer months when bacterial growth and lower water levels increased the concentration of microbes.[80]

On June 6, 1916, New York City pediatricians reported the year's first cases of poliomyelitis—found among residents of the densely populated waterfront area. By month's end, cities all over the United States were witnessing their historically worst polio outbreaks. Recognizing that they were facing an enormous epidemic, the New York City Department of Health and the U.S. Surgeon General turned to a novel solution—publicity. They reached out to the nation's newspapers, civic organizations, and schools urging hygiene as the best defense against polio. On the eve of the Fourth of July holiday the Surgeon General declared that "a state of imminent peril to the Nation" existed.[81]

The public health leaders of America did everything they could imagine to try to control the child killer. In Gotham, teams of nurses, police at their sides, scoured the tenements. And all households containing a poliomyelitic child were placed under quarantine.

All over the city signs were nailed over entry doors:

INFANTILE PARALYSIS (POLIOMYELITIS)
Infantile paralysis is very prevalent in this part of the city.
On some streets many children are ill. This is one of those streets.
KEEP OFF THIS STREET

It would be decades before scientists would understand that quarantine had no value in epidemic polio control. A child's own parents, siblings, or friends might be dangerous sources of contagion. Only a vaccine could prevent polio and that innovation would be four decades more in coming.

Though polio seemed in retreat in 1917,[82] it would resurface with a vengeance. And polio was just the first of several new challenges between 1916 and 1919 that severely undermined the nation's admiration and belief in public health. Public health's germ theory–based zenith had been reached in less than twenty years, thanks to bold political maneuvers, strong science, and equally impressive strategic planning.

Now it would begin its downward spiral.

While American men were mired in the trenches of Europe fighting World War I, on the home front, temperance leagues, largely led by Christian women's groups, successfully pushed Congress to pass the Eighteenth Amendment to the U.S. Constitution. The new law prohibiting nationwide "the manufacture, sale, or transportation of intoxicating liquors" reflected widely publicized middle-class moral indignation over what was portrayed as an epidemic of drunken fathers and husbands—generally pictured as working-class.

Though the impetus for Prohibition was not public health, it was obvious that alcoholism was unhealthy, not only for the drinker but, potentially, for the entire family.

Popular evangelist Billy Sunday predicted a rosy future as a result of Prohibition: "The reign of tears is over. The slums will soon be a memory. We will turn our prisons into factories and our jails into storehouses and corncribs. Men will walk upright now, women will smile, and children will laugh. Hell will be forever rent."[83]

To the contrary, Prohibition spawned a public health catastrophe fueled by a massive crime network. Customer demand for alcohol never waned and in cities like New York, Prohibition actually increased both alcohol consumption and the use of narcotics. And while federal authorities chased trucks loaded with bathtub gin, physicians openly prescribed as alternative sources of recreational levity medicines rich in morphine, opium, laudanum, belladonna, absinthe, marijuana, and cocaine—all of which were sold and swapped in speakeasies.[84]

Nationwide, crime rates jumped 24 percent during the first year of Prohibition. Jails filled to 170 percent of capacity. Bribery and extortion of government officials swiftly became so commonplace as to barely raise eyebrows among news readers.[85]

In 1919 the New York City Department of Health sadly reported that there were at least a hundred thousand drug addicts in Gotham, users primarily of opium or cocaine. As the era swung into the Roaring Twenties, the numbers of alcoholics and drug addicts rose. Newly appointed Commissioner of Health Dr. Royal S. Copeland fought to place all matters related to drug addiction within his department and turned Riverside Hospital into an addiction treatment center. But the police, many of whom were addicted to Prohibition-related graft, fought Copeland. By 1920 his drug treatment funds were dried up and Riverside, having managed to rehabilitate less than 5 percent of its patients, was closed.[86]

Another continuing theme of public health had emerged: the battle pitting those who would medicalize drug and alcohol addiction against those who would criminalize it. Though in coming decades public health would witness an occasional victory, Americans would generally opt for law enforcement approaches to illicit drugs. After repeal of Prohibition in 1933, concern about alcoholism would rarely enjoy such a powerful spotlight again, but anxiety about illicit drugs would swell steadily throughout the century.[87]

Bad as America's new love for addictive substances was, the real disillusionment with public health was incited not by opiates and alcohol but by another virus: influenza. The swine flu pandemic began during the summer of 1918 in Kansas and circled the planet three times in eighteen months.[88] By early 1920 the virus would have claimed an estimated twenty to twenty-five million people worldwide.[89]

In November of 1918, every one of the 5,323 hospitals in the United States was overwhelmed; nearly all of their 612,251 beds were filled. On the eve of the pandemic in 1917, the national death rate due to influenza was 164.5 per 100,000 annually. It soared to a staggering 588.5 per 100,000 in 1918 and stayed high until 1921.[90]

So overwhelmed were public health authorities that virtually all of their other activities had to yield to influenza control. With quarantine out of the question—there simply were too many flu cases—health departments had little to offer. Otherwise helpless, they counted the numbers and raced about collecting bodies. Other forces stepped in to fill the vacuum: in the absence of a clear understanding of the influenza virus, every manner of crackpot and quack sold elixirs, masks, vapors, alcoholic tinctures, and hundreds of other items.

For health officials from New York to Los Angeles, the 1918–19 epidemic was another awful slap in the face of their otherwise triumphant achievements. Polio, drug and alcohol addiction, and influenza each highlighted crucial shortcomings of the sanitarians. There were, after all, limits to their power over the microbes and the social forces of disease.

In its 1920 annual report the New York City Department of Health struck an almost plaintive note that was in sharp contrast to Biggs's braggadocio of the previous decade:

> While a very few years ago, the slogans, "Safety First," and "Health First," had been popularized to a very considerable degree, one might term the present state of affairs in practically every civilized country as showing an attitude which may be characterized as indicating consent to permit a "Health Last" policy to govern. These observations are not irrelevant as a matter of stock-taking. This low ebb of interest in social welfare activities . . . is reflected in the progress of public health activities. The trend of times makes evident the need for sane, aggressive leadership, in such things that promote human welfare. . . .

The trust citizens had placed in their public health leaders seemed somehow unwarranted. Recent triumphs over diphtheria, yellow fever, and cholera were overshadowed in the collective memory by the apparent failures.

And it was becoming increasingly obvious that even the public health triumphs of the early twentieth century were not to be universal in either their implementation or impact. Pomeroy's Los Angeles County officials quietly logged the three-fold differential in mortality rates between Mexican-American and white infants, but conducted no studies that might reveal why the disparity existed. Even in the heyday of Biggs's authority in New York City, the roughly ten-year difference in life expectancies between white immigrants and native-born African-Americans constituted little more than a set of statistics dutifully logged year after year.

For a century, health-oriented intellectuals in England and the United States had speculated upon the relationship between poverty and disease, variously concluding that it was either the squalid environs of the poor, the nature of their home life, or "familial tendencies" (a.k.a. genetics) that determined their medical misery.[91] In the United States the added factor of immigration clouded the picture, and native-born white health leaders found bigoted explanations for the poor health of recently arrived, impoverished workers. Anti-Semitism, stereotypes of Irish and Italian traits, anti-Catholicism, and other prejudiced perspectives offered easy explanations—albeit, as history would show, incorrect ones.

The spectacular monetary gap between America's richest and poorest citizens was impossible to ignore at the turn of the century.[92] The top 1 percent of America's income earners made more money in 1920 than did the bottom 50 percent. Inescapably obvious to public advocates of the day were both the painful poverty of the people on society's lower rungs and its contribution to the paucity of healthy options available to them.

But at the turn of the twentieth century it was also common in both England and the United States to subsume concern about poverty beneath the thick layer of moral indignation that ascribed alcohol and drug use, sexually acquired illnesses, and psychiatric difficulties to the moral weaknesses or inferiority of poor people.

The germ theory crusaders of the early twentieth century, however noble their cause, were also incapable of confronting the roots of racial and economic disparities in health. With the rise of social Darwinism during the 1920s, explanations for racial variations in life expectancy and health shifted from the search for moral weakness to evolution and, in primitive form, genetics.[93]

The concept of "racial immunity" to disease was a popular one among physicians and many public health advocates, but not among statisticians and demographers, who saw a very different picture in the disparate mortality rates. "I do not believe that there is such a thing as *absolute* racial immunity to any disease," wrote Metropolitan Life Insurance actuary Louis Dublin.[94] "The Negro death rates for practically all diseases in the prevention or cure of which care and sanitation are of paramount importance are much higher than among the whites: but this does not prove that the Negroes are, *inherently*, more susceptible to such diseases—or, for that matter, that they are less resistant to them. It is probable that their higher death rate is due more than anything else to ignorance, poverty, and lack of proper medical care."

In the West the gulfs between the races—Mexican-Americans, Chinese-Americans, and whites—were equally gargantuan. Mexican-Americans had, by the turn of the twentieth century, become the region's key unskilled labor force and by 1920, up to a third of all Mexican-American households in Los Angeles County had absentee fathers, and the mothers, who had more than four children on average, typically toiled in a distant Caucasian household.[95] A constellation of factors no doubt contributed to their far-higher mortality rates, compared to whites,[96] but no one in the Los Angeles County Department of Health during the 1920s had the time or inclination to study the matter.[97]

Throughout the twentieth century, American public health leaders would struggle with questions of race, genetics, ethnicity, and economic class, unable to define the relative impacts those had on individual and population health. And that debate, coupled with social exclusions from the health system, would form a critical, lasting, and shameful theme of U.S. public health.

III

By the thirties, the expansionary era had come to an end, and the functions of
public health were becoming more fixed and routine. The bacteriological
revolution had played itself out in the organization of public services, and soon
the introduction of antibiotics and other drugs would enable private physicians
to reclaim some of their functions, like the treatment of venereal disease and
tuberculosis. Yet it had been clear, long before, that public health in America
was to be relegated to a secondary status: less prestigious than clinical
medicine, less amply financed, and blocked from assuming the higher-level
functions of coordination and direction that might have developed had it not
been banished from medical care.

—Paul Starr, 1982 [98]

On October 29th, 1929, the New York Stock Exchange crashed after several days of sharp declines, hurling the world into the Great Depression of the 1930s. Paul de Kruif, a bacteriologist who had become the best known science writer of his day,[99] traveled the country in the months following that black October day. His eyes were opened to a reality of poverty and disease that he—indeed, nearly all scientists of his day—had never before seen. Nearly boiling with rage, he wrote:

> I don't know why it took me so long to see that the strength—and life-giving results of the toil of those searchers were *for sale*; that life was some-thing you could have if you bought and paid for it; which meant you could have your share of it if you'd been shrewd, or crafty, or just lucky.
>
> It still puzzles me why for so long I found excuses for our ghastly cartoon of a civilization—that's great . . . that's ruled by the Calvinistic humbug that God has predestined suffering and that suffering is good; that awards its searchers prizes, smirks congratulations at them, and allots the real benefits of their science to the well-heeled few; that turns its face from millions in pain, or hidden-hungry, or dying with an absolutely possible abundance of life-giving science all round them.[100]

De Kruif did an about-face from a public health booster who believed science would conquer humanity's worst diseases to the profession's sharpest critic. Amid national poverty on a scale America had never previously witnessed, de Kruif saw that years of ignoring the public health needs of the poor or, worse yet, blaming the poor for their own illnesses, were now undermining the very successes he had once loudly trumpeted.

In his travels across America, de Kruif saw a patchwork quilt of health;

some communities were seemingly unaffected by the Depression while others experienced resurgent tuberculosis at levels he called "murder," and crippling rheumatic fever epidemics among children (New York City's rate rose twenty-fold between 1929 and 1934). Government cutbacks had curtailed vaccination programs in many states, prompting surges in diphtheria that de Kruif decried as "damnable." There was also soaring child malnutrition.

In 1935 a *New York World Telegram* editorial[101] declared: "One hundred and thirty-five thousand pupils in New York City's elementary schools are so weak from malnutrition that they cannot profit by attendance. . . . This is almost one in every five of the children enrolled—18.1 percent in all."

Sarcastically, de Kruif asked, "Should children eat? Why keep them alive?"

Then he turned his formidable anger to birth issues, chronicling the "fight for life" in grossly substandard Depression-era hospitals.[102] All across North America, he argued, basic standards of hygiene had disappeared from hospitals. Mothers were again dying of puerperal fever at rates last seen before Semmelweis's great discovery about hand washing. Babies were succumbing to "childbed fevers" as they were tended by nurses who changed one set of diapers after another without washing their hands. Syphilis and tuberculosis rates were soaring and, according to the National Tuberculosis Association, by 1937 TB was costing the nation $647 million a year in medical care and lost productivity. Yet hospitals had no funds to combat these scourges and departments of public health were on the edge of collapse all over the country. "Let's face it," de Kruif said, "with the poverty of our hospitals and universities deepening and becoming more desperate, with our rulers, comptrollers, budget-balancers bellowing economy, there is small chance that this wherewithal will be forthcoming to train the new type of death fighter."[103]

Public health leaders, so recently America's heroes, were shunned, impotent, even forced to act as apologists for government and industry.[104] The Charles Hewitts and Hermann Biggses of the world were long gone. Into their place stepped bureaucrats.

The Great Depression killed more than lives and economies: it rang the death knell for the public health revolution. The functions of public health would be saved through federalism, creating ever-larger national programs staffed at all tiers of government by often lackluster physicians and bureaucrats.

But when the stock market crashed in 1929, the federal public health effort was a jumbled mess involving forty different agencies that answered to five different cabinet secretaries. A total of five thousand U.S. government civil servants worked in public health programs of some kind.[105] It was hardly a force equal to the challenge.

In the United States in the years following the crash every critical indicator of population health worsened, just as they would sixty years later in Eastern

Europe following the collapse of the Soviet Union.[106] Suicide rates among males soared, especially among unemployed men aged fifty to sixty-four years.[107] And suicide rates, overall, went from 12 per 100,000 men and women in 1925 to 17.4 per 100,000 in 1932—the highest rate ever recorded in U.S. history. Between 1929 and 1936 overall life expectancy for men and women combined rose slightly, but that masked a sharp decline of more than five years in life expectancy that occurred between 1933 and 1936.

During the Great Depression, the incidence of death from certain communicable diseases increased significantly nationwide, among them were scarlet fever, diphtheria, whooping cough, measles, influenza, and pneumonia. In some regions, tuberculosis and typhoid fever death rates also spiked during the 1930s. Worse, hospitals all across America went belly-up.[108] The problem, of course, was that the patients were broke and, regardless of whether they were government institutions or private facilities, the hospitals simply couldn't cover their operating costs. And with no money in their pockets, patients shunned the prestigious and private hospitals in favor of free care in government-owned facilities.

It would be difficult to overstate the impact the Great Depression had on the lives, and health, of the American people. Unemployment ran between 10 and 40 percent in most cities, with industrial centers hardest hit. Sales of consumer products and capital goods collapsed because overnight the consumer market disappeared. Farmers were forced to lower their prices so much that they couldn't cover the costs to harvest and transport their products. Over a quarter million farms were foreclosed by 1932. Construction came to a complete halt.[109]

Entire industries closed their doors. Their former employees turned to relief offices where, increasingly, the city officials in charge turned them away. City coffers were empty. Hardest hit were the African-American, Mexican-American, and American Indian populations—in their ranks unemployment ran as high as 60 to 75 percent. Also devastated were the beneficiaries of earlier public health triumphs: America's unprecedentedly large population of retired people over the age of sixty-five, which represented 5 percent of the nation's population in 1929. Few of them had pensions or sources of income during the Depression. More than ten thousand banks collapsed nationwide between 1923 and 1932.

Local governments sought all sorts of solutions to the crisis, few of which were judicious or, in the end, effective.

The alternative to suicide for many families was relocation. Between 1929 and 1940 the nation's demography shifted radically as millions of people moved from one place to another in search of jobs. Many of them had been uprooted by the devastating dust storms of 1935, a result of decades of over-farming the soils of Arkansas, Texas, Oklahoma, and the Great Plains.[110]

Many of these refugees went to California, where they were supremely unwelcome. Conservative Californians placed great faith in their native son, Herbert Hoover—the first westerner ever elected to the presidency. Even as the Great Depression worsened, most civic leaders accepted as wise policy Hoover's 1932 assumption that "it is not the function of government to relieve individuals of their responsibilities to their neighbors, or to relieve private institutions of their responsibilities to the public." It was a sentiment to be heard from California-spawned presidents well into the future.

Class war was brewing in the West. "Hoovervilles," clapboard housing slums loaded with dust bowl refugees and itinerant workers, sprang up outside every major western city. Labor organizers, from anarchists with the Industrial Workers of the World (IWW) to Eugene V. Debs socialists, found fertile soil amid the outrage. Trade unionists throughout California staged demonstrations and all manner of protests against the "capitalist bosses."

Los Angeles's leaders responded to the mounting tension by targeting Mexicans and Mexican-Americans for mass deportation, beginning in 1931.[111]

In this topsy-turvy atmosphere, all aspects of governance were strained, and public health was no exception. On the eve of the stock market crash, the County Department of Health had 400 employees; ten years later it had 419. During that time the population it was to serve swelled from about 677,000 people to 900,000, though the numbers involved some guess work, as on any given day nobody really knew how many Mexicans, "Okies," or Mexican-Americans were living in the county. Department reports from the time have a breathless quality to them, as if even the moments spent hammering at a typewriter were precious. An American Public Health Association assessment of the department's performance in 1930 found it "severely wanting," as its beleaguered staff raced about the vast county barely able to meet the populace's most basic health needs.

Even in times of prosperity during the 1920s, when Dr. Pomeroy had planned for a network of health clinics spanning the vast county, his dream had been quashed by the weighty opposition of the local American Medical Association, which would brook no competition from government. By 1935 most of Pomeroy's planned health care system lay in shreds, the victim not only of AMA assault but, probably more significantly, of attack from a new and growing group: red baiters. Provision of health services for the poor, even in times when most Los Angelenos were suffering, was considered "socialistic" by the county's elite, and they followed the *Los Angeles Times*'s lead in denouncing alleged abuse of tax-supported services by the so-called undeserving poor.[112]

In the midst of such chaos, whooping cough, diphtheria, typhoid fever, puerperal fever, maternal and infant mortality, and tuberculosis rates all rose during the Great Depression.[113] And in 1934 when polio struck hard in Los Angeles, the health department couldn't cope.[114]

This polio strain was unusual[115] in that many cases involved adults, few victims suffered paralysis, death rates were low, and most had what appeared to be encephalitis.[116]

County health officials were at a loss to explain how the disease was spreading, why it was causing such bizarre symptoms, how it could be stopped, or what treatments might work.[117]

By the epidemic's height, public health authority had completely broken down. Fearing infection (which had passed to many health workers) public hospital staff abandoned their posts, leaving remaining personnel so overwhelmed that stretchers and gurneys, laden with waiting patients, stretched around the block and for hours on end ailing children wailed and victims called in vain for assistance.

For years afterward, the L.A. County Department of Health spoke with a meek voice and was rarely able to gain recognition or cooperation from the region's political leaders, physicians, or general populace.

And it was hardly alone. Counties, cities, and states all over the United States fell apart between 1929 and 1933 as tax revenues disappeared. In some areas, physicians volunteered their services for epidemic control duty. But before the presidential election of Franklin Delano Roosevelt, most public health departments in the United States had either already shattered, as was the case in Los Angeles County, or were teetering on the brink of collapse.[118]

One significant exception was Minnesota, which swung so far to the left during the Great Depression that Roosevelt's Democratic Party became its targeted right wing. Just weeks after the stock market crashed, Minnesotans elected Minneapolis leftist Floyd Olson to the governor's seat, putting his Farm Labor Party in power. That party considered social programs, such as those for public health, of paramount importance and dismissed opposition to public welfare as part and parcel of some dark capitalist plot. "As long as I sit in the governor's chair," Olson said, "there is not going to be any misery in the state if I can humanely prevent it. I hope the present system of government goes right down to Hell."[119] To that end, public health programs gained prominence during the Olson years and were pushed toward provision of medical and disease control services for rural farmers and the urban poor.

Long after the reign of Farm Labor ended in the 1940s its impact on Minnesota politics and public health could still be felt. And for six decades Minnesota would be famous for both its high rates of graduated income taxation and strong tax-supported social programs, including public health and provision of medical care for indigent and poor working Minnesotans.

By the end of Roosevelt's nearly four-term presidency, public health in the United States would be federalized. True, each municipality and state would offer its own unique brand of health services and programs, but what was once

100 percent based on local revenues would become dependent on dollars from Washington. And with that largesse would come Washington-dictated policies and increased power and influence for the U.S. Public Health Service (USPHS).

The USPHS was initially a tiny federal force with authority strictly limited to major ports of entry into the United States—particularly New York's Ellis Island and San Francisco's Angel Island—and to national contagion catastrophes. That changed after a showdown in California in 1901, just after *Yersinia pestis*, the plague, struck San Francisco's Chinatown.[120] It was no doubt brought by sea from Shanghai or Hong Kong. Angel Island USPHS microbiologist Joseph Kinyoun analyzed the blood of Chinatown patients and rats and confirmed the presence of *Yersinia pestis*. He immediately alerted California and federal authorities.[121]

Governor of California Henry T. Gage dismissed Kinyoun's findings as hogwash. Republican Gage would brook absolutely no such obstacles to California's development and population expansion. So he simply said there was no plague in California. Period.

After an eighteen-month Kinyoun/Gage standoff, an independent review commission confirmed the presence of *Yersinia pestis*. And for the first time in U.S. history, federal health authorities took charge of an epidemic control effort, without a request from or support of state leaders (but at the urgent behest of San Francisco local health officials).[122]

In 1912 Congress granted the USPHS authority to intervene at the local level on behalf of the health of *all* Americans, not just seamen and immigrants, and gave the agency authority over basic medical research.[123] The first sweeping federal health law, the 1921 Sheppard-Towner Act gave the USPHS annual pots of money from which to dole out to states grants for well-baby programs. This set the precedent for a new model of funding that would become the dominant paradigm of the remainder of the century: money would filter from federal sources down to the states and cities and would arrive already earmarked for implementation of policies that had been decided by federal health authorities and congressional politicians.

Given that, unlike in Europe, public health in the United States had originated at the local level and matured as a patchwork quilt of very diverse infrastructures, each with different rules and authorities, the imposition of such top-down policy making was odd. It would prove impossible to come up with one-size-fits-all health policies and, over the coming decades, local public health authorities would often feel conflicted about the federal largesse: they wanted the money but might dispute the policy to which it was attached.[124]

The Sheppard-Towner Act was an indisputable boon, however, to the forty-one states that made use of the funds during the 1920s.[125]

In 1926 the National Health Council, a consortium of private medical and public health organizations, submitted a report to Congress describing public health in the United States as a feeble and disjointed array of largely leaderless efforts that fell under five different cabinets of the executive branch. Some five thousand civil servants, working in forty different agencies, played a role in setting public health policy and executing actions of one kind or another. The USPHS was hardly alone, or even in charge.[126]

At the Democratic Party nominating convention in 1932, Franklin Delano Roosevelt had called for a "New Deal for America" in which banks and finance were regulated and the state extended its charitable hand to rescue the masses from their dire straits. Upon taking office in 1933, Roosevelt surrounded himself with a coterie of advisors, swiftly dubbed "The Brain Trust" by the press, and set to work creating his New Deal. Congress passed nearly every piece of legislation the White House sent it, and by the end of 1933 America was taking the first tentative steps out of the Great Depression.[127]

The New Deal's impact on the nation's public health infrastructure was profound and would prove lasting. A dozen agencies were created between 1933 and 1938, each of which affected the health of Americans. And most of these agencies would, in some form, become permanent components of the U.S. government.[128]

No state turned its back on what the New Deal offered (not even Minnesota), but no one made better use of it than New York City's dynamo of a mayor, Fiorello La Guardia.[129]

Even before he ascended to New York's throne, La Guardia told Roosevelt that he would happily allow the president to use Gotham as a testing—and proving—ground for every New Deal program.[130] He made this promise even though his 1933 victory was not assured.

During the Roaring Twenties Tammany's grip on the health department was absolute and it played a role in Hermann Biggs's ultimate exhaustion and disheartened resignation in 1923. Dr. Frank J. Monaghan's thoroughly corrupt leadership of the health department in every way undermined the very programs that had made New York City a national public health model.

But Tammany's greed finally went too far, becoming too blatant even for remarkably corruption tolerant New York City. Private citizens' organizations dug up enough dirt to force Monaghan out in 1925 and his successor, Dr. Louis Harris, discovered still more evidence of astounding fraud, patronage, and extortion. One ring of restaurant inspectors alone had been extorting $3 million a year from eating establishment owners who were compelled to pay five dollars "protection" a week. A $1 million fund for contagion control had simply disappeared.

Harris—by all accounts an honest man—ordered a long list of firings and indictments followed. But the department's credibility with the public had eroded severely. In 1928 the private Welfare Council of New York published its *Health Inventory of New York City*, which was highly critical of the health department.[131] Nearly every program was, it said, in a shambles. The damage done by Harris's predecessor was simply overwhelming.[132]

Into this Great Depression quagmire stepped the man known as the Little Flower, Fiorello, and after 146 years in existence, during seventy-seven of which it criminally manipulated New York City and the National Democratic Party, the Tammany machine was finally vanquished.

The conversations with Roosevelt's Brain Trust paid off less than a year after La Guardia took office and a hallmark of his tenure would be his uncanny ability to match New York's needs with Roosevelt's New Deal agenda. New Deal money paid for mosquito abatement and marshland drainage, a study of New York's rising air pollution problems, and a "full-scale assault on VD."

Between 1935 and 1937 the New York City Department of Health underwent a construction boom, getting new laboratories, clinics, and offices—all thanks to federal dollars from the Public Works Administration (WPA). La Guardia boasted, "We have cleaned politics out of the Health Department in just the same way that we're chasing microbes, germs, and bugs out of our city."[133]

One New Deal–funded study revealed in 1937 that in New York City as in Los Angeles (though through different mechanisms) the Great Depression took a far greater toll on nonwhite versus white residents. Mortality rates among New York African-Americans and other men of color were 473 percent higher than among white males. And infant mortality among nonwhites was double that of white babies.[134]

In his final term in office, after the end of the Depression, La Guardia awoke to a startling realization: despite fifteen years of economic hardship for the people of New York, hospitals and doctors there had grown very prosperous—so prosperous that city employees could no longer afford health care.[135] So in 1944 La Guardia set up the first municipal health insurance program in the United States. The city covered half of all health expenses for employees earning more than $5,000 a year and fully covered costs for lesser-paid city workers.

But long before La Guardia took the nation down the path of health insurance, the AMA kicking and screaming in protest each step of the way, he and Health Commissioner Dr. John Rice used New Deal money to transform public health activities in Gotham. In the department's 1938 annual report, Rice acknowledged that the very mission of public health had changed. Though scourges of contagion, notably syphilis, tuberculosis, bacterial pneumonia, meningitis, and polio, continued to plague the population, "diseases which influence mortality rates" could no longer absorb most of the department's energies. Rather, said the rather prescient Rice, in the future public health would need to "include consideration of physical and mental disorders which affect the general health and well-being of the community."[136]

By that time one out of every five dollars spent by the New York City Department of Health was of federal origin. Given that just four years previously the city public health effort hadn't received a nickel from Washington, that was a marked change of affairs. And in 1940 the department for the first time faced a funding crisis that would prove an ominous indicator of things to come: changes in White House policies had trickled down the funding ladder through an array of New Deal bureaucracies in Washington and suddenly New York faced a 21 percent cut in WPA revenues. Doctors and nurses in many divisions saw their incomes halved overnight as they were reduced to part-time status. That, too, would prove a harbinger of future weaknesses in America's public health safety net.

Dependency can be a terrible thing, especially if the terms of a dole are dictated entirely by the donor. In coming decades public health programs would grow increasingly reliant upon Washington's largess and, therefore, more vulnerable to the whims and priorities of faraway politicians over whom they had little or no influence. Without the political savvy of a Hermann Biggs or the supportive political hustle of a Fiorello La Guardia, few localities would prove immune to periodic tug-and-pull from Washington.

The New Deal's impact on public health was, however, remarkably positive and the benefits often came from surprising sources. The health of American Indians improved as a result of changes in their land rights under the Indian Reorganization Act of 1934.[137] Mortality decreased among farmers and "Okie" farm workers as a result of New Deal agricultural programs. Rural areas saw their food poisoning rates go down as the Tennessee Valley Authority brought electricity to tens of thousands of households, allowing installation of refrigerators. Eight million workers suddenly had money with which to feed their children, thanks to employment with the WPA. Hookworm infection rates declined as southern families earned enough to provide their children with shoes.

The 1934 congressional elections swept so many Roosevelt supporters into the House and Senate that Republicans formed an impotent minority. Despite its tremendous popularity, Roosevelt's Brain Trust met its match when the administration moved to create health insurance and Social Security programs. Roosevelt's plan was to set in place a "cradle-to-grave" social insurance program that would cover every American's health, medical, and pension needs and would be financed through a payroll contribution system. FDR envisioned a system that would serve as a safety net for unemployed workers, offer prenatal care to their pregnant wives, and provide a living wage for retirees. As he conceived it, every American, regardless of race or class, would come under the U.S. Social Security umbrella.

That was going too far.

Southern political leaders said they would never vote for a law that might carve cents out of the paychecks of white workers to pay unemployment benefits to "Negroes to sit around in idleness on front galleries."[138] The Republican Party said the FDR plan was overtly socialistic and, by said definition, had to be blocked.

And, of course, the American Medical Association chimed in again, with its leaders opposing all of the health insurance provisions of FDR's Social Security proposal.[139]

In the face of dogged opposition, the finally adopted Social Security Act of 1935 compromised or defeated all of FDR's original intentions for it and was a deeply flawed piece of legislation. As the AMA had hoped, it had no provisions for health insurance.

Thus, for the second time in U.S. history, the possibility of universal health care based on compulsory insurance was raised—and defeated. And the primary force responsible for vanquishing it was, in both cases, the AMA.

Paul de Kruif, who was highly critical of the compromises struck in the Social Security Act, eventually concluded that the only hope of salvaging public health in the United States rested with further federalization and creation of a large corps of USPHS officers. He advocated creation of something not terribly unlike the future U.S. Center for Communicable Diseases.

In *The Fight for Life* de Kruif wrote:

> Why cannot our U.S. Public Health Service be entrusted with co-ordinating in the instances of these now-preventable plagues, the people's fight for life? You hear the wail that this will breed a new bureaucracy. Let this then be remembered: we have an army and a navy supported by the government, by all the people—to defend our nation against threat of human invasion that becomes real not once in a generation. They are bureaucracies, granted.
>
> But is it anywhere advocated that the army and the navy be turned over to private hands and the defense of our country be left to us individuals armed with scythes and shotguns, because the army and navy are bureaucratic? . . . Who then objects to the organization of a death-fighting army against the far more dangerous subvisible assassins in ambush for all the people—always? . . .
>
> If you allow our death-fighters—we can assure you they are competent—the money to wipe out such and such and such deaths that cost us billions to maintain, within a generation there will no longer be this drain upon the wealth of our nation.[140]

IV

There is no reason to doubt, of course, the ability of the scientific method to solve each of the specific problems of disease by discovering causes and remedial procedures. Whether concerned with particular dangers to be overcome or with specific requirements to be satisfied, all the separate problems of human health can and will eventually find their solution. But solving problems of disease is not the same thing as creating health and happiness.

—René Dubos, 1959 [141]

At 7:55 A.M. on December 7, 1941, the Japanese air force attacked the U.S. naval fleet based in Hawaii, thus compelling American involvement in World War II.

While the military economy created jobs and brought the Great Depression to an end, it also skewed government spending toward the war front. For many parts of the country, the sudden shift of federal funds away from domestic spending proved painful—local governments had grown accustomed to New Deal dollars.

The Minnesota Department of Health, for example, had planned on a 1942 budget of $764,134, of which 60 percent ($453,496) was to come from federal funds. Most of that federal contribution, however, was diverted by Washington to the war effort. In addition, tens of thousands of public health professionals—doctors and nurses—were recruited to the war effort, thus depleting domestic services of vital personnel.

On the other hand, the war propelled vital public health research, resulting in bold new programs for control of insect-borne diseases (notably typhus, yellow fever, and malaria), bacterial infections, and venereal diseases. And by the end of the 1940s, Americans would be shifting their concern from microbes to two chronic killers: cardiovascular diseases and cancer. Commensurate with that shift would come a slow change in how people in the United States viewed their physical milieu: once considered a constantly threatening miasma of germs, it began to seem controllable, even subservient, to human exigencies.

By 1941 FDR's New Deal had vastly improved the nation's health. Per-capita health spending, having plummeted in the middle of the Great Depression by 120 percent, surpassed precrash levels in 1941, reaching nearly $4,000. Life expectancies for whites rose from the despairingly low 61.1 years of 1934 to 64.8 years for babies born in 1941—a net gain of 3.7 years of life. Nonwhite Americans gained two years of life during those years, rising from a 1934 level of 51.8 years to, in 1941, 53.8 years.[142] One clear reason was food: Americans in 1941 were finally able to afford to eat as much as they had in 1929, before the stock market crash. Tuberculosis, scarlet fever, typhoid, and malaria death rates all improved markedly—the latter two were halved.[143]

After Pearl Harbor, the challenge for local authorities was to maintain 1941's rosy health picture amid wartime staff reductions and scarcities and in the face of new, war-related health crises—all at a time of enormous social movement and upset.

Roles were shifting in America as women filled employment slots vacated by drafted men and blacks, migrating en masse from the South to military production centers of the far West and Midwest, entered the industrial workforce on an enormous scale. Economic wealth followed the war industry and the number one beneficiary of World War II government spending and financial growth was Los Angeles County.[144] Most of California's $19 billion in military contracts went to Los Angeles, which by the war's end was the nation's second-largest industrial center and had the most vast and modern industrial infrastructure in the entire world.[145]

Between 1940 and 1945 the population of California grew 135 percent from 6,982,000 to 9,491,000, and most of that increase occurred in Los Angeles County.[146]

On July 26, 1943, the burgeoning, industrious, and unsettled metropolis of Los Angeles experienced Black Monday. It was the fourth day of horrible air pollution in the region and the worst Los Angeles had ever endured. As the *Los Angeles Times* described it: "With the entire downtown area engulfed by a low-hanging cloud of acrid smoke, yesterday morning city health and police authorities began investigations to determine the source of the 'gas attack' that left thousands of Angelenos with irritated eyes, noses, and throats. . . . Visibility was cut to less than three blocks in some sections of the business district."

A word was invented to describe that haze: *smog*. Though by the 1950s smog would envelop cities from Rio to New York, Los Angeles was the first to suffer its ongoing assault. On "good days" the nauseating mass was blown eastward by winds from the Pacific, but on Black Monday the cleansing winds didn't blow for days on end and the smog formed brown layers of carbon monoxide, ozone, and industrial effluent.

Three years later, when smog had become a nearly permanent feature of Los Angeles, Ed Ainsworth wrote in the *Los Angeles Times*:[147] "The recent rain washed the once-celebrated air of Los Angeles and gave Southern California an unaccustomed view of an object known as the sun . . . through the pall of 'smog' which settled over Los Angeles in 1943 and has persisted with exasperating firmness ever since, it hardly ever was visible to the naked eye."

Near the oil fields of Long Beach the peculiar haze was regularly redolent with sulfur and methane, prompting local residents to talk of "rotten egg days." Eastward toward Fontana around the steel mills, smog tasted vaguely metallic in the back of residents' throats. In the posh San Gabriel Valley towns of Pasadena and San Marino, the eyes first sensed smog's arrival, tearing uncontrollably. Children who ran and romped outdoors were soon overcome by aching lungs and powerful headaches.

In the mad haste to grow, grow, grow that had been Los Angeles's hallmark since Anglo real estate developers first began hyping it to potential buyers from the Midwest during the 1890s, the county had given little thought to the fact that it was nestled in a basin and subject to periodic, prolonged air inversions.

By 1941 Los Angeles no longer had its Big Red rail system,[148] and it was checkered with freeways, boulevards, and interstate highways that hundreds of thousands of motorists traversed daily. Long before the automobile would truly take hold in the rest of America, Los Angeles was a car commuter culture.

Black Monday and the subsequent wartime smog were the result of combined industrial and auto emissions. And, for the always understaffed and beleaguered County Department of Health, smog was a nightmare that stretched the department to its limits.

By the time the war ended, Los Angeles County would have more than 4 million residents and cover four thousand square miles. Forty of its forty-five incorporated cities contracted with the County Department of Health not only for public health but also for medical services.

Dr. Roy O. Gilbert, who took over as Los Angeles County health officer in 1945, made it clear that the primary task of public health remained communicable diseases control. Unable to obtain special funding with which to address the smog problem and lacking solid scientific evidence that the clearly irritating gases constituted a public health crisis, Gilbert simply added "air pollution" to the long list of duties for the department's Sanitation Section.

In 1947, four years after Black Monday, California enacted its first of many pieces of legislation aimed at reducing the presumed health risk of air pollution. The law gave health authorities the right to declare smog alert days. On heavily polluted days, the Los Angeles County Department of Health would issue warnings requesting that residents avoid driving, stay indoors, and keep children from running and playing. In some Los Angeles school districts, smog alerts prompted principals to ban all forms of student exercise; during recesses youngsters were told to lie down indoors.[149] Powerless to control the sources of smog and lacking funding for research on air pollution measurement, the health department could do little more.

Over the next decade researchers worldwide would analyze smog and conclude that it contained a host of chemicals considered dangerous to human health: cyclic hydrocarbons, carbon monoxides, nitrous oxides, sulfur dioxide, benzpyrene, ozone, and lead. Public anxiety about smog would increase when some of its contents would prove to cause cancer in laboratory animals. But it would be decades before the sources of smog were effectively reduced. In the meantime, public health leaders stood by helplessly, convinced, as Columbia University's George Rosen wrote in 1958, that "the atmosphere of the modern industrial community is a carcinogenic sea, polluted and made murky by many sorts of individual waste. In such an environment it is hardly possible to avoid daily contact with cancer-producing agents. . . . However, inherent difficulties have so far prevented a full epidemiological and technical solution of the problem."[150]

Air pollution standards would not be set in California until 1956, and the automobile would not formally be named the primary source of smog until so designated by the Air Pollution Control Board of Southern California in 1959. For the remainder of the decade pollution control officials, gasoline distributors, and automobile manufacturers would spar over standards for car engine design, fuel, and emissions.[151] Particularly striking was the comparatively minor role public health leaders eventually played in the struggle against smog, a battle largely waged through political and regulatory action at the federal level.

Just as it would be well over a decade before such things as chemical pollution and smog were linked to a growing public—and public health—concern about cancer, there was also a time lag after the war before the growing incidence of heart disease became alarming.

During the war years Minnesota remained a comparatively clean, if freezing cold, state where the incidences of nearly all communicable diseases continued to fall. The most dramatic mortality shift for wartime Minnesotans was due to heart disease. When the Japanese struck Pearl Harbor, Minnesotans were dying of heart disease at a rate of about 270 per 100,000. By the time the war ended and the troops had returned home, in 1947, the cardiovascular death rate had skyrocketed, reaching 309.7 per 100,000. It was the largest increase in heart disease Minnesotans had ever seen.[152]

The state's Department of Health had long accepted that heart disease was its populace's number one killer, yet did little to try to control it. In part the inaction was because, like its counterparts all over the United States, the Minnesota State Department of Health was constructed around a communicable diseases model and had little idea how to tackle chronic ailments. In addition, at the time, most physicians thought of heart attacks and strokes as inevitable components of old age. They were wrong, as the sharp increase in deaths among younger men, aged forty-five to fifty-four years, indicated.[153]

Public health leaders in the state had little knowledge at the time of the relative roles smoking, poor diet, and lack of exercise played in causation of heart disease. Minnesota was at the front end of a radical change in American lifestyles in which a host of factors were interacting to increase the risks of cardiovascular diseases. Machinery had made Minnesota's farmers more sedentary; the automobile had made most everyone more sedentary; and diets were changing. Supermarkets appeared offering processed foods high in the fat, sugar, and salt that improved sales. Treats, laborious to prepare at home, were suddenly abundant.

And tens of thousands of men had acquired a taste for chain-smoking while on the World War II battlefields. Cigarette sales soared in the 1940s and 1950s and smoking was suddenly socially acceptable in virtually every setting from offices to churches, schools to movie theaters, hospital waiting rooms to doctors' offices. Every medium, even the *Journal of the American Medical Association* and many other leading medical publications, ran cigarette ads. In truth, public health leaders in the 1940s saw no reason to attack America's love affair with the cigarette.

During the war years, the biggest source of public health consternation in all cities that served as staging and leave sites for military personnel was escalating venereal diseases rates. In New York's case, the battle against gonorrhea and syphilis consumed the city's communicable diseases control resources, leaving few dollars or health personnel to fight the old scourges of tuberculosis and childhood diseases.

Nationally, syphilis and gonorrhea rates had been rising steadily since the turn of the century and no public health agency had developed an effective strategy for venereal diseases control.[154] At the end of World War I national syphilis rates averaged 113 per 100,000. By the end of World War II average syphilis rates would reach 450 per 100,000, with the highest incidence among military men.

Gonorrhea had shown an overall rising trend since 1900, though national rates had fluctuated. During the middle of the Depression, gonorrhea averaged 121 cases per 100,000 Americans. In 1941 the rate rose to 146.7 per 100,000, and in 1944 it reached 236.5 per 100,000.[155]

From the earliest days of organized public health, Americans had exhibited a peculiar inability to cope with the conjunction of three fearsome factors: sex, disease, and death. In colonial America and later in the United States, even nonsexual diseases were traditionally framed in moralistic terms.[156] Reflecting the general American predilection for Christian moralism, social condemnation of individuals who suffered from venereal diseases was far more extreme in the United States than in Europe. And, as a direct result, individuals with syphilis and gonorrhea were more likely to hide their ailments until the diseases reached physically obvious, and completely incurable, tertiary stages. Secrecy, of course, required that there be no change in one's behavior lest a spouse question why a mate no longer desired sexual intercourse. So shame supported the spread of gonorrhea and syphilis.[157]

In the 1930s hospitals all across America had a policy of refusing to treat venereal diseases on the grounds that the patients were immoral. It was as if the alleged lack of morality was, itself, contagious.[158] Even the AMA—usually a staunch opponent of government-provided health services—offered no resistance to the creation of public health VD clinics, isolated from the hospitals and staffed by government doctors and nurses.

Congress passed the Venereal Disease Act in 1935, giving the USPHS authority to conduct research on syphilis and gonorrhea. A year earlier, New York State's health commissioner, Dr. Thomas Parran, was kicked off CBS Radio for uttering the word *syphilis* on the air. Shortly thereafter, Roosevelt appointed Parran his Surgeon General, and the New Yorker made VD one of his primary causes.

For many years the highest rates of syphilis and gonorrhea had been seen among African-American men, a fact that reinforced the white racist view of profligate, rampant sexual activity among blacks. Because of the racial stereotyping and moralism surrounding sexual diseases, African-Americans resented all discussion of syphilis and gonorrhea in their communities.

One of the highest syphilis rates in the entire world could be found in Macon County, Alabama, where in 1932 Dr. Taliaferro Clark of the USPHS discovered that 35 percent of the black population had syphilis and 90 percent of the cases had gone untreated.

The USPHS funded Tuskegee University, working under Clark, to conduct a study of syphilis in Macon County, Alabama.[159] Under the original study design, Tuskegee was to recruit four hundred black men who already had syphilis and two hundred who did not for tests and observation. No treatment was to be provided, as it would interfere with the study's two goals: to determine the long-term course of the disease in the absence of treatment and to note the peculiarities of the disease in black men. (There was widespread, mistaken belief among physicians that blacks responded differently to the disease than did whites.) Though white physicians initiated the study, over its four decades it was executed by African-American nurses and doctors as well.

In order to lure men into the study, none of the patients was told he had syphilis—rather, they learned from the Tuskegee staff that they suffered from "bad blood." And for years their continued participation was guaranteed by the provision of free transportation, hot meals, medical care for nonsyphilitic minor ailments, and burial insurance. Initially imagined as a six-month study, the Tuskegee experiment would last until 1972. In all that time, the Macon County men and their families would never be told that they had syphilis. Nor were they provided with penicillin in 1943 when USPHS researchers discovered that it could cure syphilis. For decades the USPHS would continue the study and outside reviewers would approve it, until an Associated Press journalist stumbled upon its existence in 1972. A storm of publicity followed, as a result of which study participant Charlie Pollard learned he had been duped and was dying of syphilis. He retained the famous civil rights attorney Fred D. Gray, who in 1974 brought a class action suit on behalf of all the Macon men against the USPHS. In an out-of-court settlement, each of the surviving men got a paltry $37,000 in compensation.

By then, all but seventy-two of the participants were dead, most having suffered the extremes of tertiary syphilis: infection and destruction of the brain and heart and lesions all over the skin, mouth, and genitals. Thirty had died directly from syphilis and at least seventy more of complications associated with their venereally acquired infection. Never realizing that they carried an infectious disease, by 1974 the men had passed syphilis on to twenty-two of their wives, who transmitted the diseases to seventeen children and they to two grandchildren.

The travesty of Tuskegee would continue to fester in both the public health and African-American communities, widening a credibility gap that was already vast. Eventually, the divide would become so great that in the 1990s all U.S. government public health pronouncements and programs would be viewed with hostility, even outright contempt, by African-Americans of all social classes.[160]

The legacy of the Tuskegee experiment would prove to be merely an extreme example of a larger failure for American public health. Throughout the twentieth century there would continue to be glaring differences in the life expectancies, health statuses, infant mortalities, and access to medical care for white versus nonwhite U.S. citizens. Public health leaders would, variously, prove ineffectual, apologist, blatantly racist, or simply determinedly ignorant in these matters. By the 1960s the divide between public health (both government and academic) and the nation's minority communities would be explosive.

Because the Tuskegee subjects were functionally illiterate, they never realized that they were suffering the very symptoms that, beginning in 1936, were emblazoned on flyers and notices distributed nationwide by the U.S. Surgeon General's office. That is also why they never learned, as did most Americans, about two landmark discoveries that could have cured their "bad blood."

In 1937 USPHS physician John Mahoney, while toiling in the government's Staten Island laboratory, discovered that sulfa drugs could kill gonorrheal bacteria. Five years earlier, Scottish scientist Alexander Fleming discovered a sulfa compound he called penicillin. And it proved powerfully effective in laboratory tests against a broad range of bacteria.

In 1943 Mahoney showed that penicillin and other sulfa antibiotics could also kill tough spirochetes like syphilis. And that discovery opened a new door for public health. Immediately both civilian and military physicians realized that if the promise of a cure could flush all the ashamed gonorrhea and syphilis carriers out of hiding and encourage them to name their sexual partners, it would be possible to treat all of the cases and thus halt the spread of venereal diseases.

And by all accounts, penicillin seemed the long-awaited magic bullet promised sixty years previously by Erlich. In minute doses the drug miraculously healed even advanced cases of syphilis and gonorrhea. And when supplies ran short, army doctors discovered that even the unmeasurable quantities of the drug that had passed into the urine of a treated patient could be used to cure another.[161]

Within months of Mahoney's discovery of the utility of penicillin in syphilis treatment, the New York City health department opened a special VD ward at Bellevue Hospital and distributed free penicillin to doctors and hospitals city-wide. The city also instituted contact tracing policies under which all syphilitic and gonorrheal patients were pressured to name their recent sexual contacts, who were subsequently tracked down, interrogated, and treated. When neces-sary, either because the contact's full name wasn't known or the individual re-fused treatment, officers of the New York Police Department were deployed. Biggs's old typhoid tactics of five decades earlier were resurrected for venereal disease.

Similar procedures were followed all over the United States after 1943, and U.S. average rates of syphilis fell from an all-time high of 447 per 100,000 in 1943 to 154 per 100,000 in 1950. By 1970 the U.S. syphilis rate would be 43 per 100,000.[162]

Gonorrhea rates, however, proved more mercurial. Unlike syphilis, gon-orrhea could respond to a single dose of penicillin and patients desirous of pri-vacy who could afford to see a private physician could remain outside the net of public health scrutiny. Amid widespread overuse of the new antibiotic by private physicians, penicillin-resistant strains of gonorrhea would soon emerge, further limiting successful control.[163] During the 1950s rates would fall as low as 129 per 100,000, but by 1970 they would have surpassed the 1947 all-time high of 284.[164]

Antibiotics allowed a similar transformation in public health approaches to tuberculosis. In 1944 the Mayo Clinic in Minnesota successfully used strep-tomycin to cure TB in a group of hospitalized patients and public health leaders immediately recognized that the contact tracing model could be applied to the control of tuberculosis.[165] By 1970 the national tuberculosis rate would have been cut by 91 percent, compared to its 1944 level.[166]

The primary impact of the antibiotic revolution on other bacterial diseases, such as streptococcal pneumonia and typhoid fever, was an immediate reduc-tion in death rates. In some cases the rates approached zero. Between 1936 and 1945 pneumonia death rates nationwide fell to less than 1 percent of all cases, a 40 percent drop. Though health departments continued to keep track of the bacterial diseases and distribute available vaccines, antibiotics medicalized their control. Physicians, antibiotics in hand, wrested authority over the bacterial domain from public health and would never again relinquish their power except during epidemics. This would prove in coming decades to be a serious problem, as antibiotic-resistant strains of the old killers emerged.

In 1943, even before Mahoney proved penicillin could cure syphilis, there were already more than three thousand six hundred antibiotic products in some stage of development. That figure would increase ten-fold over the next decade. So great was public excitement over the magic bullets that most of these products were ushered into clinical use after only a modicum of testing. As a result, side effects were often severe and dosages uncertain. The use of antibiotics therefore actually increased national hospitalization rates, as doctors generally urged their patients to take the miracle drugs only under close supervision. Civilian hospital admissions skyrocketed during the war, from about 10.5 million in 1941 to 14 million in 1946, and the bulk of all hospitalizations were voluntary. Thus, the antibiotic revolution increased the power of hospitals, transplanting entire fields of public health from the home or community level into the entirely physician-controlled environs of institutional medicine.[167]

Germany surrendered in May 1945 and the Pacific effort escalated that spring. And on July 16th, four months after Roosevelt died in office, a team of physicists successfully tested the world's first atomic bomb in Alamogordo, New Mexico. For three weeks the administration of President Harry S Truman internally debated use of the novel weapon, then on August 6th the *Enola Gay* dropped its payload on the Japanese city of Hiroshima. Three days later a second atom bomb fell on Nagasaki.

Japan surrendered on August 15, 1945, bringing World War II to an end.

And within nine months of Victory in Japan Day, the first children of what would prove to be the largest baby boom in U.S. history were born.[168] By the time the Baby Boom would end in 1964 the nation's women would have birthed 76.4 million babies, bringing the U.S. population up to more than 105 million.

The economy boomed, too. The U.S. gross national product increased from $100 billion in 1939 to 1945's $212 billion. Though Americans might quibble about President Truman's performance, they were passionately patriotic at the war's end and proud of the government of the United States. Federalism had served them well, ushering the country out of the Great Depression, guiding the nation to victory in battlefields all over the world, and rewarding the citizenry with phenomenal postwar prosperity.

It seemed an auspicious time to reconsider the comprehensive health plan President Truman had submitted to Congress two years earlier, only to have it languish in committee.

In 1946, however, the Republican Party gained control of Congress in national elections and Senator Robert Taft took over the relevant health committee. Taft made it clear that public health ought to be meted out to the poor as each state saw fit and the poor should accept whatever they got, on whatever terms were dictated. Period.

Some Republicans went further, charging that "socialized medicine" was all part of a Moscow-dictated Communist plan. The Cold War was getting under way both internationally and domestically and public health was caught in the crossfire.

Instead of Truman's plan, Congress passed the Hill-Burton Act of 1946, a bill designed by the AMA. Under Hill-Burton the federal government would spend, over the next three decades, more than $4 billion modernizing and building hospitals. By 1966 some 4,700 hospitals were either built or improved using Hill-Burton funds.[169] And in keeping with another aspect of AMA intent in the law, the new facilities emphasized high-technological approaches to medicine.

The Truman and Eisenhower administration eliminated or outlawed most forms of overt racially discriminatory uses of federal dollars and FDR had banned all War Department purchases from manufacturers that practiced racially biased hiring. Nevertheless, Hill–Burton money was used to build eighty-nine segregated hospitals in the South, medical facilities that barred African-Americans from entry. And some Hill-Burton–funded northern hospitals had policies that amounted to segregation, as less than 1 percent of their patients were black, though they were located in communities heavily populated by African-Americans.[170]

Increasingly, public health responsibilities and curative medicine shifted from small city clinics and private doctors' offices to the new hospitals. And, not surprisingly, expenses rose.[171]

Hill-Burton brought a critical change in the power structure of American health and presaged tensions that would prove critical forty years later. As the power of hospitals rose, and medical technology improved, hospital affiliation became essential for all but country doctors. In time such affiliations became harder to obtain.

By 1960 the medical areas most intimately connected to public health— family practice, pediatrics, infectious diseases, internal medicine, medical social work—had dropped considerably in status, garnering lower pay and less prestige. Conversely, those medical pursuits most closely associated with concepts of hospital-based curative care rose to the top: surgery, oncology, cardiology. And within those higher-prestige fields, physicians and nurses became increasingly specialized over the postwar years.

Commensurate with the growth of hospital power would be the rise of private health insurance, which was chiefly obtained by Americans as a result of collective bargaining between unions and large employers.[172] Less than 20 percent of the U.S. population was covered by any form of health insurance in 1945, and most of that offered limited protection that failed to cover key costs accrued in hospitalization. By 1960, however, about 25 percent of hospital costs would be covered by insurance.[173] After passage of the Hill-Burton Act hospital spending drove overall health costs upward at an accelerated pace.

The primary driver of private health insurance was corporate America. As the country's largest companies made concessions to labor that provided health coverage, the numbers of insured Americans rose.

But inherent in this development was a bias toward social power. Those elements of labor that were best organized, or worked in the most pivotal industries, were in position to exact superior health plans from their employers. In consequence, by the 1970s health insurance would be provided to those workers who were in the best financial position to buy their own, if necessary. The poorest workers would have no coverage.[174] And private insurance was to have a positive influence on the finances and power of hospitals, as it readily reimbursed hospital costs but played virtually no role in public health or the care of indigent patients.[175]

"Third-party coverage offered a direct incentive for care to be given inside rather than outside the hospital," observed University of Pennsylvania historian Rosemary Stevens.[176]

This trend didn't immediately render public health irrelevant in the United States, of course. There was little, if any, profit to be made in epidemic prevention and control, venereal disease surveillance, tuberculosis-related efforts, prenatal screening of poor women, and the like. These services would remain in the hands of government and charitable services. But the administrators of public health programs would, over time, see their prestige plummet, comparative salaries fall, facilities age and become technologically inferior to local hospitals, and their clientele base shift away from society as a whole toward the most indigent and socially alienated segments of the population. And as the postwar years wore on, the field of public health would become so wretchedly remunerated compared to curative medicine that its professionals were likely to be drawn from one of two pools: highly motivated altruists or mediocre scientists, doctors, and nurses.

Exacerbating this tension between public and private health care was a cardinal change in American lifestyles, as characterized by a new type of community which was created, culturally and physically designed, to exist in a kind of limbo between urban and rural life: the suburb. With a baby boom under way and with war veterans' subsidies in hand, millions of young families were seeking a way out of the cramped, polluted cities.

In the booming postwar economy 11 million suburban homes were built between 1948 and 1958; and 83 percent of national population movement and growth during those years flowed to those newly created communities, most of them generally inhabited by fewer than fifty thousand people.[177] Much of the Hill-Burton hospital construction money went to building suburban hospitals.

Suburbanization of America would continue well into the 1980s, and its impact upon public health would be multifaceted.

Suburbs were automobile cultures; air pollution created by millions of commuting cars was the immediate companion of suburbanization. With car culture came a lack of community cohesiveness. Suburban Americans nation-wide began to experience what Los Angelenos had long known: social isolation and anonymity. The combination of heightened privacy, lack of community co-hesiveness, and antipathy toward the cities they had abandoned would make suburbanites uniquely difficult for public health authorities to reach.

Abandoned by the white middle class, cities rapidly deteriorated. Without their middle- and professional-class tax bases, New York, Chicago, Pittsburgh, Detroit, and other large urban centers could no longer maintain their public infrastructures. The erosion pushed still more flight from the cities.

As early as 1949 the impact was shockingly obvious; many American cities suddenly had slums in their downtown cores. Congress saw this and approved funds for construction of 810,000 public housing units to be built in place of the recent urban squalor. But by 1955 not even a quarter of those units had been constructed and many so-called urban renewal projects were turning into eye-sores and centers of crime. By the 1960s "the projects," as they were called, and degenerated neighborhoods of most U.S. cities would be racially stratified cen-ters of explosive antigovernment sentiment, all but impenetrable to public health officials.

After World War II urban public health was still to face, and despite its deterioration often meet, some of its classic challenges.

New York City had always been the primary microbial connecting point between the United States and the rest of the world. In the 1940s immigration ceased drawing heavily from Europe, and shifted to tropical sites that offered a new set of microbial hitchhikers. By 1948 Gotham was the number one immi-gration destination for Caribbean people, particularly those from Puerto Rico.[178]

In the late winter of 1947 a tourist brought smallpox from Mexico City to New York City.[179]

Eugene Le Bar was not feeling well when he reached Gotham, but he checked into a hotel and began sightseeing.[180] Less than a week later, Le Bar died of smallpox.

New York City hadn't had a smallpox outbreak since 1902, when 310 peo-ple died of the disease. There were few doctors or nurses who had ever seen a smallpox case and the Department of Health's laboratory had to turn to the military for help, as it no longer had reagents that could be used to diagnose the disease.

After Le Bar's diagnosis was confirmed, Health Commissioner Dr. Israel Weinstein ordered the department's lab onto a twenty-four-hour-a-day vaccine production schedule. The goal was to make enough to immunize the entire population of New York City—a decision warranted by uncertainty about how long prior vaccinations might continue to afford protection. And he commanded a vigorous surveillance search for additional smallpox cases. Their task was awesome, as Le Bar had walked all over the city for days, then checked into two hospitals.

Nearly every police station, public hospital, child health clinic, labor union hall, large company, and school in the city became a vaccination center. Public health nurse volunteers knocked on doors in every neighborhood in the city, spreading the word. And three thousand volunteers from the Red Cross and a variety of other organizations were corralled into service.

By April 20th, with more than 6 million New Yorkers having been vaccinated, the health department could justifiably boast of having executed the world's largest rapid immunization campaign and limited a potentially devastating epidemic to just eleven cases with only two deaths. By any measure it was a genuine public health triumph.[181]

But as surely as one virus was vanquished, another surfaced. Just one year later: polio. The 1948 outbreak was the worst the nation had experienced since the first one in 1916, and it persisted for years. By 1950, when about thirty-two thousand people contracted the disease, acute poliomyelitis was the most feared communicable disease in the United States.[182]

The National Foundation for Infant Paralysis (NFIP), begun by FDR's friend Basil O'Connor in 1938, waged a March of Dimes campaign in the 1950s to raise funds for polio research. Nearly two-thirds of all people in the country made donations.

The foundation had a public health, not a curative medical, goal. Rather than fund the search for a treatment, O'Connor and his colleagues hoped to eliminate, via development of a vaccine, the threat polio posed to society as a whole.

But the virus was extremely difficult to study until in 1949 the Harvard Medical School's Dr. John Enders and two of his former graduate students, Drs. Thomas Weller and Frederick C. Robbins, made a pivotal discovery and created a simple way to mass produce polio viruses. For their efforts the trio was awarded the 1954 Nobel Prize in Medicine and Physiology.[183]

At the University of Pittsburgh Dr. Jonas Salk seized on the discovery and set to work making a polio vaccine. By 1953 Salk had a killed virus vaccine. But the key proved to be adding an adjuvant (a potentizer) developed by Dr. Jules Freund at New York's Public Health Research Institute.[184]

Gotham's Health Commissioner Dr. Leona Baumgartner announced the discovery of the adjuvant to proud New Yorkers in 1953, declaring the city's intention to be the first test site of large-scale human use of the Salk vaccine. In the fall of 1953 more than eighty thousand six-to-eight-year-old New York City schoolchildren rolled up their sleeves for shots of either Salk's vaccine or a placebo. In 1954 and '55 tens of thousands of children nationwide enlisted as Polio Pioneers to serve as willing guinea pigs for the vaccine.[185] And though every aspect of the Salk vaccine effort was mired in politics, ethical debates, and production and distribution snafus, there were never shortages of schoolchildren lining up for polio shots. The fear of polio was far greater than any parental concerns about the experimental nature of the vaccine.[186]

And on April 12, 1955—a date deliberately selected because it marked the tenth anniversary of the death of polio victim Franklin Delano Roosevelt—Jonas Salk announced that the polio vaccine was safe and effective. The reaction nationwide was jubilant—nearly as celebratory as on the announcement of V-J Day ten years earlier. Church bells rang from coast to coast. When commuters in Los Angeles heard the news on their car radios, thousands spontaneously began honking their horns, stopping their cars, and shouting with joy on gridlocked freeways. Schools all over the country held celebration assemblies. And every news organization worldwide spread the word in elated tones.

At that moment, few doubted that Salk's vaccine was one of the great triumphs of public health. It offered hope that similar techniques could be deployed for development of vaccines against other killer diseases.

The moment the Salk vaccine went into widespread use in the spring of 1955 polio began to disappear from North America. But Salk's key scientific rival, Albert Sabin, warned prophetically, "Everybody in the public health field knows that when you reach the point where you begin to inoculate an agent into millions of children, your problems have only just begun."[187]

Indeed, they had. One of the Salk vaccine manufacturers, Cutter Laboratories of California, failed to adequately kill the viruses from which they made vaccine, thereby causing polio in 220 children and creating a national scandal that nearly wiped out political support for the national public health effort.

What would eventually push polio down to zero in the United States was Sabin's oral vaccine, put into widespread use in 1961. Sabin had always argued that an injected vaccine might protect the individual but could and would not lower the background level of polio in the community. Therefore, he said, the risk of polio would remain, and it would reemerge as a public health threat the moment collective immunity waned. Since no one knew how long Salk's vaccine could keep someone immune to the virus, Sabin's point was worrisome.

And he had solid scientific reasons for insisting upon an oral vaccine. In the course of natural infection, polio viruses are ingested in water and pass from the intestine to the bloodstream and eventually to the central nervous system. Salk's injected vaccine caused the viruses to be destroyed in an individual's bloodstream, but as long they remained in his GI tract, they were free to multiply and be passed back out into the environment in his stools. As a result, the amount of polio present in a given community might not be diminished by that population's use of the Salk vaccine.

Sabin invented ways to keep polio viruses alive in crippled, nonlethal form. These attenuated viruses, mixed with Freund's adjuvant and a harmless liquid, could be swallowed. And, because they were alive, the attenuated polio viruses could make their way into the intestines and stimulate profound local immunity.

The new vaccine droplets began to be dripped into the mouths of schoolchildren nationwide in 1961. Despite the marginal risk[188] of acquiring poliomyelitis from Sabin's vaccine, the oral formulation had two distinct advantages over Salk's injectable one: it eliminated polio viruses from the environment and it erased all hazards of needle-borne disease.

Needles and syringes, though mainstays of medical and public health practices since the turn of the century, were well known to be capable of carrying and transmitting diseases. As early as 1933, Omaha physician Oliver Nickum had identified cases of malaria spread among Nebraskans who shared syringes for purposes of injecting narcotics.[189] By the mid-1940s the medical literature was full of reports of hepatitis, malaria,[190] and jaundice cases in hospitals where needles were reused on several patients.[191] Other diseases, such as bacterial meningitis and tuberculosis, were also known to be spread through medicinal and public health use—and reuse—of syringes.[192]

Extensive debate among physicians about various methods for sterilizing syringes between reuses clearly showed that nothing short of high heat autoclaving could do the trick.[193] Nevertheless, in the 1950s and '60s the exigencies of epidemic prevention took precedence and well-intended physicians, nurses, and public health officers routinely filled syringes with several vaccine doses at once, and then used the same device sequentially on several people. And in hospitals reuse of syringes, particularly for anesthesia drips and routine injections, was common practice.

Australian physicians reported that eight cases of polio had resulted from reuse of a syringe on fifty-three people in a 1949 diphtheria immunization campaign near Melbourne.[194] And German and Dutch physicians published word of other small outbreaks of diseases, resulting from vaccine campaigns employing reused syringes.[195]

Nevertheless, amid the euphoria elicited by discovery of the vaccine for polio (and one for measles in 1963, and for rubella and mumps in 1969), few public health crusaders, physicians, or members of the public gave the syringe issue much thought. Years later this omission would come back to haunt U.S. and global public health leaders amid accusations that reused syringes deployed in mass vaccination campaigns, particularly in developing countries, had spread everything from poliomyelitis[196] and Ebola virus[197] to monkeypox[198] hepatitis C, and the human immunodeficiency virus.[199]

In the 1950s and '60s, however, the world eagerly embraced vaccinology, and it certainly saved remarkable numbers of lives. In 1985 the U.S. Centers for Disease Control (CDC) would estimate that, for example, the combined measles, mumps, and rubella (MMR) vaccine introduced in 1968 had spared the lives of 24,600 children in the United States and saved the nation $1,385,500,000 in direct and indirect medical and productivity costs *per year* (in figures value adjusted to 1983 dollars).[200] By 1990 vaccine-preventable childhood infections—the scourge of Biggs's day—would be responsible for less than 0.1 percent of all deaths in North America, Japan, and Western Europe.[201]

Immediately following World War II, American political and public health leaders enthusiastically began exporting their achievements. When the United Nations was formed in 1946, and with it a health committee that two years later would be called the World Health Organization (WHO), it was with the strong blessing of the Truman administration. In his 1949 inaugural address President Truman announced that a key feature of U.S. foreign policy would be to "embark on a bold new program for making the benefits of our scientific advances and industrial progress available for the improvement and growth of underdeveloped areas." And by 1953 the United States, chiefly represented by scientists from the Centers for Communicable Diseases, was involved in public health efforts in thirty-eight nations.

To be sure, there had long been American health crusaders working overseas. But two new, strong motivations prevailed in the 1950s. First, leaders in the field were proud of their achievements in vaccines development, antibiotics, water sanitation, sewer design, hospital construction, mosquito control, and tuberculosis eradication. And second, politicians who focused on the Cold War saw saving children's lives as a powerful way to win allies in the nonaligned Third World. In 1955, with Cold War anticommunism in full swing, conservatives took delight in underscoring that it was capitalist America, not the Soviet Union, that had first triumphed against polio. Remarkably, given the sorry state of Russian health that would be revealed four decades later, Western leaders in the 1950s believed that the Soviets had, as they claimed, created a public health and scientific paradise that threatened to put capitalist America's to global shame.

In 1950, after straddling this Cold War fence, WHO's World Health Assembly signaled the agency's intention to tip its balance, when need be, away from the superpowers and toward the poorest nations on earth: "Public health officers have for long affirmed that economic development and health are inseparable and complementary and that the social, cultural, and economic development of a community, and its state of health, are interdependent."

The driving incentive for most American scientists, physicians, and nurses who worked with international health organizations in poor countries was not Cold War politics, but a zeal not unlike that which drove Hermann Biggs in turn-of-the-century New York City: they believed deeply in the mission of public health and in the reliability of the scientific tools at their disposal.

The Cold War escalated in 1949 when the United States created the North Atlantic Treaty Organization (NATO),[202] which openly functioned as a security alignment for Western Europe's defense against the Soviet Union. The Soviets successfully tested an atomic bomb that year, making them America's military match. And both the United States and USSR began development of an even more lethal weapon—the hydrogen bomb.[203]

Then the Cold War turned hot in Korea, where Communist North Korean forces and the United States fought between 1950 and 1953.

America's government and many of its citizens became deeply paranoid—as, unbeknownst to most people in the United States at the time, did their counterparts in the USSR. A terrible so-called Red Scare affected every aspect of life in the United States during the later 1940s and the 1950s, whipped up by such noted anti-Communists as Senator Joseph McCarthy, Congressman Richard Nixon, the House Un-American Activities Committee, and columnists Drew Pearson and Walter Winchell. By the time World War II hero General Dwight D. Eisenhower moved into the White House in 1953, suspected "Communists" across the nation were being purged from their jobs and service in government at every tier.

In such an atmosphere most overseas programs run by the U.S. government were, by necessity, caught up in Cold War politics. At WHO gatherings U.S. and USSR representatives sparred over whose populations exhibited healthier lives. Each accused the other of having CIA or KGB plants within their WHO delegations.

Even public health comments made domestically concerning international issues could land the speaker in hot water. A classic case in point: the Linus Pauling/Edward Teller debates over the public health impacts of radioactive fallout from the hundreds of surface nuclear bomb tests conducted by weapons designers in the USSR, United States, France, and China.

In the decade after Hiroshima, Americans had varied and generally confused impressions about atomic weapons. Most frankly didn't understand either the physics or the terrible power of the weapons, and few appreciated the risks of radiation.[204]

For three decades Linus Pauling had been one of the world's top protein chemists, working out of his California Institute of Technology (Caltech) laboratory on problems of protein structure. In the 1940s Pauling decided to tackle one of the most intriguing puzzles then facing biologists in the United States, namely the mysterious relationship between proteins and genetics. They knew that there was a missing link somewhere, though Lysenko's fantasies in the Soviet Union insisted otherwise.

In the 1940s a chemist at Columbia University in New York City, Edwin Chargoff, found that DNA was essentially a simple sugar and phosphate backbone that held together—in the case of human cells—four types of compounds called nucleotides. The precise and unvarying ratios among and within these compounds, Chargoff's numbers, were published in 1949,[205] instantly creating a sensation among Pauling and his many competitors in pursuit of the holy grail of genetics.

In 1951 Pauling modeled a key structure of human proteins in his lab, calling it an alpha helix. But it would be two junior scientists at Oxford University in Cambridge, England, who would figure it out in 1953. American James Watson and Britain's Francis Crick deciphered the relationship between Pauling's alpha helices and Chargoff's numbers, discovering the structure of DNA.

In 1956 Crick published what he dubbed the "central dogma," the basis of all life on Earth, delineating the precise relationship between DNA and proteins. Crick's central dogma turned on lightbulbs in the brains of thousands of scientists worldwide (except in the Soviet Union, where the information was banned), prompting a flurry of discovery that would lead to the Biology Revolution of the later twentieth and early twenty-first centuries.

Long before the structure of DNA was elucidated, researchers had shown that human chromosomes could be irreversibly damaged by exposure to various types of radiation. Once the structure of DNA was determined, it was clear to Pauling how that would occur.[206]

In 1948, at the urging of his liberal wife, Ava Helen, Pauling began speaking out against the anti-Communist purges then under way in Los Angeles schools and colleges and all repression of scientists in the United States.[207] He paid a high price for his outspokenness, losing all of his federal research grants, coming under harsh attack from the Los Angeles Times and dozens of other news organizations, and in 1951 nearly losing his job at Caltech.

For Pauling and other biologists who spoke against the bomb, it was reports of postblast illnesses that served as motivation. Gamma radiation emitted by the blast disrupted cell division and every human body function deteriorated for months after exposure. Hair fell out, blood thinned, the immune system collapsed, skin peeled and flaked off, superficial wounds festered into gaping, incurable sores.

Physicist Edward Teller, a Hungarian Jewish immigrant who had played a key role in designing Fat Man, the bomb dropped on Hiroshima, was deeply affected emotionally by the Soviet takeover of Hungary in 1948. Like most of the Manhattan Project participants, he had initially favored creation of an A-bomb in order to stop Hitler and save Europe's Jews. After World War II, it was Stalin whom Teller despised, and the Hungarian believed that defeat of the Soviet Union would require a far more powerful weapon. Teller was thoroughly convinced that without what he called a Superbomb the United States would be overrun by communism and he, an outspoken anti-Stalinist, would be thrown into a Soviet gulag somewhere in Wyoming or Montana.[208] He therefore led a team that designed the thermonuclear hydrogen bomb—the H-bomb.

On March 1, 1954, Teller's first Superbomb was dropped in the middle of the Pacific Ocean on the coral atoll Bikini. It was seven hundred and fifty times more powerful than Fat Man and it spread radioactive bits of Bikini over a radius of seven thousand square miles.

Six months later, the Soviet Union tested its first H-bomb, dropping it—incredibly—on a Russian-inhabited Siberian village called Totskoye, located just six hundred miles from Moscow.[209]

Following the Soviet detonation, several U.S. administrations perpetuated a public fantasy of survivable thermonuclear war. It put additional burdens on beleaguered health departments. They now had to teach schoolchildren of the 1950s and '60s to "duck and cover," for example (get under their desks as soon as teachers gave the signal that a "Soviet hydrogen bomb" had fallen and carefully cover their eyes lest they be blinded). Some health departments had to assume radiation and civil defense duties. New York created a Medical Emergency Division to plan a response to nuclear attack, with part of its planning designating hundreds of subway stations as bomb shelters. Families were instructed to build individual bomb shelters similar to those many English families carved out of their basements during the German bombing of London. Inside those shelters, the Atomic Energy Commission (AEC) instructed, should be sufficient provisions for the family for a year.

Pauling and hundreds of other scientists were incredulous. They felt that the U.S. government was betraying a vital public health trust with the American people by deliberately creating a sham notion of survivable nuclear war. They argued that the radiation in nuclear fallout would make any bomb site unlivable for decades, possibly centuries.

The bomb makers, of course, knew this to be so, though it would be decades before their views would be made public. In a 1940 internal memo circulated at the Manhattan Project, scientists informed the Roosevelt administration: "Owing to the spreading of radioactive substances with the wind, the bomb could probably not be used without killing large numbers of civilians, and this may make it unsuitable as a weapon for use by this country. . . ."[210]

At the end of 1954 Pauling, now the newly famous winner of the Nobel Prize for Chemistry, set out on a world speaking tour to warn of the effects of low-level radiation on human cells. The AEC's position was that whatever radiation was produced by nuclear bomb blasts—and the agency consistently low-balled those estimates—would simply add incrementally to natural background radiation, increasing the burden of atmospheric radiation by just 1 percent above natural background levels.

Few scientists familiar with nuclear fallout believed the AEC's numbers. But rather than debate that point, Pauling simply said, okay, let's suppose it is just 1 percent. Well, there are an estimated 1.5 million babies now born annually with genetic birth defects caused by background radiation. A 1 percent increase in radiation would produce fifteen thousand more babies each year who suffered such mutations.

Nuclear fallout, Pauling declared, was a public health catastrophe, and the American government was betraying its citizens by claiming to the contrary. The bomb emitted strontium-90, which would concentrate in the bones of growing children, and iodine-131, which would collect in people's thyroids, causing thyroid cancer and dysfunction, Pauling insisted. As a reward for his views, Pauling was placed under close FBI scrutiny for the rest of his life. Pauling persisted with his antinuclear campaign, in 1958 debating on national television the fallout issue with Teller and traveling to the Soviet Union to demand that they, too, cease surface bomb tests.

In 1961, newly inaugurated President John F. Kennedy invited Pauling to the White House and pledged support for a test ban.[211] The surface nuclear test ban would be formally signed by the United States and USSR on August 5, 1963. And two months later Linus Pauling would again receive a call from Stockholm—this time awarding him the Nobel Peace Prize.

It is clear from public records[212] that are now available that the AEC knew all along that any use of nuclear weapons would create a public health catastrophe.[213] Nevertheless, in the name of national security the Eisenhower administration had veiled all radiation research conducted by the AEC and the Defense Department in secrecy and misinformation. And in 1955, with creation of the first nuclear power plant, it extended that veil to cover the civilian sector.

For nearly four more decades, all information regarding the public health impacts of radiation would be rife with critical flaws. The AEC and its descendant, the Nuclear Regulatory Commission (NRC), would hide—*literally*—mountains of data and obfuscate or distort the information that was released. Employees of both government and civilian nuclear industries and plants would be compelled to sign secrecy agreements, violation of which would constitute grounds for prosecution on charges of treason or espionage. Scientists who independently studied the human health impacts of low-level ionizing radiation would be vilified, their reputations smeared. And, to be honest, their research did often prove unreliable because their access to the critical data entombed in the AEC archives was so limited.

For the rest of the twentieth century, the American public would exhibit simultaneously both abject fear of all things radioactive and adoring acceptance of microwave-emitting ovens and cellular phones, as well as the concept of nuclear deterrence. Public health sciences would largely fail to find a rational position, or even agree, on such basic concepts as safe doses of exposure, cumulative dosage effects, the threshold theory of radiation dosing, the relative safety of nuclear power plants, the differential damage produced by various types and wavelengths of radiation, or appropriate methods of disposing of and storing spent nuclear waste.

In the 1990s the Clinton administration would finally declassify many of the old AEC and Nuclear Regulatory Commission (NRC) documents, opening a window on ghastly human experiments, most of which were conducted by well-meaning civilian physicians, working in major U.S. teaching hospitals, who were largely oblivious to both the risks and ethical questionability of their actions.[214] But some of the experiments and cover-ups of public health problems would prove to have been unquestionably unethical and immoral.[215] These horrors would only see the light of day after the collapse of America's chief adversary, the Soviet Union. The public health radiation field would, at the close of the century, still be highly polarized and conflicted.[216]

Public health radiation research and government credibility and policy were, then, chief casualties of the Cold War.[217]

Although New York City Health Commissioner John Mahoney wrote editorials decrying the apathy toward civil defense he felt New Yorkers were exhibiting, by 1952 it was obvious that few of them either found his outcries credible or believed that they could, indeed even wanted to, survive an H-bomb attack by living in subway tunnels.[218] Mahoney's own staff rebelled, too: they didn't believe in the "duck and cover" message themselves and they were sick of taking on more responsibilities for paltry pay.

The salaries of Gotham's Department of Health employees had been frozen for a decade, a period when their private sector medical colleagues' incomes were swelling way beyond the rates of inflation or average U.S. salary increases. But New York City was continuing to lose its tax base to the suburbs and the department was expected to do more with less. In 1952 the American Public Health Association (APHA) assessed the performance of the New York City department:[219] "The Department of Health of New York City was once an outstanding leader in municipal affairs. It was one of the best health departments in the country. It no longer is."

The widespread play the critique got in New York's media drummed up public concern, and swept Robert Wagner Jr., a strong supporter of public health, into the mayor's office in the 1953 elections. He named Dr. Leona Baumgartner his health commissioner, and the flamboyant physician went directly to the public for support. She gave weekly health reports over the radio, speaking with a zeal New York hadn't heard from a health leader since Hermann Biggs.

Baumgartner understood the new concept of public relations. She realized that health programs could no longer simply demand or expect popular support, particularly given the competition they were getting from hospitals and private medicine. With remarkable prescience, Baumgartner decided in 1954 that the best way to reach Americans in the future was going to be via a new technology called television.

Overnight the United States had become a TV nation.[220] Over time, people in the United States would spend more and more of their life glued to what disparagers called "the boob tube," and their collective consumer behavior would reflect the barrage of TV advertising to which they were subjected. Their overall caloric intake would rise and their level of exercise would drop.[221]

By 1955, a year after it went on the air, Baumgartner's weekly TV spot was being watched by 5 million viewers nationwide.[222] She proved a very adept public health propagandist. In 1954 her department's budget was $18.4 million. Six years later it was $30.7 million. Baumgartner turned her entire department into public health proselytizers. Collectively they gave about twenty-five hundred lectures and speeches per year, made dozens of films, and addressed radio audiences every week. An entire health education department, staffed by fifty people, was needed to coordinate the enormous public relations campaign.[223]

The health of Americans was undergoing a great transition in the 1950s as the mortality impact of infectious diseases receded, to be replaced by cancer, heart disease, and accidents. Baumgartner's department recognized that in 1957, "public health and the work of the Health Department is ever-changing, for the nature of health problems change. As one is solved, another emerges."[224]

Among the least popular of the "new" problems Baumgartner and her counterparts in cities all over the United States faced was heroin. Invented in 1898 by the German company Bayer Pharmaceuticals, Inc., heroin had been in use—legally and illegally—for decades in the United States, but didn't become a major problem until 1948, when traffickers flooded the streets of New York with it. Between 1948 and 1960 the city, and most of the country's other urban centers, suffered wave after wave of what public health officials, the police, and the media termed "drug epidemics."[225] With the rise in heroin use—almost exclusively by people aged fifteen to twenty-nine years, most of them males—came hepatitis, which spread among the users through shared needles and syringes.

New York City had little idea what to do with people who had grown addicted to heroin. Though criminalization of the problem had been the longstanding approach, the health department tried its best to offer heroin users an alternative way to get off drugs short of going cold turkey in jail. But as Baumgartner said in her report to the city for 1960, "There is a growing awareness that the narcotic addict should be looked upon primarily as a sick person, not solely as a criminal. But inasmuch as the physiological basis and curative treatment of the narcotic addict are still both unknown, programs for the addict are obviously palliative and relatively ineffective."[226]

Surveys from the mid-1950s to the end of the century put the number of heroin addicts in the United States at, variously, between 300,000 and 1.5 million.[227] Some law enforcement and political leaders painted a picture of heroin use that, terrifyingly, focused not upon the very real nightmare of the lives of the addicts themselves but on their alleged antisocial, even demonic, behavior.[228] The specter of deranged heroin addicts roaming urban streets further nudged the middle class toward the suburbs. And though in absolute numbers whites always dominated the ranks of American heroin users, the middle class envisioned the dangerous narcotics user with a black face.

Indeed, heroin use did concentrate and appear more obvious in the nation's increasingly rundown African-American ghettos.

Following World War II the pace of black migration northward and westward quickened, but when southern African-Americans reached Boston, New York, Chicago, Los Angeles, Detroit, and other destinations, they found the cost of housing beyond their limited means and real estate segregation an obvious urban reality.[229] Though the administrations of Eisenhower, Kennedy, and Johnson marked a time of remarkable prosperity and economic growth for the nation as a whole,[230] more than half of the nation's black population lived in poverty throughout the 1950s and well into the 1960s. A key reason was job discrimination. And rigid segregation in schools forced most blacks to settle for second-rate educations.[231]

African-Americans during the 1950s instigated legal actions and staged a series of both spontaneous and well-planned protests that would come to be known as the civil rights movement. By 1956 Reverend Martin Luther King Jr. of Montgomery, Alabama, had emerged as its clear leader. The old gospel song that urged people to "Hold on just a little while longer / Everything will be all right" captured the spirit of determined strength that marked the civil rights movement in the 1950s. But by the 1960s, the nation's African-American populations, particularly the young urbanites, had become much more defiant and rebellious.

One hundred years after southern whites seceded from the United States to form a confederacy dedicated to perpetuation of slavery, some African-American leaders in the North were calling for black a revolution.[232]

"To be a Negro in this country and to be relatively conscious is to be in a rage all the time," writer James Baldwin said in 1961.[233]

The deep racial divide reverberated in the medical and public health systems. Dozens of blacks—perhaps hundreds, though nobody was keeping count—died because emergency rooms at white hospitals refused them treatment.[234] (Among the most famous of such tragedies was the death of blues singer Bessie Smith.) In order to obtain the right for qualified black nurses and physicians to practice medicine in Newark City Hospital, National Association for the Advancement of Colored People attorney Thurgood Marshall had to sue the state of New Jersey. Until 1940 the American Medical Association listed all African-American members with the abbreviation "Col." next to their names, indicating that they were "colored" doctors.

By the late 1950s the Eisenhower administration had made it clear to most of the states that no federally funded hospitals could deny medical care on the basis of the color of the patient's skin. Nevertheless, a new form of segregation emerged—black patients were turned away from prestigious facilities and directed to city- and county-run public hospitals, which all but the poorest whites typically shunned.[235]

Public health departments in the fifties were typically all white, or had black employees working only at bottom-level jobs. The most well-meaning of white leaders, such as New York's Baumgartner, were bewildered by the hostility that greeted their efforts in black ghettos like Harlem, East New York, and the South Bronx, even though for a decade the American Public Health Association had backed up the all-black National Medical Association's call for an end to discrimination in health and medical practices.

By 1961 President Kennedy's Department of Health, Education, and Welfare (HEW) was deluged with claims of racial discrimination practices by federally funded hospitals,[236] but legislation that would have empowered HEW to cut off funding to discriminatory medical facilities was languishing in a Senate subcommittee. So HEW did little more than catalog the complaints and mail query letters to the offending hospitals. The Civil Rights Leadership Conference called HEW's inaction "a silent but nonetheless full partner in the perpetuation of discriminatory practices."[237]

In June 1963 President Kennedy finally introduced his version of a civil rights act, Title VI, which stipulated that acceptance of federal funds would carry a quid pro quo of nondiscriminatory practices. Growing support for Dr. King and national outrage over the disgraceful actions of southern whites—particularly their political leaders—had swung the political pendulum to support for Kennedy's civil rights legislation. The time seemed ripe, at last, for change.

But on November 22, 1963, President Kennedy was assassinated on a campaign swing through Dallas.

Five days after the tragic assassination, President Johnson told a joint session of Congress that "no memorial oration or eulogy could more eloquently honor President Kennedy's memory than the earliest possible passage of the civil rights bill for which he fought so long. We have talked enough in this country about equal rights. We have talked for one hundred years or more. It is time now to write the next chapter and to write it in the books of law."[238]

Johnson's HEW secretary, Anthony Celebreeze, was immediately saddled with the hot issue of segregated hospitals. And he stalled—took no action—hoping that the Supreme Court would resolve the matter by hearing *Simkins v. Cone*, a case brought by a black man accusing Cone Memorial Hospital of North Carolina of racial discrimination.[239] But on March 2, 1964, the Court let stand a lower court decision in favor of the hospital.

Urged by Johnson to whip up support for the civil rights bill among his fellow liberals,[240] Vice President Hubert H. Humphrey specifically claimed the *Simkins v. Cone* decision as cause for immediate passage: "Racial discrimination in medical facilities is at least partly responsible for the fact that in North Carolina the rate of infant mortality (for Negroes) is twice the rate for whites and maternal deaths are five times greater."

On June 10, 1964, with bipartisan support, Johnson's Civil Rights Act of 1964 was passed by both houses. Title VI of the act eliminated all legal forms of racial discrimination in the practices of medicine and public health.

In a harbinger of the way the battlefield would shift, Arizona senator Barry Goldwater expressed disgust with the act,[241] signaling a new spin on civil rights, adopted in a political atmosphere that had made overt supporters of racial segregation political pariahs. The new tack for the extreme conservative wing of the Republican Party, then led by Goldwater, was to attack federal authority for imposing socially liberalizing laws.

In 1964 President Johnson pushed passage of two other massive initiatives that would profoundly affect public health: his War on Poverty program and Medicare. LBJ's overall goal was to create what he called the Great Society through a federal effort akin to Roosevelt's New Deal. A key difference, however, was that while Roosevelt pushed large-scale federal spending during a time of tremendous economic deprivation in America, LBJ wanted a similar level of spending for social programs at a time when most Americans were enjoying tremendous prosperity. That was a hard sell.

When Johnson declared his War on Poverty, twenty-one million people in the United States were living below the administration's poverty line. At the bottom of the heap were three social groups targeted by Great Society programs: people over sixty-five years of age who, having been cleaned out by the Depression, had little in savings upon which to live out their final years; blacks; and women who were single parents. Among the remedial programs Johnson pushed as part of his Great Society effort were Medicare, Medicaid, and Aid to Families with Dependent Children (AFDC).

The net effect of Great Society initiatives was the creation of a federal system aimed at offering the nation's poor, elderly, children, and immigrants an opportunity to join the American mainstream. Johnson's intention was for the programs to act as a sort of stepladder that would put individuals within reach of prosperity. But it would be up to the individual, on his or her own, to make the final ascent. It was never LBJ's intent to create a no-load handout system or turn the federal government into a welfare state. And his programs would no doubt have unfolded more successfully had Johnson not been irreparably involved in the Vietnam War.[242]

Spending on the war created enormous budget deficits, draining resources LBJ had hoped to use on domestic programs. Military spending rose from an already all-time high of $49.6 billion in 1965 to $80.5 billion in 1968. It was money the U.S. Treasury couldn't spare and it started America on a downward spiral into debt.

"I knew from the start," Johnson later told author Doris Kearnes Goodwin,[243] "that I was bound to be crucified either way I moved. If I left the woman I really loved—the Great Society—in order to get involved with that bitch of a war on the other side of the world, then I would lose everything at home. All my programs. All my hopes to feed the hungry and feed the homeless. All my dreams."

Except for the Civil Rights Act of 1964, Johnson did, indeed, lose most of his dreams to the war bitch. Every one of the Great Society programs he had envisioned was eventually enacted by Congress in a form unrecognizable to its designer. The programs as enacted were seriously flawed and the mistakes would have profound public health implications. Medicare and Medicaid, in particular, would completely reshape American health care and public health. And the end result would not be as LBJ had envisioned.

While Congress and the administration debated details of these social programs, the nation was ripping itself apart. Riots, demonstrations, generational polarization, racial conflict, and labor struggles were exploding in every nook and cranny of the society.

Johnson was the chief victim of the so-called credibility gap between Washington and the people of the United States, but every member of Congress felt the sting of public mistrust and attack from many sides: the war in Vietnam necessitated a draft, which fueled an already active student movement and turned millions of college students into angry protestors. Despite passage of the Civil Rights Act, life in African-American urban ghettos only worsened, prompting explosive riots. And many white, working-class Americans fought militant battles to protect the jobs and lifestyles they felt were threatened by hippies and blacks. Torn asunder, the nation was not in a thoughtful mood, and the sixties proved to be a reactive, rather than a contemplative, era.

As a result, Congress passed legislation aimed at massive U.S. crises, such as lack of health care and entrenched poverty, but did so in a piecemeal fashion that reflected the push and pull of powerful lobbying constituencies and interest groups. The goals were to eliminate poverty and increase access to health care. But few political leaders stood back and asked: How? Why? An overarching vision was lacking.

Between 1900 and 1940 average U.S. life expectancies at birth for females had risen from 48.3 years to 65.2 years, 16.9 additional years of life. Male life expectancy in that time frame increased from 46.3 years to 60.8 years, a total gain of 14.5 years. These fantastic gains were made after the germ theory revolution but before development of modern vaccines or antibiotics. They preceded most forms of treatment for cardiac disease and for cancer, short of surgical tumor removal. And the gains occurred in the absence of a vast nationwide network of hospitals.

Perhaps more striking, they were achieved in a nation that had three times declined creation of a universal health care system and, thus, had routinely denied medical care to three generations of America's twentieth-century poor and people of color. As early as 1911, when Britain created its national compulsory medical insurance system, American voters had signaled their desire to have some sort of government-ensured equity for access to health care.[244] In 1919 Californians even gave the concept their voted approval. But the AMA, using the then-new pejorative "socialized medicine,"[245] quashed that and all subsequent efforts to create universal American health care.

The great gains were made, therefore, not by medicine, but as a result of large-scale public health efforts that had sought to prevent infectious diseases through community intervention. As early as 1900 Hermann Biggs had proven that such interventions saved money and were therefore not simply matters of humane policy but also made sound fiscal sense.[246] The basic philosophy had focused on the collective: the health of individuals would be protected by raising the level of health of the community as a whole. Some of the gains were the result of economic improvements and rising standards of living. Others reflected enhanced nutritional norms.[247]

In contrast, between 1940 and 1965 (when Congress was debating Medicare) female life expectancy rose from 65.2 to 73.7 years, for a gain of just 8.5

years. Male life expectancy increased from 60.8 to 66.8 years, a net gain of just 6 years.[248] Perhaps more significant was the trend in average remaining life expectancies after Americans reached the age of sixty years. In 1900 the average woman in the United States who had managed to reach that ripe age could expect to live an additional 24.4 years and reach age eighty-four. The average sixty-year-old male faced 23.1 more years of life and would live to be eighty-three years of age.

By 1940 average additional life expectancy for sixty-year-old Americans was 33.3 years for women and 30 years for men. Serious gains had been made, adding 8.9 years of elderly life for women and 6.9 years for men. By 1965, elderly women had gained another 4.2 years; elderly men just 1.7 years.[249]

A shift was obviously occurring and the question to be asked as infectious disease crises receded in significance was, what population-based strategies might appropriately address the new era? What was to be the goal of Medicare? Was it to increase these average American life expectancies? To improve the quality of those years of added life? To equalize availability to modern medicine for all elderly Americans? To increase the size of the paying medical consumer populations? To enhance the role and size of hospitals in America? To compensate physicians for services, as few might have practiced gratis for elderly patients?

The questions were never really asked or answered. Instead, political leaders simply reflected cultural trends of the day and assumed that what everyone wanted—and *needed*—was more medical care.

Average Americans knew in 1965 that they were healthier than their parents or grandparents had been. They were taller, stronger, gave infectious diseases little thought, could have sex without fear of dying of syphilis, could swim in a public pool without pausing to consider polio, and had vast and varied quantities of food at their disposal. Newly discovered drugs or vaccines were announced almost daily. On television, doctors were portrayed as omnipresent geniuses who could save and heal the world. Overall, people living in the United States in 1965 had a remarkably optimistic, even adoring, belief in new technology.

Social problems—poverty, racism, Communist threats, the war in Vietnam, student unrest—seemed complex and controversial to Americans and there was little societal consensus on any of them. Science and technology, however, offered solutions, strategies, and miracles, especially in medicine. Americans had an almost unquestioning faith that money spent on Big Medicine was money well spent. The human body was, metaphorically, a machine that occasionally broke or, with age, deteriorated. Enough medicine could fix it.

In popular opinion, then, the goals of Medicare, Medicaid, and any other health programs the government supported ought to be two-fold: speed up the pace of medical discovery and make the fruits of that research available to all Americans as quickly as possible. Let the toolbox for broken human machines expand and build more and better body repair shops.

This perspective served physicians and hospitals well, so long as they were left to implement it with as little regulatory oversight and "meddling" from government as possible. The doctors wanted to set the standards of care and hospitals insisted their institutions should control costs. It was a de facto policy of self-regulation by the medical industry.

"Such policy is . . . acutely sensitive to even the possibility that some new drug, piece of equipment, or diagnostic or therapeutic maneuver may contribute to health," wrote economists Robert Evans and Gregory Stoddart.[250] "That someone's health may perhaps be at risk for lack of such intervention is prima facie grounds for close policy attention, and at least a strong argument for provision. Meanwhile the egregious fact that people are suffering, and in some cases dying, as a consequence of processes not directly connected to health care, elicits neither rebuttal nor response."

Comparatively weak voices (in contrast to those of organized medicine) rose from the public health community, arguing for a less simplistic, more global approach to the nation's health. They could not have foreseen how the medicalized model would eventually drive costs to the point where, thirty years later, few Americans could readily afford medical care, but they were tabulating the changing demographic face of health problems in the United States. As New York's Baumgartner put it, they recognized that ". . . technological, ideological, and social changes create new threats, new problems for man. It seems clear that the majority of man's future ills will be of his own making.

"So it is that man's goals for good health are ever changing. With the ever increasing tempo of technological change and the extension of human aspirations it seems likely that changes in the health field will now come more rapidly than they have in the past."[251]

A health transition was, assuredly, under way, but from what, and to what? And why? Many of the gains and victories made on behalf of the nation's health during the first half of the century were still inexplicable in the 1960s. Why, for example, had tuberculosis continued to decline between 1920 and 1945? That is, during a period after the social reforms responsible for the disease's primary decrease had long since had their impact, but before introduction of antibiotics.[252] Where did the devastating 1918 swine influenza come from and how likely would be the future emergence of a similarly devastating pandemic?[253] What precisely was the relationship between poverty and disease?

Though he was employed by Harvard Medical School, the bastion of American medicalization of health, infectious diseases expert René Dubos scoffed at the notion that a massive medical system could address the fundamental roots of the population's health or lack thereof. He argued in his 1961 classic *Mirage of Health*[254] that, "while the modern American boasts . . . the highest standard of living in the world, . . . ten percent of his income must go for medical care and he cannot build hospitals fast enough to accommodate the sick. He is encouraged to believe that money can create drugs for the cure of heart disease, cancer, and mental disease, but he makes no worth-while effort to recognize, let alone correct, the mismanagements of his everyday life that contribute to the high incidence of those conditions."[255]

So, by the mid-1960s the United States still had no developed health *policy*, though it certainly had health *care*. The net effects of Medicare and Medicaid would be to push more and more people into health care, always in the absence of any clear policy that placed such care in a larger context. As a result, public health's power and influence would continue to diminish, while that of the individual's health *care* would rise.

For decades—indeed, since the days of William Petty Graunt's 1662 *Bills of Mortality* for London—public health advocates had noted an intimate relationship between socioeconomic status and health. The Health Transition in post–World War II America somewhat blurred the demographic picture, as cancer and heart disease initially appeared to strike equally across social classes, perhaps even tilting a bit toward wealthier Americans. By the mid-sixties, however, most of the chronic diseases were also displaying a social gradient that brought the greatest grief to the poorest Americans.

It might have been wise to combine the War on Poverty programs with Medicare and Medicaid, creating a single strategic approach to upgrading the health and well-being of Americans.[256]

The 1965 Medicare Act was a two-part law that placed authority for the health care program under the Social Security Administration—*not* under HEW. Under Part A, hospitals were allowed to designate a third agency or nongovernmental organization to oversee their budgets and negotiate with the Social Security Administration. Nearly all hospitals in the country named the private nonprofit "Blues"—the Blue Cross and Blue Shield insurance companies. Part B spelled out physicians' rights to decide appropriate care and, also through the Blues, to bill Social Security for payment.

The federal government relinquished most of its own power to exert price controls, allowing the hospitals and the Blues to work out their own schedules of costs and prices. It also allowed hospitals to build capital costs into patient cost evaluations. Such capital costs might include, for example, the depreciation of hospital buildings that, in many cases, the federal government had paid for under the Hill-Burton Act. This arrangement was like handing every hospital in America a huge chunk of collateral with which to build more wards, buy more equipment, and hire more doctors. And overnight the megahospitals shoved smaller community and neighborhood centers into obscurity or oblivion.

For its first year, FY 1966, Medicare was expected to cover nineteen million Americans over sixty-five years of age with a budget of just $6.5 billion. It did not, however, cover even all of the health needs of those seniors. Indeed, there were so many deductibles under Medicare—and the list grew steadily—that by 1974 elderly Americans would be paying as much out-of-pocket *with* Medicare as they had in 1964 before the creation of Medicare.[257]

Medicaid offered medical coverage under a similar scheme for indigent single-parent households. Administered by states, the original intent was that federal funds would be matched locally to offer generous coverage. In practice, from the very beginning poorer and less generously inclined states put up little or no matching funds and the quality of care afforded under Medicaid varied radically across the country. In many states, Medicaid was administered out of AFDC and welfare offices, putting provision of health in the hands of social welfare agencies. And that would presage a critical danger for the future of American public health programs, which would come under attack as part of an overall rejection of welfare and "federal handouts."

The most immediate impact of Medicare and Medicaid was on patient visits to doctors and hospitals. Before these measures kicked into effect in 1966, the poor and African-Americans rarely saw doctors. Individuals living above the poverty line visited physicians 20 percent more frequently than did poorer Americans, and whites saw their doctors just 2 percent more often than did African-Americans. After 1966 all that changed radically, and by the early seventies the poor and African-Americans were actually visiting doctors more frequently than better off whites.[258]

If, then, the true measure of health was access to doctors and utilization of medical services, the Johnson-era Medicare/Medicaid programs panned out nicely.

But as early as 1967, just a year after the programs began, physicians working in inner-city areas realized that Medicaid was little more than a financing system for second-rate medicine, doled out in rundown public hospitals. Because it required often scarce state matching funds, Medicaid failed to deliver sufficient remuneration to providers to make the patients desirable to private and elite hospitals.[259]

Medicare, in contrast, was extremely attractive to both hospitals and physicians because the Medicare Act put them, along with the Blues, in the driver's seat of cost control. In 1960 the assets of U.S. hospitals totaled $10.8 billion. Four years after Medicare was implemented, hospital assets had more than doubled, reaching $26.7 billion. And by 1977 they would reach $61.1 billion. A six-fold increase in assets achieved in just seventeen years would be admirable for any industry: that hospitals had largely accomplished this by spending U.S. government money, rather than their own dollars, was awesome.[260] Not surprisingly, the hospitals and the Blues consistently found funds provided by the Social Security Administration inadequate and between 1966 and 1976 doubled the amount, per person, of their billings for the average patient's daily hospitalization. Hospital incomes also doubled, but in a shorter time span: just four years, from 1965 to '69. The costs of all basic procedures also rose.[261]

Medicare drove medical cost inflation because the Blues and the Social Security Administration accepted ever-inflating bills and paid them. Since the elderly are the medically neediest members of society and require the most invasive procedures, Medicare clients immediately constituted more than 75 percent of all hospitalized patients. That raised the goal posts, allowing the hospitals to similarly bill insured non-Medicare clients at the same prices. When questioned, the hospitals would often claim that overbilling Medicare and the privately insured covered the costs of taking in the uninsured and poorly reimbursed Medicaid patients.

The weakness in that argument was apparent to anyone who visited urban public hospitals, which by 1970 had become rundown almshouses packed to the point of housing patients on gurneys in the hallways. These were clearly the health care providers for America's poor and, not coincidentally, of African-American and Mexican-American patients. What two decades previously had been the result of segregation now was the unintended outcome of Medicaid and Medicare: striking racial stratification of health and medical services.[262] And the de facto segregation seen in the health system mirrored that which was worsening in society generally.

A case in point: the 1960 Los Angeles County census[263] designated some two hundred thousand housing units substandard or uninhabitable and most of them were located in black South Central Los Angeles or Hispanic East Los Angeles.[264] Countywide, despite phenomenal local economic growth, there were an estimated two hundred and thirty thousand families living at or below the poverty line. In the South Central and East Los Angeles slums, every single indicator of public health was far, far worse than was seen in the rest of the county. The county infant mortality rate was 19.6 per 1,000 live births—in Watts it was 33.3 per 1,000. The countywide maternal death rate was 4.5 per 10,000 pregnancies—in East L.A. it was 7.3 per 10,000.[265]

In the mid-1960s Hispanic Los Angelenos were suffering tuberculosis at a rate five times that of whites. Blacks had TB at a rate seven times that seen among whites. The risk of premature death (before age thirty-five) in these groups was four times the national average. And an American Public Health Association assessment found that some 50 percent of poor children were incompletely immunized against smallpox and measles; 64 percent had never seen a dentist.[266] In 1964 one out of every four Los Angeles babies was born into these impoverished circumstances; 26 percent of their mothers had had no prenatal care, and 80 percent of them delivered in one of two hospitals run by the county.

Though there were no Jim Crow laws in Los Angeles, the county was ranked as the second most segregated metropolitan area in the nation, just behind Chicago.[267]

On the very hot, smoggy day of August 11, 1965, an altercation broke out between a group of white police officers and a black man accused of drunk driving. As the officers swung their billy clubs, supporters of the driver poured out onto the street. Within minutes, a melee was under way: in an hour it escalated to a neighborhoodwide riot.[268] For five days, Watts burned, both with violence and from arson. It was, officially, the worst riot in U.S. history,[269] and a terrible omen of what was to come.

Los Angeles political leaders underwent a period of self-examination and scrutiny of government services. And from 1966 to 1972 most large county operations—including the Los Angeles County Health Department—were subjected to outside scrutiny. The governance of Los Angeles County had taken on a flavor and style unlike anything found elsewhere in the country, at least, found *legally*. All power rested in the hands of five men who constituted the County Board of Supervisors. The board oversaw an annual budget that exceeded that of forty-two of the states, including Massachusetts, New Jersey, and Pennsylvania.[270] It was derived primarily from property taxes and federal subsidies of various kinds. The supervisors met publicly, but few citizens or journalists ever attended their hearings or followed the men's activities.[271] So trivial was the scrutiny given their activities that supervisors were rarely compelled to step down for any reason other than ill health or death.[272]

Los Angeles County had the nation's second-largest population-receiving welfare, just behind New York City. And it had Medi-Cal, the state version of Medicaid, with more people on the rolls of publicly financed health care than anywhere else—except, again, New York City. The county's health systems were, according to the American Public Health Association,[273] "inelastic . . . fragmented and cumbersome, the orientation too rooted in past practices to permit the Health Department to meet current or future health needs. . . ." The department was rife with "inaccessibility" and "complexity [with a] multiplicity of geographic areas and political jurisdictions." There was a tremendous shortage of staff and "some needs [were] . . . totally unmet." The department exhibited "impersonality" with a "remoteness from the public served."

But the APHA inspectors were also sympathetic. They realized that the two thousand county health employees faced formidable challenges: air pollution, vast physical distances coupled with poor transportation, concentration of most health care into just two hospitals, terrible staff morale and high turnover, lack of Spanish-language skills, a cumbersome governance structure, and rising costs.

As was the case nationwide, Los Angeles witnessed a surge in hospital use and costs following federal enactment of Medicare and Medicaid. From 1961 to 1965 Los Angeles hospital prices rose about 6 percent annually. After 1966 when Medicare kicked in, hospital rates inflated 16 percent each year for the rest of the decade. And physicians' fees doubled during the two years between 1966 and '68. Most of the increase in costs was due to a rise in prices rather than to enhanced services provided.[274]

There were plenty of doctors and 745 hospitals and clinics in the county, but nearly all were concentrated in the richer, whiter sections of Los Angeles. That left just a handful of Christian charity hospitals and the two mammoth health department facilities (LAC-USC Medical Center and Harbor General Hospital) to handle all of the needs of the blacks of Watts, Hispanics of East L.A. barrios, and the poor whites of downtown's skid row.

Two trends surfaced in Los Angeles that would soon appear in every U.S. community with a sizeable population of indigent people: most poor patients came to emergency rooms for nonemergency care and the bulk of all pediatric ailments seen in the ER were minor enough to have been handled easily by a private physician. Like general use of the two already swamped hospitals, ER visits there also skyrocketed after creation of Medicare and Medi-Cal—up 16 percent in the first year. More than half that increase was for nonemergency treatments. Similarly, pediatric clinics were overwhelmed by Medi-Cal patients, most of whom suffered common, nonacute childhood infections. This trend reflected the poor community's lack of access to private doctors or smaller medical clinics.[275]

Though the county budget exceeded $1 billion in 1967, it contributed only about 1.6 percent of it to the health department's public health programs, just $16.39 million.[276] A full quarter of the department's funds came from outside the county and the department was vulnerable politically and financially to any changes in public health and medical policies that might occur in far-off Washington or Sacramento.

In addition to its heavy burden of other public health expenditures, in 1969 Los Angeles was also trying to cope with a sudden surge in the numbers of mentally ill individuals who were seeking help from county facilities. That year HEW issued guidelines calling for closure of mental asylums, medication and release of the patients, and supervision of the nation's mentally ill through small, community-based outpatient centers. Only in extreme cases should the patients live in a treatment facility. Most states followed the federal lead and swiftly closed their institutions. In July 1969 the California Mental Health Act went into effect, shifting all financial and social responsibility for the care of the mentally ill from the state to the counties.

Los Angeles County was overwhelmed. It tripled its spending on mental health efforts, putting 1970 expenditures at about $48 million.[277] Despite financial support from the state in 1970 to ease the transition, the county soon saw an increase in violent incidents and hospitalizations related to mentally ill individuals.

And in years to come the cities of Los Angeles County, like those throughout America, would see their streets fill with homeless, mentally ill individuals who were abandoned by families, which were unable to obtain support from government, and unable to cope with their relatives' abuse or violence.

As it struggled to handle such new challenges, Los Angeles was also in the midst of a huge gonorrhea epidemic, with local incidence running nearly double the national average.[278]

The task of VD control had become far more complicated for public health than anyone had imagined when the invention of penicillin had offered the longed-for magic bullet. By 1975 gonorrhea would be the nation's most common and expensive infectious disease and by 1980 there would be 2.5 million active cases of the disease reported annually in the United States.[279] Several coincident factors were responsible: public health authorities had long underestimated the amount of sexual activity among Americans and therefore grossly mistargeted their programs, ignoring most white and middle-class adults and teens.[280] Two reasons for increased sexual activity in postadolescents were the birth control pill, which was introduced into widespread use in the mid-1960s, greatly reducing the concern that sexual intercourse would result in pregnancy. Similarly, the antibiotic revolution brought young Americans to the realization that venereal diseases no longer need be viewed as potentially fatal.

In addition, a rights revolution that began with passage of the Civil Rights Act in 1964 was spurring radical cultural changes. During the rest of the sixties, the U.S. Supreme Court decided a long list of legal cases on the side of individual and group rights, giving heavier weight to the Bill of Rights and to key rights clauses of the Constitution than had any other court. Influential intellectual leaders expanded on the rights concept, embracing it for racial, sexual, labor, and student subgroups within the larger society.[281]

The right to be sexual, indeed, openly so, was also advocated by the so-called counterculture, the hippies of the late sixties, and by gay men, who were coming out of their closets of shame by the late 1970s. Between 1960 and 1971 venereal diseases rates in San Francisco would jump from 3,869 total reported cases to 17,928, with nearly all of that increase being among gay men.[282] Even in comparatively staid states like Minnesota, rates of sexually transmitted diseases (STDs) rose in the sixties and kept increasing into the next decade.[283]

Despite apparently high rates of sexual activity among teens and young adults in the United States, the country certainly wasn't ready for an open discussion of sex, and public health officials generally had to confine themselves to merely making VD documentaries for school viewing and tallying the grim numbers. There was no clear national strategy for attacking the problem.[284]

The summer of 1968 found the nation rocked by youthful protest, primarily focused on opposition to the Vietnam War. The "Happy Warrior" from Minnesota, Vice President Hubert Humphrey, ran a desperate campaign against California Republican Richard Milhous Nixon. Few domestic issues—certainly not health—figured prominently in the campaign. In November Nixon beat Humphrey by just 500,000 votes, or 0.7 percent of the votes cast.

When Nixon was sworn in as president in January 1969, the nation was more deeply polarized than at any time in the twentieth century. He called upon the "Great Silent Majority" of Americans to stand behind his policies. The war in Vietnam continued. National tensions rose. And new public health issues came to dominate American debate. With the problems of the microbial miasma seemingly solved, people in the United States were now concerned about the chemical miasma around them. When the terms *safe water, healthy air,* and *natural food* were used in the 1970s, they didn't refer to the absence of germs but of pollutants.

A quiet, unassuming marine biologist from New York's Long Island had first focused the nation's attention on the environment in 1962 with publication of her landmark book *Silent Spring*.[285] The public was particularly struck by her evidence of the pesticides' impact on human health, their potential as carcinogens, and their effect of thinning birds' egg shells, leading to marked diminutions in some bird populations. Rachel Carson's concerns proved highly contagious, becoming sources of great angst for an entire generation of Americans. "The current vogue for poisons," Carson wrote, "has failed utterly to take into account these most fundamental considerations [of ecologies]. As crude a weapon as the cave man's club, the chemical barrage has been hurled against the fabric of life—a fabric on the one hand delicate and destructible, on the other miraculously tough and resilient, and capable of striking back in unexpected ways."

The late 1960s and early seventies saw health and environmental concerns blend in U.S. public opinion, spawning new realms of government regulation, academic pursuit, commerce, and political activism. By the end of the Nixon administration on August 8, 1974, the environmental movement in the United States would be enormous. Its impact on government could be felt by at least six federal agencies.[286] It influenced numerous fields of public health and, to a lesser degree, medicine, including toxicology, epidemiology, health statistics, oncology, and occupational health. Environmentalist thinking would have both polarizing and radicalizing effects on public health, eventually pushing many leaders in the field into confrontation with corporate interests. While public health had always been a voice for society's poor, it would now also join a large U.S. chorus protesting—largely on behalf of a middle-class constituency—corporate polluters.

With every passing 1970s day, another chemical was implicated, another pollutant named. Public panic rose and, in the end, that would leave public health vulnerable to a large, and often effective, assault on its credibility.

Well before the public began paying attention to cancer, the nation's death rates had been steadily climbing. In 1900 deaths due to cancer claimed 64 of every 100,000 Americans. By 1940 that rate had nearly doubled to 120.3 per 100,000. In 1950 it hit 140 per 100,000. And in 1969 the U.S. annual cancer death rate was 160 per 100,000.[287] Though far more people died of heart diseases (500 per 100,000 people annually in 1969), cancer created a unique level of concern. Only about one out of every twenty-five Americans in 1900 died of cancer. By 1969 the figure was about one out of every seven, and both cancer and heart disease morbidity and mortality rates had steadily climbed since World War II.

The major cause of those rising death rates was not, however, some mysterious environmental pollution. It had been recognized and named long before the 1970s: tobacco smoking. In 1956 Deputy Director of the National Institutes of Health Dr. Luther Terry, impressed by then-mountainous evidence that smoking increased lung cancer, called upon the nation to "Stamp Out Smoking."

Terry became Surgeon General in 1961 and launched an aggressive effort to confront the role of cigarettes in disease. He appointed a blue ribbon tobacco study panel and in January 1964 he told a televised, standing-room-only press conference of its conclusions: "Cigarette smoking is causally related to lung cancer in men. The magnitude of the effect of cigarette smoking far outweighs all other factors. The data for women, though less extensive, points in the same direction."[288]

The report caused an immediate sensation both within the medical profession and on Capitol Hill.[289] At Terry's urging, the Johnson administration ordered health warnings placed on all packs of cigarettes.

The tobacco industry waged a vigorous "public health campaign" of its own, supporting members of Congress whose constituencies included tobacco growers whose healthy well-being, the industry said, was imperiled by antitobacco laws.

Clandestinely the industry funded the Tobacco Institute, a quasi-independent center that for decades published studies finding few or no ill effects associated with cigarette smoking. Remaining unpublished were the institute's revelations not only of the ill effects from cigarettes, but of a powerful addictive response to the tobacco stimulant, nicotine. It would be nearly thirty years before the institute's documents would see the light of day.[290]

In the 1970s many public health advocates and their attorneys tended to downplay tobacco's contribution to cancer and heart disease.[291] They did so not because they disbelieved evidence of tobacco carcinogenesis, but in reaction to the chemical industry, which consistently explained away cancer cases found among people exposed to their products by referring to the victim's cigarette smoking. Both sides were being less than candid.

Though tobacco use and its public health consequences became increasingly politically partisan issues, there never was a good reason why. Surgeons general ranging from left-liberal to ultraconservative consistently followed Luther Terry's precedent in striking out against the tobacco industry. Indeed, the loudest voice would prove to be that of Ronald Reagan's appointee to that post, Dr. C. Everett Koop, a notorious social conservative who was considered the darling of the 1980s American far right. But he had a powerful public health conscience and was the cigarette industry's arch-nemesis. "How," he asked, "could the tobacco industry dare to dismiss as unfounded and unproven the absolutely clear connection between smoking . . . and a dozen or more serious, debilitating, exhausting, expensive, and humiliating diseases? How could it do that? The answer was—it just did. The tobacco industry is accountable to no one. . . . The tobacco lobby is overwhelmingly powerful."[292]

Most of tobacco's protectors on Capitol Hill were Republicans and Southern Democrats, who justified their opposition to smoking-related public health measures on two grounds: job protection for tobacco farmers and industry employees and philosophical opposition to any regulations that fettered free enterprise—including health laws aimed at saving tens of thousands of lives every year. The politicians were less open about reason number three for their staunch support of tobacco: money. The industry spent between $500 million and $1 billion every year from 1969 to 1999 on advertising and made generous campaign contributions. In contrast, public health had paltry advertising resources during the 1960s and 1970s, and few of its leaders appreciated—as New York's Baumgartner did—the power of Madison Avenue. Even in the mid-1980s, federal antismoking advertising spending would amount to a mere $70 million a year compared to the more than $900 million annual protobacco ad dollars.[293]

In 1964 Surgeon General Terry could cite more than seven thousand studies demonstrating a link between tobacco and human morbidity and mortality. By 1988 Surgeon General Koop would be able to point to ceiling-high stacks of documents, more than sixty thousand studies, proving links between tobacco and dozens of diseases in both smokers and so-called passive smokers—people who shared airplanes, offices, and homes with smokers and breathed their exhaled tar, nicotine, carbon monoxide, and other insidious chemicals. These studies demonstrated clearly why and how tobacco exerted its lethal effects.

Bad as the biochemical effects of burning tobacco were, they would surely have had only minimal public health impact had it not been for nicotine. Without nicotine's addictive qualities, far fewer beginning smokers would have gotten hooked. The immediate pleasurable stimulation the smoker feels is the result of nicotine's attachment to receptors located on the synapses of the brain's nerve cells. Normally, these synaptic receptors are used by the most critical neurotransmitter, acetylcholine, to send the messages that are the essence of how the mind thinks. Nicotine competes with acetylcholine to saturate these receptors. The sensation for the smoker is pleasure. Nicotine also binds hormone receptors that control release of adrenaline, one of the most powerful chemicals in the body. When adrenaline surges into the bloodstream, the stimulation can be extremely dangerous to smokers' already taxed hearts, but the smoker, paradoxically, feels more pleasure.

Neurostimulation is a greedy mistress. The brain wants more and more of it: the longer a smoker uses cigarettes, the more the brain actually changes physically, adapting to nicotine stimulation so thoroughly that it can not readily function without it.[294]

"That is what we are really talking about: not smoking, not tobacco, but nicotine addiction. Most smokers are drug addicts," Koop would conclude. And tobacco companies he would add, were pushers.[295]

Tobacco smoking was estimated to have caused, during the later quarter of the century, four hundred thousand deaths each year in the United States, resulting in the loss of five million years of potential life.[296] After the Surgeon General's 1964 report was released, researchers established that a long list of cancers and other ailments was associated either with cigarette smoking or with sharing a home for years with a smoker.[297] The USPHS estimated that smoking was responsible for almost a third of all cancer deaths in the United States (nearly nine out of ten lung cancer deaths), and for one out of every five deaths due to cardiovascular diseases.[298]

Despite their comparatively minuscule budget for raising public awareness, public health leaders tried to combat Madison Avenue's pitch for cigarettes through education campaigns, primarily in schools. But early campaigns seriously underestimated the power of nicotine addiction. The most health-conscious smokers heeded the educational warnings and quit, but several legal measures would ultimately play critical roles in thinning the ranks of U.S. smokers. The Federal Communications Commission banned broadcast advertising of tobacco products and most local and state governments eventually abolished smoking in public. Heavy taxes were levied on cigarettes and in the final years of the century, lawsuits filed by the families of lifelong smokers who died of cancer won phenomenal multimillion-dollar cases against tobacco giants, and, through legal discovery, opened doors on long-covert data gathered by the To-bacco Institute.

Between 1964 and 1989 the numbers of American smokers would fall from more than 40 percent to 29 percent of the population. Most of the quitters would be white, middle-class adults. Still smoking in numbers exceeding a third of their populations would be African-Americans and American Indians.[299]

Tobacco offered unique challenges to both public health and medicine during the 1970s. Public health had yet to find effective ways to alter human behavior when the dire outcomes of their actions were both well in the future and less than certain. It was one thing to mobilize five million people to take a specific action in the face of an immediate threat, e.g., getting vaccinated against smallpox. It was quite another to get the same five million people to alter a behavior that most of them found quite pleasurable, particularly when the odds were relatively low that a given individual would face ill consequences. The new public health era called for just such interventions, however. Heroin injection, addictive use of prescription drugs, behavior that spread sexually transmitted diseases, routine consumption of distilled alcohol, and smoking were all features of American lifestyles in the 1970s that, for health reasons, needed to change. And few public health leaders had any idea why these behaviors were so prevalent in society or how they could be altered.

It was in this cultural and political miasma that the Environmental Protection Agency (EPA), the Occupational Safety and Health Administration (OSHA), and the National Institute of Occupational Safety and Health (NIOSH) were born. In 1970 Congress passed laws creating each of these agencies. The EPA's crucial guiding law, the Federal Insecticide, Fungicide, and Rodenticide Act (FIFRA), also gave the agency national chemical regulatory powers. With passage of the 1970 Clean Air Act, the EPA was granted powers to also set national ambient pollution standards.

The EPA was organized by Congress as both a public health and environmental protection agency—a sometimes contradictory mandate, as standards for one might not be ideal for the other. It was designed to function as both a research and a regulatory agency, which would put the EPA in the uncomfortable position of using its own research to decide and then enforce regulations that might cost an industry millions of dollars.

OSHA, in contrast, was just in the business of setting and enforcing work-place safety regulations. NIOSH was a separate research agency that supplied data intended to inform OSHA's policy decisions.

Like the much older Food and Drug Administration (FDA), OSHA and the EPA were regulatory agencies that could essentially take one of four positions on any drug, chemical, or hazard that came up for their review: order more research; ban the compound or hazard; restrict the use of the compound or hazardous material/machine/tool to specific situations or doses; or take no action at all.

Public health advocates had reason to focus on all of these agencies, as there were clear health implications involved in the use of pesticides, air and water pollutants, pharmaceuticals, petrochemicals, and most of the other items that came under the agencies' jurisdictions. But many other interests also had cause to pay close attention to OSHA, EPA, and the FDA, including organized labor, the affected industries, farmers, environmentalists, organized medicine, research scientists, and disease interest groups such as the American Cancer Society. Their needs and interests were often on collision courses, alliances and compromises proved elusive, and eventually all three agencies would be overwhelmed by interest groups' lawyers. Further aggravating matters, most states created counterpart agencies which set their own standards of regulation and enforcement. While these standards could not legally be weaker than those set at the federal level, they could be stricter.

Though there were many facets of pesticides, pollutants, and pharmaceuticals about which the public could be concerned, the phobia of the day was cancer. And it was exceedingly difficult to demonstrate irrefutably whether or not any given drug or chemical could, when used in a designated manner or dose, cause cancer.

Of the agencies that turned their attention to this problem, the FDA was guided by the toughest, and ultimately most unworkable, principle: the 1958 Delaney Clause. The House Select Committee Investigating the Use of Chemicals in Food and Cosmetics, led by New York Democrat James Delaney, had held hearings during the 1950s that were heavily influenced by the testimony of Dr. William C. Hueper of the National Cancer Institute.

Hueper pioneered the use of laboratory mice and rats to test the cancer-causing effects of various compounds. In the 1950s he established that various chemicals similar to beta-Naphthylamine could cause tumors in rodents.[300] He extrapolated beyond his data, however, concluding that Americans were awash in chemical and radiation carcinogens that were producing a massive cancer epidemic. He incorrectly concluded that 90 percent of all human cancer was caused by environmental and occupational carcinogens. When he came before the Delaney Committee, Hueper insisted, persuasively, that there was no safe limit of exposure to a carcinogen.

In legislation passed by the Delaney Committee in 1958, the FDA was ordered to ban or forbid licensing of any food additive or compound used on foods that caused cancer in human beings or laboratory animals. The language of the Delaney Clause stipulated that there could be *no safe limit* for carcinogens in foods.

By 1970, saddled with the Delaney Clause,[301] the FDA had three problems. First, many foods that have no additives were found to contain powerful carcinogens, such as the tars formed by barbecuing meats and aflatoxins in peanut butter. Second, many industry people were attacking the relevance of laboratory rodent studies to human exposure to potential carcinogens. And third—the legally most difficult point—nobody knew how to interpret the Delaney Clause in light of new technology. When it was enacted in 1958, scientists measured the presence of potential carcinogens at parts per million levels, but by 1970 technology could detect chemicals at parts per billion level; in some cases, parts per trillion. Were such levels dangerous to human health?

For their part, the EPA and OSHA assumed that there were, indeed, tolerable or safe levels of exposure for most compounds. They set legal limits (called tolerances at the EPA), and those became the enforceable standards for exposure. Consumers could, for example, be sold fruit with X amount of malathion on its surface. Public water supplies could contain Y levels of toluene.

Throughout the 1970s, the various interest groups would fight over these tolerances and standards, both at the federal and state levels. With so many constituencies to please, the EPA, OSHA, and FDA would grow increasingly bureaucratic, alternately functioning like castles under siege or angry cops out to get industry. Rarely would any of the interest groups be happy with either the quality of the science upon which decisions were made or the outcomes of all the wrangling.[302] And nobody could say to what degree the public's health benefited from the regulatory triad.

The biggest winners, critics agreed, were lawyers, as most EPA and OSHA issues ended up being settled in litigation.

In 1990 the U.S. Department of Health and Human Services would look back on twenty years of environmental health efforts and conclude: "We are just beginning to understand the full range of health effects resulting from exposure to environmental agents. . . . Only a small percentage of thousands of commonly used chemicals has been adequately tested for the ability to cause or promote cancer. Even fewer have been evaluated for effects on critical organs, such as the neurologic, immunologic, and reproductive systems. At present, little is known about chemical mixtures, which is how most chemicals present themselves to humans."[303]

By the time that DHHS assessment would be made, the national mood, as well as the thrust of U.S. public health, would have shifted 180 degrees: by 1990, the country would see the world in much more individualized terms, and public health would have turned its priorities from things external to questions of personal lifestyles and choices.

During the 1960s and seventies the FDA had its mettle tested, with mixed results. The first challenge began in the 1950s, with a positive outcome for the agency in 1962. A drug in common use in England, Canada, and Australia was awaiting licensing for sale in the United States. It was said to be very effective, but some researchers within the FDA had reservations about okaying an agent for use by pregnant women without further clinical scrutiny. Senator Estes Kefauver was holding hearings in Congress concerning pharmaceutical fraud and the FDA leadership realized that for the first time since their agency's creation, legislators were giving their activities serious scrutiny. It seemed prudent, therefore, to go slowly.

And that proved a wise policy. The British drug under investigation was thalidomide. It was intended to prevent miscarriages and was recommended for all pregnant women who were over thirty-five years of age or who had previously suffered a spontaneous abortion. In congressional hearings, FDA leaders announced that their investigations had led them to deny the drug company a license to sell thalidomide because it was causing terrible birth defects. Realizing that the FDA could justifiably say that its caution had spared thousands of U.S. babies from such a fate, the Kefauver Committee was moved in 1962 to amend the old 1938 Food and Drug Act to expand the public's trust invested in the FDA. It gave the agency powers to dictate the terms of clinical trials on experimental drugs and to determine, as a condition of drug licensing, whether the product actually did what the manufacturers claimed.

Squeaking in under the wire for drug approval just before the new law took effect was Enovid, an oral contraceptive manufactured by G. D. Searle: the Pill. In early 1962 the FDA had already received reports of more than 132 cases of severe health problems among women who took the Pill. In 1963 FDA investigators concluded that the Pill was clearly dangerous to women over the age of thirty-five. Under severe industry pressure, the committee withdrew that claim six weeks later.

In the mid-1960s the World Health Organization also investigated the then-global allegations of deaths and cardiac injuries caused by the Pill. Under pressure from other United Nations agencies involved in limiting the growth of human populations, WHO demurred and issued no condemnation of the Pill. In 1968, however, Britain's Dunlop Committee on the Safety of Drugs released a landmark report demonstrating that the Pill caused formation of blood clots that clogged the circulatory system, producing a long list of damages to the cardiovascular system.

Investigative journalist Barbara Seaman, a New York City freelancer, took interest in health outcomes associated with the Pill and in the FDA's apparent foot-dragging. Her 1969 book, *The Doctor's Case Against the Pill*,[304] proved a powerful indictment of the product, its manufacturer, and the FDA. And it became a rallying cry for feminists in the 1970s who believed that women's trust was uniquely betrayed by government: their gender's health needs weren't given the same level of scrutiny and deliberation as were those of men.

When Seaman's book was published, some eight million women in the United States were on the Pill.

As evidence mounted[305] implicating the Pill's principal hormones, progestin and estrogen, in the wide array of disorders, manufacturers lowered the hormonal dosages incrementally throughout the 1970s and 1980s. The FDA's only action had been to order manufacturers in 1968 to put warnings of the apparent risks into Pill packages. The manufacturers' voluntary dose reformulation made the Pill far safer and deaths attributable to the contraceptive became extremely rare occurrences.[306]

Women would find more cause to question the FDA during the 1970s as revelations mounted about the U.S. alternative to thalidomide, diethylstilbesterol, or DES. It, too, was intended to prevent miscarriages in high-risk pregnancies and had been on the market since the early 1950s. By 1958 it had become wildly popular among OB-GYNs. Between 1958 and 1965 fully half of all pregnant women in the United States were given DES prescriptions.[307]

Following the 1962 thalidomide episode, the FDA decided to use its then-new powers to review the safety and efficacy of more than four thousand drugs it had already approved, including DES. Issued in 1967, the report found DES only "possibly effective" and "not harmful."

Then in 1971 evidence began to mount of extremely rare vaginal cancers in young women whose mothers had taken DES while pregnant with them.[308] The issue of "DES babies" was explosive. In the fall of 1971 a congressional subcommittee held hearings on DES, each day bringing forth a new revelation: DES was used in livestock; it was fat-soluble and stayed in the animal and human body, causing ill effects, for years; high doses of DES had been used experimentally on Michigan coeds as a "morning-after" pill to prevent pregnancies.

And throughout it all, the FDA took no action. It needed more data, FDA Commissioner Charles Edwards told the incredulous subcommittee. Under rebuke from Congress, the FDA sent a warning letter to all physicians in 1971. And DES would still be on the market, with FDA approval, during the Reagan administration, despite the now clear evidence that the estrogenic drug was causing breast and testicular cancers in the offspring of DES moms.

The FDA took incremental actions against DES throughout the 1970s and eighties as evidence mounted of increased risk of vaginal and breast cancer and of abnormal genital development in both male and female DES babies. It issued warnings, changed labeling, and mailed updated alerts to physicians, but the agency did not really sound an alarm, or come right out and say, "Don't use this drug." So doctors would continue prescribing DES "morning-after" pills well into the 1980s. In 1988 the manufacturer, Eli Lilly and Company, itself changed the recommended uses and admitted the dangers of DES.[309]

By 1990 it would be estimated that some two million baby boomers had been exposed in utero to DES. By any measure, DES was a public health disaster, fueled by FDA inaction. "One cannot look back at the history of DES without being struck by the consistent and often flagrant failure of regulatory agencies— notably the FDA and USDA—to carry out their mandated responsibilities," concluded Stanford University medical policy analyst Diana Dutton.[310]

In responding to the rising public anxiety about cancer, President Richard Nixon was more inclined toward solutions that were curative rather than regulatory. He was convinced that a well-financed, all-out "War on Cancer" would yield scientific breakthroughs that would diminish, even eliminate, cancer mortality in America. During his administration, the National Cancer Institute enjoyed handsome increases in its research budget.

Nixon pursued a very aggressive military policy in Vietnam, widening the war and declining in peace talks to make concessions to the government of North Vietnam. His positions on domestic policy reflected an odd jumble of progressive and traditional policy initiatives, and certainly his handling of the economy did not appear to be his strong suit.[311]

Unemployment climbed steadily from 3.6 percent when Nixon was elected in 1968 to 4.9 percent in 1970. In 1971 the United States had an unfavorable trade balance for the first time since 1893. Wall Street coined a term for the administration's fiscal policies: *stagflation*. Between 1971 and 1973 the dollar fell steadily in value compared to the Japanese yen and German mark. Nixon responded with price controls. They were useless. In 1973 the economy went into a tailspin amid falling productivity, rapidly raising inflation. By 1974, unemployment hit a fourteen-year high, topping 7 percent. And then came the crushing blow of the 1973 to '74 oil embargo against the U.S. by the Organization of Petroleum Exporting Countries (OPEC).

For the remainder of the Nixon administration, and on through the Ford and Carter years, the U.S. economy suffered double-digit inflation and had negative productivity growth coupled with high unemployment.

And there were very worrying signs that amid such economic and governmental strain public health was betraying many of its core responsibilities.

In 1970 national incidence of measles (rubeola) rose, indicating that child vaccination rates had fallen. That year, more than forty-seven thousand children contracted measles, double the number in 1963 when the rubeola vaccine was first put into large-scale use. And 1971 saw seventy-five thousand more measles cases. While these numbers were well below the half million cases per year the

U.S. had experienced in the 1950s before the existence of vaccines, they bore sad evidence of a breakdown in access to routine pediatric care for many Americans.

In the winter of 1971, with his reelection campaign already under way, Richard Nixon gave a speech to Congress that caught every politician, health planner, and medical organization in the country off guard. The last person anyone expected to hear call for national health insurance was a man as conservative as Richard Milhouse Nixon.

Nixon introduced a set of bills that were designed to completely overhaul access to health care for all U.S. citizens. He told Congress that a radical change was needed because of the staggering increases in spending on health care: "For growing numbers of Americans, the cost of care is becoming prohibitive. And even those who can afford most care may find themselves impoverished by a catastrophic medical expenditure."[312]

Within hours everybody on Capitol Hill was forming interest groups and alliances with various health-related camps and formulating alternative health plan proposals. With the first presidential primary just eleven months away, Nixon's health care plan—a fluid proposal, the details of which would metamorphose over the next three years—was a catalyst for vigorous debate and power struggle. It was the fifth time in the century that the nation's political leadership tried to address American health policy in a sweeping manner. Public health would, sadly, once again prove to be a very minor player in the first serious revisiting of national health care issues since the Truman administration. And, as always, the AMA and American Hospital Association would try to block all congressional and presidential efforts to create a national health care financing system. They particularly opposed any clauses obliging them to provide care to poor Americans. But this time their voices would be drowned out by a chorus of other constituencies with different agendas, including organized labor, corporate employers, and insurance companies.

The reasons health had reached center stage again, after a twenty-five-year hiatus, were three-fold, Harvard health economist Rashi Fein argued in 1970.[313] First, cost. In 1965 the nation had spent a total of $39 billion on health; by 1969 that spending topped $60 billion.

The second reason was Medicaid. Costs for government financing of health care for the poor were skyrocketing even faster than the already outrageous inflation rate for medicine as a whole. Total public spending on health had jumped from $3.1 billion in 1950 when two-thirds of all health dollars came from non-government coffers (private insurance, patients' own pocketbooks) to $22.6 billion in 1969. And by 1969 some 60 percent of all health spending was based on government dollars—either federal or state. If that trend continued, Fein said, the country would end up with a government-financed national health care system, whether or not it intended to have what the AMA labeled "socialized medicine."

The third reason the country was ripe for national health debate was that many governors and state legislatures, feeling the fiscal pinch, were already entertaining once-radical ideas for solutions to their health financing crisis. Nixon and Congress were merely reflecting at the national level debates that had already been going on at local levels for a couple of years.

The battlefield and players had changed since the Truman era, as had the relative strength of the players. The American Public Health Association and its constituencies at local levels found themselves singing a sad chorus to which almost nobody listened. Public health interests came closest to being met by Senator Edward Kennedy's Health Security proposal, which had strong support from the AFL-CIO and organized labor. Health Security offered coverage for all Americans through a system of payroll deductions, inflation caps, employer contributions, and federal allocations to local governments.[314]

Nixon's plan also intended to move the United States toward universal coverage, but through a radically different mechanism. It was modeled on systems already in place in Minnesota and California that Dr. Paul Ellwood had dubbed "health maintenance organizations"—HMOs. Ellwood, executive director of the American Rehabilitation Institute, was the number one HMO booster in the nation and, as a die-hard Republican, had the Nixon administration's ear. Ellwood argued that traditional fee-for-service medicine and standard health insurance "perversely" rewarded doctors and nurses for ignoring all preventive care and overutilizing procedures that were costly and might not prolong patients' lives. HMOs, Ellwood said, did just the opposite.

Though they weren't called HMOs, the first such health organizations had surfaced in the state of Washington around 1906 to service the lumber industry. Two doctors dreamed up a scheme for lumber workers to prepay fifty cents each month and in exchange get whatever medical care they needed. By 1920 there were a couple of dozen such prepaid health groups scattered across Oregon and Washington, generally organized around particular pools of workers. During the Great Depression, desperate doctors and patients naturally gravitated to the idea and more prepaid systems emerged.

Wherever such plans arose, they were staunchly opposed by the AMA, which booted the physicians involved out of the association and put pressure on the states to revoke those doctors' licenses. In the AMA's view, any system of preset patient payments for health care would constitute unfair competition for private practitioners and would drive down prices.[315]

By 1971 Kaiser-Permanente, offered to the general public in Los Angeles and Northern California since the 1930s, was the nation's largest HMO, with 4.6 million members.[316] There were about thirty HMOs operating in the United

States in 1970. Nobody had data that could prove such systems were superior, either in terms of cost or quality of care, to fee-for-service medicine. Nonetheless, the complex original Nixon plan included a request for $23 million in seed money and another $300 million in loan guarantees to promote creation of more HMOs to meet the health needs of 90 percent of the population.

Both the Nixon plan and Kennedy's Health Security proposal ultimately failed in Congress. In 1971 and '72 they were caught up in presidential election campaigning and no less than four alternative plans were offered by legislators working with the insurance industry,[317] the AMA,[318] the American Hospital Association,[319] and a host of others.

Conspicuously absent from the debate were the patients.

Electioneering stalled everything until 1973. And then the Watergate scandal[320] so paralyzed the Nixon White House in 1973 to '74 that it was unable to defend the president's health care proposal. Congress eventually passed a bill containing some of Nixon's ideas: it lent modest support to HMOs, spurring some development in that area. But by 1985 the nation would have just 323 HMOs, a far cry from the sixteen hundred Nixon had envisioned.[321] Finally, the economic tailspin of 1973 to '74 killed all hope—once again—that Congress would create a comprehensive plan to provide health care for Americans. There simply was no money to spend.

In order to slow health care inflation caps were put on all federal reimbursements for hospital and physician's costs. The administration started a phase-out of Hill-Burton (which would cease in 1976) and allowed recipient hospitals to lower their mandatory charity work from 5 percent of total patient clientele to just 3 percent. All general medical and infectious diseases research funds to the NIH were slashed by millions of dollars, though cancer and heart disease research budgets rose. Community health centers—which had been hallmarks of public health, offering preventive care to underserved areas—were closed. Most subsidies for science and medical education and for advanced training were cut to the bone. Some Medicare costs were shifted away from the federal government; the patients expected to pick up more of their tabs.[322]

The United States ended up taking a trajectory on health care that was almost the exact opposite of the one Nixon had initiated in 1971. Instead of emphasizing collective health and disease prevention, the path now would lead to further medicalization and individualization. Sadly, the data would later show that America was thereby exiting the period of her greatest health improvement since the Biggs era. Between 1968, when LBJ's programs were in full swing, and 1975, when budget cuts had whittled such programs to the bone, the overall U.S. annual death rate had dropped 14 percent.[323] Every health indicator had shown remarkable improvement. Cardiovascular deaths: down by 23 percent. Infant mortality: dropped 38 percent. Maternal mortality: plummeted an astounding 71 percent.

That was the legacy of an aggressive war on poverty and expansion of health services for the poor. It occurred in a period that was denounced by the AMA and American Hospital Association as "regulated," a code word meaning "very bad" or even "socialistic" in the New Right circles of rising political superstar California governor Ronald Reagan.

The nation's new mood was characterized by strong regional differences in both the structure and financing of health care. And many parts of the country would see tremendous diminutions in care for the poor, the uninsured, rural residents, and those living in inner-city slums.

President Nixon's general health plans may have gone awry, but he had a striking and lasting impact on one critical area of public health: use of illegal drugs. During his 1968 campaign, Richard Nixon had delivered at Disneyland a key speech on drug abuse.[324] "As I look over the problems in this country," he said, "I see one that stands out in particular: the problem of narcotics." Drugs, he averred, "are among the modern curse of the youth, just like the plagues and epidemics of former years."

The solution, the Republican candidate insisted, was more cops, more FBI, more special military forces, more customs agents. The drugs Nixon feared— marijuana, psychedelics, heroin, amphetamines—were, in his rhetoric, characterized as problems among hippies, radicals, and blacks.[325] In his published diary of 1969, Nixon aide H. R. Haldeman noted that the president "emphasized that you have to face the fact that the whole problem is really the blacks. The key is to devise a system that recognizes this while not appearing to."[326]

A series of law enforcement bills constituted the basis of the administration's War on Drugs. The key elements were an eight-fold jump in the budget of the Law Enforcement Assistance Administration, which trained and supplied local police departments; new authority to shut U.S. borders if necessary to close off drug traffic; and greater powers for the Federal Bureau of Narcotics and Dangerous Drugs.

At the time, 1971, the total U.S. illegal drug trade was estimated to be worth $2 billion, with marijuana, thanks to some forty million pot smokers, constituting the bulk of the market. In contrast, the numbers of heroin users were thought to be quite small, amounting to fewer than three out of every one thousand people.[327] And over the years the relative use rates of most drugs, and deaths associated with them, would remain fairly stable.[328]

On a per-capita basis, there was more narcotics use in inner-city areas than in white suburbs, though even well-manicured suburbia had its share of heavy drug use and heroin overdoses.[329] This was no coincidence. Mafia narcotraffickers who brought processed heroin into the United States during the 1950s, sixties, and seventies deliberately targeted African-American and Hispanic urban communities. Further, by 1969 the cheapest high-grade heroin in the world was sold on the streets of Saigon. Black and Hispanic men disproportionately served in the military in Vietnam, and it is estimated that up to 20 percent of the war's veterans came home addicted to heroin.[330]

The Nixon administration's War on Drugs was not, however, limited only to law enforcement. The perspective guiding the administration was an adaptation of contagion models of disease. Nixon's staff thought that heroin users committed crimes in order to obtain drugs and that neighborhoods that festered with crime became drug-permissive environments. The heroin user, then, had to be broken of his habit in order to prevent the contagious spread of drug abuse.[331] So in 1971 the administration allotted funds for creation of methadone and counseling treatment centers nationwide, directed by a Special Action Office located inside the White House.[332] It was a public health approach, taken in tandem with classic law enforcement tactics. Given the austere conditions dictated by the economy at the time, however, the administration phased out federal support of methadone and treatment centers beginning in 1973, intending that the states would pick up the burden. As it turned out, few states would be able or willing to carry the onus, and by 1980 treatment programs would have seriously deteriorated, even disappeared. Nationwide there was far more popular support for incarceration, versus treatment, of drug addicts.

First in the world to offer free methadone to heroin addicts had been New York City. The program was pioneered in 1963 by health department physician Vincent P. Dole. Four decades later his basic storefront clinic model would still form the basis of chemical treatment for heroin addiction.

The nonmethadone treatment model, based on group support and heavy counseling, rose out of Los Angeles County, from the privately funded Synanon Center in Santa Monica. Though the Synanon approach would undergo many refinements over coming years, it, too, would essentially still be the basis of the nonchemical mode of treatment four decades later.

Much of the funding and energy behind the treatment efforts dissipated with Nixon's resignation in August 1974. Never again would the federal government play as aggressive a role in the public health aspects of addiction.[333]

Vice President Gerald Ford, a Michigan Republican, took over the White House and served as president until January 1977. His brief tenure was marked by the emergence of startling new infectious diseases issues.[334]

Though most people in the United States who thought about health trends in 1975 had their eyes on chronic diseases, it was the golden age for the Centers for Disease Control in Atlanta. All over the world the CDC was leaving its imprint, notably in battles against malaria, smallpox, yellow fever, and newly recognized hemorrhagic fever diseases in Latin America. Key to the CDC's success was the Epidemic Intelligence Service (EIS), the brainchild of the agency's Dr. Alexander Langmuir. It attracted the world's top infectious diseases specialists for scientific and advanced crisis intervention training. The CDC then deployed the young recruits to handle microbial outbreaks from California to Calcutta. Langmuir mentored a whole generation of EIS officers who, by the mid-1970s, were stamping out epidemics all over the world.

In 1976 America celebrated its Bicentennial in what would prove to be the busiest, and politically hottest, year the CDC would ever face: a mysterious killer virus emerged in extremely remote parts of northern Zaire and southern Sudan. The Zairois government—a critical U.S. Cold War ally—requested CDC assistance. The CDC's Dr. Karl Johnson headed up an international team that intervened in what was the first recorded epidemic of the Ebola virus.[335] A group of American Legion members celebrating the Bicentennial in Philadelphia suffered, and many died, from a previously unknown disease that commanded the laboratory resources of the CDC for much of 1976 and '77. And the agency came to fear that the 1918 killer flu, swine flu, had returned and might claim millions of lives.

Sadly, Legionnaires' disease, as it came to be known, and the fiasco triggered by the swine flu scare would so dominate public concern and attention in 1976 and '77 that few people in the United States would even realize that the CDC and WHO had achieved the greatest public health victory of the twentieth century: they had wiped out smallpox.[336]

That victory wasn't, however, what made the CDC a household acronym in America. Rather, it was the scandals, and America was quite fixated on scandal in 1976, having just weathered the Watergate debacle and a rather sorry end to the Vietnam War.

In the case of swine flu, the CDC and the U.S. Army appear in hindsight to have overreacted to a single death and a handful of secondary cases attributed to a new strain of influenza that struck a military base in New Jersey in the winter of 1976. And the White House, for its part, leapt way beyond the evidence, sending the country into a real public health fiasco.[337] The three most important outcomes of the swine flu affair were demonstration of the inadequacies in the U.S. vaccine system; loss of public faith in the CDC and, more generally, in public health leaders; and an insurance legacy that would impede vaccine efforts for the rest of the century.

Consider this, the CDC told HEW secretary Forrest Matthews, *if*, just *if*, this strain of swine flu is as lethal as the swine-type flu that killed more than twenty-five million people worldwide in 1918 to 1919, wouldn't an epidemic be far worse today? After all, we have global air travel and far more people on earth.[338]

President Ford had to make a command decision based on a "what if." He opted for rapid production of a vaccine and mass immunization of the U.S. population.

And that's when the limitations of the U.S. vaccine production system were revealed. Once, to meet such crises, Hermann Biggs and Leona Baumgartner could order mass production of vaccines out of their New York City laboratories. Once, Truman and Eisenhower had been able to rally manufacturers to mass produce vaccines for U.S. soldiers. Once, Jonas Salk had made a discovery and a few months later millions of kids were getting polio shots.

But by 1976 the vaccine industry was shriveling as drug companies found pills and medicines to be far more profitable markets. A few lawsuits, particularly those related to the Cutter Laboratory polio incident, had sent chills through the pharmaceutical industry. Companies that still had vaccine production facilities were loath to get involved in a rush job without protection from litigation. And private insurance companies balked at the prospect of insuring them.

President Ford asked Congress to pass a bill making the federal government liable for the vaccine. This essentially put HEW in the position of indemnifying the drug companies.

The drug companies had a hard time meeting the CDC's goal of having 100 million doses of vaccine ready in time to vaccinate Americans in September, before the typical October flu season commenced. One company misinterpreted its instructions and made the wrong vaccine.

And as the vaccine became available, skeptics drew sizeable media attention, arguing variously that there was no swine flu, that the vaccine was dangerous, or that the entire effort was a fiscal boondoggle. Then some vaccinees fell ill with Guillan-Barré syndrome, a neurological disorder that might have been linked to the vaccine,[339] and the public turned its back on the immunization campaign.

By the time the dust settled, former Georgia governor Jimmy Carter was president, HEW was flooded with lawsuits alleging all sorts of vaccine-associated problems, and no epidemic had materialized.

The swine flu fiasco would still resonate in the vaccine industry and in public health circles three decades later. It would render Congress unwilling in the future to consider carrying any liability for lifesaving vaccines and generally skittish about having the federal government involved in the business of making vaccines.[340]

The three most devastating flu epidemics of the twentieth century had caught public health officials by surprise. The best guess on the costs to the United States of the 1918–19 epidemic was at least six hundred thousand lives and $100 billion in medical care and lost productivity. A 1957 Asian flu claimed seventy thousand U.S. lives and cost $4 billion. And the 1968 Hong Kong flu killed nearly thirty-five thousand people in the United States and cost $3 billion.[341] By 1976 an international flu surveillance network was in place, run by the World Health Organization. Its goal was to spot new influenza strains as early as possible, giving vaccine makers plenty of time to generate new, safe products.

The swine flu fiasco heightened industry concerns about safety and litigation,[342] and put additional pressure on the WHO surveillance network. But the WHO network had many limitations and would continue to be vulnerable to surprises throughout the century. There were major gaps in surveillance in Asia, especially China, where nearly all influenza strains seemed to originate.[343] Further, even at the end of the twentieth century much about influenza would remain elusive, including an understanding of how to predict which particular strain of the virus might prove to have epidemic potential.[344]

As there was no obvious way to make flu prediction more certain and thus increase the lead time between first recognition and a full-fledged epidemic, the public health focus would remain for the rest of the century entirely on the side of vaccine development.[345] Only three countries in the world, however, had mass flu vaccine production capacities: Russia, France, and the United States. (Minor vaccine production capacities existed in a few additional countries.) And by 1990 the Russian system would have deteriorated to the point where few outsiders trusted the reliability and safety of the product. If there were an emergency, even France and the United States—both of whose vaccine production capacity was privatized—would fail to meet the immunization needs of even their own populations.

The 1976 swine flu fiasco did serve to awaken U.S. public health leaders, give them a dose of humility, and allow them to recognize the weaknesses in their public health safety net. Despite surveillance and vaccine efforts every year after 1976, influenza would remain a major killer for the rest of the century. In any given year about one hundred thousand Americans, mostly elderly, would die of influenza or the bacterial pneumonia that was flu's opportunistic companion. Each year, between eighteen and forty-two million people in the United States would seek outpatient care for their flu and another twenty-one to fifty million would suffer at home and never seek medical treatment.[346] But those numbers would have been far worse were it not for annual vaccination efforts. Studies by the CDC showed that mass vaccination each year reduced flu rates among elderly Americans by 31 to 45 percent, even in years when the strain of flu that ultimately hit the United States only weakly resembled the one to which the vaccine was directed.

In 1995, after years of review and planning, Dr. Peter Patriarca of the FDA concluded that there was little that could be done to enhance public health preparedness for a truly devastating flu pandemic. "And we're not talking about an Andromeda Strain that's coming down from outer space," the FDA planner warned. "We're actually talking about a reasonably probable event."[347]

Reflecting on the swine flu fiasco, Dr. Walter Dowdle, who was a key player at the CDC at the time and one of those who advised mass vaccination, said, "Nineteen seventy-six was a vaccine in search of a pandemic. . . . And [it] was really a dry run for the next great pandemic. To me, the big lesson . . . was the desirability of more clearly separating the process of scientific decision-making from the political process. . . . All of the big programmatic decisions were political."[348]

At least equally political was the response to the emergence of Legionnaires' disease in 1976.[349] For four days during the July '76 U.S. Bicentennial, members of the American Legion frolicked in a cluster of Philadelphia hotels. Within days some of the Legionnaires and their wives would fall ill: by summer's end, 182 of them would have symptoms of the same mysterious disease, and twenty-nine would have died of it.

Because the cause of these deaths wasn't immediately explicable by the CDC, all manner of theories arose, some reasonable, but many outrageous. As the months wore on without an answer to the Legionnaires' puzzle, members of Congress became agitated and called hearings to denounce the CDC. Claims of cover-ups arose from members of the public inclined to think in terms of conspiracies. And with the public health agency already under attack over its handling of swine flu, the Legionnaires' mystery further fueled the fire of popular suspicion that, at best, the CDC was inept, and at worst, there was something sinister going on.

Such accusations were grossly unfair, of course. The CDC was faced with an unknown microbe that was of a class of germs not previously considered particularly pathogenic. And it was spread by a means that hadn't previously been a source of disease. Such novelty is rarely subject to swift analysis. In January 1977 the CDC announced that the culprit was a bacterium they dubbed *Legionella*, and it was spread through air-conditioning systems. *Legionella*, it turned out, was a scum bacterium that grew in the biofilms that formed at the interfaces of air and nonsalty water. Air conditioners, showers, misters, humidifiers, and similar devices that sprayed moist air were rife with biofilms, and if the device was not cleaned regularly and filtered, those scum layers would grow and become *Legionella* breeding grounds.

Once the organism was discovered, the CDC and the state public health agencies set to work testing human samples saved from past, mysterious pneumonia outbreaks. It turned out that 235 people in the United States had suffered Legionnaires' disease at two different locations in 1976. And for years thereafter the numbers of newly identified cases would rise—there would be 1,615 cases in 1994.[350]

Two days after the CDC announced the discovery of *Legionella*, Jimmy Carter was inaugurated as thirty-ninth president of the United States. He inherited a nation still suffering from stagflation and reeling with disappointment in its political leaders. The national debt was the largest in U.S. history: $66 billion.

In some localities—notably New York City—the economic situation was far more serious than mere Nixonian "stagflation." New York in 1977 was pennies shy of having to declare bankruptcy.

Everything in Gotham deteriorated. The city streets were full of uncollected garbage, plows were slow to clear the impassable streets after snowstorms, entire neighborhoods were ruled by gangsters. The public health laboratories likewise fell apart. Aging equipment went unrepaired and, when truly broken, unreplaced. Basic biological and chemical supplies were underpurchased. Personnel hemorrhaged out of the system as their long-stagnant pay rates were rendered ridiculous by rising national inflation. The caliber of replacement personnel was so poor that many dedicated top-level professionals in the department quit in disgust. Public health clinics became so seedy that only the most desperately poor New Yorkers crossed their thresholds.

In the same 1976 elections that swept Jimmy Carter into the White House, Ed Koch was elected mayor of New York City.

The Carter administration had nothing but disdain for Koch and his handling of Gotham's affairs. The White House worked directly with Governor Hugh Carey and Felix Rohatyn, head of New York's Municipal Assistance Corporation, offering whatever assistance it thought might pull New York City out of its all-but-official state of bankruptcy. But Gotham's sagging public health system garnered few federal grants or support, thanks to the feud between Koch and Carter.[351] Eventually, while Koch and Rohatyn tackled the city's financial disaster, national stagflation also eased, and by 1980 New York City was beginning to see a light at the end of the long, dark tunnel of fiscal gloom.

On March 28, 1979, a nuclear power plant outside Harrisburg, Pennsylvania—just over one hundred miles from New York City—suffered a near-meltdown. An accident in the reactor caused the plant to shut down and its nuclear core to overheat.[352] Radioactive fallout was released. It was the worst nuclear accident in U.S. history, though it would pale compared to the 1986 Chernobyl catastrophe in the Soviet Union.

Departments of health throughout the Northeast were deluged with inquiries from anxious residents who were convinced they had suffered dangerous radiation exposure. In the days following the Three Mile Island accident, Americans heard claims from every manner of supposed public health expert that ranged from certainty that the incident would cause a massive future increase in the U.S. cancer and birth defect rates to "there was no real accident." Because the debate begun decades earlier by Pauling and Teller had never been scientifically or politically resolved, the American people were left to panic or yawn according to their own inclinations. The Nuclear Regulatory Commission (formerly the AEC), EPA, White House, HEW, and public health departments all over the country sought to calm the public. But distrust was high, credibility low. Many Americans disbelieved the NRC's most basic information, such as details of the amounts and types of radiation released in the accident. And if that data could not be trusted, all subsequent assumptions regarding human exposure and health effects were suspect.[353]

Years later most health-related details regarding Three Mile Island would remain murky. Pennsylvania governor Richard Thornburgh complained from day one that he couldn't get any straight answers out of the Met Ed Company, which ran the reactor. Later that year, Met Ed officials were found to be lying about key details in congressional testimony. Crucial radiation detectors that should have been in place on and around the power plant either had never been installed or were missing by the time independent investigators reached the site. At NRC hearings, some of the plant's engineers admitted to a series of preaccident failures and prior radiation leaks at Three Mile Island.

When the accident first occurred, Met Ed officials told the media that a cloud of fallout radiating at 40 rads an hour had been released and was heading toward local towns. We will never know how accurate that statement may have been and almost nobody who heard that news even knew what it meant. Even a physicist would have had a hard time calculating how 40 rads of radioactive energy, rems of human exposure, the dose received by an individual, and relative risk all interrelated. What could be said—and was said by Governor Thornburgh—was, it was a lot of radiation and it was dangerous. Thornburgh ordered evacuation of thirty-five hundred children and pregnant women living around the plant; what followed was a stampede of two hundred thousand panicked Pennsylvania citizens.

When, years later, Three Mile Island's disaster was long-forgotten by most Americans, scientists would still be debating how many people may, or may not, have suffered cancer as a result. Ten years after the accident the cleanup bill topped $1.2 billion and it wasn't over. The contaminated plant and its nuclear waste aren't scheduled for final burial and cleanup until 2020.[354] On April 10, 1999, TMI was sold for $100 million to the British-owned company AmerGen.

Like the swine flu fiasco of 1976, the mixed messages Americans received regarding the health impact of Three Mile Island profoundly undermined the credibility they granted to government health officials. Though they certainly had not been responsible for the incident, and, in light of the Cold War coverups at AEC and NRC, could hardly be blamed for their lack of clarity on radiation risks, public health leaders suffered nevertheless.

Meanwhile, the energy crisis that had begun with the OPEC embargo during the Nixon administration continued into Carter's presidency, exacerbating economic woes and pushing development of alternative sources of energy, such as nuclear power. Rising Middle East tensions would only worsen the situation and ultimately doom Jimmy Carter to a single term of office.[355]

Such periods of economic strain are, historically, perilous times in which to initiate controversial policy maneuvers. Nevertheless, President Carter, like Nixon before him, was convinced that the American health system was out of control. Like his predecessors who had visited the issue, Carter never questioned the basic premise that good *health* was synonymous with good *health care*. The underlying principles of public health versus those of medicine weren't debated. Rather, as had Truman, LBJ, and Nixon, Carter set out to broaden access to all medical treatment while, at the same time, controlling costs:[356]

> Although American medical skill is among the best in the world, we have an abominable system in this country for the delivery of health care, with gross inequalities towards the poor—particularly the working poor—and profiteering by many hospitals and some medical doctors, who prey on the vulnerability of the ill. From the enormous profits, unnecessary hospital facilities can be built; the cost of the empty beds and underutilized equipment is financed by the public through higher taxes to pay for Medicaid and Medicare, plus bigger hospital bills and insurance premiums for private care. Normal competitive restraints on excessive costs are almost nonexistent.
>
> Few Americans realize how much we are paying each year for this inefficiency. Major studies conducted in 1978 revealed that per-capita cost of health care was almost $1,000 per year, and these costs were doubling every six years!

The Carter administration plan called for creation of federal standards of care that would constitute the legal minimum package employers could offer their employees. Federal subsidies would assist small businesses in meeting these costs for their employees. Employers would shop around to insurance providers, all of whom would have to offer at least the federal standard of minimal care. Carter assumed that competition would force providers to spice up their packages with additional benefits for the same rock-bottom price.

Shortly before Carter's bills were introduced in 1979, Senator Edward Kennedy, who still held to his dream of Canadian-style Health Security, convened a press conference denouncing the White House scheme. Kennedy's opposition came from Carter's left and represented the outcry of constituencies of the poor and labor unions. But when the Carter plan died days later on Capitol Hill, it was the victim not of Kennedy's opposition, but of a well-organized assault from

Carter's right. Carter insisted that his plan "would have saved the American people more than $50 billion (!) in the first five years—after leaving the hospitals free to raise their prices 50 percent faster than the prevailing inflation rate."[357]

Carter's plan—and Kennedy's—were running headlong into a new trend in U.S. health care: the moral center of the debate on health had shifted. When the decade had opened, few political or medical leaders dared publicly challenge the basic principles of access and physician independence that had guided health reform arguments since the Roosevelt era. The basic premise of all Roosevelt's New Deal programs was that America could not recover from the Great Depression unless *all* Americans had access to the fruits of prosperity, including health care. By the end of the Carter administration, however, "the prevailing assumptions about the need to expand medical care were reversed: the need now was to curb its apparently insatiable appetite for resources. In a short time, American medicine seemed to pass from stubborn shortages to irrepressible excess, without ever having passed through happy sufficiency," wrote medical historian Paul Starr.[358] "Rising costs brought medical care under more critical scrutiny, and the federal government, as a major buyer of health services, intervened in unprecedented ways."

Enter corporate medicine.

It lurked all around the edges of congressional debate. It rendered both the Carter and Kennedy plans irrelevant. When *Fortune* magazine, the leading platform of conservative capitalism, started an editorial rampage against medicine in 1970, anyone reading corporate tea leaves should have seen it coming. Medicine in the United States was a mess, *Fortune* opined, a "helter-skelter" system, "inferior in quality, wastefully dispensed, and inequitably financed."[359]

For years physicians had been able to dictate not only their fees but also consumer demand. It wasn't the patient or the insurance company that said, "let's run another test on that gall bladder." It was the doctor. And the doctor decided how much to charge for the time he or she spent studying the test results and treating the patient. From the point of view of economists, this was insane. It meant consumers could not *behave* as consumers, shop around, choose not to buy, or to buy elsewhere. And doctors induced demand. In other words, the supplier manipulated demand.[360] After creation of Part B of Medicare, the trend spiraled completely out of control.[361] This constituted a market failure because there was no genuine competition and consumers could not "vote with their feet and paychecks," opting out of treatment.

In the 1960s and 1970s the U.S. government tried to create more physician competition by easing immigration procedures for foreign doctors. And the doctor-to-patient ratio jumped: from 136 doctors per 100,000 Americans in 1960 to 197 per 100,000 in 1980 to 245 per 100,000 by 1990. The increase in doctors did improve the quality of medical care, especially for public hospital users, by shortening waiting times in ERs and clinics, but it completely failed to bring down costs. The immigrant physicians quickly learned how native doctors worked the system and set their prices accordingly.

In 1970 New York State's health department tried to control doctor-induced inflation by saying, "Okay, we'll reimburse eight dollars per Medicaid visit. That's it. End of story." There was great confidence that this would hold costs to a reasonable level. But six months later, physician fees had exploded, costing the state 20 percent *more*. Why? Compelled to hold the line at $8 per visit, physicians shortened their average time per patient to five minutes, crammed more cases into each workday and billed for larger net sums.

Physicians, of course, were only one piece of what economists saw as an irrational system. A 1976 study by the National Center for Health Statistics[362] found that total physician costs in the U.S. for 1972 were $16.9 billion. Hospitals charged a total of $34.2 billion. And pharmaceuticals added $5.6 billion. The total tally was about $133 billion, or 8.6 percent of the U.S. GNP. During the time Congress was debating the Carter and Kennedy plans, costs soared further and by 1980 the tally was $249 billion—9.5 percent of GNP. By 1981 it was $286.6 billion—9.8 percent of GNP.[363] In terms of per-capita expenses, Americans were putting out $358 a year for medical care (and just pennies for *public* health) during the Nixon administration, $604 a year during Ford's presidency, and by the time Carter yielded the White House to Ronald Reagan per-capita health care spending would be $1,225 a year.[364]

Dorothy Rice of the National Center for Health Statistics in Washington, D.C., discerned other key trends in U.S. health spending. She noticed, for example, that in 1950 just shy of two-thirds of all medical costs were paid out of pocket by patients—only 9 percent was covered by insurance and 22 percent subsidized by federal and local governments. By the end of the Carter administration, just under a third of health care costs were out of pocket. Private insurance picked up 26.2 percent of the tab. And, crucially, government paid out the lion's share—40.4 percent.[365]

Rice's data verified that the increase in health care expenditures was almost entirely a matter of rising prices, which, in turn, were the result of physician billings, wage increases for hospital personnel, and rising costs for high technology tests. The latter, Rice thought, had received too much blame and attention. Physicians and hospitals were the key to pricing.[366]

And by 1980 it was obvious that Medicare had shifted American health resources in the direction least likely to affect public health: toward increased expenditures in the final days of life. The most dramatic gains in life expectancy in the United States were made between 1800 and 1930 when infant and child death rates plummeted steadily—at one time half of all annual deaths in New York City, for example, had been among children under fifteen years of age. By

1980 public health interventions and improved standards of living had brought child deaths down to less than 5 percent of all annual mortality.

But by 1980 Medicare was paying out most of its dollars for treatments to extend by days, maybe months, usually inevitable deaths. Rice saw, for example, that the average female (aged six months to sixty-four years) spent $431 a year on health care, about half of that on intestinal, digestive, and OB-GYN problems. In contrast, the average woman aged sixty-five or more years spent $1,707 a year on health care, with half those dollars going for cardiovascular treatments, strokes, heart attacks, hypertension, and the like. For males, the pattern was quite similar.

As hospitals filled with elderly, dying patients, death itself became a less dignified and private process.[367] Thus, Medicare was driving cost inflation for U.S. health care in general,[368] and undignified treatment of dying elderly patients was pushing Medicare's upward spiral.

The ethical implications of this observation were too overwhelming for Congress, Carter, or the nation to face: who could possibly deny their mother or grandfather every conceivable chance to live a longer, pain-free life? Even if the odds that modern medicine could fulfill such a hope were less than 10 percent, on an *individual basis* the need for treatment seemed undeniable, even morally mandated. So if, on a *population basis*, this appeared to be little more than an irrational waste of resources, no politician dared whisper, "Pull the plug."

But by the end of the 1970s corporations saw the profit potential in this irrational system and began buying and consolidating hospital chains, and by 1990 more than 40 percent of the nation's most prestigious hospitals would be investor-owned. At the same time, large employers were panicking over mounting medical expenses. The Fortune 500 companies gravitated toward health care plans that offered cost controls management styles similar to those used in the corporate world. Efficient health management was the target; the goal was to stop runaway costs—but without denying grandma a heart transplant.

It would prove to be both an impossible task and a mandate that had little if anything to do with public health. Indeed, time would reveal that such approaches to medical care management often ran contrary to the essential exigencies of public health.

It was in this shifting climate of health costs and concerns that Carter's plan failed in Congress, leaving Carter bitter and disheartened. The defeat exacerbated tensions and mutual disrespect between the White House and Congress. "In the final showdown," Carter charged,[369] Congress "was flooded with money, in the form of campaign contributions from the health industry. . . . [T]he American Medical Association alone . . . contributed an average of more than eight thousand dollars to each of the two hundred and two members of the House of Representatives who voted against the bill! Of the fifty members who accepted more than twice this average amount, forty-eight voted with the health industry. They prevailed, and the American people lost. The fight for equitable health care was one of my major efforts and one of my great disappointments."[370]

But the Carter administration's HEW did take two important steps on behalf of public health. The first targeted refugees, the second, all Americans.

Between 1975 and 1980 the United States absorbed nine hundred thousand refugees from Southeast Asia. The so-called boat people poured out of Vietnam, Laos, and Cambodia, fleeing communism, defeat, or retribution for their perceived or real past collaboration with U.S. troops. Many were held for months in squalid, disease-ridden camps in Thailand and neighboring Asian nations before reaching the United States. In addition, as part of Carter's call for global human rights, some one hundred and twenty-five thousand Cubans and fifteen thousand Haitians were granted legal residence in the United States during his tenure.

The Carter administration created the Office of Refugee Health, placed within HEW. Its purpose was to screen incoming immigrants for a host of communicable diseases and to serve as a cultural bridge for their entry into the mainstream medical system. Many of the Southeast Asian immigrants had never previously seen a hospital or undergone an allopathic medical exam. The main public health purpose of the refugee effort was to prevent introduction of tuberculosis into the communities in which the immigrants settled. Refugees found to have tuberculosis were put on antibiotics to clear their lungs and render them noncommunicable.

The second initiative, *Healthy People*, was published in 1979 and 1980. The two-volume report was the brainchild of Surgeon General Julius Richmond, who believed it was time to inaugurate a "second public health revolution." (The first had been the bacteriological revolution at the opening of the twentieth century.) In Richmond's vision, the new public health targets were related to personal behavior: diet, smoking, drug abuse, exercise, accidents, and safety. Under Joseph Califano's leadership, HEW's *Healthy People* laid out precise 1990 goals for the United States.[371] They included reducing infant mortality by 35 percent; an overall mortality decrease of 25 percent; and a 20 percent reduction in the number of days people over age sixty-five spent bed-bound by illness. If strategies for achieving those ambitious goals appeared weak or vague in the reports, few objections were raised.

After all, at long last U.S. public health actually had some goals.

V

Money's too tight to mention.
I can't get no loan extension.
Money's too tight to mention.
Oh, money, money, money!
We're talking about Reaganomics,
Oh Lord, down in the projects.
They're passing all kinds of bills
From down on Capitol Hill.
Money's too tight to mention.
Cut back!

—Simply Red, 1988[372]

Is it a coincidence that over the last fifteen years these public health reports
have emphasized personal responsibility at a time of conservative government?
These are "blame the victim" approaches. It's clearly cheaper than funding
public health.

—William H. McBeath, executive director, American Public Health Association[373]

On January 20, 1981, Ronald Wilson Reagan was inaugurated as the fortieth president of the United States of America. In his speech that day, Reagan proclaimed that "government is not the solution to our problem; government is the problem."

And he set the tone for his leadership, as well as for America in the 1980s (and beyond) by continuing: "It is my intention to curb the size and influence of the federal establishment and to demand recognition of the distinction between the powers granted to the federal government and those reserved to the states or to the people. All of us need to be reminded that the federal government did not create the states; the states created the federal government."[374]

The former governor of California was reflecting views quite popular in his home state, birthplace of the New Right. Reagan, who swept the national elections in a breathtaking landslide, was the New Right's icon and visionary. In both actions and rhetoric, Reagan reflected an agenda originally outlined by Arizona senator Barry Goldwater in his losing bid to defeat LBJ in 1964. But Reagan added one additional nuance—front-burner importance was given to conservative and fundamentalist Christian values, with a correspondingly adamant opposition to abortion. The time hadn't been right for Goldwater, but it was definitely ripe for Reagan.

In 1978 Proposition 13 was passed by California's voters by a two-to-one margin. It rolled back rates to a total of one percent and froze assessments at 1978 levels. Taxes could only increase when property was sold and thereby reassessed. Homeowners or investors who held onto their properties, however, need never again pay more taxes than they had in 1978. The five supervisors of Los Angeles County, as well as the governing bodies of every other part of the state, lost their major source of revenue increases—*snap!*—just like that. And, thanks to inflation and Prop. 13, never again would any of the counties of California seem to have enough money to cover the costs of their schools, hospitals, public health operations, sheriffs, jails, and buildings and roads maintenance.

This didn't bother many Californians when Reagan espoused strong support for Prop. 13 during his campaign swings through the state in 1980. On the contrary, when government officials squealed in fiscal pain, most voters took it as just desserts for years of pork barrel spending.

In 1980 Los Angeles County's population was, officially, 7,477,657. The off-the-books count of unregistered immigrants from Mexico and Central America put the census at somewhere between 7.8 and 8 million. There wasn't much open land left in the county.

The biggest public health problem for Los Angeles residents was their absolute dependence upon automobiles. Los Angeles had an astounding death rate from car accidents of 1,043.2 per 100,000 annually. Statewide, the figure was 949.6 per 100,000. The national motor vehicle death rate in 1980 was just 24 per 100,000.[375]

Also, thanks to the area's glut of autos, in 1980 Los Angeles County suffered 181 days of smog that exceeded federal air safety standards, or half the days of the year.

The county health department had swelled into a bureaucratic behemoth, employing nearly twenty-five thousand people. Yet, judging by its own data, the massive department wasn't doing very well and would be hard-pressed to meet the federal *Healthy People* goals for 1990.

Between 1971 and 1981 Los Angeles acquired at least half a million more people. The white population, however, was shrinking,[376] having fallen by 10 percent between 1960 and 1980 as a result of declining birth rates and a striking slowdown in immigration to Los Angeles from the East and Midwest. In contrast, the Latino and African-American populations rose. Combined, they made up more than 40 percent of the L.A. county's population and demographers forecast that whites would be in the minority by 1990.[377]

But the health department clearly had not figured out how to reach most of the nonwhite population.

For example: Los Angeles County's overall infant mortality rate was lower in 1980 than the national average (11.9 per 1,000 live births versus 12.5 nationally).[378] But the low-average infant death rate masked striking ethnic differences and clear public health failures. Skewing the average downward were white and Asian Los Angelenos, with rates of 10.8 and 6.2, respectively. In contrast, Latinos suffered an infant mortality rate of 15.4 per 1,000 babies, and the truly terrible rate among Los Angeles's black population was 21.4 per 1,000, double that of whites and more than triple the rate for Asians.[379]

Key to this huge disparity in infant mortality was the fact that African-American women in Los Angeles were more than twice as likely to give birth to undersized and/or severely premature babies weighing less than 2,500 grams.[380] Low birth weight babies were at high risk for death, mental retardation, vital organ dysfunction, and virtually every other life-threatening ailment known to afflict newborns. The factors responsible for low birth weight were well known and included maternal age (less than eighteen years), poor maternal diet, lack of prenatal care, and maternal alcoholism. All of these factors were playing a role in the African-American population of Los Angeles and could have served as targets for public health action.

To put the numbers in perspective: the infant mortality rate among L.A. African-Americans in 1980 was equal to that of the former Soviet Republic of Georgia in 1994, during its post-Communist collapse, and was well above the average of 17 per 1,000 live births in industrialized nations.[381] And although Los Angeles's rate of 79 percent completion of childhood immunizations[382] was about equal to the world average in 1980, it was well below not only the average 90 percent immunization rates achieved in Western Europe that year, but also below vaccine achievements in much of Asia and Latin America.[383]

In 1980 Los Angeles County also had one of the highest gonorrhea rates in the nation, at 683.7 cases per 100,000 Los Angelenos, compared to a U.S. rate of 443.3 per 100,000. And syphilis rates in Los Angeles rose from 16.6 per 100,000 in 1970 to 27.8 in 1980, nearly three-fold greater than the U.S. rate. Hepatitis B was prevalent at a rate well above the national average as well—12.2 per 100,000 in Los Angeles versus 8.4 per 100,000 in the United States as a whole. Black Los Angelenos had even more astonishing levels of gonorrhea and syphilis, well exceeding the county's already abysmal overall rates: for gonorrhea, 2,068.6 per 100,000; for syphilis, 160.1 per 100,000.[384]

The racial divide in Los Angeles continued to have a striking impact on the health of the county's population. In 1980 the white population was far more likely to be employed, well educated, and have access to one of the 192 private hospitals and hundreds of clinics in the county. In contrast, African-Americans and Latinos were more apt to be unemployed or working in the lowest-paid jobs and to rely for health care upon one of the seven hospitals run by the county's health department.

While the county's five supervisors pondered how to pay the bills after enactment of Proposition 13, the health department was growing increasingly dependent on outside revenues from Medicare, Medi-Cal (California Medicaid), and numerous state health programs to carry costs.[385] And even with those revenues, there wasn't enough money to cover the enormous budget for the L.A. County Department of Health. In 1981 the supervisors decided to cut it back, laying off twelve hundred health department employees and closing eight neighborhood health centers. The budget cut also forced reductions in services at the seven large county hospitals and clinics.

That wasn't nearly enough slashing, however, to balance the budget, particularly given increased county spending on crime control. So the county hospitals quietly increased their billing rates to Medi-Cal and Medicare. Los Angeles County's public health system was, then, extremely vulnerable. If appropriations dropped in Washington or in Sacramento, the county's health complex could crack.

And the nation had just elected a president whose avowed priority was to reduce government spending.

On February 5, 1981, President Reagan addressed the nation. The topic was the sorry state of the "stagflated" U.S. economy. In his campaign, Reagan had spoken of supply-side economics, a vision he adapted from the work of University of Chicago economist Milton Friedman. The concept boiled down to reduced government spending, elimination of the nation's budget deficit, tax relief for industry in order to prod sagging national productivity, and tax relief for citizens in order to boost their consumer power. In his two terms in office, Reagan would actually increase federal government spending, eclipsing the one trillion dollar mark, largely through rising military expenditures.[386] The budget deficit at the end of Reagan's presidency would be $200 billion, for a per-capita debt approaching $13,000. (By comparison, when Richard Nixon took office in 1969, the budget deficit was $25 billion.)[387]

Nevertheless, on that February evening in 1981 Ronald Reagan told Americans that they were "in the worst economic mess since the Great Depression. . . . It's time to try something different, and that's what we're going to do."

Reagan went on to say that his council of economic advisors was drawing up a budget cuts plan that would affect "virtually every department of government."[388] Reagan planned to tear down all of the domestic programs created by Democrats Kennedy, Johnson, and, especially, Carter.

For those concerned about health, there was a lot of holding of breath for the next seven months, waiting to hear which federal programs were facing major fiscal surgery.

August 1981 was the beginning of what Columbia University health policy scholar Eli Ginzberg called, "what is likely to be the greatest upheaval in the American health system since World War II."[389] On August 13, Reagan signed the Omnibus Reconciliation Bill, which, over three years, cut $130.5 billion from the federal budget and would reduce tax revenues by $787 billion over the same time span. Five weeks later he called for an additional $13 billion to be excised from the 1982 budget. By October 56 percent of the U.S. voters polled said that they opposed the Reagan administration's budget plans.

Too late. The ball was already rolling down Capitol Hill and couldn't be stopped.

The public health impacts of the Reagan administration's budget and tax cuts of 1981, 1982, and 1983 were far-reaching and profound. Every conceivable aspect of public health in the United States felt the pinch.

First, the tax law changes, coupled with reductions in various social welfare benefits, had the effect of radically shifting wealth in the United States from the poorest to the richest in the society. Political economist James D. Savage of the University of California summarized the effect as follows:[390] "The act, which enforced the FY 1982 budget cuts, was found to increase the total poverty rate during that fiscal year by 2 percent, and by 2.9 percent among children. The increase in childhood poverty was largely caused by the budget reductions that removed 493,000 cases from the Aid to Families with Dependent Children program."

The public's health had always worsened when the gap between rich and poor widened, which, between 1981 and 1985, it did considerably. By April 15, 1985, for example, the poorest U.S. households—those that survived on less than $10,000 a year—were $2,490 poorer than they had been in 1982. In the same time span, the upper middle class, earning $40,000 to $80,000 per year, gained $8,620, and wealthy households taking in more than $80,000 a year netted $24,270. Expressed another way, the poorest Americans lost 9 percent of their wealth in three years while the wealthiest gained 9 percent.

By mid-1982 U.S. unemployment rates reached a post-Depression high of 10.8 percent.

In the budget cutting, many Health and Human Services (HHS, formerly HEW) programs were severely slashed or eliminated. Shut down entirely were the Public Health Service Hospitals, the Public Health Service Corps (physicians deployed to rural and inner-city areas), and federally subsidized health care for civilian seamen.

Overall, 25 percent of the HHS budget was eliminated by bills passed from 1981 through 1983 (though some of the cuts didn't phase in until 1985). Programs such as the Indian Health Service and the Office of Refugee Health that served small, needy constituencies were the most drastically affected.

Native Americans had suffered the poorest health seen in North America ever since Columbus landed in Dominica in 1492. Waves of European plagues obliterated upward of 90 percent of the original populations, driving many tribes to extinction. The poverty, forced relocation, and humiliation that followed their defeats in the Indian Wars left most Native Americans desperately vulnerable to tuberculosis, sexually transmitted diseases, diabetes, heart disease, and alcoholism.

Congress had created the Indian Health Service (IHS) in 1955, placing it under the control of HEW. And in just five years IHS had lowered infant mortality among Native Americans by 25 percent and the tuberculosis death rate by 50 percent. But by the 1980s unemployment among Native Americans topped 40 percent, and at least one-third of all Native American households lived below the poverty line. A full two-thirds of the 1.1 million tribal people who lived on or near reservations had no health insurance. And the IHS was their sole provider.

Reagan's IHS cuts came in both direct and indirect form. Since most of the doctors who worked on the reservations were members of the Public Health Service Corps,[391] the elimination of that organization meant that IHS clinics and hospitals were immediately understaffed. Some administrative cuts were intended to be picked up by local tribal governments: in most cases, the tribes couldn't afford the burden. And cuts in AFDC and Medicaid hit hard for those Native Americans not qualified for IHS care.

At the close of the Reagan administration in 1988, one-third of all deaths among Native Americans would hit people less than forty-five years of age, and they would be 438 percent more likely than the rest of the U.S. population to die of ailments related to alcoholism. They would also be 400 percent more likely to die of tuberculosis, 155 percent more likely to die of diabetes, and 131 percent more likely to die in accidents of one kind or another.[392]

As the impact of budget cutting increments hit HHS sharply during Reagan's second term, the agency was forced to define "Indian" in a manner that narrowed the pool of people IHS served. As of 1987, only members of federally recognized tribes who resided on or near a reservation could receive IHS care, a ruling that cut nearly half of the estimated two million American Indians out of IHS's care.[393]

Pay cuts and deteriorating hospitals prompted many doctors to abandon IHS and the agency was forced to hire physicians with felony records, even a man wanted for homicide.[394] Admission rates plummeted at IHS hospitals and clinics as Indians realized that the facilities and staff quality had both deteriorated. In 1978 112,203 people were admitted to IHS facilities; by 1986 that number had fallen to 96,886.[395] Between 1970 and 1986, in both IHS and tribal facilities, the average daily number of clinic visits alone fell by about a thousand patients per day.

At the Gallup, New Mexico, IHS hospital in 1987 pediatrician Gary Escodero surveyed the ER, showing a visitor the facilities. Patients waited, patiently, on hard plastic chairs in a sterile room. Escodero shouted over the sound of a passing train that rattled the building.

"This looks like a bus station," his visitor noted.

"No frills," Escodero said with a shrug. "This is not a nice place to wait. About all you can say is you can sit down. And quite a bit of the time you have people standing around here because it's too crowded. No frills, but the job gets done."

One of Escodero's colleagues and a nurse were busy suturing a prone Navajo man whose clothing and body were drenched in fresh, red blood.

"That's a helluva laceration," the visitor said, noting that the patient's chest was sliced from just to one side of his heart all the way around to the middle of his back.

"Yeah, right," Escodero agreed, leaning in to examine the suturing work under way. "What had happened was he was crossing the street and got hit by the mirror of one pickup truck, which spun him around into the path of a truck coming in the opposite direction and it torqued him. And he was hemitransceted."

Both the patient and the pickup truck driver had been drunk when the accident occurred.

In Albuquerque later that year, Dr. Ben Muneta of the Navajo Nation Health Service acknowledged that "yeah, alcoholism is a problem" among his people. And spending money on a public health campaign aimed at the roots of the alcoholism issue would be a lot cheaper than sewing up hemitransceted trauma patients. But budgets for public health education were down.

The shy, thirty-three-year-old, Stanford-educated Muneta said it was hard enough patching people up and trying to fight the alcohol problem. But now new problems were cropping up. Syphilis, gonorrhea, haemophilis influenza, tuberculosis, and a new virus—HIV—were all claiming huge tolls among his Navajo people.

"Various tribes have gone through various epidemics that have wiped out up to 90 percent of the tribe," Muneta recalled in a near-whisper. "A lot of traditional healers feel there are diseases like these that break the order of things. The disorder is attributed to taking too much out of nature, destroying the jungles of the world and other ecological systems. Where there are diseases, there's a loss of checks and balances. And this is one of Nature's ways of telling us we're not as great as we think we are."

Meanwhile, at the IHS hospital in Fort Defiance, Arizona, the peeling paint and the holes in the walls vividly bespoke entropy.

"Yeah, we let it go," a doctor shrugged. "No money anymore."

In 1983 a modern, new IHS hospital opened in Chinle, Arizona, in the middle of the Navajo nation. It was built with money provided by the Carter administration and opened just before the Reagan IHS cuts would have frozen further construction. Chinle Hospital was everything the Fort Defiance and Gallup hospitals were not: clean, airy, modern, and comfortable. But the effects of budget cuts could be seen there, too: most of the mothers on the obstetric ward hadn't had any prenatal care because home visit services for obstetric nurses had been cut. As a result, more than half the births were high risk. And for babies born with disabilities related to difficult births, the Chinle doctors had to practice triage, handling the life-threatening problems first and putting the less severe cases on a three-to-four-month waiting list.

In Washington, Dr. Everett Rhoades, director of the IHS, said that budget cuts had "absolutely" forced triage and rationing of care. His 1987 budget left him $600 per capita per year for treatment of American Indians.

"A pretty fair comparison would be to compare that six hundred dollars to the approximately one thousand four hundred dollars spent on health care per capita for the rest of the U.S. population," a grim-faced Rhoades said. About 30 percent of the health needs of American Indians were going unmet, he continued, and that figure applied only to Indians on reservations. For urbanized Indians, Rhoades said, "that's a one hundred percent unmet need."[396]

Things were a lot worse over at the refugee health centers, where by 1987 nothing was functioning and the doors were closed. With federally funded refugee clinics no longer in operation, some nine hundred thousand Indochinese and thousands more Cubans and Haitians had simply joined the ranks of Medicaid patients. Refugee tuberculosis screening, in particular, was a key public health loss that would soon come to haunt the nation.

And, thanks to another set of sweeping Reagan administration changes, caring for the newly medically disenfranchised was thrown into the hands of states and counties. That's because, following his 1982 State of the Union address, Reagan fulfilled his promise to "with a simple, bold stroke" turn billions of dollars worth of federal programs over to the states. It was, Reagan said, "new federalism."

"Government," Reagan said, "doesn't solve problems, it subsidizes them."

Government—or, at least, *federal* government—was bad, the president said. Programs should be handled at the more accountable local level. If people locally didn't want to pay for them, well, that's democracy. "Meanwhile," wrote political historian Lou Cannon,[397] "the great social concerns of education and public health became back-burner issues for the Reagan administration. Reagan was not interested in the complexities of regulatory reform and he drew no distinctions between regulations restraining economic competition and regulations designed to enforce laws protecting the environment or the health and safety of Americans."

The Reagan administration sought to move most public health programs that targeted the needs of the poor to the states. And those programs that stayed at the federal level were marked for reductions in size (e.g., the CDC), weakening of their regulatory authority (e.g., FDA, EPA, and OSHA) or cost control (Medicare).[398]

The initial Reagan administration plan, announced in October 1981, called for huge cuts in Medicaid and Medicare spending. And twenty-five federal health programs were designated for consolidation into two massive block grants to the states. The overall budget for all of the programs would fall from $1.9 billion in 1981 to $1.4 billion in 1982. One of the block grants would combine ten preventive health services into a single $242 million effort. The second grant, for health care services to the poor, would meld fifteen federal programs into one big $1.138 billion effort. Each state's share of these two block grants would be proportional to the health funds they had previously received from the federal government. Essentially, the block grant money would go to the states' governors' offices to dole out as they pleased within the limits of the federal program's design and each state's own legal constraints and health strictures.

Congress settled for a slightly modified version of the block grant idea. Instead of two megagrants to the states, Congress created four, folding the existing federal programs into Primary Care (funded at $246 million for FY 1983); Maternal and Child Health ($347.5 million); Alcohol, Drug Abuse, and Mental Health ($432 million); and Preventive Health ($81.5 million). The final category covered most traditional public health activities, meaning that public health was allotted just 7 percent of the health budget.

Under the Reagan plan the states and counties were to administer Medicaid, AFDC, and dozens of specific public health programs. And where federal dollars were found inadequate, the states would make up the difference, if their constrained budgets would allow.[399] The key problem was that since the FDR days the federal government had increasingly encouraged state dependence upon Congress for such programs: the average state had gone from receiving less than 1 percent of its public health budget from the federal government in 1950 to more than 35 percent in 1978. Further, over those decades the states had shifted their own spending priorities and the average state now spent less than 5 percent of its public health budget on local programs.[400] Worse still, by 1978 the average local health department derived only 1 percent of its revenues from local sources, such as city taxes or fees charged to Medicaid patients. Most local health departments had grown addicted to county property taxes or federal dollars.[401]

"The first question of most local governments is how much of the federal cuts will be offset by state funding increases. The answer given by most states—

none—is not the answer that local governments want to hear," University of North Carolina analysts concluded in 1982.[402]

Putting aside the harsh economic straits, many state legislatures and governors had political or ideological objections to some programs (for example, family planning and venereal diseases education) and refused to implement them according to federal guidelines.[403]

Under the 1981 Omnibus Budget Reconciliation Act, Medicaid was cut by 3 percent in 1982, 4 percent in 1983, and 4.5 percent in 1984. Given that the nation was in an overall inflationary period and health care was the most rapidly inflating sector of the economy, in real terms these cuts amounted to a more than 18 percent slash in Medicaid expenditures. To make the pain of compensation slightly less odious for the states, the administration redefined eligibility for Medicaid, excluding all dual-parent households and, through other mechanisms, dropping one million people from Medicaid rolls.[404] Medicaid never had covered all of those in America who lived below the poverty line—now it would cover even fewer. During the Nixon administration nearly half of the impoverished in the United States were disqualified from Medicaid.[405]

In the case of Medicare the White House and HHS tried to cut costs by creating Diagnosis Related Groups (DRGs), representing a new approach to categorizing medical costs and billings. DRGs lumped billings by diagnosis, say, hypertension or diabetes. Any billings for treatment or services that were not on a preset list of covered items for that diagnosis would not be reimbursed. By the late 1980s and early 1990s the DRG system would be producing yelps of fiscal agony at hospitals all over the United States.

First, hospital occupancy rates plummeted (from 78 percent of all beds in 1984 to 62 percent in 1993) because DRGs set stiff limits on how many days patients could spend in the facilities. Hospitals that traditionally served poorer clienteles (rural facilities, inner-city hospitals, public hospitals) starved for cash because they had grown accustomed to covering the costs of treating poor patients by overbilling Medicare, i.e., passing those costs on and forcing the federal government to meet the needs of the poor through backdoor financing. DRGs rendered such backdoor financing impossible.

The result: hospitals shut down. According to the Government Accounting Office, between 1980 and 1991, 309 rural and 294 urban hospitals went out of business. For those hospitals that stayed open, Medicare losses—uncovered payments—totaled 12 percent of all costs by 1987.

Public hospitals were especially hard hit by DRGs. Their beds were full, their waiting rooms packed, mostly with patients no one else wanted: Medicaid recipients, the uninsured, and the underinsured. As the ranks of these patients swelled, so did local government debts. Cities and counties were forced to pick up tabs that the federal government, the states, and private insurance were unwilling to cover. In 1991, for example, sixty-six of the nation's one hundred public hospitals took in $12.2 billion in revenues but still owed another $15 billion.[406]

In New York City the public hospitals were in such dire shape by 1988 that they had become frankly dangerous. Patients were robbed as they lay helpless in their beds; drug addicts raided the pharmaceutical shelves; and homeless people moved in, blending in among the patients and sometimes picking pockets and stealing food from hospital cafeterias and patients' meal trays. Pay rates fell so sharply that poorly trained nurses and doctors were hired from overseas, with resulting catastrophes due to language and cultural misunderstandings over patients' needs. Thousands of pap smears were "lost" by overworked staffers who simply let samples and paperwork pile up while telling physicians their patients were "fine." As a consequence, some women were never notified that they had precancerous cervixes. By the end of the Reagan years some doctors would view working inside those hospitals as a matter of conscience, a sort of badge of charitable honor.[407]

The New York City problem was exacerbated by the almost complete lack of primary care options for the poor. At least one out of six of all patients treated in the public hospitals could have been better handled on an outpatient basis.[408] Similarly, nationwide, public and inner-city hospitals experienced a 24 percent increase in emergency room visits between 1985 and 1990, according to the American Hospital Association.[409]

Ironically, DRGs failed to control costs. Many private hospitals figured out how to bill inappropriate diagnoses, thereby getting around the system, and costs continued to rise.[410] The door opened wide for entrepreneurial medicine. It was a matter of survival. Hospitals started running more and more like companies—forming chains, eliminating "inefficient departments," merging with other facilities, and opening "Doc-in-a-Box" centers, as the small drop-in clinics located in shopping malls were called.[411]

Even with the constraints of DRGs, these private hospitals harvested record profits during Reagan's second term. How? In 1982 Reagan pushed another law through Congress called the Tax Equity and Fiscal Responsibility Act—TEFRA. It allowed hospitals to earn profits off Medicare and Medicaid patients, and any losses incurred treating Medicare cases could be written off on the hospital's taxes. Such tax incentives were of little value to public hospitals but were tremendous privatization incentives. Further, if a hospital managed to treat a Medicare patient for *less* than the DRG cost, TEFRA allowed it to keep the difference.

As a result hospitals located in areas rife with wealthy Medicare patients, such as Miami, Tucson, Palm Springs, and much of the Sunbelt, turned huge profits and drove up the overall costs of medical care in America.[412]

Meanwhile, the Reagan administration cut the Medicaid rolls; the states cut them further. The ranks of the uninsured swelled. The size of copayments required from those who did have insurance ballooned. All of this proved deeply disturbing for advocates for the poor but not for the society as a whole.

University of Wisconsin ethicist Daniel Wickler felt that the growing acceptance of market forces in the health care arena was a symptom, not the disease. The moral disease, Wickler argued, was the "personal responsibility for health" movement. For more than a decade the model of public, or collective, health that was espoused by Hermann Biggs had subtly yielded to a far more individualistic model in which each person was considered responsible for his or her own health status. The new view had arisen from two directions: left-wing "New Age" thinking and right-wing moralism, Wickler said.[413]

In the New Age view, individuals were encouraged to look at their lives holistically, devoting attention to all of the factors that might contribute to their physical and "spiritual" well-being, e.g., diet, fitness, meditation, positive outlook, and smoking/drinking/drug habits.

From the Right, Wickler insisted, came a sort of paternalistic moralism that condemned smokers, drinkers, the obese, and the exercise-averse for being morally weak and posing a burden to society. That burden would be in the form of the bill society would eventually pay for treating the ailments allegedly caused by the "bad" behaviors.

In both cases, Wickler argued, the result was a "blame-the-victim" perspective that absolved government and employers of their moral duty to provide health (both medicine and public health) to the *whole* society.

The "blame-the-victim" outlook had overtones of both class bias and racism: "It is one thing to explain a junkie's poor diet by his mental state and unopposable drives; it is quite another thing to blame a wide variety of lifestyle elements on a factor as undifferentiated as 'ghetto life,' " Winkler insisted.

Thus, during the Reagan years three critical public health themes developed in parallel: emergence of new contagious threats to health; skyrocketing numbers of uninsured Americans; and a heightened sense of individual, rather than community, responsibility for disease.

In 1978, however, there were twenty-five million Americans who could not afford private health insurance but did not qualify for Medicaid or Medicare and another sixteen million Americans lacked insurance for part of that year.[414] By 1984 the number of full-time uninsured had risen to thirty million and, due to higher copayments and deductibles required by both private and public health insurance, a new class had surfaced: the "underinsured." These were individuals who would be unable to afford payment for any health care that wasn't covered by their inadequate insurance, Medicare, or Medicaid. They were estimated to number another 55.7 million.[415] And the numbers would just keep mounting.[416]

Even before the Reagan era swelled the ranks of the uninsured, there was ample evidence that lack of insurance led to poorer public health outcomes. The CDC found in 1978, for example, that insured children were much more likely to be fully immunized than were uninsured children.[417]

The insurance gap widened even further in the 1980s because more Americans lost their jobs in the bad economy and states were unable to make up the difference created by shortfalls in the Reagan block grant programs.

In Los Angeles County, for example, Prop. 13 and the decline in Medicare revenues were already creating pain, even though government defense contracts were pushing a fiscal boomlet in the region. Then the California state legislature, unable or unwilling to conjure funds to offset federal Medicaid reductions, ruled in 1982 that 270,000 childless, impoverished adults could no longer receive Medi-Cal. The state decided that it was up to the counties to find ways to handle these patients. For L.A. County that meant absorbing 87,000 impoverished patients, beginning January 1, 1983.

Los Angeles County didn't have the money. For six months, UCLA's Dr. Nicole Lurie tracked a cohort of 186 newly disinsured patients, comparing their health to a group of two hundred patients who remained qualified for Medi-Cal. Over that time little changed for the two hundred on Medi-Cal. But the disinsured had a mean increase in blood pressure of 10 mm of mercury, which Lurie found "extremely significant. It's clinically very meaningful. . . . That kind of increase increases your chance of dying of heart disease by 40 percent."[418]

One such patient did die. Having suffered hypertension for years, and now unable to afford either medical visits or her medication, she had a fatal brain hemorrhage. In all, Lurie saw two deaths in the disinsured group that she ascribed to lack of health care and several other patients suffered seizures and other disorders as a result of no longer receiving medications.[419]

While the ranks of the uninsured swelled, evidence mounted connecting cancer and heart disease prevention to diet and exercise. This would lead to and fuel what Wickler had labeled the "personal responsibility movement."

Working in East Africa, British physician Denis Burkitt had discovered a form of lymphoma cancer that now bears his name. He also found a relationship between high-fiber diets and lowered incidences of cancers of the bowel and colon.

"Visualize water coming from a tap, the basin overflowing," Burkitt said of cancer prevention in 1981.[420] "Now, how are we going to keep the floor dry? We could mop the floor rather than turn off the faucet. I've been mopping for years. Doctors give testimonials to mopping. I mopped for years in Africa. *No* impact. I think with cancer it's better to turn off the taps. Of course, one can get rich mopping. The car parks of hospitals are full of Lincolns—the moppers."

Burkitt felt certain that most cancer was preventable: the tap, he said, could be shut.

"See here, if we modify the way we eat we can decrease cancer by a third. Eliminate smoking and you're down another third. Turn off the tap, that's what it is," Burkitt insisted. His message was, ultimately, quite clear: eat more fiber and less fat.[421] "All you must do to avoid cancer is to revert back to what your ancestors ate. It's as simple as that," Burkitt concluded, referring to prehistoric diets. (Critics pointed out that in prehistoric times our ancestors rarely lived long enough to develop cancer.)

At the National Cancer Institute (NCI) in Bethesda, Maryland, Dr. Vincent De Vita's focus was on treatment, not prevention. He oversaw budgets that had swelled faster than most malignancies, thanks to the on-going War on Cancer that had begun during the Nixon administration. De Vita predicted in 1981 that "fifty percent of all cancers will be curable within ten years."[422]

True, the NCI was noting new problems associated with drug-resistant types of tumors—cancer cells that mutated into forms that could thrive in the presence of powerful chemotherapeutic agents. That was bad news for treatment; but the NCI had come to realize over the previous five years that most cancers had their roots in genetics and that fact could be very good news in terms of preventing tumor development.

De Vita was dismissive about the prospect of shutting off Burkitt's "taps" and was disinclined to take a strong public health stand on dietary issues such as fat, beta-carotene, artificial estrogens, and other factors found to be associated with either cancer promotion or prevention.[423] He was busy overseeing an intellectual revolution that was approaching the cancer problem on the molecular level. It had begun in 1975 with development of genetic engineering techniques that allowed scientists to manipulate DNA and RNA and observe which changes prompted transformation of cells. And in just five years a host of oncogenes were discovered—on/off switches in human DNA that, when triggered, prompted the wild cell growth that is, ultimately, cancer.[424] In 1981 any links between these molecular observations and the sorts of population-level macrodiscoveries Burkitt made were purely theoretical.

But by the mid-1980s the pace of discovery had accelerated dramatically, pulling the two seemingly unrelated positions closer together. Scientists discovered that some oncogenes' switches were exceedingly vulnerable to specific carcinogens or viruses. For example, Burkitt's lymphomas were usually caused by Epstein-Barr virus. And an oncogene in lung cells was deregulated by chemicals in cigarette smoke. Other oncogenes appeared vulnerable to estrogens, testosterones, and other hormones.

Also, higher specific cancer rates had been observed in populations that ate large amounts of pickled or barbecued foods, and this led to chemical analysis of pickling agents and tars.[425] Epidemiologists also claimed to see higher cancer rates in heavy coffee drinkers,[426] alcoholics, and individuals who ate a great deal of saturated fats such as were found in butter and bacon.

Some public health advocates, insurance companies, and physicians raced ahead of such data, however, telling Americans what they should and should not eat long before the scientific evidence supporting their recommendations was clear. In the "blame-the-victim" atmosphere of the 1980s, the dietary commandments seemed to come down as if from Mt. Sinai. But unlike Moses' tablets, the pronouncements about diet and cancer were frequently revised and the public was told, "that's not what we meant—what we *really* mean is. . . ." Fiber and colon cancer,[427] high-fat diets and breast cancer,[428] caffeine and cancer,[429] alcohol and breast cancer[430]—the houses of cards that supported all these theories would fall in the late 1990s. Indeed, even Burkitt's claimed connection between high-fiber diets and lowered cancer risks would be proven completely incorrect in 2000.

The strongest personal responsibility messages during the 1980s came from the American Cancer Society and Surgeon General Koop regarding cigarettes, and from the American Heart Association, which attacked both tobacco and cholesterol.

In truth, the U.S. heart disease epidemic that had begun after World War II was already abating by 1980; between 1970 and 1985 deaths due to heart disease plummeted by 48 percent.[431] Every Western industrialized society and Japan witnessed the same trend; an upsurge in heart disease and cardiac deaths between 1945 and 1970, followed by a marked downturn. Nationally, each year from 1969 to 1990, death rates from cardiovascular disease declined by 2.6 cases per 100,000 people.[432]

The reasons for improvement in heart disease rates and death incidences were many, but the full picture was, ultimately, elusive. Whatever the cause(s), it had to have been present as early as the late 1960s to exert such a powerful impact in the 1970s. During that time, cigarette smoking was declining among men but rising among women in the United States. That made it hard to ascribe the downturn to tobacco avoidance, given that decreased cardiac disease was seen in both genders. The effect could not be demographic, either, as population changes in the United States actually ought to have increased heart disease. The population was increasing, aging, and becoming racially more diverse, reflecting a broader gene pool of those potentially at risk. It would also be hard to credit diet, as Americans ate loads of fatty foods during the 1960s.

The improvements in heart disease rates during the 1970s and 1980s were not universal. During most of the 1980s, for example, African-American adults had high blood pressure rates that were well above those of their white counterparts, and higher cardiovascular death rates as well. African-American life expectancies at birth actually declined during the Reagan years.[433]

The American Heart Association and numerous medical and public health groups went on the "personal responsibility" offensive during the 1980s, driving home dietary and exercise themes related primarily to lowering cholesterol levels.[434]

In the 1980s researchers all over the world discovered a striking, but complex, correlation between heart disease and cholesterol. Men who died of heart disease were, they found, more likely to have consumed diets rich in fats, especially high-cholesterol animal fats. There was enough cholesterol evidence in hand by the mid-1980s to prompt strong dietary recommendations from on high. Government reports, cookbooks, and nutrition guides all entreated Americans to eat much as Burkitt recommended: less fat and more fish; banish butter, eggs, and bacon; avoid cream; eat loads of oats; and increase overall carbohydrate intake while lowering the amount of protein in the diets.[435]

To a remarkable degree, Americans got the message—sort of. Americans *decreased* the percentage of their diets that contained fat and cholesterol, but generally *increased* their overall caloric intakes. In the mid 1980s about a third of U.S. adults were overweight, by the late 1990s that figure had risen to half.[436]

Public health advocates had never presented a uniform, clear set of dietary recommendations. Indeed, each week in the 1980s and 1990s seemed to bring new evidence that fish protected the heart—no, wait, not all fish. Maybe this fish. Forget fish. But oats are great—well, maybe. In the 1970s the U.S. public was deluged with dubious public health information on the "carcinogen of the week." In the 1980s it was the dietary recommendation of the week that sowed public confusion and discontent.

In 1989, however, the American Heart Association expressed little public doubt and put its icon on "heart healthy" products as its seal of endorsement. The intent was to provide consumers with a public health shopping guide. And the AHA felt confident that the scientific evidence was solid and adequate enough to warrant putting the association's credibility on the line with specific product endorsements.

But the cardiologists and scientists who attended the AHA's annual convention in 1989 didn't present a particularly united front on the matter. Scientists who worked on cholesterol chemistry warned that such an approach was overly simplistic. "It's not clear cut," Alan Chait of the University of Washington in Seattle cautioned. "I say yes, doctors should keep an eye on the research. But it's really not ready for widespread practice."[437]

Dr. Dean Ornish of the University of California San Francisco thought the public health focus on cholesterol was dangerous, as it offered Americans a false sense of security. To really protect one's self against heart disease, Ornish argued, "you need a complete lifestyle change. Diet, alone, will never do it."

A much easier solution was offered by medications. Anticholesterol drugs could bring cholesterol levels down by as much as 30 percent in a year without severe dietary or lifestyle changes. At the 1989 AHA meeting a physician, upon hearing a speech describing such drug efficacies, shouted from the audience, "Sounds to me like the best public health option would be to put those drugs in the public drinking water!"

Such schemes being neither *true* public health nor in the realm of reality, public health advocates instead resorted to exhortation and scolding, paternalistically chastising Americans for failing to eat right. But they were up against the slick, expensive, and far more pervasive advertising dedicated to persuading the nation to consider the alternative: A fork laden with "delicious, moist chocolate cake" fills your television screen. When it pulls back, one bite is missing. Are you tempted?

"The great struggle to come, already emerging, is that between public health and personal responsibility, on the one hand, and the market on the other," bioethicist Daniel Callahan wrote.[438] "The market can, and does already, overshadow both 'genetics medicine' and public health. It sets the stage and the social context, and thus has a commanding and still-rising power. The ultimate struggle I have in mind is between the population perspective of public health and the individualist perspective of the market."

Insurance companies and HMOs, both of which were well aware of the power of the market, grew more aggressive. If, indeed, getting all their clients on "heart healthy" diets could lower cardiac surgery bills, it made sense to push principles of prevention.

It certainly made good business sense.[439]

And perhaps good public health sense, too. In 1950 the annual age-adjusted national death rate was 841 of every 100,000 Americans: 48 percent of that mortality was due to cardiovascular disease. By 1990 the age-adjusted death rate would be 520 per 100,000, with 34 percent of those deaths due to cardiovascular illness. So it appeared that over forty years the national death rate plummeted, and a 14 percent decline in heart-related mortality was the chief reason.[440] But was America's dietary change—from high-fat and moderate caloric intake to lower-fat but far higher overall calorie consumption—the cause of this improvement in heart health? Could it, in other words, be considered a public health victory? And did it follow that a greater emphasis on personal responsibility (and, in its absence, on guilt) would lead to greater improvements in population health?

Skeptics offered three lines of reasoning. First, the downturn in the "heart disease epidemic" well predated the national anticholesterol drive. Second, the number of smokers in the United States fell dramatically during the same period and tobacco exerted at least as powerful a deleterious effect on the heart as did

LDL cholesterol. And finally, in the nineties many of the "heart healthy" messages of the 1980s would be overturned in light of further science.

Margarine, for example, would turn out to contain dangerous transfatty
acids that increased heart risks not by raising LDL levels, but by lowering HDL
levels. Vitamin E's heart benefits turned out to be minimal, perhaps nonexistent.[441] Eggs would turn out to contain less cholesterol than originally thought
and to pose much less risk. Diets rich in folic acid and B vitamins would turn
out to have such powerful benefits for the heart that they could outweigh such
"sins" as moderate red meat intake.[442]

Could the public be blamed for its confusion?

The focus on diet may have been misplaced as a public health effort. It
was perhaps more appropriately a component of medicine, with its mechanistic
view of a clogged and cancerous human body. Further, an individual's nutritional needs and how he or she understands them may not be well addressed
by wholesale appeals to society. Given America's propulsion into obesity, it
would seem that interpretation and implementation of dietary messages is a
complex matter.

During the Reagan era, then, health insurance access declined and the
personal responsibility movement rose. Public health programs were severely
strained by both increased burdens (as responsibilities shifted from federal to
state to local levels) and decreased budgets.

And new public health challenges loomed: toxic shock syndrome (TSS),
food-borne and antibiotic-resistant illnesses, the human immunodeficiency virus (HIV), and crack cocaine.

Toxic shock syndrome revealed a new kind of vulnerability that clearly was
not related to personal responsibility, insurance, or any of the health topics then
on the agenda. It was about new product designs, emerging diseases, and failures in the public health safety net.[443]

During the mid-1970s a strain of *Staphylococcus aureus* emerged that carried genes for an unusually powerful toxin. In doses so small as to be nearly
unmeasurable, this bacterium could so radically upset the human immune system as to cause death from shock. The emergence of this new form of staph
coincided with novel product designs for tampons that could remain inside a
woman's vagina for six hours or longer during her menstrual cycle. The FDA
had given the products approval without much scrutiny as the agency exercised
little authority over devices (tampons), as opposed to foods and pharmaceuticals.

As it turned out, these superabsorbent tampons provided ideal ecologies
in which the new, highly toxic strain of staph could thrive. Beginning in small
numbers in 1975, then in an avalanche by 1980, women all across North Amer-

ica (and wherever else the U.S.-made tampons were sold) contracted, and died of, TSS.

The Centers for Disease Control, FDA, tampon industry, and various private researchers got bogged down in disputes about the cause of the national epidemic of tampon-associated staph deaths. One tampon product, in particular, seemed to be associated with more cases, so the FDA targeted Rely, pushing it off the market.

It would turn out that TSS wasn't *caused* by any tampon but by a bacterium and that puzzle was ultimately solved not by federal public health agencies or regulators but by the Minnesota State Department of Health and a University of Minnesota scientist. Two researchers were key: State Epidemiologist Dr. Michael Osterholm and university microbiologist Patrick Schlievert.

The duo was able to crack the toxic shock case because Minnesota had arguably the best state health surveillance system in the nation, providing Osterholm with an ideal window on the evolving epidemic. The Minnesotans had other advantages as well: good collaboration between local academic and public health scientists, an excellent state health laboratory network, a strong statewide infrastructure, and few confounding health problems in Minnesota's female population that could complicate diagnoses.[444]

During the 1980s Minnesotans were the healthiest of all Americans and among the healthiest in the entire world.[445] While social welfare and public health spending was declining nearly everywhere else in the United States, Minnesotans generously supported these programs, offering one explanation for their remarkable collective wellness. Between 1980 and 1993 the state's spending on health rose 90 percent and public health spending consistently held at about 3 percent of the overall health budget. Spending for health care, HMOs, nursing homes, and other health institutions rose and was adequate to ensure access for every single Minnesotan. The state offered MinnesotaCare for all uninsured children and medical assistance to all indigent adults.[446]

Amid the national economic gloom Minnesota's 1985 unemployment rate was 12.6 percent, versus a national rate of 14 percent. Most of Minnesota's adults had completed high school and had had additional college or trade school courses, making them one of the best-educated populations in the United States. And most Minnesotans shared similar cultural and social values, as more than 96 percent of the population was white, and in excess of 90 percent of the white population was descended from German or Scandinavian immigrants. A key value shared by most Minnesotans was that of community, or collective, problem-solving and commitment. It was an ideal cultural environment for support of social programs that were aimed at the population as a whole.

In 1968 the Minnesota Department of Health's budget had been terribly dependent upon federal dollars. For every one dollar the department got from state and local sources, it received $1.30 from the federal government.[447] By 1985, when the full impact of the Reagan administration's cuts and block grants could be felt, the state and federal contribution to the budget were much closer.[448] And by the end of the 1990s state and local contributions would exceed federal contributions, bringing in $1.12 for every federal dollar.[449]

Despite budget constraints, the staff of disease investigators working under Osterholm was increased from 28 in 1980 to 144 by 1990. There was no alternative: epidemics were suddenly breaking out all over the otherwise remarkably healthy state. In addition to the toxic shock syndrome epidemic, Osterholm's staff had their hands full with unusual outbreaks between 1981 and 1987.

In 1986, for example, a *Giardia lamblia* diarrheal epidemic broke out in a rural Minnesota community. Months of investigation revealed a very complex pattern of the protozoa's spread, involving a child care center, a nursing home, and food.[450]

During the 1981–87 period the state epidemiology team also investigated numerous respiratory, diarrheal, and chickenpox outbreaks in child care centers. (By 1985 nearly half of all preschoolers in the state were in such centers—a steadily increasing trend that reflected the growing ranks of working mothers in Minnesota.[451]) And the team demonstrated that another new, dangerous microorganism was spreading in child care centers: *Escherichia coli* 0157:H7.

E. coli is one of humanity's ancient microbial companions and a bacterial cause of diarrheal disease. Usually, *E. coli* infections are only dangerous to babies, as people swiftly develop immunity to the bacteria. Every adult's intestinal tract typically harbors small colonies of the bugs, kept in check by the immune system.

But in 1982 a new form of *E. coli* emerged, dubbed 0157:H7. It contained an unusual toxin that caused hemolytic uremic syndrome, or bloody diarrhea.[452] Outbreaks of *E. coli* 0157:H7 occurred all over the United States in the 1980s. In at least nineteen of them particularly severe illnesses resulted, causing hospitalization of 24 percent of the infected individuals and killing 1 percent. By the end of the 1980s, the CDC would be getting twenty thousand *E. coli* 0157:H7 case reports a year and the new organism would have become the primary cause of bloody diarrhea in the United States and Canada.[453]

An Osterholm/CDC retrospective study identified a total of 117 hemolytic uremia syndrome cases that had occurred between 1979 and 1988. Most were sporadic or seemingly unrelated to one another, but every group or cluster of cases was connected to a child care center. The sporadic cases, Osterholm's group found, all could be traced to hamburger meat.[454] And the bacterium not only was drug resistant but also released more of its deadly toxins under drug stress. Drug treatment could actually hasten death.

By the mid-1990s the United States would have exported *E. coli* 0157:H7 to countries all over the world, either in beef or in foods that had absorbed the deadly bacteria via exposure to cow manure. Vehicles of export spread included salami, beef jerky, venison, pasteurized milk, potatoes, lettuce, apple cider, alfalfa sprouts, and radish sprouts.[455]

What nagged at Michael Osterholm, a tenacious bulldog of a scientist, was that the number of food-related outbreaks in Minnesota was increasing and—more important—they were getting harder to track because of the increasing complexity of food production and marketing. *E. coli* grew in the gastrointestinal tract of cattle, but it was impossible to track any particular batch of meat to a certain site of original contamination because by the 1980s the hamburger production industry combined the meat from hundreds of cows into single batches.

It was becoming obvious to Osterholm that the federal safety apparatus couldn't handle the problem.

"We have a grossly inadequate public health infrastructure," Osterholm concluded, and he realized that it no longer was enough just to work hard in Minnesota: he was going to have to find the time and resources to start agitating at the national level.

In Los Angeles County Dr. Shirley Fanin was reaching the same conclusions. In 1985 her communicable diseases division at the county's health department was overwhelmed by *Listeria* food poisoning incidents. With careful detective work, her staff had traced the outbreaks to Mexican cheeses being sold to the county's swelling Latino population. Though *Listeria* was treatable with antibiotics, some children were ending up with life-threatening illnesses. Finding and treating the ailing youngsters and informing the public about the dangerously contaminated cheese products were tasks made all the more difficult by the radical demographic changes under way in Los Angeles.

"Who would have thought," the brassy, outspoken Fanin said in 1985, "that we would be dealing with an epidemic caused by Mexican cheese eaten by Salvadorean war refugees."

The world was shrinking and public health risks reflected the new paradigm.

Shortly after taking office, President Reagan had ordered a combination of covert and overt operations in support of pro-U.S. forces throughout Central America: the anti-Sandinista Contras in Nicaragua and the governments of Guatemala, Honduras, and El Salvador.

As the brutal wars and repression spread, hundreds of thousands of Central Americans fled to the United States, most settling illegally in Florida, Texas, Arizona, and California. Between 1981 and 1988 Los Angeles County absorbed the largest number of these illegal immigrants, variously estimated to have totaled 350,000 to half a million. (When, by 1991, the wars had largely ended, few of these refugees returned to Central America.)

Most of the Salvadoreans who reached Los Angeles during those years were traumatized and terrified of deportation back to what they felt would be certain death or torture. Unlike the Mexicans and Chicanos in Los Angeles, the Salvadoreans kept their heads down, tried to be invisible, stayed away from anyone connected to government, and avoided even the health care system except in emergencies. Since they did not qualify for Medi-Cal, the county had no choice but to provide them with gratis medical care, holding out no hope of state or federal reimbursement.

This greatly exacerbated the L.A. County Department of Health's already awesome list of problems. By 1984 the Board of Supervisors had taken to mortgaging government buildings in order to raise funds for its payroll. Cutbacks in Medicare and Medi-Cal revenues came as the patient burden increased.

Just five months after Reagan's inauguration, doctors in New York, Los Angeles, and Washington, D.C., publicized word of odd deaths occurring in gay men and IV drug users. Parasitic pneumonias, once-rare skin tumors, types of lymphoma usually seen only in elderly men—suddenly, previously healthy young men were turning up at hospitals with these diseases and dying there.

It was, of course, the beginning of what would become the twentieth century's second worst pandemic (after the 1918 influenza), caused by the human immunodeficiency virus, or HIV. By the end of the century, just nineteen years after the first cases of the disease were reported, more than thirty-four million people worldwide would have become infected with HIV. At least half of them would have developed the end-stage syndrome called AIDS and at least twelve million would have died of the disease. It would have spread to every corner of the planet, defying both public health efforts and the scientific pursuit of genuine cures or vaccines.

There could be no greater evidence of the need for a new, global approach to public health. But when the first IV drug users suffering from AIDS staggered into New York City public hospitals and initial handfuls of ailing gay men begged for help from doctors in San Francisco and Los Angeles, the public health response was abysmal, even nonexistent.

Though a tiny cadre of epidemiologists, scientists, and physicians struggled at the CDC and in San Francisco, New York City, Los Angeles, and elsewhere in the United States, as well as in Europe, to understand the new threat, their efforts were ignored or rebuffed by government.

At the top, the Reagan administration seemed utterly incapable of getting past the fact that most of the first cases of AIDS involved homosexual men. It was the first administration in the White House that had campaigned on a Christian fundamentalist platform and Reagan's constituents were avidly antigay. According to his personal physician, Reagan thought AIDS was something like measles: a virus that was passing through but would soon disappear without any special effort on humanity's part. That this was an inaccurate understanding of measles—a virus controlled through vigorous public health efforts—was one thing. Worse, it was a dangerously wrong perception regarding HIV.[456]

It seems clear from the record that Reagan never fully understood that a true pandemic of an incurable disease was unfolding on his watch. And though many of his aides did appreciate the scale of the epidemic, they agreed with the assessment of the Moral Majority's Reverend Jerry Falwell that the disease was God's retribution for immoral, sinful, homosexual behavior. Some members of Congress shared that view and openly opposed virtually every piece of public health AIDS legislation that reached the House or Senate.

Within the Department of Health and Human Services, the medicalized view of public health predominated during the Reagan years. So in response to AIDS classic public health measures were shunned in favor of a completely un-supportable belief that laboratory science would swiftly solve the problem—by the turn of the century, that still had not come to pass.

Within HHS, Surgeon General C. Everett Koop was the most outspoken—often the sole—voice in favor of public health approaches to the HIV crisis. He recognized that in the absence of scientific "magic bullet" solutions, there was a crying need for public education. Armed with accurate information about how the virus was spread and how individuals could best protect themselves, the American people would, Koop reasoned, make proper choices. But the infor-mation had to be fairly explicit to be useful. And sexually active adults had to be advised to use condoms.

The mere idea of promoting condoms was anathema in the White House and within the Republican Party. Throughout U.S. history, whenever moralistic issues got in the way the public's health suffered. This had been especially true in the case of sexually transmitted diseases and drug abuse issues. By the time HIV surfaced in the United States, the incidence of gonorrhea, chlamydia, syph-ilis, hepatitis B, and other sexually transmitted diseases had been escalating for decades. Americans opposed sex education in schools, discussion of condom use, and education about birth control, particularly for adolescents.

On October 22, 1986, in the largest public health mailing in U.S. history, Koop issued his Surgeon General's Report on AIDS to 107 million U.S. house-holds. Though the report fell short of containing the explicit discussions of ho-mosexuality advocated by many AIDS activists, it nevertheless came under harsh attack from the Moral Majority, the Right to Life movement, and the right wing of the Republican Party—all of which interpreted it as an endorsement of the sins of premarital and extramarital sex and homosexuality.

In retrospect, what was more remarkable about the Koop mailing was not its contents but that it occurred five years *after* the epidemic was recognized and more than two years after HIV was discovered, proving the disease was contagious. There clearly was foot-dragging in Washington on every public health measure related to HIV: funding for basic research, public education, antidiscrimination legislation to protect infected individuals, and health care coverage.

Because nearly all of the epidemic's casualties were young adults or their children, HIV hit the very demographic groups that were most likely to fall outside the health care safety net after the Reagan administration's changes in Medicare, Medicaid, and special public health programs went into effect.

AIDS activists, who were for the most part white gay men in their twenties and thirties, made the search for a cure and antidiscrimination legislation their top priorities. As the toll of HIV cases and deaths rose, and many died never having received quality care, Dr. James Curran of the CDC called out for "human resources to care for the people who are already infected."[457] But doctors and dentists all over the United States declined to treat HIV patients on the grounds that those individuals posed a threat. The same health providers willingly worked with patients who carried far more contagious microbes, such as hepatitis B and drug-resistant forms of staphylococcus and streptococcus, but the specter of AIDS prompted them to break all of the primary tenets of physician ethics.

From a public health point of view, the key AIDS priorities in the 1980s should have been: number one, identify the cause of the disease; number two, determine exactly how the organism was spread from person to person; number three, stop that spread; number four, initiate vigorous research in pursuit of both a cure and a vaccine.[458]

The record shows that number one (identification of the cause) and number two (modes of transmission) were achieved very quickly, in large part through the efforts of U.S. federal agencies. The CDC, working closely with epidemiologists in San Francisco, Los Angeles, and New York, swiftly identified the means by which AIDS was spread and proved that the disease was caused by some form of infectious microorganism. Within months of the May 1981 recognition that a new, fatal disease had emerged among gay men, Curran's team at the CDC had determined that it was spread via anal and vaginal intercourse, contaminated IV needles, and contaminated blood. A little later in the epidemiology, they noted mother-to-child transmission. The bottom line, the CDC said in 1982, was exposure to contaminated blood.

Even in the absence of discovery of HIV, appropriate public health measures (number three) based on those observations would have involved widespread education about how every American could avoid blood-to-blood exposure and concrete steps to decrease such risks: screening of the U.S. blood supply, basic protective gear for hospital and clinic employees, promotion of condom use by sexually active adults, ensuring that all injections—medical or for illegal drug use—involved use of sterile needles and syringes, and closure of or strong admonishments against social settings that encouraged behaviors that put people at risk of blood-to-blood exposure.

Rational as that list appeared, implementation of every one of those measures ran up against a wall of political, social, economic, and civil libertarian obstacles. Indeed, by the end of the century incidents of blood-to-blood exposure would still be commonplace in U.S. society, and several measures that might have mitigated against HIV exposure would remain blocked. In some instances, the right laws may indeed have been passed and appropriate public health steps taken, but that happened only after much delay and argument.[459]

The nation's most prestigious medical science body, the Institute of Medicine, issued everything from memos to tomes begging—in plaintive, nearly supplicant tones—for a viable public health response to the epidemic.[460] In 1988 the institute urged "the federal government to take the lead in developing a comprehensive and coherent national plan for delivering and financing care for HIV-infected and AIDS patients." It insisted that "present funding is insufficient for public health approaches to stem the epidemic." And it decried the "gross inadequacy of federal efforts to reduce HIV transmission among IV drug abusers. . . ."

By the time those statements were released, some eighty thousand Americans had developed AIDS and forty-five thousand had died of the disease. It was far too late to close the proverbial barn door: simple public health measures would no longer be sufficient.

What had gone wrong?

Bigotry against homosexuals and injecting drug users had blinded the general public, politicians, the medical community, and, sadly, many public health leaders to the urgency of responding to AIDS when effective action might have had a profound impact: between May 1981 and the end of 1984. Those health leaders at the CDC, and in New York City, San Francisco, and other hard-hit cities who did voice concerns and try to implement appropriate measures were thwarted by community resistance that was both complex and overwhelming. From the Right they faced outright hostility. From most tiers of government they received shrugs or snubs. From the industries most involved in blood products and related equipment they heard cries of government interference and economic woe.[461]

Nor did public health leaders get much support from mainstream America, which continued to be woefully ignorant about AIDS and frighteningly prejudiced. A *New York Times*/CBS poll in 1988 found that more than 75 percent of respondents had "no sympathy for homosexuals suffering from AIDS." A shocking 19 percent said they had no sympathy for AIDS patients *regardless of how they acquired their HIV infection,* even if the individuals were infants or transfusion recipients.[462]

How did public health leaders counter such public hostility? In general, by identifying with the populations of Americans who had AIDS or were at greatest risk for HIV infection, even to the extent of adopting issues that served only to distract the nation from the primary health issues involved.[463] All disease surveillance and identification of infected individuals was made confidential or anonymous, thus protecting individuals from societal discrimination. And HIV infections were never reported; only full-blown AIDS cases were tracked, amid clearly justifiable concerns about protecting the civil liberties of outwardly well, HIV-positive individuals.

Thus, nobody truly knew at any given moment how large the public health catastrophe was, where and in which communities it was spreading, whether any public health interventions were actually slowing that spread, or if such programs might be failing and the millions of dollars spent on them wasted. The snapshots public health leaders got of the epidemic were, by definition, out of date. Epidemiologists in the 1980s and 1990s were forced by political and technological limitations to use slow-motion tools to decipher the epidemic's nuances. It was terribly crude.

And it opened the door to policy decisions based as much on political and emotional issues as on science. For example, as late as 1986 in New York City it was Department of Health policy *not* to tell individuals who donated blood that their sample had tested HIV positive.

"We should not share test results with people whose blood is tested," the city's Dr. Joyce Gaynor told blood bank officials in 1985. "We should refrain until we know the significance of such a finding."

Elsewhere in the United States, some public health officials blatantly lied to donors, telling those who turned up positive that their blood was rejected because it contained hepatitis. Some refused, even as late as 1986, to test blood at all.[464]

There would not be a nationally uniform FDA blood products policy until 1989, and the parameters of general testing (both of individuals and donated blood and plasma) would never be made nationally uniform. As a result, each state would decide its own policies regarding who might be tested voluntarily, versus under legal mandate; whether individuals who tested positive would be so informed; in what context that awful information would be dispensed; how— or even if—the identities of HIV-positive individuals would be tracked or codified; and what systems would be in place to track the names of those who advanced to AIDS or died. It would evolve into a hodgepodge system full of epidemiologic flaws and fraught with policy confusion.

In states in which gay activists were vocal and well organized, the toughest civil libertarian restrictions were put in place. And in states with little vocal gay activism, civil libertarian protections were typically far weaker. Jesse Helms's home state of North Carolina, for example, kept records by name of all HIV-infected individuals and their sex partners. This meant that it was easiest to track the unfolding epidemic in states with the smallest HIV-positive populations.

And it meant that public health authorities working in the hotbeds of HIV at the time—New York City, Los Angeles, San Francisco, Newark, Washington, D.C., Miami, and Chicago—were operating largely in the dark.[465] For example, in 1984 all of these cities hotly debated whether to close gay sex clubs and bathhouses in order to minimize spread of HIV. At the time, Curran's CDC staff had word of only 6,122 cases nationwide and 2,800 deaths. Overall, Curran concluded in 1984, "it is estimated that two hundred to three hundred thousand people in the U.S. have been exposed to the virus."[466] Though the virus that would later be dubbed HIV had been discovered by then, widespread use of HIV blood tests was not yet in place and epidemiologists had to do seat-of-the-pants reckoning, often in the face of open hostility from the gay community that they sought to protect.

While the bathhouse issue was under debate, epidemiologist Andrew Moss of the University of California San Francisco told that city's health commissioner, and later the superior court: "What we expect to see is that this growth will continue until the disease has saturated the population—that is, until most of the people who are susceptible to the disease get infected—and at that point we will see the number of new cases trailing off."[467]

The remarkably prescient Moss said that public health policy on AIDS should emphasize at least two other factors: "One is to make it clear to people what the truly terrifying nature of the disease is, how grave and serious a disease it is. The second is to attempt to support what you might call serially monogamous lifestyles—that is, cutting down by changing from a lifestyle with a very large number of sexual partners to a lifestyle that is closer to serial monogamy."

Public Health Commissioner Dr. Mervyn Silverman did decide to close the city's bathhouses and Superior Court Judge Roy Wonder upheld his decision. In New York City, Health Commissioner Dr. Stephen Joseph confronted similar difficult decisions and reached analogous conclusions.

Both men faced attempts to oust them from office as a result.

Silverman came under attack from gay activists who thought his actions discriminatory and homophobic and from Mayor Dianne Feinstein who felt he had moved too slowly and not taken drastic enough measures. Silverman was asked to resign. Joseph survived activists' attacks, but Mayor Koch did little to defend his health commissioner.

In New York the debate over how to limit spread of HIV in the gay community was ultimately decided at the state level.[468] On October 24, 1985, after months of hearings and debates, State Health Commissioner Dr. David Axelrod sent a memo to Governor Mario Cuomo: "I have concluded that establishments which allow, promote, and/or encourage sexual contacts that produce blood to blood or semen to blood contact are a serious menace to the public health and must be prohibited. . . . It applies to any establishment that caters to dangerous heterosexual or homosexual sex."[469]

Governor Cuomo, a liberal Democrat, followed Axelrod's recommendation to close sex parlors and bathhouses and stated, "Until the scientists find a cure for AIDS, education is our only vaccine."[470]

Which brought America, finally, to public health step number four: institute vigorous research. There was a tremendous blind faith that Science would, indeed, find a cure for AIDS. It just needed some nudging. Many top NIH scientists, particularly at the National Cancer Institute, professed great optimism. More practical scientists, such as National Institute of Allergy and Infectious Diseases director Dr. Anthony Fauci and his circle, assiduously avoided use of the word *cure*. They believed it highly disingenuous to offer hope that science could, indeed, cure a disease caused by a virus that hid inside human DNA. How could such a microbe be excised without destroying the individuals' genes in the process?

The thrust of AIDS activism, however, was focused on the search for a cure. As more of the estimated 700,000 to 1 million men and women in the United States who were infected with HIV came to realize that their time was running out, the activists' ranks swelled and militance increased. Certain a cure could be found, given an all-out effort, they attacked the drug companies, the FDA, the NIH, the White House, HHS—any institution thought to be dragging its feet regarding AIDS.[471]

It was a first among infectious diseases: the patients were living long enough and being well enough organized to set the relevant public health agenda. Given that their lives were on the line, the agenda's number one item was a medical goal. Classic public health aims took a distant second place.

With one possible exception: needle exchange programs. The drive to push government to supply, or at least legalize, sterile syringes for injecting drug users was a major focus of both activism and of pressure from the public health community from the second Reagan term through Bush and on throughout the Clinton administration. By 1988 some 38 percent of all injecting drug users in New York City, for example, were HIV positive, and it seemed clear that the prevalence there among drug injectors would soon surpass that seen in gay men. Further, because many injecting drug–using women worked as prostitutes, there was considerable concern that through them HIV would reach the larger heterosexual society.[472] Many health advocates believed that provision of clean needles was the key to slowing that part of the epidemic. These needles could be provided either through simple distribution of syringes or through street exchange programs (in which users traded used syringes for an equal number of sterile ones), legalization of over-the-counter sale of syringes, legalization of the possession of drug-use paraphernalia, or a combination of all of the above.[473]

Of these approaches, needle exchange received by far the most attention and also faced significant public health obstacles. First, it would be opposed by Congress not only during the Reagan administration but by the Bush and Clinton administrations as well.[474] Many state legislatures and governors were similarly disinclined to weaken in any way their restrictions on the activities of illegal drug users.

The second obstacle was an already very high HIV rate in the injecting drug–using population.[475] Needle exchanges would probably have had a powerful impact from 1981 through 1984 when the incidence of HIV in that community was still manageable. But by Reagan's second term, many cities were reporting HIV rates of 35 to 60 percent among injecting drug users.[476]

Yet another impediment was the methadone and treatment crisis.

In June 1982 Reagan delivered his War on Drugs speech, declaring, "We're taking down the surrender flag that has flown over so many drug efforts. We're running up a battle flag."[477]

The Reagan strategy marked a 180 degree turnaround from the Nixon years. Gone was any serious commitment to methadone or other treatment options aimed at reducing the demand side of America's drug problem. Reagan, who promoted supply-side economics, favored an all-out attack on drug supply with no particular discrimination among drugs based on their public health impact. Nixon had clearly targeted heroin because his administration felt it had the greatest public health and criminal consequences. Reagan, however, favored an indiscriminate and equal assault on everything from drugs like heroin and methamphetamines, which had powerful public health impacts, to marijuana, LSD, and hashish, drugs whose minimal public health impacts were far exceeded by those of alcohol and tobacco.

In 1984 Congress passed the administration's Omnibus Crime Bill which granted the FBI and local police departments unprecedented powers of drug supply interdiction. Indeed, the act, as implemented under the Reagan and Bush administrations, gave government powers of search and seizure not used in the United States, colonial America, or England since the days of the Magna Carta.[478] Agencies as diverse as the L.A. County Sheriff's Department, New York Police Department, U.S. Forest Service, INS, and FBI were granted the rights to make military-style assaults and raids upon private property based on no more than suspicion of the presence of a few marijuana plants or vials of cocaine.[479]

Meanwhile treatment programs, which already were grossly underfunded, were slashed. And the number of drug-related deaths in the United States doubled during the Reagan years—due to AIDS, suicides, and overdoses, in that order.[480] Federal funding for methadone programs was completely eliminated by the White House in 1982. In its place was yet another block grant program: the states were given much-reduced funds to be used as they saw fit for drug abuse education, prevention, and treatment programs. Further, drug abuse research grants to the NIH were cut by 15 percent.[481] Reagan's "Drug Czar," Carlton Turner, supported the "gateway theory of drug addiction," which saw marijuana as the gate through which all addicts first passed. Close that gate, he argued, and such nasty business as street methadone clinics will disappear because there will be no new heroin addicts.

So treatment programs—methadone and all other types—saw their budgets shrink steadily from 1982 right through the Reagan and Bush administrations. Just as HIV hit the injecting population, two ways of escaping it were shut off: increased police targeting of drug users made carrying sterile needles a very dangerous proposition; and getting off drugs through treatment became nothing more than a pipe dream. In the last year of the Reagan administration there were an estimated sixty-seven thousand drug addicts on waiting lists for treatment centers all over the country and only one out of every five drug users who sought treatment was able to get into any program.[482] The Institute of Medicine estimated that by 1989 there were 14.5 million Americans in need of drug abuse treatment for cocaine, heroin, amphetamines, or other illicit compounds, with 4.6 million having "clear and probable need" due to heavy substance abuse.[483]

When 44 percent of all newly diagnosed HIV cases in New York City were seen among injecting drug users, the New York Academy of Sciences issued an unprecedented statement of alarm.[484] The report noted that there were 242 storefronts and clinics in New York City offering various types of addiction treatments, most of them poorly funded. Yet only a handful offered their clients HIV-prevention services of any kind.

And the tragedy for public health was that drug abuse treatment programs worked. They were proven—better proven, in fact, than needle exchange efforts. Numerous studies demonstrated that regardless of the type of treatment programs offered or to what sort of drug(s) an individual was addicted, simply having an environment in which to address his or her problem successfully weaned the user from drugs 40 to 50 percent of the time, with a recidivism rate of 20 to 30 percent. Second-time treatment clients had higher rates of success and lower recidivism rates. Heroin programs successfully weaned addicts 74 percent of the time. And the efforts were highly cost effective.[485] When the societal costs of HIV and other infections spread via contaminated needles were factored in, the cost effectiveness of treatment was calculated to approach fifty dollars saved for every one dollar spent.[486]

But during the Reagan administration a form of cocaine that seemed to defy any attempt at treatment surfaced: crack. The crystallized rock form of cocaine that made a *crack* sound when lit and smoked was a marketing ploy— a phenomenally successful one. During the height of the 1970s disco scene, powder cocaine was all the rage among movie stars, top athletes, rock musicians, and young wannabes. The coke snorter then was, typically, middle class or affluent, white, urban or suburban, and college-educated. Cocaine in powder form, however, was very expensive. Users found they could escalate their intake by smoking pure cocaine that was fired up with a gas torch: a process called freebasing. But freebasing, too, was expensive, and it was dangerous, as Americans learned when celebrity Richard Pryor accidentally set himself afire.

By the time Reagan took office in 1981, cocaine use was already fading out, with the drug having become both unaffordable and unenticing to most Americans. However, Troy Duster of the University of California Berkeley argued that when the Reagan administration began its War on Drugs in 1982, targeting marijuana, the street economics of drugs changed overnight. An expert on the socioeconomics of drug use, Duster found that the escalated attacks by law enforcement on marijuana growers and suppliers drove the price of that drug up from a typical 1980 price of $80 an ounce to a 1990 cost of $250 to $300 an ounce.[487]

That left a drug access vacuum on the streets, in colleges, and at high schools. In 1984 drug traffickers devised a cheap five-dollar coke high.[488] Crack was nothing more than a cut-rate version of the cocaine crystals that had bankrupted so many stockbrokers and movie stars in the 1970s. Chemically, it was the same stuff, though less pure and likely to be heavily adulterated. Duster argued that narcotraffickers were able to flood the streets of U.S. cities with crack precisely *because* there was a War on Drugs under way and many scholars agreed with his perspective.[489]

A significant indicator of increased cocaine use could be found in emergency room admissions data. In 1977 just 1 percent of all ER cases nationwide was related to smoked cocaine; that figure reached 5 percent in 1986. (Overall government surveys of hospitals showed that serious drug-related emergencies, involving any narcotic or stimulant, increased radically during the Reagan War on Drugs, as did drug-related deaths.[490])

The emergence of crack cocaine coincided with acute economic depression in urban African-American and Latino neighborhoods. Reaganomics took a toll on most nonwealthy Americans, but its sharpest cut was into inner-city areas. In 1981 unemployment among males aged twenty to twenty-four years was over 11 percent for whites, versus 24.4 percent for African-Americans. Blacks disproportionately filled the ranks of the nation's swelling population of people who had no homes in which to live and survived on the streets, in governments shelters, along train tracks, and wherever else they might find nightly havens. In 1982 between 64 and 73 percent of New York City's homeless population was African-American; 10 to 15 percent was white. Most of the homeless were unemployed men.[491] Thousands of these lost souls roamed the semiabandoned lunar landscapes of the South Bronx, Harlem, Brownsville, and Bedford-Stuyvesant where fire department stations no longer existed and infernos routinely swallowed up one housing project or slum after another.[492]

The black and Latino former residents crammed into already-dense bordering neighborhoods, turning parts of Harlem and Brooklyn into places—akin in human density and poverty to Lung Block, the late-nineteenth-century locus of tuberculosis described so dramatically by Jacob Riis.

For many youngsters in those neighborhoods, there seemed few options open for bettering their lives. The business interests behind crack found an eager army of youth for whom racism, their often terrible educations, and the lack of sources of self-respect created a deep alienation from the larger society. Selling crack opened a door to unparalleled wealth, esteem, and power.[493]

By the end of 1985 the National Institute on Drug Abuse (NIDA) said there were five million crack/cocaine users in America, and one of every six of them lived in Gotham. At least twenty-two million people in the United States had tried crack or cocaine, NIDA said.[494] In 1985, however, crack still hadn't overwhelmed New York City—or anywhere else. In fact, the numbers of crack smokers were small and represented only 6 percent of Gotham's cocaine-using population, according to the city health department's chief epidemiologist, Dr. Blanche Frank. By 1988, however, 66 percent of all cocaine used in New York City was smoked crack and 11 percent was injected.

In 1986 two well-known athletes (Len Bias and Don Rogers) died of crack overdoses and the mass media suddenly was full of lurid stories about "the new drug epidemic." Using the police and Reagan administration officials as primary sources, the media reports framed the crack situation as a catastrophic "plague" that was sweeping across America and claiming the nation's teenagers. It was not. It never would be.

What followed was a media feeding frenzy in which the extent of crack use and its dangers were grossly exaggerated.[495] The images presented of crack and the crack user were fiendish. The drug was said to be the most addictive substance on earth; it drove users to unparalleled heights of violence; using women gave birth to addicted, even malformed babies.

The U.S. budget for the War on Drugs soared from less than $2 billion in 1981 to more than $12 billion in 1993. The budget for the Drug Enforcement Administration (DEA) quadrupled between 1981 and 1992.[496] Law after law was signed at the national, state, and local levels as politicians sought to "get tough on drugs." In 1986 Congress passed the Anti-Drug Abuse Act, which increased mandatory sentences for drug-related crimes. And, as noted, Congress approved every requested increase in law enforcement funds.

At the state level, the antidrug fury seemed to know no bounds. Minnesota, for example, passed legislation in 1988 imposing penalties for possession of crack that were twenty-five times stiffer than for possession of an *exactly equal amount* of cocaine in powder form.[497] Though Minnesota's population was more than 96 percent white, most of the individuals arrested in 1988 and 1989 for crack possession under the new law were African-American.

Though the Minnesota law was overturned in court,[498] it underscored a fundamental, yet unstated, aspect of the nation's response to crack: race. The War on Drugs had become a war on youthful male offenders of color.[499]

Minnesota was only mirroring a national trend. The percentage of the U.S. prison population that was black jumped from 37 percent in 1960 to 47 percent in 1989 after Reagan's War on Drugs began, and it would continue to climb. Latinos, too, saw their representation among the U.S. incarcerated climb from a mere 2 percent in 1960 to nearly 14 percent by the end of Reagan's presidency.

And it soon got much, much worse after Vice President George Bush was elected president by a margin of seven million popular votes and 314 electoral college votes (he took 426 of 538).[500] Nine months after taking office, Bush gave his first speech to the nation to address "America's number one problem." That problem wasn't unemployment (running at about 6 percent) or the enormous $10 billion trade gap. It was crack.

Holding a Baggie full of crystals up to the camera, Bush told his "fellow Americans" that it contained crack that had been "seized a few days ago in a park across the street from the White House."[501]

Crack, Bush said, was turning American cities into murder zones, in which children killed children. The solution he proceeded to outline basically took Reagan's War on Drugs, which had focused primarily on marijuana, doubled its budget, and aimed the full force of law enforcement at small-time crack cocaine dealers and users.

Public health solutions to drug problems—however exaggerated those problems may have been—were completely ignored. The public's perception, contrary to all evidence, was that crime was increasing; and in the collective mind's eye the perpetrators all wore the face of a black crack head. That perception was catered to. Bush named arch-conservative William Bennett his Drug Czar. Bennett believed that crack was so addictive, and produced such violent behavior in users, that the only hope for stemming a tidal wave of drug-induced horror was mass arrests.

Ninety percent of all incarcerations for drug offenses made at the state and federal level during the Bush administration (1989 to 1992) were of African-

Americans or Latinos.[502] African-American men, in particular, were targeted by law enforcement: though they comprised only 7 percent of the U.S. population in 1992, they made up half the population of prisoners.[503] Police forces clearly targeted ghettos and slum areas for drug enforcement.[504] There were no DEA raids with heavy police artillery waged against colleges, Silicon Valley, hangouts for high fashion models, private white clubs in Manhattan, or the latest chic club for movie stars in Malibu, though drug use was a prominent feature in all those settings.

"An extremely disturbing current in public policy debates of the past decade is the tendency to identify the causes of problems confronting minority communities as the failings and inadequacies of black people themselves," the Drug Policy Foundation observed.[505] "From the policy analyst's point of view, the root of black communities' poverty and hopelessness seemed to be nested in a pathological set of self-defeating and destructive behaviors, a group pathology unprecedented in its persistence and incidence among black people.

"Were the adherents to this view racists and bigots? Were those who shared this vision all right-wing conservatives? No. Respected scholars at major research universities embraced this perspective. The mainstream black press ... embraced readily the self-help rhetoric. And black churches, particularly the more fundamentalist in orientation that bloomed in the 1980s, unhesitatingly adopted this stance."

It was, critics charged, another blame-the-victim perspective: if African-Americans were arrested and imprisoned more frequently for drug-related crimes, it must signal an inner, collective weakness in character, genes, community structures, or families. The Bush administration's ultimate target was not, in fact, the drugs: it was deteriorating moral and family values that were said to be the root cause of drug abuse.[506]

Drug-related violence, however, was the result of turf battles between drug dealers and gangs. Little—in some communities, *no*—crack violence was deliberately directed at the general citizenry.[507] The majority of all cocaine users during the Reagan and Bush years were white; but arrests were overwhelmingly black. And by 1993 four million Americans, most of them African-American, would have lost their right to vote due to criminal drug convictions.[508]

To justify the criminal sweeps and even calls for shooting or beheading crack users,[509] politicians and law enforcement officials cited scientific papers regarding the physiological effects of crack and cocaine.

"Crack is definitely a unique compound, compared to regular cocaine," said psychiatrist Scott Lukas of Harvard School of Medicine. "It's been marketed well, and it's cheap. A drug like crack, which induces a profound change very quickly, is likely to be more reinforcing (addictive) than any other."[510]

But cocaine, in *any* form, is powerfully addictive. It doesn't have to be smoked. Animal studies of cocaine use gave a frightening picture of the drug's powerful impact.

In 1985 Michael Bozarth and Roy Wise of Concordia University in Montreal stunned the medical community with the results of research comparing cocaine and heroin use in rats. Either heroin or cocaine was put in water bottles attached to small levers. By pressing the lever, a rat could obtain more of whichever drug had been assigned to it. The rats with access to heroin quickly developed a routine, consistently taking the same amount of the drug, eating normally, and staying well-groomed. Although they were less active, the heroin-addicted rats were basically healthy.

In contrast, the rats with access to cocaine took the drug as often as possible; one half died of cocaine overdoses. Most became self-destructive, stopped eating regularly, and lost a third of their body weight. Many suffered seizures. The rats' health and appearance deteriorated and their behavior was completely erratic.

The researchers concluded that "cocaine is a much more toxic compound than heroin."[511]

During the Bush administration a new dimension of alleged health effects of crack surfaced: "crack babies." Researchers claimed evidence that the babies born to crack-using mothers (all of whom in these studies were African-American or Hispanic) were more likely to be tiny, abnormal, and show signs of cocaine addiction. The studies rarely controlled for racial disparities in infant mortality and birth outcomes seen in the United States absent drug exposure. And in claiming that there were "crack babies" but *not* "cocaine babies," the scientists were on thin ice. The studies would not hold up over time and, when controlled for race, no genuine differences between the babies of crack- versus cocaine-using mothers would persist. But the "crack baby" myths were powerful during the Bush years and prompted such dubious legal actions against crack-using women as mandating their sterilization and taking away their babies.[512]

The National Criminal Justice Commission and many local health departments favored public health approaches to the crack problem. In their models, a combination of careful public education about the hazards of crack, plentiful treatment centers, and enhanced employment opportunities in inner-city areas constituted the strongest solution.[513]

In 1989 New York's Mayor Koch proposed a $1.2 billion five-year plan to, indeed, provide treatment for every crack and cocaine user living in the five boroughs. Health Commissioner Joseph, however, argued that until an equivalent to methadone was found for cocaine, treatment would prove exceedingly difficult.[514]

In the absence of quick medical fixes for the much-hyped crack problem,

New York and most other large cities followed the White House lead and waged military-style forays into the "crack-infested neighborhoods."

In New York City the murder rate skyrocketed in 1988, increasing 13 percent over the previous year with most of the excess killings related to drug turf battles.[515] The murder escalation occurred during the toughest police crackdown ever experienced in Gotham's history; 48 percent of the city's arrested blacks and Latinos ended up serving time compared to just 18 percent of arrested whites.[516]

Drug sales clearly continued and Koch's proposed $1.2 billion treatment program never materialized.

In the 1989 elections Manhattan Borough President David Dinkins defeated Koch, becoming the first African-American mayor in New York City history. Dinkins immediately ordered a decrease in police activities and an increase in public health approaches. But he failed with both. The police had only one mind-set relative to drugs: arrest as many small-time dealers as possible. Dinkins ordered a shift in focus to arresting major cocaine suppliers. But many NYPD officers were unable or unwilling to comply and the streets remained saturated with cocaine.[517]

Los Angeles followed a route similar to New York City's, virtually ignoring the public health aspects of drug use in favor of police assaults on alleged dealers and users.[518] Even liberal city and county officials favored strong police action to break up gangs and stamp out crack. LAPD Chief Daryl Gates told a U.S. Senate committee in 1990 that "casual drug users should be taken out and shot."[519]

Sadly, crack did, indeed, represent a public health catastrophe on at least three fronts.

First, the intense police war on drugs forced users into seedy, even disgustingly derelict, "crack houses" where users and dealers congregated, protected by children who stood watch in the neighborhood for police and undercover agents. Because cocaine had an aphrodisiac effect that increased users' sexual appetites, the crack house settings also fueled the exchange of sex. In addition, women who were desperate for cocaine prostituted themselves in exchange for a hit.

The result was a jump in the U.S. incidences of heterosexually acquired HIV and other sexually acquired diseases.[520]

Further, in some parts of the country crack was bypassed for injected cocaine, which, unlike heroin, required repeated injections over the course of a day. In cocaine shooting galleries users frequently shared syringes with resultant spread of HIV.[521]

And perhaps most significantly, the War on Drugs put up to a quarter of the nation's African-American young men in jails and prisons where, whether they liked it or not, they were behaviorally "homosexual." Sodomy and rape were commonplace in prisons and jails.

Once released, most of these young men returned to heterosexual life, often to a waiting wife or girlfriend. The mass incarceration of black men and Latinos created a unique HIV amplification system: it spread through forced homosexual activity in a prison or jail setting where condoms had officially been declared illegal. As the black male population cycled in and out of this prison milieu, HIV soared among African-Americans. By 1998 AIDS would be the number one cause of death for black men and women aged twenty-five to forty-four years and the CDC would estimate that some one hundred thousand African-Americans were HIV positive. That year, though blacks comprised just 13 percent of the U.S. population, they would represent 48 percent of all new AIDS cases reported to the CDC.[522]

When public health officials reached out during the early 1990s to warn and educate the African-American community about the risks of HIV, they were stunned by the hostility and suspicion that greeted them. Tuskegee, the War on Drugs, racial hospital segregation—these legacies had built a mountain of resentment in the black community against organized medicine and government health authorities. Many African-American leaders declared HIV a racist conspiracy, claiming that the virus had been manufactured specifically to kill members of their race. Though prominent African-American public health leaders would try to counter these ideas, there was an overwhelming sense in the community that the soaring incidence of HIV in their ranks simply could not be a coincidence. It had to be deliberate. They had been victimized.

By the end of the decade, as the twenty-first century dawned, public health would still be scrambling to gain the confidence of African-Americans. And though the surgeon general and the leader of the CDC's AIDS program were both African-American, it would prove a formidable challenge. Suspicions ran high.

Decades of failing to address the needs of minorities in the United States, particularly of African-Americans, were now undermining HIV prevention, drug abuse education, and other vital public health efforts.

"Systems that increasingly focus on problems that most people do not have or that are not remediable, and in the process draw resources from relieving those problems they *do* have, may find their constituencies eroding (and with good reason)," wrote a group of Canadian health analysts.[523] Though their comments were focused on Canada's failings, they could just as well have applied south of their border. In the absence of any sense that they had a stake in the larger community's health—or that it was in any way concerned about their health—marginalized populations saw no reason to cooperate for the greater good. Which, of course, undermined what analyst Daniel Callahan called the primary tenet of public health:[524] "Good public health can and will raise the health status of people as a group but it will not necessarily help me as an individual. . . . Generic public health programs do general good, but they may not do individual good except indirectly."

If individuals cannot perceive a personal or community interest in public health goals, Callahan argued, the institutions of health and medicine will be viewed by those alienated groups with the same disdain and hostility as is directed toward other government institutions, such as the police, FBI, CIA, and the military.

The validity of that insight became horribly obvious—but, sadly, was ignored—when there was a resurgence of two ancient human nemeses in the United States during the Bush administration. Both had long since been considered vanquished in the United States, and their control had been marked as classic cases of public health triumphs. And both would emerge most powerfully between 1990 and 1993 in beleaguered New York City.

The first was measles.

Thanks to very effective child vaccination campaigns during the 1960s and 1970s, annual measles tallies had fallen from typical 1950s levels of more than two hundred thousand to fewer than one thousand.

But from 1989 through 1991 the United States experienced a measles epidemic larger than any then seen in the Western Hemisphere, Europe, and most of Asia—only sub-Saharan Africa (and, unbeknownst to the outside world, the USSR) could rival the scale of the U.S. outbreak. At least 55,467 youngsters came down with measles, 11,251 of whom suffered severe cases that required hospitalization. A total of 136 children died.[525]

The epidemic first emerged in New York during the Koch administration and then spread nationwide when Dr. Woodrow Meyers was the city's health commissioner and Dinkins was mayor. It was obvious to those two African-American leaders that the majority of the measles cases and deaths were occurring in their own black community and, to a lesser extent, among Puerto Ricans and other New York Latinos. Most of the youngsters who contracted measles were unvaccinated, came from impoverished homes, and lacked full access to health care.

Drastic cuts in federal support for health care programs for the poor, coupled with the Medicaid block grant shift to the states, meant that fewer children in New York City even saw doctors, and those who did were less likely than in the pre-Reagan era to get properly vaccinated against measles or other child killers. New York's underfunded Medicaid system reimbursed physicians just two dollars per measles vaccine. This failed to cover either the vaccine's cost (over ten dollars) or the doctor's time and overhead (averaging fifty dollars per visit).

"Thus, vaccination of a Medicaid child in New York may well have inflicted an obligatory fiscal loss on a provider, creating an incentive not to vaccinate," researchers concluded.[526]

About 20 percent of the city's Medicare kids under the age of five years were unvaccinated, compared to 10 percent of the poor who sought care in city-run public health clinics, and less than 5 percent of children whose parents had private health insurance.

In less extreme form the same pattern was seen all over the United States in 1990 and 1991. The nation's measles epidemic stopped when public health officials found the means to boost immunization rates—generally via large, free vaccination programs and heavy publicity directed at pediatricians and primary care physicians. By 1992 the numbers of measles cases in the United States had fallen to 2,234, and by 1997 that number was down to just 138 cases.

Sixty-six percent of the 1997 measles cases would be white children, most of them from fully insured households. They would be part of a new, 1990s anti-vaccination mood among Baby Boom parents who mistakenly believed that the risk of vaccination was greater than the dangers posed by the diseases.[527]

In the white community—particularly in the western states—failure to fully vaccinate children was largely the result of conscious parental decisions. The reverse was true in minority communities where it generally reflected lack of access to health care. Thus, ranking at the bottom of national immunization rates in 1995 would be affluent San Diego and Santa Clara counties in California and inner-city areas of acute poverty such as those in Detroit, Newark, and Chicago.[528] And 60 to 70 percent of all child cases of measles, whooping cough, and tetanus in the United States in 1997 would be among unvaccinated white children.[529]

"Most [measles] cases reported in 1998 were associated with importation [of the virus], including short chains of indigenous transmission of measles that occurred following international importation of measles," the CDC would conclude in 1999.[530] Which meant that the United States remained vulnerable to new measles epidemics if, as had occurred in 1989–91, immunization rates fell, and as long as measles continued to be epidemic in many other countries.

In the age of global travel, then, U.S. defense against the virus was intimately linked to UNICEF's ongoing, global child vaccination campaign. If the agency's lofty goal of 90 percent global immunization could be attained, the United States might be able to let down its guard against measles. Until then, however, any future slackening in child immunization rates would surely lead to another epidemic.

Barely had the measles epidemic died down in 1992 when whooping cough rates surged upward in the United States, with more than half of all cases occurring among unvaccinated children. In 1976 the United States hit its all-time low in whooping cough cases, with fewer than one thousand reported. But thereafter vaccination rates declined and the numbers of whooping cough cases rose. In 1993 there were 4,989 cases in the United States, 2,218 of which were infants. It was the largest number of cases seen in American since 1967.[531]

Though these epidemics were brought under control, others would follow. And U.S. vaccination rates would continue to rank low when compared to the rest of the industrialized world.[532]

The Bush administration's international perspective in 1990 and 1991 did not, however, embrace health. Such issues as where the United States stood in the worldwide race to achieve 90 percent vaccination rates among earth's children by 2000 never registered on the president's radar screen.

What did register, with the 1989 fall of the Berlin wall and the pending collapse of the Soviet Union in 1990, was what Bush called "a new world order." It was a new realpolitik in which the United States was the sole planetary superpower, able to flex its military muscles at will in the service of global political and economic "stability." It was in that context that, during the fall of 1990, the administration mobilized the largest allied force deployed anywhere since World War II and prepared for war against Iraq.[533]

The new world order was, critics charged, nothing more than Bush's pursuit of the status quo and preservation of foreign and domestic power structures that dated back decades.[534] Domestically, Bush's policies on health, drugs, AIDS, and environmental issues could be called Reagan lite. During his four-year presidency, Bush repeatedly exercised White House veto power to stymie any health effort that could enhance access to abortion or birth control, mandate health care benefits of any kind, or bring about a return of federal involvement in local public health. In his 1990 State of the Union address, Bush vowed to control rapidly inflating health costs. But for a solution, he offered only an antisolution: "All we have to do is to say that the Democrats are for socialized medicine and we're not," his staff explained.[535]

During Bush's single term in the White House the budget deficit increased from 22 percent of the GNP to 25 percent, topping $1.5 trillion. Though, like his predecessor, Bush claimed to oppose "big government," his administration added more regulations to federal law than had any before him—sixty-eight thousand in 1991 alone. And regulatory spending rose by 20 percent. These funds did not make their way to basic public health programs, however, and Reagan's DRG and block grant programs remained in place.

So money-starved New York City continued to struggle under the weight of its many burdens: crack, measles, police crackdowns, racial disparity, and a deteriorating urban infrastructure. Then, beginning in 1989, all of New York's problems converged in the state's and city's crowded jails.

Packed with African-American and Latino men caught in drug raids, the facilities were filled way above capacity. And vigilant public health researchers noted that amid such crowding, tuberculosis was spreading rapidly and was proving particularly dangerous for HIV-positive inmates.[536] Between 1900 and 1975 tuberculosis incidence had fallen steadily, both nationally and in New York State. But after 1975 it began a slow resurgence, with the numbers of TB reports rising like a rocket from 1980 to 1989.

"We should sound the alarm," the NIH's Dr. Stan Vermund said at a 1990 meeting of the American Association for the Advancement of Sciences. "This requires immediate attention. . . . There is an association between the HIV epidemic and the rise in the number of TB cases. We should be vigilant in screening people . . . and giving maximum support to our public health departments in providing resources in following up on tuberculosis cases."

Mincing no words, Vermund added, "No one should die from TB. A tuberculosis death is an indicator of a failing health care system." It was indeed failing—especially in New York City where, in 1990, one out of five of the nation's TB cases surfaced.[537]

When a New York State prison guard died of TB in 1991, the somnambulant public health authorities awoke. And lab work done in New York City's Public Health Research Institute (PHRI) showed that dangerous antibiotic-resistant strains of *Mycobacterium tuberculosis* were circulating in the jails and on the streets. One strain, dubbed "W," was resistant to so many drugs that it was essentially untreatable.

That put medicine back in the nineteenth century.

As the crisis surfaced, New York City Commissioner of Health Meyers resigned after a brief tenure, apparently overwhelmed by his job. He was replaced by Dr. Margaret Hamburg. At age thirty-seven, Hamburg was the youngest person ever to serve as commissioner and only the third woman. Though she lacked a public health degree, Hamburg was uniquely qualified to meet the city's awesome challenges. Trained at Harvard Medical School, Margaret Hamburg had served under Director Anthony Fauci at the National Institute of Allergy and Infectious Diseases during the early stages of the AIDS epidemic and had gained a reputation for her strong advocacy of HIV research, executed with political savvy and sharp diplomatic skills.

Hamburg had barely stepped inside the headquarters of New York City's rundown, seedy health department just down the street from City Hall in June 1991, when her staff voiced its concern that Gotham was on the verge of an all-out tuberculosis epidemic.

But nobody had faced down a TB epidemic in the United States since the turn of the century and most contemporary doctors had never diagnosed a TB case—or confronted the personal threat of acquiring the disease from their patients. Hamburg reached out to the CDC for help. And she turned to history, reading the TB control papers of Hermann Biggs. One key Biggs phrase from 1914 truly resonated: "Public health is purchasable. Within natural limitations a community can determine its own death rate."

National spending on tuberculosis control had steadily declined during the years in which TB staged its resurgence. And though the CDC had been requesting sizeable TB funds, the White House under Reagan and Bush typically had granted less than a third of what the agency said it needed.[538] New York City was spending less than $2 million in 1988, only about $200,000 of which came from the federal level. At that spending level the city could barely staff a TB office, much less aggressively track down and treat tuberculosis carriers.

By early 1992 Hamburg's staff, assisted by the CDC's Dr. Thomas Frieden, concluded that the city's epidemic was evolving as follows: First, untreated cases had gone unnoticed in the poorest neighborhoods of the city during the late 1970s when New York was reeling from its near-bankruptcy. Then the growing racial alienation from the health system, coupled with drug abuse and homelessness, engendered a striking dropout rate from treatment programs. By 1989 some 88 percent of all TB patients treated at Harlem Hospital, for example, disappeared before being cured. Those patients stopped their antibiotics as soon as they felt better, but before the bacteria were completely gone from their systems, thus allowing drug-resistant tuberculosis strains to emerge. When their illnesses returned, the patients came back for more antibiotics, and then again disappeared once they felt better. The cycle repeated over and over until at least a third of all active TB cases in New York City in 1990 were drug resistant. By then the War on Drugs was in full swing and about a quarter of all young African-American men had spent time on the city's Riker's Island or in one of the state prisons. In the densely crowded cells, the recalcitrant TB patients, 55 percent of whom were African-American and 45 percent of whom were homeless, unwittingly spread their tuberculosis to cell mates. When the infected prisoners were discharged to the streets, they, in turn, passed the disease on to family members and acquaintances.

This cycle arose during the late 1980s, in parallel with HIV's emergence in the city's minority communities and jails. In 1992 all the components hit New York hospital AIDS wards at once—homeless individuals, ex-convicts, highly socially alienated individuals, gay HIV patients, and a deteriorating public health infrastructure—and the results were explosive. In three New York City hospitals TB spread like wildfire on the HIV wards, killing 85 percent of all AIDS patients who acquired it and doing so with terrifying rapidity. Most died in less than eight weeks—non-HIV cases typically suffered years of TB. Tests of hospital employees revealed that up to half the doctors and nurses on these wards got infected. Some took ill. Some died.

"I would be a fool not to find it overwhelming," Hamburg told a visitor to her humble city office in March 1992. "A lot of people here are not sleeping at night."[539]

Joint CDC/New York City Department of Health studies in 1992 revealed that 39 percent of the 3,811 active TB cases identified in the city carried drug-resistant strains. It took even the highest-tech labs six weeks or more to determine to which drugs the various strains would respond. Investigations uncovered fantastic lapses in hospital infection-control practices, including allowing patients who harbored multidrug-resistant TB to wander about the hallways.

At PHRI a genetic nightmare was revealed: the dreaded "W" strain of TB that could resist nearly every available drug was not homegrown. Rather, it had originated in Russia in the final years of the Soviet Union. And as early as 1988 fully a quarter of all New York City TB cases had been among foreign-born individuals.[540]

By the end of the 1990s the world would be facing a massive tuberculosis pandemic, with drug-resistant strains of the microbe spreading from one corner of the planet to another. Fully 20 percent of all TB in the world would have some degree of drug resistance and more people would die of the disease in 1999 than did in 1899. The World Health Organization forecast 48 million active TB cases globally by 2020—a 41 percent increase over 1998 levels, which already constituted the largest case load in world history.[541] These global cases all posed continuing threats to Americans—no TB strain was too remote at the millennium to reach Kansas or Idaho. Indeed, since Reagan had eliminated the Refugee Health Service, there wasn't even a veneer of protection left to safeguard against the arrival of foreign strains.

By 1997 Hamburg's department brought the size of New York City's epidemic down by 54.6 percent and reduced the multidrug-resistant TB incidence by 87.3 percent. Though tuberculosis would remain a serious concern in the city for years, the threat of a major epidemic was past—at least for the moment. The cost of this achievement was extraordinary: easily $1 billion.

It was Czech scientist Karyl Stiblo's directly observed therapy (DOT) approach that was key: compelling patients not only to start multidrug therapy, but to stay on it for eighteen months until every last mycobacterium was cleared from their bodies. The health department in New York City hired squads of DOT workers who chased down a long list of TB patients, including the homeless, every day and watched to make sure they took their medicines.

To control spread of TB in New York jails, a multimillion-dollar isolation facility and screening center was constructed at the city's Riker's Island jail. Every inmate was X-rayed and screened before entering the prison population and active TB cases were placed in the medical isolation unit.

Hamburg couldn't simply order such measures with the wave of her hand, as Biggs could have done a century earlier. There were civil liberties issues to consider and the legal powers of her department had eroded over the years (as they had at most counterpart agencies nationwide). Before implementing DOT, which involved forcing patients to take drugs and isolating and restraining recalcitrant patients, Hamburg's legal department had to thrash each measure out in the courts.[542] Authority was eventually granted, but there were some anxious legal delays. By 1995, however, a total of 96 percent of all New York City TB patients would successfully undergo DOT.[543]

The trick after 1995 would be to maintain vigilance and a TB infrastructure, not only in New York but nationwide. In the past, successful control of disease all too often had led to collapse of the victorious infrastructures. Global travel now ensured that new TB strains (and other microbes as well) would continue to surface in the United States and offer public health challenges.

Indeed, in 1995 a frightening new tuberculosis strain would emerge in Tennessee.

"I can't tell you how scary the potential is for this hypertransmissable tuberculosis," Minnesota's Michael Osterholm said in a speech before the annual meeting of the Infectious Diseases Society of America held in San Francisco in 1997. Described in chilling detail by CDC officials at the meeting, the supercontagious TB grew one thousand times faster in laboratory cultures than normal tuberculosis bacteria and it spread between people whose contact was limited to such casual moments as standing together outdoors in a line to buy burgers.[544]

A CDC team led by Dr. Sandra Valway figured out that the original case was a forty-one-year-old male in rural Tennessee. He had contracted the virulent TB in 1994 and unwittingly spread it to a remarkable 82 percent of all the people he shared air space with at work, at home, or in social settings. Another man with the same TB strain unintentionally infected 94 percent of his coworkers, friends, and neighbors. And eight of thirteen health care workers involved in treating these cases got infected. Fortunately, it was easily treated with antibiotics. At least, so far.

In contrast, the drug-resistant "W" strain of TB that swept New York City moved slowly, infecting highly vulnerable individuals, and there was no evidence that it spread in casual settings, such as on subway cars.[545]

Commissioner Hamburg detected a common thread among New York's tuberculosis, HIV, measles, and other public health crises: the return of contagion and infectious diseases. She felt certain that once-vanquished microbial threats were making a comeback, accompanied by new scourges that hadn't previously afflicted humanity. Influencing Hamburg's thinking was her old family friend, Nobel laureate Joshua Lederberg, whose tireless work on bacterial resistance had given him a healthy respect for the evolutionary capacities of microorganisms. At the height of the medical optimism of the 1960s and 1970s,

Lederberg had warned that the microbes were always lurking in the human environment, ready to seize any opportunity to reproduce and spread.

In 1989 Lederberg, an imposing senior figure at Rockefeller University, had been gingerly approached at a university cocktail party by junior faculty member Stephen Morse, a virologist. Was it his imagination, Morse asked, or was HIV simply the most successful of a whole raft of new pathogens? A similar notion had, indeed, occurred to Lederberg. Emboldened by Lederberg's concurrence, Morse pushed his case: We need a meeting, he argued. We need to gather the world's experts on each category of viral agents and ask them to address the question.

Lederberg agreed without hesitation and in May 1989, under the auspices of the New York Academy of Sciences and the National Institutes of Health, Morse's meeting took place. For three days the great minds of virology assessed mounting evidence of increased microbial assault on humanity and their collective concern rose with each passing hour.[546] During breaks, scientists who retreated to the roof of the conference hotel to sip hot coffee had a fine view of the White House and the Senate. At that time, the Senate was interrogating Colonel Oliver North and other former Reagan administration insiders who had allegedly engineered an exchange of U.S. arms for hostages in a complicated scheme referred to as Iran-Contra. To most of the nation, that scandal was the most pressing issue of the day. But less than a half mile away, a small group of scientists was seriously questioning the very survival of the human race.[547]

The 1989 "Emerging Viruses" conference was the second stage of a dramatic reappraisal of public health—a process that had begun a year earlier with the release of the Institute of Medicine's report *The Future of Public Health*.[548] After interviewing more than three hundred and fifty public health experts, surveying the status of health services in every state, and contrasting the U.S. experience with that in Canada, the Institute of Medicine in 1988 described public health as a "government responsibility" that had been betrayed, leaving only a "shattered vision." And it reached some distressing conclusions:

> The current state of our abilities for effective public health action, as documented in this report, is cause for national concern and for the development of a plan of action for needed improvements. In the committee's view, we have slackened our public health vigilance nationally and the health of the public is unnecessarily threatened as a result.
>
> An impossible responsibility has been placed on America's public health agencies: to serve as stewards of the basic health needs of entire populations, but at the same time avert impending disasters and provide personal health care to those rejected by the rest of the health system. The

wonder is not that American public health has problems, but that so much has been done so well, and with so little.

The IOM committee discovered a complete absence of shared mission among public health agencies: no common definition of public health or agreed upon list of its duties existed from state to state or even county to county within a state. Worse, "in too many localities, there is no health department. Perhaps the area is visited occasionally by a 'circuit-riding' public health nurse—and perhaps not."

Though it was *1988*, not *1888*, the IOM concluded that much of America had yet to achieve the public health standards set by Hermann Biggs a century earlier:

> Lack of agreement about the public health mission is also reflected in the diversion in some states of traditional public health functions, such as water and air pollution control, to separate departments of environmental services, where the health effects of pollutants often receive less notice. . . .
>
> Such extreme variety of available services and organizational arrangements suggests that contemporary public health is defined less by what public health professionals know how to do than by what the political system in a given area decides is appropriate or feasible.
>
> Tension between professional expertise and politics can be observed throughout the nation's public health system. . . . [Public health professionals'] aim is to maximize the influence of accurate data and professional judgment on decision-making—to make decisions as comprehensive and objective as possible.
>
> The dynamics of American politics, however, make it difficult to fulfill this commitment. Public decision-making in public health as in other areas is driven by crisis, hot issues, and the concerns of organized interest groups. Decisions are made largely on the basis of competition, bargaining, and influence rather than comprehensive analysis. . . .
>
> The impact of politics is clearly evident in the rapid turnover among public health officials (the average tenure of a state officer is now only two years); in a market shift toward political appointments as opposed to career professionals in the top ranks of health agencies; and in the gradual disappearance of state boards of health, which have dwindled by half (from nearly all states to only 24) in only 25 years.

The populaces it served perceived public health as little more than bureaucracies full of paper shufflers who harassed companies, hospitals, small businesses, and schools with forms and red tape. Anything really "important"—such as Medicaid—was taken away from public health offices and put in the hands of "more business-savvy" agencies. As their stature and authority diminished, the IOM found, public health officials did little to defend themselves or their missions. The report bemoaned the fact that "many public health professionals who talked with us seemed to regard politics as a contaminant of an ideally rational decision-making process rather than as an essential element of democratic governance."

The greatest tensions for public health rose out of the relationships between its advocates and organized medicine, which had "always been uneasy," but by 1988, the report concluded, were fraught with "confrontation and suspicion."[549]

Some observers, such as sociologist Lawrence Weiss, put all of the blame for the sorry state of public health on medicine. "In fact," Weiss argued, "public health as commonly institutionalized at the local and state level, even at the national level, is a wan actor in the shadow of an imposing role. The practice of medicine, once significantly guided by the leadership of public health, has come to totally dominate the field of health care, overwhelming an emaciated public health sector."[550]

That "inferior position" of public health, as compared to medicine, Weiss continued, "has kept public health in a condition of anarchy—balkanized among the states and scattered about a number of federal agencies. Today the nation's public health apparatus is barely able to respond to the epidemics of the late twentieth century such as tuberculosis, AIDS, and measles, much less play a leadership role in health care planning and reform."[551]

At the time the IOM report was released there were 22 million Americans who had no health insurance, 38.8 million whose coverage was so poor that they couldn't easily obtain health care, and 43 million who didn't have a primary care physician or regular clinic that oversaw their care. Nearly all of the nation's health care for the poor and the underinsured was handled by just 10 percent of the country's hospitals, most of them facilities run by local governments.[552]

The IOM report was not without its critics,[553] but it was generally accepted among public health advocates as an accurate rendition of their sad state of affairs.[554]

The only health initiative to come out during the Bush presidency was *Healthy People 2000*, his administration's 1990 summary of goals for the future. The report, which was massive in size and scope, detailed the number of the targets the Carter administration had set in *Healthy People 1990* that had been hit (almost none), and laid out future strategies for U.S. public health.[555] Remarkably, voluminous as *Healthy People 2000* was, it made no reference to the crisis in access to health care, to rising numbers of Americans lacking insurance, or to the future financing of Medicare and Medicaid. At the 1990 annual meeting of the American Public Health Association, the organization's executive director, Dr. William McBeath, brought down the house with a strident attack upon the Reagan and Bush administrations, the *Healthy People 2000* report, and the state of the nation's commitment to public health.[556]

"The potential of *Healthy People 2000* is sold short by the administration's timidity to address the tough issues involved with implementation. In the 672-page document, no space is found to call for increased funding. . . . As it stands, *Healthy People 2000* may be filled with good stuff; but it is a cup half empty," McBeath cried out over the thunderous applause of some six thousand public health professionals gathered in New York City's Madison Square Garden.

"Wanting," McBeath continued, "is an action plan for implementation to achieve the goals and objectives set. The document seems to draw us a picture of the 'Emerald City,' but never shows us a 'yellow brick road.' The objectives themselves deserve more."

McBeath decried three Republican terms in the White House which, he argued, witnessed "a broad scale retreat of government from public health" and "neglect of support for America's public health infrastructure." He blamed the Ford/Reagan/Bush era for "continuing erosion of local public health support in this country."

Particularly galling, McBeath insisted, was the emphasis the conservative Bush, Thatcher, and Mulroney administrations in the United States, United Kingdom, and Canada all were placing on "personal responsibility" and "individual health promotion."

"Is it coincidence that over the last fifteen years national prevention initiatives emphasizing individual responsibility have paralleled the rise of conservative governments seeking to reduce public expenditures and privatize, even commercialize, the delivery of health services, e.g., in Canada, the United States, and the United Kingdom? In a time of rising health care costs and tight budgets, it may seem cheap and expedient for governments to 'blame the victims' by preaching individual lifestyle change. It certainly would be more demanding to adopt 'healthy public policies' that make 'the right choices, the easy choices.' It's also clearly more expensive in the short run to adequately funded health services programs."

McBeath told a reporter at the APHA meeting that the Bush administration had "allowed ideology to interfere with policy," particularly in its opposition to all forms of family planning, gun control, and sexual diseases education.

Public health leaders at the 1990 meeting condemned the lack of access to health care for millions of Americans and the War on Drugs, and they echoed the sentiments of APHA president Myron Allukian: "Health is the bottom line for the survival of the nation. And we are an ailing nation."

In defense of the Bush administration, HHS assistant secretary Dr. James

Mason told the hostile audience that "none of us can ignore the fact that the benefits of health care are not shared equally by all Americans. . . . It is clear to you, me, the president, and Congress that people must have access to the medical services that they need. But we must be cost-effective, . . . I would not suggest the federal government will ride in on a white horse with bags full of money to solve every public health problem."

Vigorous debate ensued over every aspect of public health and health care. The debate would build until health became the number one issue in American politics and swept little-known Arkansas governor William Jefferson Clinton into the White House in 1993—the first Democrat to hold that position since Jimmy Carter. The debate over the future of health in America would dominate the political landscape after the end of the Persian Gulf War in 1991 and through 1992 and 1993, only to die ignominiously in 1994. Many pieces of the health puzzle would converge briefly in 1992 and then fall apart, each thereafter to follow its own political course.

As debate unfolded, some public health officials advocated that their agencies exercise control over medicine in America, making the health insurance industry, hospitals, doctors, and the entire health care infrastructure accountable to public health boards and citizen's committees.[557] Many favored creation of community health partnerships that would meld medicine, government public health, local political interests, and private sector concerns at the local level, allowing these constituencies to jointly define their goals and strategies in the populace's search for health.[558]

For the first time many public health advocates found allies among economists, who argued that disease prevention was almost always more cost-effective than the medical interventions aimed at correcting a health problem once it surfaced. This was a position *strongly* backed at the international level by the World Bank and the World Health Organization.

Key to tallying the costs of diseases and the savings realized by their prevention was the economists' computation of Disability Adjusted Life Years. DALYs represented an empirical way to describe the impact on society not only of deaths but of short-term and chronic illnesses. Computation of DALYs took into account the individual who had an illness, the cost of treating the ailment, the impact at that individual's workplace of his or her absence, the impact on the family, the potential for contagion, and other issues that, in sum, constituted the full cost of disease.[559]

Global economic analysis revealed that pubic health interventions—clean water, safe food, vaccinations, family planning, sexually transmitted disease prevention—were far more cost-effective than the bulk of medical care efforts, whether considered individually or in toto.[560]

In the United States, of course, health spending by 1992, when the issue was paramount in presidential election debates, was skewed in precisely the *least* cost-effective direction. Less than 1 percent of all private and public spending on health in the United States that year was directed to public health, 99 percent was spent on medical care. As the health debate reached the boiling point in 1992, the number of Americans lacking health insurance topped thirty-seven million, or 15 percent of the population. The number of uninsured and underinsured Americans topped thirty-seven million. Annual health care spending averaged $2,349 for each American under sixty-five years of age, and an astounding $9,125 for those over sixty-five years of age.[561] The situation had deteriorated throughout the Bush administration, without any apparent attempt on the president's part to address spiraling medical costs and rising numbers of uninsured Americans.[562]

Conjuring estimates of the numbers of uninsured and underinsured Americans had become such an overwhelming problem that hundreds of academics and government demographers were preoccupied with little else. The rates were highly fluid and were exacerbated by the dramatic changes occurring in the overall economy. With most insurance traditionally linked to employment, tens of thousands of Americans might, on any given day, suddenly have no health coverage because workplaces were disappearing—*snap!*—overnight.[563] The workers, on their own, couldn't afford private health insurance. The experts could see the trend and count some numbers, but the dismal situation was so fluid that estimates of both the numbers of uninsured Americans and the overall costs of health care grew increasingly mushy.[564]

Economist Kathy Swartz of the Urban Institute felt that thirty-seven million was a reasonably hard number to apply to the pool of uninsured in 1990. She estimated that 29 percent of them were living on incomes below the national poverty line, but the rest had incomes well above it: 18 percent were earning more than double the poverty level, and 22 percent more than triple that level. (Poverty for a family of four in 1990 was defined as earning less than $14,000 per year.)

Though the pool of America's uninsured had indeed expanded during the Bush years to embrace many middle-class families, fully a third of the poor had no insurance, could not qualify for Medicaid, and had no possibility of buying private sector coverage, Swartz said.

Most alarming, 50 percent of the nation's uninsured were between the ages of newborn and twenty-four years. Twenty-six percent were children under seventeen years of age. Among the uninsured adults, all but 1.2 million had jobs; they simply didn't earn much.

An increasing trend, Swartz discovered, was the exclusion by insurers of "medically uninsurable individuals"—people who had been diagnosed with cancer, heart disease, or any of a list of hundreds of other chronic ailments *before* applying for coverage. Swartz felt that, when the numbers of uninsured and underinsured were tallied, the total exceeded eighty million Americans, or more than a quarter of the nation's population. Another 30 percent of the population was covered by Medicare/Medicaid or other government programs, leaving just 45 percent fully covered by some form of private insurance.

In other words, 12 percent of the U.S. GNP was being spent on a system that wasn't adequately addressing basic public health needs and utterly failed to meet the medical exigencies of a quarter of the population. And the nation was spending $832 billion for this mess.

Other critics charged: "A society that spends so much on health care that it cannot or will not spend adequately on other health-enhancing activities may actually be reducing the health of its population."[565]

Spending so heavily on last-ditch surgery for terminal patients had to be taking a toll somewhere. Rich as the United States of America was, resources weren't unlimited.[566]

And new costs arose. By one estimate, in 1991 the United States was spending about $600 million annually on pre-AIDS treatment and more than $1.5 billion on AIDS care.[567]

A striking twenty-five-year survey of insured and uninsured Americans who were followed from 1971 to 1987 proved the intuitively obvious: namely, that lacking medical insurance was bad for one's health. In the study, insurance status was a more powerful predictor of life expectancy than social class. The results, the researchers said, "are consistent with the study hypothesis that a lack of health insurance is causally related to a higher mortality rate, because of decreased access and lower quality of care. . . . The findings support a policy imperative for universal health insurance to reduce both financial barriers to care and the risk of premature mortality."[558]

Unlike its Canadian and Western European counterparts, the United States had come to see health not as an individual "right" or as a duty of government but as a "good" or "product" that, like hamburgers or houses, could be bought and sold. Health was a "marketplace" in which patients, physicians, hospitals, pharmaceutical companies, and insurance providers bought and sold goods. It was billed as "free enterprise"—except that it wasn't.

In short, in a truly free enterprise health market, without the hundreds of different forms of government regulation in place, only healthy or wealthy people would be "cost-effective" enough to have insurance and the uninsured would be left to die, untreated, by the millions every year. In economists' terms, medical care could never function, then, in a truly unregulated marketplace because none of the standard rules of supply and demand applied to the health "product." The health insurance market, for example, acted increasingly not as "insurance," but "assurance"—as in a business that picked and billed its clients in a manner that assured that it would never carry bona fide risk on their behalf. Suppliers manipulated and controlled demand: only very rich clients who paid for Cadillac-quality health coverage could actually demand that certain medical procedures, particularly elective ones, be performed.

Most public health advocates thought it was therefore immoral to make health a business enterprise. Though since ancient times people had paid their doctors, these critics argued that the marketplace concept was a new, American one.

Canadian Robert Evans, for example, said that "every society faces the problem of containing steady pressure for expansion of health care. The American system has gone out of control because it lacks the structural features—universal coverage and political accountability—that have permitted some degree of containment in other countries. . . . Over the longer term, however, health care may be an even greater threat to our future capacity to create the wealth which seems so evidently linked with the health of populations. It may stunt our growth."[569]

Canadian scholars took dim views of the U.S. health quandary and most shared Evans's perception that south of their border far too much attention was paid to *medicine* and far too little to *health*. It was, they argued, as if the United States of America had become a nation of gullible fools who bought every gizmo a door-to-door huckster proffered, without ever asking, "But do I *need* this thing?"[570]

This wasn't a uniquely Canadian view. California political scientist Michael Reagan observed: "The *public* good is nonrival: your consumption of it does not prevent me from also using it. National defense is a classic example. Not even Bill Gates can purchase defense privately, and when government provides it, everyone benefits. Mosquito abatement works the same way. Defense and mosquito control share another trait: they are nonexcludable. If you pay your income tax and if I do not, we will both be defended. The mosquito does not know who paid a share of abatement taxes and who did not, so the 'free rider' escapes its bites, just as well as the good citizen taxpayer.

"Is health care a public good? No. So what is it?

"Health care is a *mixed* good. It has the properties of a private good—rivalry and excludability. But because U.S. society generally thinks no one should go without needed medical care, Americans have a problem with simply selling health care like other private goods."[571]

U.S. citizens may not have been ready in 1992 to embrace the Canadian national health system as a model,[572] but they clearly were fed up with their existing nonsystem and ready to consider alternatives. The time was uniquely ripe for change—at last. Surveys and opinion polls revealed a phenomenal transformation of public attitude, from the laissez faire sentiment that had dominated health reform talk during the first Reagan term to a willingness to pay up to $1,000 a year in additional federal taxes if the government would cover all health care costs.[573] Seventy-five percent of American voters ranked health as a "very important" concern determining their voting choices in 1992.[574]

Another telling shift was in the public's perception of links between poverty and health. When asked to agree or disagree with the statement "Poor people are able to get needed medical care," fully 48 percent had agreed in 1982. By the end of 1992 only 26 percent agreed. And most felt that the responsibility for providing care to the poor rested squarely on the federal government. By the end of 1991, however, satisfaction with the U.S. health care system had fallen to an abysmal 6 percent of all voters. Fully 42 percent were prepared to throw the damned thing out and start all over again with something like federally funded universal health care.[575]

Most observers concluded that health reform had an absolute mandate from the American people, even if Bill Clinton personally did not.[576]

VI

It is hard to believe that if the U.S. health care expenditures are not appreciably constrained by the market changes that are under way—and there is little or no reason to expect that they will be—the American people and Congress will remain wedded to their anti-governmental bias and pay the dual penalty of lack of universal coverage and much higher levels of health care spending. We may decide to do just that, but not without a renewed confrontation over national health reform, a confrontation that might lead next time around to a different outcome.[577]

—Eli Ginzberg, Columbia University, 1996

[S]ome of the most important contributors to human capability may be hard to sell exclusively to one person at a time. This is especially so when we consider the so-called public goods, which people consume together rather than separately.

    This applies particularly in such fields as environmental preservation, and also epidemiology and public health care. I may be willing to pay my share in a social program of malaria eradication, but I cannot buy my part of that protection in the form of "private good" (like an apple or a shirt). It is a "public good"—malaria-free surroundings—which we have to consume together.[578]

—Amartya Sen, recipient of the 1998 Nobel Prize in Economics

D ays after his inauguration in 1993 Bill Clinton appointed attorney Hillary Rodham Clinton to head up a health care reform effort. She was, of course, his
wife, the First Lady. And her husband gave her a deadline of one hundred days
to map out a strategy for complete reform of the U.S. health care system, with
two key goals in mind: control costs and cover every single American.

Rodham Clinton organized a committee of five hundred advisors that for
months convened secret meetings notable for who was *not* allowed in: the insurance industry and managed care companies. The bulk of the committee was
drawn from academia, though key foundations and think tanks had presences
as well. As rumors leaked regarding the direction the committee was likely taking, alarm bells rang in the corporate headquarters of the health industry.

Aggressive lobbying ensued to lay the groundwork for opposition to the
White House plan in Congress and in households across America. Lobbyists for
every possible interest group swarmed through the halls of Congress during 1993
in unprecedented numbers, among them beleaguered, poorly funded public
health advocates.[579]

If the goal was to improve the health of the American people, they argued,
it would have been wise to begin by reviewing the relative importance of public
health actions versus medical care in achieving that aim. But improving the
health of Americans *wasn't* the goal. In the White House, on the GOP and Democrat sides of Congress, and even from the lobbyists and interest groups collaring
the politicians, the aim was to pay for medical care and, as a corollary, to control
medical costs.

"Why has the debate about health care reform neglected public health?"
asked public health leaders Phyllis Freeman and Anthony Robbins.[580] "Health
insurance is a necessity for every American. It buys medical services and avoids
personal financial disaster. The ultimate purpose of health care reform as currently debated in the United States is to pay for insurance against the costs of
illness. This narrow focus on sickness insurance misses opportunities to improve
health, yet it is perfectly tuned to the concerns of the public."

Who could blame the citizenry for feeling first, and foremost, worried
about paying medical bills? But it was government's responsibility—a piece of
its social contract with the citizenry—to think beyond individual needs to those
of the whole. And the collective public, Freeman and Robbins argued, would not
be served by *any* of the reform proposals floating around Washington in 1993
to 1994.

Many economists argued in the 1990s that so long as treatment had priority, both in terms of stature and funding, over prevention of illness, *no* finance
or regulatory scheme could control costs. Thus, by starting from a cost-
containment perspective, and then ignoring public health, Washington was un-

dermining any hope of achieving its most ardent aim: cost containment.[581] The only conceivable way to hold down costs in a medically driven health system, experts insisted, was by rationing care in ways that ultimately denied poorer and socially less powerful constituencies procedures that were readily available to those who could afford to pay extra to obtain, for example, an untested bone marrow transplant for breast cancer treatment or a third liver transplant.[582] But the mere specter of rationing—which was, in truth, no phantom but a hard reality for Americans in the nineties—was enough to prompt knee-jerk reactions from politicians, all too often shifting federal funds *from* public health *to* medical budgets. It was utterly irrational.

"Public health practitioners should ingest a healthy dose of skepticism regarding the current national health care debates, while intensifying their efforts to enhance the delivery of properly designed and prioritized public health and environmental health and protection services delivered through our varied and complex system of state and local health agencies," warned Larry Gordon.[583] "[W]e should circle the wagons in the name of public and environmental health and protection and understand, explain, promote, market, sell, interpret, propose, advocate, and communicate the need for improved public health and environmental health and protection services."

Nearly every public health department in the nation was suffering by the time Congress debated health reform in 1994. Surveys demonstrated that years of dwindling funds and increased burdens of providing health care had all conspired to severely weaken the capacities and performances of most of the nation's public health services. Worse, the range of services that departments were expected to provide had grown to include everything from seat belt use campaigns to teen pregnancy counseling, HIV prevention to domestic violence intervention, refugee screening to alcoholism counseling—a list so long as to entirely dilute any clear sense of a public health mission. Nowhere in the nation did public health departments report that they were successfully meeting the needs of their communities in the 1990s. They couldn't.[584]

In 1992 Minnesota's Osterholm became president of the Council of State and Territorial Epidemiologists. In that position he surveyed health departments in all fifty states and the U.S. territories to see how the nation's public health infrastructure was faring.

What he found was chilling.

Combined, the states and territories were spending just $74 million on disease surveillance—more than half of that going for HIV and sexually transmitted diseases. Spending nationwide for monitoring for drug-resistant bacteria and viruses was merely $55,455. For surveillance of *all* diseases (other than TB, STDs, and HIV) the states and territories were spending $11,559,055.

Counties and cities were funding most of their non-HIV disease monitoring entirely from local tax revenues. That meant that most American resources available for protecting consumers from contaminated foods, children from school epidemics, and households from bacterially infected water were subject to local political whims and tax rates.

A total of just 1,608 people were on state and local payrolls for disease surveillance efforts, half of them funded by federal "soft money" (grants and temporary program funds).

And the real shocker: Twelve states had *nobody* on the payroll at the state or local level who was responsible for monitoring disease-causing microbes in food or drinking water. Thirty-four states employed such food- and water-monitoring professionals at a ratio of 0.01 to 0.9 surveillance workers per million residents of the state, Osterholm said. Only five states had one or more water/food–surveillance professionals per million residents.[585]

The status of public health laboratories across the country was equally grim, with most so poorly staffed and supplied that they could not handle processing of samples during even small bacterial epidemics.[586]

To make matters worse, Osterholm said, the "almost defunct infrastructure," as he called the nation's disease surveillance system, was facing the emergence of new microbes about which Hamburg, Lederberg, and Morse had warned. From 1990 through 1993 his staff in Minnesota handled outbreaks of herpes simplex virus,[587] *Salmonella* food poisonings,[588] *Shigella* diarrhea,[589] hepatitis B and C viruses,[590] and measles.[591]

Just three weeks before the 1992 elections the Institute of Medicine released its landmark *Emerging Infections* report.[592] Inspired by Lederberg and Morse's virus meeting of 1988, the institute examined the full gamut of infectious diseases from viruses to parasites. And it concluded that "humankind is beset by a greater variety of microbial pathogens than ever before."

The United States was defenseless against the new microbial threats, the institute argued, because it had "no comprehensive national system for detecting outbreaks of infectious disease."

A host of key factors—most of them global—had conspired to create this new threat to public health: human and animal travel, international distribution of foods and plants, increasing urbanization of human populations, lack of safe drinking water, terrible health infrastructures. This novel onus was being heaped upon a U.S. health infrastructure that no longer was able to meet even its traditional burdens.

The Institute of Medicine report hit the public health community like buckets of ice water, waking it up but leaving it shivering in its impoverished, unheated facilities, unable to muster the energy to tackle the problem. The specter of emerging diseases would not shake up government and the general public until 1994, following the plague epidemic in India and during the 1995 Ebola outbreak in Kikwit, Zaire. Both events coincided with a flurry of movies, books, and television news specials on frightening and deadly new diseases (notably Richard Preston's *Hot Zone* and the hit Dustin Hoffman movie *Outbreak*).

In response to concern among scientists and, for more sensational reasons, in the general public, the Clinton administration in 1994 issued an action plan for CDC responses to newly emerging and reemerging disease threats.[593] The gist of the plan was a call for vigorous surveillance and monitoring of disease trends throughout the United States, as well as overseas—especially in developing countries. That would, of course, be an impossible goal given Osterholm's findings regarding the sorry state of state and local surveillance capacities in the United States, years of public health budget cuts, and ongoing tensions in Congress regarding foreign aid—even aid intended to prevent global epidemics.

After the Ebola epidemic in Kikwit, the World Health Organization—for the first time in its history—endeavored to create a rapid response capability for epidemics and outbreaks and restructured itself to better reflect the restored prominence accorded microbial diseases.

And in Washington the White House issued every federal agency an executive order to review the Institute of Medicine and CDC concerns about emerging diseases with one key question in mind: Does this constitute a national security threat? In July 1994 Undersecretary of State Timothy Wirth announced the results of that governmentwide survey: emerging infectious diseases represent "a national security threat. . . . We are once again losing the battle against infectious diseases in many parts of the world, indeed in many parts of the United States. These diseases know no boundaries."

Once any concern was added to the list of official threats to the security of the United States of America, departments throughout the government were obliged to create offices directed to that issue. Suddenly, what had been an ignored public health worry was elevated within the Clinton administration to parity with global warming, international arms sales, the global narcotics trade, human rights, and military/political instability. Emerging diseases became a strategic concern and events such as the appearance of multidrug-resistant TB in Siberia, spread of HIV in sub-Saharan Africa, and expansion of dengue virus territory in South America commanded the attention of agencies never previously interested in such matters: the State Department, CIA, National Security Council, Department of Defense, Department of Commerce, Federal Emergency Management Agency, and others. For some agencies, the connection was straightforward: if U.S. troops hunkered down in trenches somewhere suddenly started dying of disease by the thousands—as happened during World War I as a result of influenza—the nation's security would be imperiled because its soldiers could not fight in its defense. And security experts noted that there really was no way to distinguish a naturally emerging disease threat to soldiers from one that was deliberately set loose as an agent of biological warfare.[594]

Analysts accustomed to thinking in geopolitical terms framed the emerging diseases issue in much the same way as Thomas Homer-Dixon, Paul Kennedy, and Samuel P. Huntington delineated the national security threats posed by environmental degradation, resource scarcity, and religious conflicts: each was said to contribute to instability on both the national/state levels and in a borderless international sense.[595]

The gist of the emerging diseases/security arguments was that globalization and human encroachment into previously remote ecologies offered unprecedented opportunities for the appearance and spread of pathogenic microorganisms that could have devastating impacts on humans, their crops, or livestock.[596] Because such events were by definition unpredictable, elevated global vigilance was necessary to spot emergencies before they led to epidemics. That required global cooperation and recognition that microbes freely crossed international borders and were far less likely in the twenty-first century, compared to the mid-twentieth century, to remain confined to any specific country or world region.

Pandemics could be destabilizing and economically devastating, as HIV's catastrophic impact upon most of Africa proved. Global disease prevention was both necessary and cost-effective.[597]

The 1995 report presented by Undersecretary of State Wirth to President Clinton, commonly referred to as the "CISET Report,"[598] argued that for these and hundreds of other reasons, "the effort to build a global surveillance and response system is in accord with the national security and foreign policy goals of the United States."

Absent any new microbial threats, the CISET Report stated, infectious diseases were already costing the United States more than $120 billion a year in direct and indirect expenses, and at least 10 percent of that financial burden was the result of microbial problems that had emerged only since 1980. Some twenty-nine previously unknown human disease pathogens arose between 1977 and 1994, the report stated, and the pace of disease emergence was quickening.

"There's not a single panacea. Not a single remedial measure," Lederberg told the CISET gathering on July 25, 1995. "It's rather a matter of reinforcing a fabric of public health that has existed; a fabric that has become rather threadbare. But I have some bad news . . . it's going to take some money."[599]

About $500 million a year, to be precise. The funds, according to the CISET Report, would be used to salvage the anemic U.S. surveillance and public health laboratory system and to build up such capacities in key areas of Africa, Asia, the former Soviet Union, and Latin America.

Though the CISET Report proved pivotal in elevating concern about emerging diseases both inside the White House, in the executive offices of WHO, and at the highest levels of government in several nations (notably the United Kingdom, Canada, Australia, Germany, Jordan, Brazil, Egypt, and Israel), its budget requests of the U.S. government were DOA.

As Lederberg had predicted, "without a champion in the halls of Congress, I think this report hasn't much of a chance of getting appropriate attention."[600]

The problem? The Clintons' health care reform package had been slaughtered by Congress, the president was personally besieged and weakened by sexual, management, and real estate scandals, the administration was trying to retire the enormous national deficit that had largely accrued during the Reagan and Bush administrations, and antifederalism fever was sweeping the nation.[601]

When Rodham Clinton's health reform package finally hit Congress in October, 1993, it landed with a loud *thud*—all thirteen hundred pages of it. It was as indecipherable as it was weighty. Even specialized congressional staffers who had dedicated their careers to medical issues couldn't figure out much of it. Submitting any proposal in such a format to a hostile Congress was an astounding mistake, severely compounded by months of excluding from the planning process the very industry representatives that stood to gain or lose the most money from health reform.

Further exacerbating the political ineptitude was an almost total White House silence in response to the medical insurance industry's fantastically effective TV campaign, warning viewers that the Clinton administration was going to force nasty "government medicine" down the country's throat. This would, the ads said, create a system of rationed care, terrible quality, no patient choices, and inadequate access to most types of treatment, all driven by demands for cost control. That, as it would turn out, is exactly what America would get, but in privatized form. The Clintons would lose, the health industry would win— and the horrors envisioned in the ads would be visited upon America by private enterprise.

The much-bungled White House proposal exacted so much hostility from Congress that many politicians declared it dead before it was read. However, the Congressional Budget Office reviewed the proposed bill, dubbed the Health Security Act, and concluded that the Clinton plan was extremely complex, but could work. And if it did succeed, it would save the nation billions of dollars in coming years, thanks to medical cost controls.[602]

But the Republicans pronounced the plan to be nothing more than another example of the Democrats' dastardly penchant for "big government programs,"[603] and it died along with several counterproposals for health reform that were debated in 1994. Their defeat would flavor Congress's attitude toward nearly all health-related initiatives for the rest of the nineties. America was to face the twenty-first century without any coherent system of health care provision and with an ailing public health infrastructure hobbled by lack of funds. Even the much hoped for $500 million for emerging diseases programs failed to materialize.[604]

Defeated in its attempts to perform major surgery on the nation's health system, the Clinton administration would spend the next six years slapping Band-Aids on the patient.[605]

In November of both 1993 and 1994 the Republicans enjoyed spectacular election results, emerging with control of both the House and Senate and the governor's seat in thirty states. Newt Gingrich, a Georgia conservative and key author of the New Right platform, the "Contract with America," became Speaker of the House for the 104th Congress. Federalism, as America had known it since the Great Depression, was dead. In its place came more block grants, à la Reagan, in which spending for public health and welfare programs was left up to the states. The new Congress hailed Reagan as its icon and Gingrich as his interpreter.

"What Congress is doing that is *unfamiliar* is giving back what had previously been centralized. At a time when the nation is coming to grips with the politics of retrenchment, Congress is exercising its historic option of leaving matters to the states—thereby alleviating its own burden of making hard financial and policy choices," argued University of Virginia government affairs expert Martha Derthick.[606]

For example, when the GOP-dominated Congress sent block grants to Arizona governor Fife Symington in 1995, the conservative fellow Republican said thanks very much and here's what I intend to do with the cash, don't get in my way. He increased police, prison, and highway spending levels in Arizona by, respectively, 18, 15, and 8 percent. And he cut education by 5 percent, reduced aid to the poor by 17 percent, and decimated public health, lashing its budget by an eye-popping 43 percent. His legislature, which was also Republican-dominated, killed funding that would have provided health care to 150,000 poor Arizonans; eliminated a Women, Infants, and Children (WIC) nutrition program; and cut hundreds of children off the welfare rolls.[607]

In most states the cutting was more incremental, building over a few years to amount to a serious hacking of public health.

"As the scientific case for public health becomes stronger, political and popular support has not kept pace," argued Hastings Institute analyst Daniel Callahan. "Public health programs in the United States—and the situation is similar in many other countries—are either not being improved or, in many cases, are being allowed to wither. . . . Between 1981 and 1993 there was a 25 percent decline in funding for public health programs as a proportion of the American health care budget. Some twenty-two state health agencies saw a decline in state funding, and another thirty-three saw cuts to services in 1992. Nothing has improved since then. . . . Overt resistance to public health care is rare. On the contrary, public health has been subject to the death of a thousand cuts, some of them noticed, others not."[608]

Whether cuts were wholesale or incremental, the news for public health seemed terribly grim after the 1994 defeat of reform. The American people had been ready for radical change in 1992—by 1994 they were resigned to allowing the marketplace, rather than the government, decide the fate of health. And that situation was unlikely to change, argued Massachusetts General Hospital's Dr. David Blumenthal, unless the numbers of uninsured Americans topped sixty-five million or there was "a catastrophic societal event, such as a depression like that of the 1930s or another world war. A disease pandemic (one dwarfing the AIDS epidemic) could also hasten such a change in public sentiment. These would certainly be high prices to pay for attaining long-sought health care goals."[609]

Barring such horrors or a complete failure in the health care market, Blumenthal thought it unlikely Americans would again entertain the notion of universal health care until sometime in the mid–twenty-first century.[610]

Indeed, for the first time since it was adopted in 1948, the Democratic Party in 1996 dropped its call for universal health care from the party platform. And even longtime congressional supporters of universal health care, such as Congressman Henry Waxman of California and Senator Edward Kennedy, fell silent on the issue.[611] Downsizing and "reinvention"[612] became the name of the game at the Department of Health and Human Services, as HHS struggled to identify its role amid such a hostile environment.

The most obvious change after 1994 was a continued increase in the numbers of uninsured Americans, reaching 44.3 million, or one out of every six Americans, by 1998.[613] Even 12.2 million households in which annual earnings exceeded $50,000 lacked health coverage.

The second major change involved employers, whose costs for employee insurance had inflated by 218 percent between 1980 and 1992. They continued to offer insurance to employees, but under increasingly restrictive conditions.[614]

Given the relative weakness of unions and the many sectors of the economy that weren't unionized at all, observers thought strikes over this issue unlikely. More probable was a cycle in which greater numbers of uninsured Americans spiraled into debt trying to pay their share of premiums and deductibles, possibly returning to work prematurely following illness, and, as a result, becoming less healthy.

Few tears were shed among Washington insiders. The GOP leadership washed its hands of health care—block grants shifted funds to the states, so if Rhode Island's populace wanted universal health care, well, fine, they could have it.

But could they? A 1997 Rand Corporation survey found that few, if any, of the fifty states could sustain the sort of tax increase that would be necessary to supply health coverage to all their citizens. Without substantial federal assistance, expanded access to medicine seemed unlikely—indeed, more probable was rising *non*insurance in every state in the United States.[615]

What was public health to do? How could it survive if America was unlikely to entertain another fundamental reassessment of its health goals until a catastrophe or financial failure occurred? Many argued that if you can't beat 'em, after three hundred years of fighting maybe it was best to join 'em: it was time for public health to work with medicine. The goal was to make managed care emphasize preventive medicine (a.k.a., "personal responsibility"), promote such services as immunization, and allow doctors to carry out public health activities within the private sector.[616]

As successful as some such collaborations proved, private sector medicine could not keep drinking water safe, stop air pollution, encourage condom use, ensure that pharmaceuticals and alternative treatments were what they claimed to be. . . . In short, those fundamental aspects of public health that were about *collective*, not *individual*, well-being were simply not amenable to such attempts at private sector collaboration.

It recalled the ancient dichotomy between Hygeia and Panakeia: In Greek mythology, the god Asklepios had two daughters. Panakeia was the healer and she invented cures for all manner of ailments. Asklepios's other daughter, Hygeia, taught Greeks sensible ways to live so that they would stay healthy and have no need of Panakeia's healing. Both daughter's names have lived down through the ages. Hygeia in English is hygiene, and even schoolchildren of the 1990s still learned that proper respect for hygiene would enhance good health. Panakeia has been transformed over time into a longed-for, but futile, dream—a cure-all, a universal treatment, a panacea.

Hygeia's modern followers were the practitioners of public health. Panakeia's were medical professionals. And just as the sisters had their mythical fights, more than two millennia later their adherents, too, could still fail to see eye to eye.

By the end of the nineties, however, it wasn't clear that either Panakeia or Hygeia was well served in America.

Certainly not in Los Angeles.

When stagflation and recession had soured life in the rest of the United States, Los Angeles had prospered, thanks to a steady supply of multibillion-dollar defense contracts. But the Pentagon sugar daddy turned its back on California after the fall of the Berlin wall and collapse of the Soviet Union. As the East and the Rust Belt gingerly began their fiscal recoveries in the early 1990s, Los Angeles sank into the deepest recession the region had experienced since the Great Depression. By February 1993 the state's unemployment rate exceeded 10 percent. Its budget deficit reached an all-time high of $15 billion.[617]

Beginning in 1992, Los Angeles County suffered a series of one-two punches: An all-white jury acquitted four white police officers of any crimes committed in connection with the brutal, videotaped beating of Rodney King, an African-American motorist they had pulled over on suspicion of drunk driving. Within seconds of the verdict, riots erupted throughout South Central Los Angeles and spread citywide. When the riots ended three days later, some fifty-three people were in the morgue and two thousand were hospitalized, fifteen hundred buildings were ash heaps, and property damage was estimated at $1 billion.[618]

Then, at the end of the six-month dry season that began right after the April '92 riots, L.A. County was again engulfed in flames—hot Santa Ana swept brushfires across the county from mid-October to early November, destroying an estimated $1.4 billion worth of homes and property.

The county had finally cleaned up after the fires when an earthquake measuring 6.8 on the Richter scale hit it on January 17, 1994. When that final tally was made, sixty-one people were dead, more than ninety-three hundred had been hospitalized, forty-five thousand apartments and homes were too damaged to be occupied safely, three major freeway arteries were unusable because of collapsed overpasses, and Governor Pete Wilson declared that the calamity had caused $15 to $30 billion worth of damages.

Los Angeles was shell-shocked, its populace left wondering about the seemingly biblical proportions of their collective tragedy. For the first time in L.A. history, the flow of immigration reversed.

By the summer of 1995 L.A. County was teetering on the brink of the largest municipal bankruptcy in the history of the United States. The county's government had just until November 1 to cut its budget by more than $2 billion or be forced to default on all its loans and face fiscal collapse. (Proposition 13 meant the county couldn't raise property taxes to cover the huge deficit.) Though the county budget covered many other functions besides health, the health slice of the pie was enormous—and more vulnerable politically than any other piece.

There was deep trouble in Tinseltown, so deep in September 1995 that the Los Angeles County Medical Association declared that "the county's sky is falling!" The complexion and the future of all of Los Angeles County were about to change more dramatically than had any other U.S. metropolitan region since the end of World War II.[619]

At the core of the crisis propelling Los Angeles toward a much-diminished stature in the new millennium were issues that threatened to evoke comparable crises in many other major American counties, including New York's Suffolk, Nassau, and Westchester; Florida's Dade; Illinois's Cook; Texas's Dallas–Fort Worth; Massachusett's Boston; and the District of Columbia. Fueling these crises, and in turn taking the brunt of the burden of repairing them, were the nation's underfunded local health care systems for the poor and uninsured.

On June 20, 1995, Los Angeles's five supervisors were "stunned and shell-shocked," as one of them put it, by a budget memorandum from the county's chief administrative officer, Sally Reed. The county's operating budget for 1995–96 was $13.1 billion, Reed said, but actual revenue could not possibly be expected to exceed $11.1 billion. Twenty percent of the county's workforce would have to be laid off immediately, some of the six county hospitals would have to be closed permanently. "There will be painful results," Reed declared.[620] "The structural budget deficit has grown so large that any attempt to solve it with anything less than permanent adjustments is extremely risky. . . . The bond rating agencies and investment community have stated their concerns with a county budget that does not address the imbalance between revenues and expenditures in a meaningful way."

Reed's "meaningful" solution? LAC-USC Medical Center closed immediately, diverting an astonishing 372,300 annual inpatient days of hospitalization and 871,300 annual outpatient visits to other, presumably private, medical facilities. With its first clinic dating to 1879, LAC-USC Medical Center was the largest medical facility in the world and trained more physicians and nurses than any other medical institution.

LAC-USC was the primary health and medical provider for Los Angeles's estimated 9.75 million residents in 1995. About three-quarters of a million of these residents were undocumented and 4.1 million were considered medically indigent (without insurance or Medi-Cal coverage).[621] By 1995 Los Angeles County had the highest percentage of uninsured and state-covered individuals in the nation.[622]

Reed's call for closure of LAC-USC Medical Center sparked immediate protest from the county's twenty-two thousand licensed physicians, from the Los Angeles County Medical Association (LACMA), and from the private hospital system. The hospitals and private doctors cried that they couldn't possibly absorb the patient burden.

"We said sudden death for any acute care hospital is a bad idea," health task force leader and former California legislator Burt Margolin explained hastily to an inquiring reporter for whom he had crammed a few scant minutes into his twenty-hour-a-day schedule.[623] "Because it's irreversible. You could never reopen LAC-USC or any other county hospital because once it was reopened, it would have to meet new earthquake codes. And there is no way those facilities could affordably be brought up to code. So closure is permanent, irreversible."[624]

The task force's solution was one that Margolin found only slightly less distasteful: shutting down all but eleven of the county's forty-five public health clinics.

In late August, the County Board of Supervisors appointed Margolin "Health Czar," made the Health Crisis Task Force a permanent feature of the government, and gave the private sector until September 1 to submit proposals for privatizing parts of the county's public health system. The pace was feverish—the deadline for being declared insolvent was October 1, the beginning of the county's new fiscal year.

"Our long-term vision of where the county should be is based on the assumption that there is too much money tied up in hospitals," the weary Margolin explained. "We want to move money from the hospitals eventually into community-based primary care. But in the meantime, we've had to cut back on the public health system. That means less screening for tuberculosis, less control of communicable diseases—the threat of spread is real. There will be a significant decrease in primary care to the poor and uninsured. Therefore, they will be at greater risk of getting sick and spreading disease. As people think about that it frightens them. But people with insurance don't think about it. They say, 'That's not me.' They're wrong, of course. Because when we lose the public health safety net, when you talk about the collapse of the health care system, of trauma care, of nine-one-one . . . there's no room for ideology or complacency here."

Department of Health Services director Robert Gates put things more bluntly: "I don't see in the current trend that there won't be people who lose their lives as a result of these cuts."

In the waiting room of L.A.'s Hudson Comprehensive Health Clinic, uninsured widow Mary Coleman said the pending closure that had been proposed for Hudson would be "disastrous" for her: "I would just get sicker, I guess." Medi-Cal recipient Edna Humphrey said she couldn't afford the deductions and medication costs that private care centers levied, so for ten years she had traveled two hours by bus to Hudson for treatment. The African-American grandmother had "absolutely no idea" where she would go if Hudson closed. Former farm worker Luis Ferral capped the dispirited discussion by saying in Spanish, "I don't really know how my medical care will be resolved [if Hudson closes]. Where am I going to go? If we continue paying our taxes, why won't they give us services? The government wants to wash its hands with the people."

The Hudson clinic's executive officer, Nancy Delgado, shook her head sadly when she described the layoff list recently posted for her staff and the grim prospects for the patients served by the clinic. "I've been in Kenya, working in medical services," Delgado said, "and I really wonder how long it will be before we look like Kenya or Zaire."[625]

The complex of events and decision-making that had conspired to create the L.A. disaster had its counterparts all over the country, though in less dramatic forms. Experts said L.A. was simply first to reach the brink of disaster because it had been presented with the most extreme set of circumstances. And worse was to come, for none of the crises L.A. experienced in 1995 as yet reflected the impact of severe cuts in Medicare and other medical services then under debate in Washington. Combined, those cuts were expected to take at least an additional $1.5 billion from L.A. County's federal revenues over the next five years. And the county had become addicted to these now disappearing federal dollars.[626]

"When we first saw this unfolding a few years ago, we saw that the state had a dramatic shortfall. But then we were able to go to the federal government and generate new revenue streams," Gates explained. "But essentially that golden goose stopped laying eggs. The elections of '94 brought in a different attitude in both the state legislature and Congress. It wasn't that long ago that Clinton was talking about universal health care and now here we are."

Gates, demoralized and exhausted, had lost the spirit to fight against such overwhelming odds: he'd tendered his resignation effective November 1, 1995. In the final analysis, Gates said with a sigh, "people just seem less concerned about health care for the poor. Everything they're talking about doing at the federal level, such as cutting Medicare, only worsens our problems. And we haven't even factored for that."

Zev Yaroslavsky represented most of the affluent county residents Gates felt "didn't care" as a member of the Board of Supervisors. A liberal Democrat and newly elected to the board, he pinned most of the blame on his fellow supervisors.

"I think that the county could and should have seen this coming," Yaroslavsky insisted. "They should have known. But the county officialdom was in a state of denial. Now you have people wandering around pontificating that the federal government screwed us. Nobody screwed us. We did it to ourselves."[627]

In July fellow supervisor Gloria Molina and Yaroslavsky went to Washington to beg Congress and the White House to save Los Angeles. Though they received a warm reception at the White House, Congress appeared decidedly disinterested in the plight of the nation's largest metropolis.

"We were amazed at how little the legislators understand about the local consequences of their actions. It just boggles the mind. And we're just in the first wave of all this," Yaroslavsky groaned. "There are three or four bigger waves—block grants, Medicare cuts, and so on—still to come from Congress. And that's real scary. Think of it: this is the easy part!"

Most immediately, this all meant that the estimated fifteen thousand people who lived on the streets or in the single room occupancy accommodations (SROs) of L.A.'s Skid Row were going to lose the only medical clinic designed to serve their health needs. Located just east of downtown, Skid Row—its official moniker since the 1920s—was a sixty-six-square-block area sprinkled with lean-tos; tents; cardboard box houses; and occupied, nonfunctioning cars. At its hub was the Winegart Center, a privately funded SRO and service center for the homeless. Within the center was a county-funded medical clinic that was scheduled for closure on or about September 15. According to Winegart's director, Paul Tepper, closing the clinic would also take down satellite operations inside Winegart that dealt with tuberculosis and HIV/AIDS. And the clientele, most of whom had drug, alcohol, and/or mental illness problems, would not be welcome at other medical clinics or hospitals.

Eloquent thirty-two-year-old Matthew (who declined to give his last name) had lived on Los Angeles streets for years before moving into the Winegart Center, and by his own admission had "a serious attitude problem. I was mean." Workers in the clinic discovered that Matthew had tuberculosis when the young man came in for treatment of an infected foot. The doctors immediately put him on antibiotics, telling him he had to take the drugs every day for eighteen months.

"I gave them a real hard time. I was belligerent," Matthew recalled one afternoon while strolling along Skid Row. "But gradually they wore me down and I took those drugs. And now I have to thank them for my life."

Asked where he would go for TB drugs after September 15, the stunned young man stopped in his tracks and pondered the question. "I have no idea," he said. "That's a good question."

Another homeless man ambled by as Matthew spoke, took a gulp from a bottle inside a paper bag, and demanded to know what was being discussed. When told that the county was facing bankruptcy and might soon close its public health facilities, he cried, "The county is out of money? No way! Somebody's putting money in their pockets. They gonna shut this place down? No. That's about somebody gettin' rich."

Like many of Winegart's residents, the anonymous street-corner politico was HIV positive. His medical needs were covered in large part by federal Ryan White Act funds that were intended to offset the burdens of AIDS care in hard-hit cities like New York and Los Angeles. But Congress was withholding $31 million in Ryan White funds from L.A. and would not release it unless the county generated $57 million in matching money by October 1. Nobody in the county seemed to have the slightest idea where those funds would be found.

Since 1989 Los Angeles had witnessed a steady rise in tuberculosis[628] and AIDS rates. It went through several large-scale food contamination incidents involving bacteria such as *Salmonella* and *Listeria*. It experienced a large measles epidemic. And bubonic plague cases had just surfaced in the mountainous northeastern area of the county when the 1995 budget battle was under way.[629]

For twenty years responsibility for infectious diseases control in the county had fallen on the shoulders of Dr. Shirley Fanin. For years she had watched her budget and power be subsumed beneath the politically stronger hospital services side of the DHS. And she now had to figure out how to prevent epidemics in a county that would no longer offer meaningful primary care for its poorest residents.

"I think there's something totally out of control here," the robust Fanin exclaimed. "We're facing cuts of more than 20 percent in public health, but those are on top of losing greater than half our assets over the last two years. So the real cut is 50 to 70 percent. In 1973 we had one hundred district health officers— MDs. Today we're down to fourteen who have to cover a county that is larger than forty thousand square miles. We're not serving any community adequately now, even before they shut down thirty-four of our forty-five clinics. If things get cut any further, we'll just have to fold up our tents and forget about the public's health."

Fanin predicted a scenario that she thought would unfold over the next three years: The current vaccination rate of L.A. kids under age five was only 58 percent, but Fanin forecast a dismal drop in even that appalling rate. As a result, she opined, childhood epidemics of measles, pertussis, and diphtheria would erupt. In 1990, for example, L.A. immunization rates had slumped to 42 percent of all children under age five and as a direct result L.A. had had a measles epidemic that put one thousand seven hundred kids in the hospital and killed forty. Tuberculosis, too, would soar, as would emergence of drug-resistant strains of TB—especially as more poor Los Angelenos would self-medicate with black market antibiotics.

Fanin also foresaw the collapse of AIDS education efforts, resulting in a rise in unsafe sexual practices, an outcome of which would be a rise in all sexually transmitted disease rates. And finally, microbes brought into the county by immigrants or traveling residents would go unnoticed due to what Fanin predicted would be the nearly total collapse of disease surveillance capacity. As a result, the county could see outbreaks of such things as cholera, Korean hantaan viruses, yellow fever, even hemorrhagic fever viruses.

"I think what we're going to be facing is both unthinkable and unavoidable," Fanin concluded.

White Memorial Hospital was also worried, but not about undesirable clientele. Located just a half mile from LAC-USC in the midst of El Barrio, Los Angeles's Latino center of poverty, White was operated by the Seventh Day Adventists as a nonprofit charitable facility. Licensed for 377 beds, White handled three thousand ER patients a month, many of them victims of local gang violence. Its intensive care and neonatal units already ran to capacity and at any given time 65 percent of the beds in the eighty-two-year-old building were filled—an unusually high rate of occupancy in a city where most private hospitals filled only about 45 percent of their beds.[630]

White's CEO, Beth Zachary, was working around the clock trying to find ways to prevent the tsunami of patients she expected would engulf her facility when nearby clinics and some parts of LAC-USC closed.

"It's hard to know how to quantify the potential," the slightly frazzled Zachary said.

All of this was also rough for the University of California Los Angeles (UCLA) and the University of Southern California (USC), which, combined, trained more of the West's physicians than any other medical schools west of the Mississippi. USC's students were trained at LAC-USC Medical Center and UCLA's students learned medicine at the county's Long Beach hospital. Even before the crisis hit, both medical schools were having a hard time covering their costs, as research and training expenses had for years been offset by submitting higher bills to insurance companies. By 1995, however, half of all insured people in the county were in an HMO, most of them in Kaiser. And the HMOs refused to cover the bills that were padded with medical school expenses. If the county couldn't pull its weight in running the hospitals, UCLA and USC certainly couldn't make up the difference. Indeed, as part of the University of California system, UCLA was facing cuts from Sacramento where legislators were hacking at the higher education budget.

Further compounding the California crisis was Proposition 187, which was voted into law in 1994. Its goal was to decrease the taxpayers' burdens by denying social services to all illegal immigrants. In practical terms, it was specific to Spanish-speaking immigrants from Mexico and Central America. And its chief tactic was to lower public health costs by denying the Latinos all but life-and-death emergency care. When Prop. 187 was passed by popular vote, physicians and public health workers cried foul: it would violate the Hippocratic oath to deny needed care. And how, they asked, are we to know which Spanish speaker is a legal versus an illegal immigrant? Do we demand to see proof? If the patient is comatose, do we leave him untreated until residency documents can be found?

Rather than saving money, it was obvious by the summer of 1995 that Prop. 187 was creating new, larger expenses for L.A. County. There were two reasons for this: First, the private hospitals used the law as an excuse to deny care to uninsured patients, dumping most Spanish speakers into county-run facilities. Second, the immigrants themselves, fearful of legal repercussions after passage of the law, stayed away from hospitals and clinics until their conditions were dire. Child vaccination rates fell and catastrophic illness rates rose.

In 1995 challenges to Prop. 187 were working their ways through the state courts and the outcome was uncertain. This left the health of 3,351,242 Hispanic Los Angelenos in limbo—especially the 54 percent of them who weren't citizens or legal immigrants. Hispanic Los Angelenos, from 1994 through the rest of the nineties, responded to the threat by shunning even legally available services, such as Medi-Cal, for their children.[631]

Though the legal challenges resulted in a 1998 decision in favor of providing essential health care to all immigrants, that didn't solve all the problems highlighted by Prop. 187. In 1996 Congress ordered that all noncitizens be eliminated from Medicaid programs, even if they were legal residents and U.S. taxpayers. Though that restriction, too, would be softened by 1999 court challenges, the message to Latinos in the United States was that they were not welcome in America's medical system. By 1997 Hispanics were more likely than any other population group in the country to lack health insurance, have no regular physician, use emergency rooms of public hospitals for all of their health needs, and delay treatments until their problems had become emergencies.[632] At the close of the century the private Commonwealth Fund determined that 40 percent of California's Latino population lacked any form of health insurance, and a quarter of the nation's uninsured were Hispanic. Overall, by 2000 Hispanics were two times more likely to lack health insurance compared to other Americans, regardless of where they lived or worked.[633]

Two weeks before the October 1 bankruptcy deadline, Health Czar Margolin ordered layoff notices sent to fifty-two hundred employees of the Department of Health Services. And Democrats Molina and Yaroslavsky increased their pressure on the White House. They were greatly aided by the considerable leverage exerted by John Sweeney, then president of the Service Employees International Union, who promised Clinton that organized labor would remember whether or not the Democratic party let public health die in Los Angeles.[634]

The clock ticked. Tensions rose throughout the county government. Republican leaders in Sacramento stopped returning panicked phone calls. Regional banks prepared new assessments of the value of Los Angeles bonds. The Board of Supervisors and Margolin burned midnight oil, desperately searching for a way to save public health and the public hospitals.

On September 22, with just eight days to spare, President Clinton came to the rescue. He declared the county a Medicaid Demonstration Project, to be funded with $364 million to transform it into, in Clinton's words, a "model for the nation." The money would be used over a five-year period (to end September 30, 2000) to re-create the entire Los Angeles County public health and health care system, shaping it according to a strategy designed jointly by federal, state, and county health authorities.[635]

But the bailout didn't put an end to belt-tightening. A year after federal money arrived, another thirty-nine hundred county health employees had been demoted or laid off in what was undoubtedly the most radical restructuring of public hospital and health care in U.S. history. Over the next four years the county had to completely transform its services and, it hoped, do so without imperiling the health of its 1.6 million Medicaid recipients, 700,000 Medicare patients, and 3.1 million uninsured individuals not covered by the federally funded programs.

By 1996 the county had the country's highest percentage of uninsured residents—31 percent of the population under the age of sixty-five years. In addition, estimates were that at least 700,000 of L.A.'s undocumented residents were using the county public hospitals and clinics. And despite Prop. 187, the numbers of illegal Hispanic immigrants flooding public hospital ERs rose from 1995 to 1996.[636] A key reason for that increase was what had happened in the two counties that formed a buffer between L.A. and the porous Mexican border. San Diego County had simply gotten out of the business of providing health care, electing instead to pass county funds on to the private hospitals in hopes that they might accept the burden of care for the indigent. And two years after its own official bankruptcy in 1994, Orange County was shutting down most of its public health and hospital facilities in its on-going struggle to become solvent. So poor people—whether or not they were legal U.S. residents—headed north to L.A. County for health care. At LAC-USC Medical Center they often queued up for ten to fifteen hours waiting for treatment for anything from a sore throat to major trauma.

Meanwhile, county officials looked back at the frantic days of September 1995 as a nightmare. They referred to the period as the "nuclear meltdown," the "nervous breakdown," or the "near-death experience." Joel Bellman, staff aide to Supervisor Yaroslavsky, summed up the period between the summers of '95 and '96 as "a genuine catastrophe being averted by a deus ex machina from Washington."[637]

In August 1996, after just four months at the helm, L.A. County Director of Health Services Dr. Mark Finucane was oddly ebullient about L.A.'s task and future. "There is no question that Los Angeles has become a laboratory not just to the Clinton administration but to a variety of other entities—teaching hospitals, schools of public health, insurance providers, local government leaders nationwide," Finucane told a visitor on a cool late summer day. "In fifteen years people will ask, 'Where were you during those years?' L.A. will be it. This is *the* laboratory for public health. We have the most competitive managed care environment here in the entire world. It's *it*. It's a seminal time. And when you contrast it with what's going on in New York, it's night and day. There's the great twin towers of public health in the U.S. One [New York City] is being dismantled.[638] Whereas here we made a decision to rebuild. I see in New York the systematic selling off of assets. And that's quite a contrast to what we're doing here. I think a lot of people in public health are looking left and right and watching what's going on in the two cities right now," Finucane concluded, clearly satisfied that history would show the Los Angeles solution to be superior.

The Clinton administration didn't rescue L.A. County by just handing it a fat check. On the contrary, Washington's solution carried high risks for L.A. and virtually guaranteed the county would be bankrupt by 2001 if radical restructuring and cost-saving measures weren't rapidly put into place. The seemingly magical $364 million in federal funds was "found" by front-loading expected federal Medicaid revenues. The administration estimated how much in Medicaid funds, based on 1994 patient loads, would flow into L.A. County coffers over the next five years and fronted the county most of that money in the form of a huge payout in October 1995. This meant, of course, that L.A. would receive dramatically less money each of the next four years. The October 1995 layoffs and cuts, coupled with the White House funds, had reduced the county's health services debt from $655 million to a manageable $7.1 million.

At least, for the moment.

But if Los Angeles hoped to continue to avoid bankruptcy still deeper cuts—approaching the health department's bone marrow—were necessary.[639]

"The challenge to the county is enormous," Supervisor Yaroslavsky acknowledged. "We have developed a good partnership with the Clinton administration. . . . But they've not given us a bail out. We're on a short leash. The county is going through withdrawal treatment at the Betty Ford Center for Chronic Overspenders. And the Clinton administration is the staff of the clinic. It's in our interests organizationally and politically to take our shots, keep getting our boosters to make sure we innoculate ourselves against going back to our overspending ways."

Yaroslavsky was well aware that by doing so he and fellow Democrats who brokered the deal had placed Los Angeles under the microscope. "Look, the big bananas are Los Angeles and New York City," he explained. "And when L.A. County sneezes the rest of the counties across America catch cold. What we do will impact the rest of the country. Unfortunately for us, there aren't a lot of examples of this kind of restructuring for us to turn to, so we're writing the book.

"The real question for counties like New York or Los Angeles," Yaroslavsky insisted, "is what does this country think it owes its citizens? What do we owe our people? Nationally we're just rearranging the chairs on the *Titanic*. Because of changes at the federal level [in Medicaid, Medicare, and funds for hospital improvements] what you're asking counties to do is provide more health care to more people, with less money."

It sounded impossible.

Los Angeles shifted its health focus from individual hospitalizations and curative medicine to disease and illness prevention. This entailed further reducing the numbers of hospital beds managed by the county and transferring thousands of doctors and nurses from treatment facilities to primary care and public health clinics. The assumption was that much of the burden of tertiary illness would decrease due to proper primary and preventive interventions. When surgery or intensive care was needed, the hope was that the patients would be accepted into private hospitals. The exceptions would be emergency and trauma care, which would continued to be a county responsibility.

It was risky. In the short run the county would lose still more money as it divested itself of responsibility for high-price-tag tertiary care of Medicare and Medi-Cal patients. Billings for such things as open heart surgery, orthopedic treatments, and intensive care represented a significant source of income for the beleaguered county, accounting for hundreds of millions of state and federal dollars. But maintaining the aging, bloated hospital empire necessary to offer such care was clearly bleeding the county dry.

Finucane wanted the people of sunny Los Angeles to stop basking in the glow of Medicare and Medi-Cal dollars and turn instead to a longer-term view of medical cost containment through prevention—the essence of public health. If fewer people in L.A. got sick enough to require costly tertiary medicine, he reasoned, in the long run everyone would save money.

"We have to begin to think of hospitalization not as a revenue source, but as a failure to prevent that hospitalization," Finucane insisted. "The first day that I started [as director] I just announced that I would make no reductions in public health. Period. What are we in government going to do that no one else does? The answer is public health. . . . I've challenged my public health managers: in three years I want to be able to say I've got the best public health system in the United States."

But after years of being treated as the pathetic stepchild to the powerful public hospital system, L.A. County's public health department was in sorry shape. For two decades the hospital administrators managed to make "stealth-like cuts" in the public health budget, said the department's chief, Jonathan Freedman.[640]

There were no such "cuts" in public health challenges: for the first time in more than fifty years, a case of locally acquired cholera surfaced in Los Angeles in 1996. The victim was a homeless man who had lived in the county for ten years without traveling outside the area and his illness was taken to signal dangerous microbial contamination of the local water supply. In addition, at least fifty thousand Los Angelenos under the age of five years were unvaccinated, according to Freedman, and represented a dangerous "reservoir of infectious disease."

And waiting times at all public health and hospital facilities had increased since October 1995. According to LACMA president-elect Johnson, nonemergency waits routinely exceeded six months. "You have a sixteen-month waiting period for [the] neurology clinic at Drew-Memorial-Martin Luther King Hospital," Johnston said. "And Antelope Valley Clinic was running one-hundred-and-ten-week waits for pediatric appointments. No wonder people don't get their kids immunized."

For example: Dr. Mary Abbott, the new medical director of the Hudson Comprehensive Health Center in downtown L.A., lost 10 percent of her physician slots in October 1995, though Hudson was spared the complete shutdown that had been planned. About half her remaining staff quit, however, or was transferred. Their replacements came from LAC-USC Medical Center, which had been ordered to shut down some of its adult medicine outpatient clinics. The cases from those closed clinics were transferred to Hudson.

"In May 1995 we saw twelve hundred to fourteen hundred patients per month in the adult medicine clinic. We are now seeing twenty-six hundred a month," the visibly exhausted Abbott said. By late 1996 Hudson's hallways and lobby were crowded with anxious patients and their families, most speaking Spanish. These urgent care adult patients had to wait an average of two and a half hours—previously, the wait had been thirty minutes.

For Hudson CEO Carolyn Clark, the change was heartbreaking. Clark, who grew up just blocks from the clinic, had devoted more than a decade to Hudson. "I think people believed, falsely, that the voters wouldn't stand for this system being shut down. I thought there would be an outcry from the community," she said.

But when Clark had instructed her staff and patients in September 1995 that Hudson would probably be shut down, the response was muted. Though the clinic's existence had been temporarily extended by the White House Medicaid Waiver, Clark had learned a lesson: don't count on the people of Los Angeles to stand up for the health of the poor.

Johnston echoed Clark's sentiments: "I'm concerned about the public mood. The public doesn't want to take care of the poor. . . . I can't imagine a physician saying with a straight face, 'It doesn't matter how long you wait for services.' But that seems to be where we're headed, for probably half the population of the county."

At the UCLA Center for Health Policy Research Michael Cousineau was packing his bags. An expert on L.A. County health care, he was joining Finucane's staff, hoping to guide the county through the transition. His number one concern was that the newly installed managed care approach to public medicine could destroy decent care for the poor.

"We have to make sure managed care doesn't kill the whole party," Cousineau said. He listed several examples: Will longer waits lead to needless heart attacks for lack of access to open heart surgery? Can basic TB control services survive with fewer clinics to dispense medicine? How can the county keep track of disease trends, stop potential epidemics, and get all of its children immunized if the infrastructure falls apart?

By late 1996 Los Angeles County's public health experiment was openly opposed by many physicians who argued variously that it would destroy trauma care for the poor,[641] that the health status of individuals was being sacrificed on the altar of cost containment, or that not enough financial constraint was on the system to allow its survival after the end of the federal bailout in 2000.[642]

To meet the terms of its 1995 agreement with the White House, Los Angeles County had to have reduced its total inpatient burden by 30 percent and increased preventive outpatient services by 50 percent by the end of the five-year Medicaid Demonstration Project. In early 1999 it still had a long way to go, but Yaroslavsky and his fellow supervisors were confident that when the federal largess disappeared after September 30, 2000, they would have a surviving system. And they remained so as the countdown continued in 2000. The county's future seemed reasonably well assured. The general economy had bounced out of its recession and into a full-fledged boom. New leadership in Sacramento looked upon the county's fiscal and public health plights with more generosity. And severe cuts and restructuring had brought the health budget out of the red for the first time in well over a decade.

When the federal checks stopped, county officials said, with much relief, the local ship of state would still float. At least until the next catastrophe.[643]

In faraway Minnesota the Los Angeles crisis worried Mike Osterholm. He had cause to realize that weakness in any segment of the nation's public health infrastructure imperiled the entire system. Public health surveillance, Osterholm insisted, was only as effective as its weakest link, and he had highlighted those weaknesses at the CISET gathering in Washington in 1995. With just over 1,600 surveillance personnel employed full- or part-time to protect the country's 250 million people against microbial contamination, that meant there was only one surveillance person for every 162,500 U.S. residents.

In Minnesota, Osterholm insisted, the biggest problems were food and "snow birds"—the local slang for Minnesotans who escaped the winter's Arctic freezes by vacationing somewhere warm, often south of the Mexican border. There, the Minnesotans often picked up microbial hitchhikers that made their way north when the travelers returned home. Increasingly, Minnesota's foods came from distant places as well, places where safety standards were minimal or nonexistent.

Osterholm told the CISET audience, "my governor served pineapple from Costa Rica to the state legislators, and we had an outbreak of *E. coli.*" Between July and September of 1994, more than 270,000 Americans suffered diarrhea as a result of contaminated ice cream from Minnesota, illustrating that food contamination wasn't only an imported phenomenon. But it worried Osterholm that 70 percent of all produce consumed in the United States by the mid-1990s was imported, largely from Mexico, Central America, Chile, Argentina, and Brazil. Was that a dangerous trend? Probably, Osterholm concluded. In addition, he noted ominously, his group in Minnesota had reviewed the medical records of three thousand Minnesotans aged one to forty years who died prematurely in 1994 of nonaccidental causes: "We could not characterize the cause of deaths of 10 percent of them. Our best guess is that infectious diseases were responsible for most if not all of those deaths."[644]

An amazing finding, given that in the mid-1990s Minnesotans still held their position as being among the healthiest people in the world. While Los Angeles and New York City struggled with catastrophes and health access crises that left upward of 20 percent of their populations uninsured, only 9 percent of Minnesotans lacked insurance in 1995, and two-thirds of the population had private insurance or HMO enrollment. (Minnesota was the most heavily HMO-enrolled state in the nation—with HMOs covering half the population.) The total government burden (Medicare, Medicaid, and uninsured) was just 34 percent of the population—a far cry from the scale of government responsibility faced by the nation's more populous, heavily urbanized states.[645]

With a population by the end of the 1990s of just 4,725,500 people, Osterholm's statewide safety net needed to cover only about half as many people as did Los Angeles County or the city of New York. While Los Angeles clawed its way out of recession and its riot- and natural disaster–induced fiscal calamities, Minnesota suffered the exact opposite problem: too much of a good thing. With the lowest unemployment rate in the nation (4 percent in 1996 and 2.2 percent in 1999) and a booming economy, Minnesota's companies continued to be starved for workers. More than 40 percent of all companies were having trouble filling jobs. And one of the gravest shortages was in the health sector, as private hospitals and medical researchers offered huge salaries, even stock options, to top nurses, doctors, and scientists—and *still* couldn't fill the vacancies.[646]

The public health outcomes of this situation were two-fold. First, key health positions all over Minnesota went unfilled in the nineties, with the gap becoming acute by the turn of the century. That meant that there were fewer doctors, nurses, and laboratory scientists; and those who were working had less time for filling out public health records and assisting Osterholm's investigators.

Meanwhile, as salaries in the private sector skyrocketed, Osterholm and his staff saw their public sector wages decrease: the state legislature froze their already pathetic salaries for eight years (1990 through 1997) while the economy inflated by a total of 14 percent. By 1997 Osterholm's senior scientists were earning $15,000 less a year than entry-level junior public health officers in Iowa, and only 10 percent of what their private sector colleagues made. Most of his staff were having a hard time paying their home mortgages and meeting basic family expenses. And because Osterholm's staff had published more major scientific papers in prestigious medical journals over the years than any other group of state epidemiologists in the nation, most of them had been offered far better-paying jobs elsewhere. As John Hottinger, chair of the Minnesota State Senate's Health and Family Security Committee, recalled, Osterholm had pleaded every year for better salaries but was rebuffed by the legislature until late 1997.

"Mike, who really is one of four indispensable people in our government, made public he was going to leave because his top people weren't getting anywhere what the market would bear," Hottinger said.[647] "There was a virtually unanimous response: 'We'll break our rules to give these people what they deserve.' "

By putting his own job on the line, Osterholm got raises for his disease-fighter staff. But when the money materialized in 1998, it proved to be a paltry, even insulting, sum. It galled Osterholm that his top scientist, Dr. Craig Hedberg, who had commanded more than one hundred food-related epidemic investigations in Minnesota, earned only $62,000—*after* the legislature gave him a raise.

"I sometimes feel we're trying to run the O'Hare airport control tower with cans and strings," Osterholm told colleagues in late 1997.[648] "Ninety-four percent of our budget for infectious diseases control is soft money [grants and temporary funds] in Minnesota."

Meanwhile, Osterholm continued, globalization was bringing record numbers of diseases to his northern state. Invasive group A *Streptococcus*, popularly known as "flesh-eating bacteria," suddenly surfaced around 1992, and its incidence had risen steadily since, attacking 3.2 per 100,000 Minnesotans in 1996. The state logged 140 cases of the dreadful disease in 1996; one in four proved fatal. The same year, a visitor from overseas brought measles to Minnesota. And the number of TB cases had risen between 1986 and 1996—by the latter year, 80 percent of the cases were among foreigners or travelers who initially became infected in other countries but developed tuberculosis once they settled in Osterholm's territory.

Osterholm was seeing all sorts of other changes that also worried him, including a rise in pediatric *Salmonella* in his state. He realized that the kids were catching the bacteria from imported pet iguanas, which seemed odd until he learned there had been a thirty-fold increase in iguana importation to the United States between 1987 and 1997. He was stunned to discover that in an eight-month period of 1996 nearly 885,000 exotic amphibians, reptiles, and rodents were legally imported through the Port of Miami alone. There were dozens of other import sites and federal authorities estimated that only 18 percent of all such animals were brought into the United States legally. The bulk of the exotic animal trade came from South American rain forests. "What microbes are hitchhiking in those live animal cargos?" Osterholm wondered aloud.

But Osterholm continued to insist that "the new national trend" to keep an eye on was food-related illnesses and the arsenal of information he gathered on it grew each year. "The number one cause of emergency room visits last year," he told colleagues at the 1997 meeting of the Infectious Diseases Society of America, "was GI tract problems and diarrhea. Food-borne illnesses resulted in 200 million episodes last year. In Minnesota we had 122 food-borne outbreaks between 1990 and 1996. Thirty-seven percent of them involved fresh produce."

With food importation on the increase, he insisted, all Minnesotans should now follow at home the classic warning to travelers: boil it, peel it, or don't eat it!

"Today you don't need to leave your home to acquire traveler's diarrhea," Osterholm said. When he gave public speeches, the Minnesota epidemiologist illustrated that point with a slide of a Minneapolis supermarket. Under an enormous banner heralding FOODS OF THE WORLD, were row upon row of neatly stacked papayas, mangos, kiwis, melons, berries, and exotic vegetables seducing snow-bound Minnesota shoppers in February. In 1996 Osterholm's group had done detailed laboratory analyses on 570 samples of *E. coli* 0157:H7 and *Salmonella* (of the *enteritidis, typhirium,* and *sonnei* species) bacteria that were involved in human illnesses in Minnesota. He discovered that 181 completely different strains were present in just those four bacterial species. In 1997 the lab studied the same four species and found 206 strains. That was evidence of globalization, Osterholm argued, as strains from all over the world were infecting Minnesotans in the 1990s.[649]

Twenty years earlier, Osterholm and his counterparts in the other forty-nine states had few food-related outbreaks on their hands. Instead, they saw isolated food poisonings, usually related to improper storage of mayonnaise, leftover foods gone bad, or poorly processed canned foods. In the late nineties, however, fresh foods were the problem. On June 2, 1998, for example, 152 people came down with acute campylobacter diarrheal disease after eating salads made at a particular restaurant using imported lettuce. In August of that year, 210 Minnesotans came down with dangerous *Shigella sonnei* infections, causing GI pain and diarrhea, after eating restaurant food containing contaminated, imported parsley. These were merely two of thirty-two such outbreaks Hedberg's food group investigated in the state in the first ten months of 1998.

Even more disturbing to Osterholm than the numbers of outbreaks and the great diversity of bacterial strains involved was the microbes' increasing resistance to available antibiotics. The *Salmonella* and *Shigella* strains his lab scrutinized, for example, were more likely to be resistant to ampicillin, chloramphenicol, ciprofloxacin, tetracycline, trimethoprim sulfate (TMP/SMX), or combinations of those drugs in 1998 than they had been in 1995.[650]

It was, Osterholm insisted, "a slow-motion catastrophe in the making."

By the fall of 1998 Osterholm had some serious soul searching to do. For fourteen years he had put in sixty-hour weeks for the people of the state of Minnesota.

He was tuckered out. The whole department was exhausted. And underpaid. And feeling underappreciated. The November election results had been the coup de grace.

The people of Minnesota, who had for more than a century elected some of the most progressive governments and individuals to take office anywhere in America, had suddenly zigzagged across the political map, shocking not only Osterholm but the nation. Following their traditional bent, they had elected middle-of-the-road Democrats in sufficient numbers to control the state Senate. But the voters stacked the state's House of Representatives with anti–Big Government, Newt Gingrich–esque Republicans. That split the legislature into a seemingly unworkable imbalance. To confuse matters further, the voters gave a third-party candidate the governorship.

But not just any third-party candidate. Minnesotans—at least, 37 percent of those who voted—chose six-foot, four-inch former professional wrestler Jesse Ventura of the Reform Party.

Ventura vowed to reduce the size of government, return most or all the state's $3.3 billion budget surplus directly to the tax payers, craft a property tax law similar to California's Prop. 13, and "get government off our backs."[651]

In making a distinction between the government and the people who elected it and whom it was supposed to serve, the Minnesota political leadership was reflecting a trend in American thinking that traced back to Goldwater. It wasn't antifederalism, however, but antigovernmentalism, fueled largely by the perception that Minnesota had become a welfare state for "them"—African-Americans, Native Americans, immigrants, and poor "white trash" recently arrived from other states.

Since 1969 white-haired Don Samuelson had held the most powerful positions in the state Senate, chairing first the Appropriations Committee, then the Health and Family Security Committee. In better, earlier days, Samuelson said, budget setting had been a bargaining process that started, in the case of public health, by the senators agreeing upon the "untouchables," as Samuelson called them—services like child immunization and communicable diseases control. Once that chunk of the pie was sliced, the politicians set to bargaining over the remainder. It worked for more than thirty years.

"But not anymore," the sad-eyed politician said. "Now, every time I've introduced the [health] budget on the floor, the press and other senators say there's gonna be an 18 percent increase in the welfare budget [if it passes]. And I say, 'It's not welfare! It's health!' It just bugs me."

The reaction against welfare and social services was powerful and complex, Minnesota House member Lee Greenfield said. "In this country we've moved away from the public good fight to individual rights," Greenfield said. "And when you do that it becomes harder to build the public health protection in."

Over in the state's Vital Statistics Office, its director, John Oswald, summarized the dilemma neatly: "We have great health indicators for the entire population, but disparities for white versus minorities are among the worst in the country."[652]

State Demographer Tom Gillaspy agreed with Oswald's assessment, noting that of the roughly 4.7 million Minnesotans in 1998, just 378,000 were minorities, and their health—like their incomes and arrest rates—was far, far worse than that of whites. For example, the 1995 infant mortality rate for white Minnesotans was 6 per 1,000 babies; for black Minnesotans it was nearly triple that figure—17.6 per 1,000.[653] African-Americans and American Indians were also far more likely than whites to die of injuries, homicides, suicides, cirrhosis, strokes, or diabetes.[654]

Statewide in 1999 minorities still constituted just a tiny fragment of the population, but in Minneapolis a third of the populace was African-American, American Indian, Hispanic, or Asian. And in that city "the health disparities between whites and blacks are the greatest seen in the entire country," explained Dr. Edward Ehlinger, chief health officer for the University of Minnesota. "I think it's due to all those classic public health issues. It's not medical care. It's economics, housing, transportation, risk-taking, lifestyle choices. All of those public health things that we've ignored."

Ehlinger argued that by pointing out the racial disparities and people's needs, "public health is acting as the conscience of our health care system. . . . Public health equals social justice. I truly believe that. Aristotle said if there are differences that are overwhelming, you either have to get rid of those disparities or get rid of democracy."

But addressing the disparities would be no simple matter, especially in the Twin Cities. Most of the state's minority populations were in Minneapolis/St. Paul, as were the bulk of Minnesota's petty and violent crimes, welfare population, teen pregnancies, HIV/AIDS population, and injecting drug users. At a time of unprecedented prosperity, white residents of the Twin Cities felt threatened and they perceived the source of their anxiety to be people of color, whom they often categorized as criminals on welfare.

Senator Hottinger thought that politics in Minnesota started changing during the 1980s, as the complexion of the state began to transform and its crime rates rose. That was when the local media and politicians became fixated on crime stories.

"Right now in Minnesota," the dog-tired Hottinger said, "there's not a lot of sympathy for people who have needs. At least, not in the sense of government. *Personal responsibility* is the watchword. We've used those words as excuses to forget about sharing and feeding the hungry. . . . I have seen a big shift in the debate in Minnesota. The old tradition here of communalism isn't being well vocalized. The debate about government and public service is terribly one-sided. It's just, 'There's too much.' And no one vocalizes the value you get from government."

Hottinger found out just how changed the word *government* was when in 1998 he sponsored a bill to create a registry of child vaccinations so that public health workers could remind parents to get their kids immunized. It was an enormous issue in the Twin Cities, where less than half of all five-year-olds were fully immunized by the time they started kindergarten. Decried as a "government registry," the proposal died on the Senate floor. The pendulum had swung away from all sense of community, Hottinger argued, and would kill public health politically in Minnesota.

"The next time there's a meningitis epidemic in Minnesota and a couple of kids die and there aren't enough public health personnel to stop it quickly, then the public's view will change," Hottinger forecast. "It's when the people in need are not 'like me' that people aren't there. But when people see people like themselves in need, then they're there for them."

In 1998 a private policy group, headed by the Heritage Foundation's Dr. Kenneth Heithoff, drew up a master plan for reforming Minnesota's public health system. The plan reflected the policy group's general schema for the whole nation.[655] The key elements of the conservative think tank's plan called for privatization of many public health activities and levying of fees, rather than taxes, to cover the costs of such things as water safety testing. Data amassed by local health agencies, the think tank advocated, ought to be contracted out to the University of Minnesota for analysis. Pollution analysis, too, ought to be handled on a contract basis, and the state should eliminate most laboratories and staff then covered by local and federal tax revenues.

Epidemiology, such as the work Osterholm's group conducted, "needs to stay a government function with the qualifier that there may be parts of it that might be privatized," the group's vice chair, Elisabeth Quam Berne, argued. "Certainly there are parts that could be privatized."

Much of public health education could be privatized as well, Quam Berne argued: AIDS leaflets, teen pregnancy information, vaccination pamphlets—all these sorts of things could be contracted out to private companies and the state employees currently responsible for their production and distribution could be laid off.

"It's market-based philosophy and practicality," she insisted. The think tank further recommended that all of the public health laboratories statewide be consolidated into one central facility. In times of overload, such as during epidemics, that central facility could farm work out to private, for-profit labs. The public health system, then, would be a stripped-down, streamlined version of its current self, Quam Berne explained, with nearly all of its activities, from provision of primary care for the poor to epidemic control handled in part or full by private contractors. The remaining state-employed public health staff would be overseers who would guarantee the reliability of the data and of actions taken by private companies.

"Public health officials need to be challenged," Quam Berne charged. "But a strong public infrastructure is part of the reason we have excellent health in Minnesota."

Such talk appalled Osterholm: "Public health *has* to be a government activity because it's by and for the people," he insisted. Sure, he acknowledged with a shrug, some government agencies were doing a lousy job. "When I look at what's happening in the food safety agencies right now, I can't believe how embarrassing the incompetence is. I feel like some days we're carrying around dead bodies here."

But limited as some state and federal public health agencies were, Osterholm continued, "you can't have a private company that has the right to intercede in disease outbreaks—you can't. . . . I have the ability to take action against companies if they fail to be good citizens."

How could the public ever feel safe, Osterholm wondered, if its food, water, health care infrastructure, air, schoolchild health—if all key aspects of public health—were handled by private companies that had no accountability, needed to make profits off the process, and possibly had conflicts of interest? If, for example, an ice-cream manufacturer in Minneapolis had caused thousands of food poisonings by distributing *Salmonella*-contaminated products, would a private investigating company be likely to cut a deal with the offender to cover up the contamination? As such private firms couldn't legally act as enforcers of the law, might they instead be likely to gain profits through "helping" offenders to "come within compliance"? Osterholm insisted that whether such a privatized public health system flouted the law or not, the perception of diminished credibility would be there and public trust would erode.

The infectious diseases laboratory nestled inside a plain, brick health department building in Minneapolis had a staff of twenty-seven scientists and technicians in 1999. In an average year they processed a quarter of a million tissue, blood, food, and water samples.

"You absolutely can't privatize [lab work]," said lab director Norm Crouch adamantly. "If you go down that road, you're going to lose the public health infrastructure. Who's going to pay for it? There's not going to be profit in it. . . . We need to have outbreak capacity. How can a private sector lab make money waiting for an epidemic to happen?"

Crouch and microbiologist John Besser had a lab capable of responding to several small, simultaneous outbreaks or to a large epidemic involving all but the top security—Biohazard Level 4 organisms—those that are highly contagious and incurable, such as the Ebola virus. Were such horrors ever to surface in Minnesota, they would be handled by the CDC's lab in Atlanta. For all else, Besser beamed, "We're ready!"

But would the lab and the department stay ready?

Even though such talk of privatizing public health didn't gain full favor in the Minnesota legislature, cutbacks did, and in early 1999 Aggie Leitheiser, director of the Department of Disease Prevention and Control, informed Samuelson's Senate committee that the department faced a budget shortfall of $5 million for the year and anticipated far greater problems for 2000–2005. The key reason, she said, was that Congress had steadily reduced block grants as well as special funds for HIV prevention and a host of core public health activities. For decades Minnesota had grown increasingly dependent on those federal funds. And if the state didn't pick up the tab, the programs would fall apart.

Already feeling the financial pinch and fading public acknowledgment for their work, the department staff's morale was sinking in 1998. It plummeted after the elections when Ventura signaled his low opinion of public health. When asked what he would do for the health of children born to unemployed adolescent mothers, the new governor said those teen moms should live with their parents and government had no responsibility for providing health services for the babies. Later, he added that he opposed state-subsidized public health programs for children.

Those comments prompted Osterholm and his staff to begin reading their tea leaves. Before Christmas, Osterholm, Hedberg, and most of the top staff involved in disease control and prevention had decided to throw in the towel. In early 1999, one by one, they left the Minnesota State Department of Health to take university and private sector jobs. On February 1, 1999, Michael Osterholm left the tiny office that had been his command post for fourteen years and created Infection Control Advisory Network, a private company providing disease intervention services to food manufacturers and cities in need of consultation and advice.

For each of them the decision to resign from public service had been agonizing: they were public health zealots, true believers. But when the people you are serving, at considerable personal sacrifice, don't believe in your mission, it's hard to ignore personal exhaustion and financial pressures.

Looking at his staff three weeks before his good-bye party, Osterholm sighed. "This section is a model program for the world, yet it holds together with a string. Minnesota will have gone overnight from an internationally known program to just any other state. That's how fragile it is. The citizens' health should not be dependent on just two or three personalities."

It wasn't just that departments like Osterholm's were having a hard time finding support for their traditional efforts: the problems were new and expanding. Globalization coupled with microbial evolution was presenting public health workers at the close of the twentieth century with a scale of difficulty and complexity for which they were totally unprepared. Osterholm's number one concern was the nation's food supply, but there were also new, unanticipated public health threats in water, hospitals, and numerous other ecological niches of U.S. society.

In late 1999 the CDC confirmed that Osterholm's heads-up messages about food-borne illnesses earlier in the decade had been on the mark, concluding that such illnesses had become so serious a problem in the United States that seventy-six million residents suffered food poisonings annually. For 325,000 of them, the infection was serious enough to require hospitalization; 5,000 Americans each year would find ingesting contaminated foods to be fatal.

"While the U.S. food supply remains one of the safest in the world, these new findings further support what we have said all along: the public health burden of food-borne disease is substantial," said HHS Secretary Donna Shalala.[656]

Orange juice and alfalfa sprouts had *Salmonella* contamination; British meat was contaminated with bizarre disease agents called prions that caused an ailment commonly called mad cow disease; hepatitis A viruses were found in frozen strawberries. The list was long.

And the cost was high. In 1997, when the CDC estimated there were just thirty-three million food poisoning incidents in the United States, the agency estimated that combined costs, reckoned as DALYs, totaled $34.9 billion.[657] When the tally had more than doubled to seventy-six million cases in 1999, costs certainly exceeded $50 billion annually.

Some of the problem was homegrown, but much of it was imported: Osterholm's "Foods of the World." U.S. outbreaks during the 1990s were linked to Peruvian carrots; Mexican scallions, cantaloupes, and strawberries; Chinese mushrooms; Israeli snacks; and Guatemalan raspberries. By 1996 upward of 50 percent of some types of produce consumed in the United States was grown in foreign countries.[658]

Retired FDA commissioner Dr. David Kessler said that the U.S. food inspection system hadn't been designed to be a global safety net. The FDA simply couldn't keep up.

In fact, as food import rates skyrocketed during the 1990s (from an annual value of less than $20 billion to more than $50 billion by 1997), the FDA, having undergone ten years of budget cuts and congressionally mandated industry deregulation, *reduced* its food inspection testing. The number of imported items screened dropped from about forty thousand in 1990 to about fifteen thousand in 1997. Food was flooding in at an accelerated pace in part because the United States had lifted old protectionist bans on their import, having conceded such restrictions under the terms of the North American Free Trade Agreement (NAFTA) and World Trade Organization negotiations. The United States could not resurrect old food import barriers without facing severe trade and diplomatic consequences.

There was by 1999 simply too much food coming in and too few people in the public health system paid to inspect it. It was, they said, as if a few dozen people scattered around the country each were given a thimble full of water from which to derive the microbial contents of the entire Pacific Ocean. Unless safety laws were enforced in the countries in which the foods were grown, the United States would simply see its gastrointestinal diseases and death tolls rise in the twenty-first century.

There would always be surprises, however, that even vigilante inspectors couldn't anticipate, especially when crops were grown in ecologies that bore *no* resemblance to those in which the plants originated.

That was certainly the case with cyclospora.

The first time anyone ever saw, and named, the *Cyclospora cayentanensis* parasite was in Papua New Guinea in 1977. Part of the parasite's life cycle entailed passing its eggs into water, where they were absorbed into plants or imbibed by animals. Once inside an animal, the parasite matured into an organism that caused highly irritating intestinal and bowel infections. This prompted diarrhea, which, in turn, passed eggs, repeating the life cycle. The parasites favored destination was the epithelial cell lining of the animal's small bowel.

Experts in Florida had seen an unusual diarrhea outbreak in 1990 and after three years of painstaking lab work had isolated *Cyclospora* from patient samples. Florida had another cyclospora incident in June 1995, the same month fully a third of the guests took ill at a wedding party at a country club just north of New York City in Westchester County.[659]

When unusual diarrheal disease cases turned up in New York City hospitals in May 1996, Dr. Marcella Layton of the health department ordered cyclospora tests. By June 11, 1996, her department had identified 161 cyclospora cases and a full court press was on to find the source of the infections.

Layton was struck by the fact that interviews with the patients revealed the predominantly male group was mostly white and well to do. That was very curious, as most infectious disease outbreaks in Layton's experience emerged in impoverished communities.

Her department conducted a case control study, matching cyclospora patients with individuals in their social circles who hadn't taken ill. And bingo!— the cyclospora sufferers were more likely than nonsufferers to have recently dined at parties or in restaurants where desserts topped with raspberry or strawberry sauces were served. At weddings where such desserts were served, up to 80 percent of guests who ate them contracted cyclospora illness.

Soon, public health departments all over the United States were buzzing with the news and discovering similar clusters of diarrheal diseases among groups who ate strawberry- or raspberry-topped desserts. By July the CDC had reports of fifty-five such clusters nationwide involving more than fifteen hundred laboratory confirmed cyclospora cases. The CDC announced in late June that initial investigations pointed to strawberries from California. The impact on California agriculture was immediate and profound and more than $20 million worth of the berries rotted for lack of buyers.

Further investigation showed, however, that 72 percent of the cyclospora patients had consumed raspberries, not strawberries. And the raspberries had been grown in Guatemala.

No similar berries are indigenous to Guatemala and raspberries naturally grow in far cooler climates that get snow in the winter and experience summer heat snaps. That hardly described Guatemala.

International food corporations first introduced raspberries to Guatemala in 1987, where they were grown during winter and early spring. Five large Guatemala farms exported 162,000 flats of raspberries to the eastern seaboard of the United States in 1996. Investigators in Guatemala found that the raspberry fields were irrigated with feces-contaminated water that, due to the subtropical climate, provided perfect conditions for *Cyclospora* growth.

In 1997 other U.S. cyclospora outbreaks were linked to Guatemalan- and Mexican-grown raspberries, mesclun lettuce, and basil in commercial pesto sauce. After trying in vain to prevent the parasites from being absorbed into the plants—where they could not be rinsed off—Guatemalan and Mexican authorities reluctantly agreed to block further export of the products. By 1999 the precise ecology of the *Cyclospora* cycle in Mexico and Guatemala remained a mystery.

A related organism, *Cryptosporidium*, was turning up with increasing frequency in U.S. water supplies. The largest outbreak, in 1993, caused diarrheal disease in two hundred thousand residents of Milwaukee, hospitalized in excess of four thousand, and killed more than one hundred. Subsequent outbreaks in New York City, Washington, D.C., and other U.S. metropolises prompted health departments to issue summer warnings to boil water before drinking it.[660]

Authorities hadn't had much cause for concern about the integrity of U.S. water supplies since World War II, but *Cryptosporidium* had managed to thrive despite chlorine and filtration systems. In 1995 the American Academy of Microbiology convened an international meeting in Guayaquil, Ecuador, to assess the safety of global drinking water supplies. Their conclusions were grim.[661]

"Increases in population over the past century have placed tremendous pressures on water resources of both the developed and developing world. These pressures include direct contamination from domestic, industrial, and agricultural wastes and less direct effects caused by climate change and ecological disturbances. The result is a contaminated and often increasingly scarce global resource, which in turn is contributing to a rise in water-borne disease outbreaks worldwide," their final report stated.[662]

Worldwide, such water-borne pathogens as *E. coli* and *Legionella* were becoming chlorine-resistant. Parasites like *Cyclospora* and *Cryptosporidium* already were able to resist chemical treatment. Antibiotic-resistant strains of bacteria, particularly cholera, were turning up in drinking water supplies of Latin America, Asia, and Africa. The experts concluded that even the richest countries in the world were ill-prepared for these developments and needed to develop new or augmented filtration systems to protect their water supplies. In addition, standard water safety tests, based on total "coliform" (or *E. coli*–like) biological contamination, were missing such new threats as *Cryptosporidium* and *Cyclospora*.

In the United States, twenty-two outbreaks of drinking water–borne illnesses occurred in thirteen states in 1995 to 1996. They involved 2,567 people, none of whom died.[663] Seven of the outbreaks were due to industrial chemical contamination of water; the remainder were microbial. None of the outbreaks involved community water systems that were substandard: rather, they occurred *despite* the state-of-the-art filtration systems.[664]

Home water filters, which were all the rage in the United States, offered little protection. Some were only able to remove the taste of chlorine. Only very expensive systems effectively removed microorganisms.[665] And bottled water, though immensely popular in the United States, was generally drawn from tap water as well. Even genuine spring water might not be any safer—and who would know? In the United States commercial bottled water was subject to less surveillance and scrutiny than most community tap water.[666]

The chlorine question posed an interesting dilemma for public health. On the one hand, chlorine was clearly the most efficient water disinfection method, particularly when coupled with filtration mechanisms; and the absence of chlorination was responsible for cholera outbreaks in Latin America and the former Soviet Union during the 1990s. On the other hand, environmentalists challenged chlorine use on two grounds: first, it is a very mild carcinogen; and second, free chlorine ions in the earth's atmosphere contributed to weakening of the ozone hole.[667]

As increasing numbers of microbes acquired chlorine-resistance capacities, the complexity of the debate increased. Clearly, drinking water safety was going to be a major dilemma for the twenty-first century.

By the end of the twentieth century, microbial resistance to both chlorine and drugs was a problem on all fronts, especially in the case of antibiotics used to treat bacterial infections. The reasons for emergence of drug-resistant strains were multitudinous,[668] ranging from inappropriate use of antibiotics in livestock to outbreaks of superbugs inside hospitals. Over time, an intricate web of human activities had been directly promoting the evolution of bacteria and their resultant resistance to precious antibiotic drugs.

In general, the trend internationally was toward increasingly sloppy infection control practices in hospitals and rising disinfectant resistance among microbes, allowing ready in-hospital spread of the microbes.[669] And the microbes acquired powers of drug resistance because antibiotics were highly overused worldwide, misprescribed, and, in nearly half of all common infections, prescribed to treat viral rather than bacterial infections. Further, fear of lawsuits and other difficulties were driving U.S. physicians to prescribe powerful, broad-spectrum antibiotics when cheaper, simpler drugs such as tetracycline or penicillin would do. Use of broad-spectrum drugs promoted wider-ranging drug resistance.[670] And widespread use of antibiotics in the livestock industry provided further pressure for evolution of superbugs.

The primary use of antibiotics in livestock was not for veterinary medicine; rather, for reasons not clearly understood, the drugs acted as growth promoters, and chickens, turkey, cows, pigs—all livestock—fed antibiotic-laced feed were 3 to 4 percent larger by adulthood than their untreated counterparts. This offered a powerful incentive for use of the drugs, for some farmers and ranchers, 4 percent could be the margin of their profits.

As early as 1969, however, the Swann Committee in Great Britain had recommended a full stop ban on the use of therapeutically significant antibiotics as animal growth promoters on the grounds that resistance acquired by bacteria in those animals would spread to human beings.[671] Sadly, the report was largely ignored in the United States. In 1970 the United Kingdom banned use of human therapeutic antibiotics as growth promoters and the European Community followed suit a few years later. However, closely related compounds that still promoted medicinally relevant resistance continued to be permitted for agricultural use.

By the mid-1990s antibiotic production and use in the United States, and globally, was largely about livestock management: human medicinal and public health use of the "magic bullets" accounted for just 0.01 to 10 percent of some antibiotic uses (varying by drug class).[672]

Barely were new drugs on the market when their counterparts went into use in livestock. Soon resistant microbes emerged in the animals[673] and spread to people. The connection between growth promoters and antibiotic resistance in both the animals and in human consumers was clear.[674]

The fundamental problem: whether the drug was called an antibiotic or a growth promoter, it was a member of a finite group of some 250 antibacterial agents that attacked their targets in just six different ways. If a bacterium developed resistance to one particular agent, it was actually insensitive to all of the antibiotics that relied on the same attack mechanism.[675] Worse yet, the ability to resist one or more of those six (and only six) ways that antibiotics targeted bacteria could be carried from one microbe to another aboard genetic rings, called transposons. These pieces of genetic information were part of a vast DNA and RNA lending library from which microbes readily borrowed and shared information as they swam through their soupy environs. An animal microbe that was harmless to humans could acquire resistance as a result of growth promoter use in, say, chickens, and then share its resistance transposons with human pathogens it encountered in the gut of a person dining on undercooked chicken or runny eggs.[676]

The Institute of Medicine issued a report in 1998 on the catastrophic scale of antibiotic resistance, declaring that both the scope of resistance and the pace at which microbes were acquiring such capacities was accelerating. "Antibiotic-resistant bacteria generate a minimum of $4 billion to $5 billion in costs to U.S. society and individuals yearly," the report stated,[677] "and in 1992, the estimated 19,000 deaths directly caused by hospital-acquired infections made [drug-resistant diseases] the eleventh leading cause of death in the U.S. population."

Nine out of ten staph infections in 1998 involved bacteria that were completely resistant to penicillin and all related compounds. (Forty years previously, all staph infections were curable with moderate doses of inexpensive penicillin-class drugs.) Similarly, 40 percent of all pneumococci, the chief cause of bacterial pneumonia and ear infections, was resistant to penicillins.

And one out of five staph infections involved so-called MRSA strains—that is, they were resistant to methicillin as well. MRSA strains could only be treated with the last-ditch, and expensive, antibiotic vancomycin, thus raising average treatment costs from $27,700 to $31,400 per case and increasing staph death rates from 8 percent to 17 percent.[678]

The pace of acquisition of resistance among disease-causing pathogens was "pretty rapid!" said Dr. Jim Hughes, director of the National Center for Infectious Diseases in Atlanta.[679] "Look at MRSA, vancomycin-resistant enterococci, the strains of *Staphylococcus aureus* in Japan with decreased susceptibility to vancomycin—these are a real wake-up call."

According to the IOM report, "The problem of antimicrobial resistance extends beyond science and public health into a domain of sizeable legal and regulatory challenge. Globalization has permitted microbes to move freely around the world, yet attempts to globalize a coherent public health response are constrained by national borders and concepts of sovereignty."

The task was daunting, particularly so given the almost complete lack of alternative drugs in the wealthy world and of laboratory equipment for resistance testing in the world's poorest countries. Nevertheless, the IOM wanted to see development of a global surveillance network with laboratories spotting resistant strains in every nation, and the report called for massive education campaigns aimed at reducing doctor prescription of and patient demand for antibiotics.

The IOM report came on the heels of studies and resolutions released in 1997 by the World Health Organization and in 1995 by the American Society for Microbiology. Both of those reports reached conclusions similar to those the American IOM adopted,[680] each emphasizing the global scale of the problem. The United States public health community would have a hard time catching up with its European counterparts, which, in turn, were finding it difficult—perhaps impossible—to catch up with the evolving microbes. But at least they were trying. For example, in 1997, the European Union banned all livestock use of avoparcin, which was chemically nearly identical to vancomycin. As a result, by early 1999 the percentage of *Enterococci* isolated from animals that proved resistant to vancomycin had fallen from 14.6 to 8 percent.[681] And as a general principle the European Union nations had long held with the 1969 Swann Commission suggestion that no human therapeutic drugs be used as livestock growth promoters.

In 1999 the U.S. FDA gingerly dipped its toes into those waters, suggesting that America ought to adopt antibiotic use standards similar to those in Europe. FDA leaders cited work done by Michael Osterholm's Minnesota team in 1996 demonstrating that use of fluoroquinolone growth promoters in chickens led to drug-resistant *Campylobacter*, which, when ingested by people, caused antibiotic-resistant intestinal infections. Some 88 percent of all randomly selected chicken samples on sale in Twin Cities supermarkets were contaminated with *Campylobacter* by 1988, the group found. One in five of the supermarket chickens carried drug-resistant forms of the bacteria.[682]

Bad as that was, food-acquired bacterial infections involving resistant microbes were rarely fatal. It was when such supergerms arose in hospital settings that outbreaks of lethal infections occurred.

In April 1997 Dr. Margaret Hamburg resigned as New York City commissioner of health. After seeing the city through its TB, HIV, and drug-resistant bacterial epidemics, Hamburg had hung on in the Giuliani administration for two years because her staff, as well as community representatives of health constituencies, had begged her to do so.[683] But as the last Democrat in a top position in New York City, Hamburg had eventually reached one too many impasses with the Republican mayor. For two years she had struggled to protect the health department's budget while the mayor ordered cuts in every single health program. Despite a booming economy in New York City and record-low crime levels, Giuliani had slashed most of Gotham's social sector spending and increased police expenditures. Under his administration, negotiations over laboratory leases for the Public Health Research Institute had fallen apart, forcing New York's critical lab to flee the city in favor of lower rents across the Hudson River in New Jersey.

Once Hamburg was out of the picture, Giuliani merged the mental health and public health services and put former mental health director Dr. Neal Cohen in charge. The mayor also created an Office of Emergency Preparedness, giving it authority over many city crises, including epidemics.[684]

By 1997, New York State had 3.1 million uninsured residents and another 4.9 million individuals who were covered by either Medicaid or Medicare. Thus, 43 percent of the state's population either had no health coverage or was insured by the federal government.[685] Less than half the population of Gotham had private insurance.[686]

Republican governor George Pataki decried Medicaid as "wasteful" and, despite the rising numbers of uninsured New Yorkers, cut New York State spending on health care for the poor by $266 million in 1999 (down to an overall $9.5 billion).[687] As Medicaid and Medicare reimbursement rates to doctors and hospitals fell even further in the second Clinton term, New York's medical community predicted that the death knell would toll for several hospitals by 2005.[688]

Yet the hospitals got little sympathy from government as, combined, Gotham's medical facilities earned a $739 million profit in 1997, up 42 percent from the previous year. If there ever had been a time when the hospitals could afford a little charitable behavior, 1997 seemed to be it. Yet to a person the hospital administrators sang a litany of economic woe and doom.[689]

There was reason for woe, but it wasn't hospital income. The shoe Hamburg had been anticipating was about to drop: drug resistance emerging in new forms. First, in the mid-1990s *Streptococcus pneumoniae* strains in patients along the East Coast were found to exhibit increasing amounts of resistance to cefotaxime, putting more pressure on last-ditch use of vancomycin for acute strep infections.[690] The incidence of penicillin resistance had more than doubled in Gotham since 1993, with the bulk of all clinical cases involving children under four years of age.[691]

Meanwhile, *Staphylococcus aureus* was becoming increasingly resistant to methicillin, thereby *also* increasing pressure for last-ditch use of vancomycin. In the mid-1990s MRSA in New York City remained the daunting hospital problem detailed at the opening of this chapter and accounted for about 12 percent of all serious nosocomial infections in the United States.

In 1997 a French medical team examined an MRSA strain in a two-year-old cancer patient, discovering that it was resistant to vancomycin. Strikingly, the girl had *never* previously received vancomycin.[692] The French child had barely recovered when a four-month-old baby boy in Japan got an MRSA infection along sutures from his recent surgery. Analysis of the staph found in the boy's wound showed that it, too, was vancomycin resistant.[693]

That same year, three such staph cases appeared in the United States. The first involved a Michigan man suffering from small-cell carcinoma and chronic diabetes. Every imaginable combination of drugs was given to him, including high doses of vancomycin. But he died of staphylococcus infection of his heart in January 1998. The second case, also a diabetic, died of staph in New Jersey. As had been the case in France and Japan, these two men had infections that were not only vancomycin resistant but were in previously unseen genetic forms.[694]

The third 1997 U.S. case surfaced in the United Hospital Medical Center located outside New York City. New York State Department of Health scientists scoured the patient's hospital looking for the source of the new bacterium. Although they found a patient and a doctor who carried MRSA, their strains were different. So when the man died of his incurable staph in March 1998, the origin of the superbug remained a mystery.[695]

The new organisms were dubbed Vancomycin Insensitive *Staphylococcus aureus*—VISA. The CDC was at pains to note that all of the new superbugs remained somewhat vulnerable to vancomycin, which was small comfort for the dead patients.

As other VISA cases emerged in New York City and elsewhere in 1998 and 1999, anxiety rose considerably in the public health community. Swiss researcher Dr. Francis Waldvogel discovered that the plastic material in catheters actually increased the probability that a colony of staph growing at that site would acquire powerful drug-resistance capacities.[696] At Rockefeller University

Tomasz detected particular strains of MRSA taken from patients in the city's hospitals that had evolved switch mechanisms that flipped on under pressure from vancomycin in the bacteria's environs. The bacteria were then able to bind vancomycin molecules harmlessly to their cell walls, rendering the drug impotent.[697] The Japanese team that treated the VISA-infected baby used sophisticated methods to detect these switch-prone bacteria in MRSA samples, finding that 9 percent of all MRSA bacteria in Japan were capable of converting to VISA microbes.

"The outlook is grim," concluded Switzerland's Waldvogel.[698] The emergences of VISA, he insisted, "seem to me to be a chronicle of a death foretold. The adaptive potential of the microbial world is such that for each new antibiotic that is introduced, several escape mechanisms are soon devised. The action of antibiotics and resistance to these drugs are linked like light and shadow: one does not exist without the other. It was naive to believe for forty years that vancomycin could remain an exception to this law. Vancomycin resistance could have been predicted, since *S. aureus* has been surrounded by vancomycin-resistant enterococci and vancomycin-resistant coagulase-negative staphylococci, and because enterococcal vancomycin-resistant genes have been transferred in vitro to *S. aureus*. Now, we may need the strategic powers of a Julius Caesar to conduct a major war against the misuse of antibiotics."[699]

In Minnesota and North Dakota the next shoe dropped at the close of the century with four children dying of *community*- (not hospital-) acquired MRSA.[700]

Careful detective work[701] revealed that none of these children had been previously hospitalized or treated with methicillin. They had caught their MRSA strains from somebody, but the sources couldn't be pinned down, though in the search more than two hundred people were, alarmingly, identified in those states who carried the same MRSA strain. That the cases were spread out over a large area and had no apparent direct or indirect connection with one another implied that MRSA was far more ubiquitous in the U.S. environment than anyone had imagined.[702]

And in 1998 vancomycin-resistant *Streptococcus pneumoniae* emerged in communities all over the world, causing severe meningitis and pneumonia.[703] The resistance was due to a chromosomal—not transposon—mechanism that rendered vancomycin useless against the organism. Surveys of clinical samples from Memphis and Stockholm patients revealed that the bacteria were surprisingly common.[704]

The new superbugs undoubtedly originated in hospital settings, but they had made their ways into American schools, day care centers, restaurants, airports—into the community. Lack of infection control in medical settings had, as Lederberg predicted, resulted in a public health danger; one that possibly would become catastrophic.[705]

In contrast to this grim bacterial picture, by the end of the nineties New York City and other HIV hot spots in the United States had some good news: the death rate among people infected with the virus had plummeted.[706] And fewer people infected with HIV were progressing to full-blown AIDS. That meant that the pool of immunologically compromised New Yorkers had shrunk, making management of tuberculosis and other institutionally spread, drug-resistant microbes easier—at least in theory.

From 1997 to 1998 the U.S. HIV death rate dropped by 20 percent (from 21,222 deaths to 17,047). And that was after a 42 percent AIDS death rate decline from 1996 to 1997.[707] The national AIDS death rate fell to 4.6 per 100,000 in 1998—a 70 percent decline since 1995. In 1995 HIV was the number eight cause of death in the United States: by 1998 it didn't even rank in the top fifteen.[708]

And national syphilis rates had dropped so dramatically during the 1990s that the CDC forecast U.S. eradication of the disease in 2005. By 1998 the nation's syphilis rate was a minuscule 2.6 cases per 100,000 U.S. residents, with more than half the cases occurring in just twenty-eight counties. (New York was not one of those counties, but Los Angeles was.) Syphilis rates were highest among African-Americans living in Baltimore, Chicago, Memphis, Nashville, Phoenix, and Detroit.[709]

Combined, these findings pointed to a dramatic set of public health achievements in control of sexually transmitted diseases.

"Any reduction in the numbers of Americans dying from AIDS is good news," said CDC director Dr. Jeffrey Koplan.[710] "We should pause and fully recognize the tremendous public health accomplishment that has been achieved by reducing AIDS-related mortality from fifty thousand deaths a year in 1995 to an annual rate of just under twenty thousand."

But was it truly a victory for public health, as opposed to one for medical care? Fewer Americans were dying of AIDS, yes, but the pace of new HIV infections hadn't flagged. The triumphant decline in mortality was achieved through widespread use, beginning in 1996, of an innovative set of treatment cocktails that held the virus at bay, but at tremendous cost. The drugs, coupled with necessary medical supervision and tests, cost successfully treated patients (or insurers, or the government) more than $20,000 a year.

Might the HIV situation at the close of the twentieth century, skeptics asked, constitute a grave public health challenge, rather than a triumph?

Internationally, HIV continued to rage out of control, having infected 47.3 million people by December 1998, 33.4 million of whom were alive in 1999. Fewer than 5 percent of the living could possibly afford to take the life-extending drug cocktails that had proven to so impressively affect mortality rates in America. Cumulatively, HIV had killed 13.9 million people in eighteen years, outstripping the Black Death's toll in Europe from 1346 to 1350 of between 9 and 11 million people. By 1999 AIDS was the number one killer in Africa, having surpassed the continent's ancient nemeses of tuberculosis, measles, malaria, and other tropical diseases. In ten African countries more than 10 percent of the population (of all ages, combined) was HIV positive. Globally, HIV was the number four killer and the number one infectious disease in 1998.[711]

Given mounting evidence that HIV originated in Africa decades prior to its discovery among gay Americans,[712] it seemed prudent to assume that as long as no affordable, effective treatment or vaccine was available for the people of that beleaguered continent, the virus would be reintroduced in the United States, Canada, and Europe repeatedly in the future. Thus, it made no sense in the Age of Globalization to imagine that a slowdown in AIDS deaths in one place on earth heralded a public health victory.[713]

But even limiting a rosy view of the HIV situation just to the United States merited warnings of hubris. A 1997 CDC survey of gay men in several U.S. cities[714] found that the rate of new infections was still dangerously high: 6 percent of gay men became newly infected each year, despite mountains of safe-sex education. Even more alarming were seroconversion rates among fifteen- to twenty-two-year-old gay males in America: in 1998 7 percent of that group was found to be already infected and 3 percent were thought to become newly infected each year. Nearly half the young gay males surveyed by the CDC in several cities[715] admitted to having had sex without using a protective condom at least once during the first six months of 1998.[716]

Nationally, at least 40,000 people were becoming infected with HIV every year during the late 1990s. That was a fraction of the 150,000 annually in the early 1980s, but in those days nobody had realized that HIV existed. Nineteen years later, after hundreds of millions of dollars' worth of HIV education efforts, hundreds of thousands of Americans were still taking dangerous sexual risks.

The problem was pop mythology. The myth: AIDS was over.

The reality: the number of HIV-positive Americans was growing daily.[717] And it was almost impossible to predict which of the infected would stay healthy and strong and which would die. Twin brothers Eric and James proved that.[718]

In 1987, at age twenty-six, Eric died of AIDS. Most HIV patients did perish back then, for treatment was, at best, a crap shoot. His passing drove his twin brother, James, to join AIDS activists in the group ACT UP. Thanks in part to the often militant voices of James and his fellow activists, the pace of HIV science quickened in the 1990s, FDA approval of new medicines was put on a fast track, and a raft of novel, seemingly miraculous, treatments reached local pharmacies in 1996. Taken in combinations of three or more different medicines, the new anti-HIV cocktails, dubbed HAART, or Highly Active Anti-Retroviral Therapy, brought the first genuine hope in the epidemic's grim history.

James, a thirty-five-year-old New York Ivy-Leaguer, jumped onto the HAART bandwagon in early 1996. A few months later Steve, the love of James's life, also started HAART. And it was immediately obvious that one of them was going to be among the successes on science's scoreboard and the other was not. While Steve thrived, James got sicker and was hospitalized twice in 1998 with AIDS-related ailments.

In September of that year James complained of grogginess. Two days later he was hospitalized with sepsis. Three days later he was dead. Steve still felt healthy.

James died when more than 250 different combinations of drugs for HAART were available and many Americans and Europeans had declared the epidemic over. Though thousands like James still suffered and died of AIDS, in the wealthier world of Western Europe and North America the sense of plague emergency disappeared post-HAART, AIDS acute care facilities closed, HIV-positive individuals began worrying about their retirement funds, and gloom no longer pervaded gatherings of gay men and their physicians.

The key class of then-new drugs, called protease inhibitors, blocked the ability of HIV to package its progeny into viable infectious form. Taken alone, the protease inhibitors had proven worse than useless: they were toxic agents toward which HIV quickly mutated and became resistant. But when taken in combination with other anti-HIV drugs of classes that targeted different aspects of the virus's life cycle, protease inhibitors seemed to elicit miraculous results in the small numbers of patients observed in prelicensing drug studies.[719]

On November 10, 1996—just six months after James started taking his HAART cocktail—HIV-positive author Andrew Sullivan wrote a controversial *New York Times Magazine* piece entitled "When Plagues End: Notes on the Twilight of an Epidemic," and *Newsweek* ran a cover story headlined "The End of AIDS?" *Science* magazine closed 1996 by declaring HAART the "breakthrough of the year," and *Time* magazine named Dr. David Ho, a key player in HAART development, its Man of the Year. By usual American media standards, a revolution was officially declared.

But if so, Steve said, it had cruelly passed by James and thousands of other Americans on HAART. By late 1998, more than a third of all individuals who started HAART during the exciting days of mid-1996 had failed on the therapy.[720]

A few weeks after James's death, Steve talked, with emotional difficulty, about the loss of his lover and the new reality of HIV. "I'm a scientist by training," Steve explained, "so I'm always looking for evidence. Things are different, yes, but people are still dying. Another close friend died a week ago. I'm not convinced that this [HAART] will keep me going until I'm seventy. But I'm forty-one now and I think I could live to fifty. But God knows what these medications are doing to us. Are we all going to need liver transplants?"

Steve appreciated that anybody who had taken the HAART cocktails for more than eighteen months was living in a sort of Twilight Zone of uncertainty. The doctors and patients did creative battle with the virus on a daily basis, having no long-term experience or signposts to guide their extraordinary complex strategies. While some declared victory, most HIV experts and seasoned AIDS activists recognized the truth: HAART was buying time, but it offered neither a cure nor even a tolerable long-term holding pattern.

Before this realization set in, however, there had been a period of euphoria. At the summer 1996 International Conference on AIDS in Vancouver, word spread of Lazarus-like recoveries by AIDS patients taking early forms of what would become known as HAART. Top HIV researchers from all over the world gathered to cautiously discuss one new possibility: eradication. If eradication were achieved, HAART would represent *both* medical and public health victories.[721]

Propelled by the jubilant news, tens of thousands of Europeans and North Americans started taking HAART soon after the Vancouver conference. And when the international AIDS community reconvened two years later in Geneva, results, overall, still looked great as the dramatic drop in AIDS deaths attested.[722]

By the late 1990s some scientists were beginning to see beyond the starry-eyed optimism. "Even if you take someone who has a successful response to HAART," said Dr. Neal Nathanson,[723] "my sense is that it won't be possible to keep someone on HAART for a lifetime. . . . I don't think the drugs alone are going to be like insulin and diabetes."[724] In 1998 Nathanson took the reins of the National Institutes of Health's Office of AIDS Research (OAR), overseeing a scientific budget of $1.7 million annually. He stepped to the helm just as doubt about HAART began to surface.

"My view is that every death that didn't occur in 1997 is not a cure, it's just a postponed death," Nathanson said, well aware of the gravity of his comments. "I don't hear much optimism. . . . I'm afraid that the death rate may start to climb back. . . . The decline in mortality, where the graph looks like it's going to zero, that could be used to argue that we should cut back in our research. And that would be a disastrous message."

Disastrous, Nathanson said, because he foresaw that there would soon be need for fundamentally new treatment strategies for HIV disease, yet most of the drugs in development at some twenty-five companies targeting the $5 billion U.S. AIDS market were simply variations on the basic HAART themes. No pill-form drug that targeted HIV in an entirely novel way, and no vaccine, were likely to find their way to the marketplace before 2005 to 2020.[725]

"For the next few years," Nathanson opined, "the only thing one can anticipate is refinements on the same drug themes."

"I think we're probably as far away from treatment cures as we are from vaccines," said Peter Young, vice president of HIV therapeutic developments for the Glaxo Wellcome pharmaceutical corporation.[726] The image that came to his mind was of "a lot of people filling up sandbags" to bolster the weakening HAART dam.

An unabated stream of new HIV cases was continually flowing into a large pool of infected people—a pool that hadn't existed prior to the HAART revolution of 1996. The drugs created a dam, however, holding the HIV stream inside an ever-expanding pool, rather than allowing them to flow on to AIDS and eventual death.

"If you were trying to graph the prognosis for the [HIV] population, clearly we're not at a point where we can say we've leveled this graph off," Young concluded with regret. "Maybe we changed the rate of flow up to that dam. But it's a work in progress."

Many researchers—including those originators of the eradication hypothesis of 1996—said four years later that the reservoir of hidden HIVs in apparently successful HAART patients was large and long-lived. David Ho thought patients would have to take the difficult drugs for twenty-five to thirty years to eliminate those hidden viruses. Some scientists put the figure even further out at forty to fifty years.[727]

Regardless of the number, it was too long. The HAART drugs involved a complex and difficult regimen, were expensive and difficult to take, and increasingly were seen to cause a range of nasty, even life-threatening, side effects.[728] With at least 250 different combinations on the market in early 1999 and a host of new HAART drugs scheduled for future FDA approval, physicians needed to keep track of a long list of dos and don'ts.[729] For the patients, taking HAART could become a full-time job. Some drugs had to be taken six times a day, some once, some twice. Some had to be ingested on a full stomach, others before eating. And all well-managed HIV patients also took a host of prophylactic drugs that prevented common opportunistic infections.[730]

And HIV developed resistance to antiviral drugs roughly the same way bacteria became resistant to antibiotics: by exploiting inappropriate human use of the drugs. But HIV did it in orders of magnitude faster than that seen with bacteria.[731] Any use, followed by an interruption and later reuse of the same drugs, gave HIV the opportunity to mutate and clone an enormous colony of resistant viruses. And in the case of HAART, very brief interruptions, on the order of days, were enough to shift the advantage to the deadly viruses. Companies responded by developing quick resistance tests that physicians could perform routinely on patients' virus samples. If a patient was found, for example, to have HIVs that had mutated to resist indinavir, the physician might then switch the client to a cocktail that had a different protease inhibitor.

Until the virus was resistant to *all* protease inhibitors.[732]

Time alone might eventually work against the HAART dam. Each time patients changed their cocktails, resistant strains seemed to emerge more quickly and they might pass those resistant strains on to their sexual or needle-sharing partners.[733] Eventually, like James in New York, patients would run out of effective options.

Some physicians reacted to HAART failure by giving patients extraordi-narily complex cocktails of up to eight antivirals, at a cost of over $60,000 a year. "And," said Manhattan HIV specialist Dr. Howard Grossman, "it's really well tolerated. It's amazing."

This "mega-HAART," as Grossman called it, was by 2000 remarkably com-mon therapy among patients who had failed standard treatment due to the emergence of drug-resistant HIVs.

As physicians like Grossman ventured into ever wilder frontiers of HIV treatment, the grand HAART experiment was rushing forward without any guid-ing data. No one was keeping track. Indeed, convinced the rhetoric stressing that "the plague is over" was valid, most AIDS service organizations saw donations drop in the late 1990s. So they had cut back on their policy and research staffs. And all over America acute AIDS care facilities shut down, breaking up teams of scientists, physicians, and nurses that used to monitor patient outcomes on a scale that offered statistically relevant information.

One of the few such facilities remaining intact in 1998 was at the University of Alabama in Birmingham, where Dr. Michael Saag supervised state-of-the-art research and care on more than fifteen hundred patients.

By the end of 1998 Saag's massive data pool was yielding heartbreaking numbers.[734] He could see that May 1997 had been the nadir for AIDS and deaths in his population, but since that time death rates were "clearly on the rise. They aren't dying of a traditionally defined AIDS illness. I don't know what they're dying of, but they are dying. They're just wasting and dying."

The data had caught up with "cure" and "eradication"—by early 1999 both concepts were dead. The new buzz word was *remission*, a term taken from an-other dismal field of medicine, cancer care. By 2000 even that word had disap-peared from the HIV lexicon.

At Northwestern University in Chicago, Dr. Steven Wolinsky analyzed viral genes found in his most successfully treated patients. His findings were abysmal: virus was always there and it seemed to mutate over time.

"The virus is not gone—it's still there years out. So the question is, is this an evolutionary question? Is there ongoing replication? Why do we always see [viral] RNA? The virus is telling me something, but I'm not smart enough to see it," Wolinsky shrugged. "Is the sky falling?"

"Is it?" he was asked back.

"I wish I knew," he concluded. In other words, was the human immunodeficiency virus following the same tragic public health route as had the bacteria that became known as MRSA, VRE, and VISA?

Emilio Emini, head of the Merck Research Laboratories in West Point, Pennsylvania, once a leading HAART optimist, agreed in 1999 that there was "no doubt about it at all" that HIV replicated and mutated in seemingly effectively treated patients. It was a shared overall consensus reached in 1999 among HIV scientists: the virus *will* reproduce and mutate. Period.

"We've said from the beginning this is a nasty little virus," Emini insisted. "My fundamental hope is that in the end we'll be able to make a sincere shot at a vaccine here."

Meanwhile, said gay author and well-known New York activist Michelangelo Signorille, outside a few scientific circles, a sort of mass denial had set in. "People were furious, . . . enraged that I would be saying that AIDS did not go away. People accused me of causing panic, being hysterical. People are embarrassed to talk about the fact that the drugs aren't working for them and even to say that their lover recently died of AIDS. Because of that sense of failure."

By late 1999 there was mounting evidence that the sort of denial Signorille declaimed was leading to a resurgence of unsafe sexual activity in the gay community, posing a potential public health threat.

Researchers at the CDC developed a test that, for the first time, offered public health authorities the chance to handle HIV the same way that they had long handled syphilis. The test allowed researchers to tell who was recently infected with the virus versus who had been carrying HIV for years. Before the test, called a detuned ELISA,[735] was developed, public health workers had no way to trace the spread of HIV in their communities. It had simply been too hard for anyone to recall the names and addresses of all of their sexual partners, spanning years of their lives. But the detuned ELISA could pick out newly infected individuals[736]—those who had caught HIV within the last 120 days. And nearly everyone could remember whom they had had sex with over the last four months.

Armed with such an itemization, public health authorities could, theoretically, track down individuals who appeared to be spreading HIV and interrupt the chain of transmission. The idea, then, was to do for HIV what for years had been done with gonorrhea and syphilis.

"It's brilliantly simple," said Dr. Willi McFarland of the San Francisco Department of Public Health. "When we heard about this we were just ecstatic because this opens up the possibility of answering questions we never could address before."

In 1999 San Francisco was the only city in the world that routinely used detuned ELISA tests. And after about nine months of detuning thousands of Northern Californians, McFarland and his colleagues were thoroughly convinced of its utility as a research tool.[737]

About nine thousand San Franciscans got an HIV test in a city clinic every year and McFarland's colleagues in neighboring Alameda, Marin, and San Mateo counties had also been administering limited numbers of detuned ELISAs in cooperative studies in 1999. What they found, McFarland said, "blew our minds." Despite several thousand HIV tests, not a *single* woman turned up positive for recent acquisition of HIV. Not one. *None* of Northern California's injecting drug users who were tested turned up positive for recent infection except those who were gay. *All* of the newly infected San Franciscans were gay men, most of them white and in their thirties.

McFarland wanted to learn more about those men, especially who their partners might be. But unlike New York and a dozen other states, California had no contact tracing law for HIV. And according to McFarland, any attempts to elicit partner information from the state's mostly gay, male HIV population were greeted with cries of "sex police!"

"It raises a lot of issues—political things—and the memory of Typhoid Mary," McFarland said. "We were baffled by the tremendous resistance to naming names. Undermining our whole effort is community resistance."

The AIDS service organization Gay Men's Health Crisis conducted a survey in 1998 in Manhattan of seven thousand gay men, finding that 80 percent had undergone an HIV test within the previous three years: 13 percent were HIV positive. That infection rate was a far cry from the 50 percent HIV-positive rate that was presumed to be in the New York City gay community in 1980. That was the good news. The bad news was that 39 percent of the respondents admitted to having had unprotected (without a condom) anal intercourse within the previous year.[738]

The reason? "Now people mistakenly feel that AIDS is over," GMHC director Joshua Lipsman said. Because of HAART's apparent success, "the misimpression in the public is that you pop a pill and you're fine."

Five years before, the ravages of AIDS had been visually obvious even to casual observers strolling through gay urban centers. Along the streets, in the cafes, one could see young men who painfully leaned their frail bodies on friends, on their canes, against doorjambs. And for uninfected gay men, every day brought obvious reminders of the dangers inherent in having sex without latex protection.

Since 1996, however, and widespread use of HAART, gay neighborhoods had completely transformed. They were full of healthy-looking, muscular men—whether they were HIV positive or not—who worked out in local gyms, took growth hormone and testosterone, and looked a lot more like Arnold Schwartzenegger than stick figures leaning on Death's door.

"I do think that the lessening of fear about death and AIDS has resulted in a decrease in fear about contracting HIV," said Dr. Mitchell Katz, the director of the San Francisco Department of Public Health and himself a gay man.

Meanwhile, gonorrhea incidence in gay men rose 74 percent between 1993 and 1996 in a national survey of twenty-six cities. Seattle, Washington, reported that the number of syphilis cases in gay men had increased in that city by 60 percent and gonorrhea by 76 percent since 1996. Chicago saw syphilis, which had disappeared from its gay population, suddenly resurface in 1998 in a North Side homosexual neighborhood. And gonorrhea incidence among gay Chicagoans doubled.[739]

According to the New York City Department of Health, Gotham's gonorrhea rates had not risen. But syphilis rates had. Overall (in all population groups, gay and straight) there were about eighty active syphilis cases in New York City in 1998. By mid-1999, the case numbers were well ahead of 1998 and the department forecast more than one hundred for the year.[740]

San Francisco's troubling trends were more obvious, according to its health department. In 1994 less than 1 percent of the gay men who were diagnosed with gonorrhea also had HIV. In 1998 the number of gay HIV-positive men with gonorrhea had risen to 16 percent, meaning, McFarland said, that more HIV-positive and HIV-negative men in the city were having sex without protective condoms.

Dr. Kimberly Page-Shafer of the University of California San Francisco and Dan Wohlfeiler of the local Stop AIDS Project surveyed 21,857 gay men between 1994 and 1997. They found a steady rise in the number of gay men who admitted to having sex without a condom, until, in 1997, it was reaching fully a third of the respondents.[741]

Another UCSF study, conducted by scientist Ron Stall,[742] saw that by the end of 1997 fully half of more than five hundred men who had been questioned repeatedly since 1993 were having unprotected intercourse. "What's remarkable about this study is that for the very first time in the history of the epidemic we are seeing very large increases in unsafe sex," Stall explained. "This is *new*. And it's on the order of a 50 percent increase over the last two years. About half of the risk-taking is unprotected anal intercourse where the men either knew their partner had a different [HIV] serostatus or didn't know their partner's serostatus."

"What's new is people were supposed to feel remorse about having unsafe sex," Katz said. "And now there's this small minority saying, 'Yes, I did, and I'm not sorry.' "

It was called barebacking, UCSF medical sociology graduate student Michael Scarce said.[743] Scarce had interviewed 826 gay men nationwide who considered themselves barebackers. Most were white and the average age was thirty-six. They knew everything that the CDC and groups like GMHC and the Stop AIDS Project had to say about HIV yet they rejected the prevention campaigns, calling public health officials and prominent gay leaders "safer sex police" and "condom police." They were, Scarce insisted, "public health outlaws," and their popularity was rapidly increasing.

"And it never would have happened without the Internet," Scarce maintained. "Barebacking was born on AOL. It was through the anonymity of the Internet that gay men were able to be honest about what they wanted and connect with one another to get it." Scarce had identified more than 150 list servers on the Internet dedicated to barebacking.

In 1999, Ron Stall said, the "$100,000 question" is whether gay culture had entered a radically new paradigm that called for dramatically different approaches to disease prevention.[744] So how would the CDC's detuned ELISA contact tracing plan figure into such a picture? Scarce predicted that "a war is coming between gay men and public health if they do contact tracing."

As the twentieth century neared its close, it looked as if HIV would, indeed, follow the sorry courses of MRSA, VRE, multidrug-resistant tuberculosis, and chlorine-resistant microbes in drinking water.

Three different research teams published proof in 1999 that drug-resistant strains of HIV were spreading among sexually active people in the United States and Europe.[745] The findings raised deeply troubling reservations about both HAART and the future of public health control of the epidemic. Since all three research groups discovered highly multidrug-resistant forms of the virus that had surfaced within the previous eighteen months, the fear was that observers were witnessing the beginning of a trend that could render anti-HIV treatments useless to people infected in the future.[746]

At a 1999 National HIV Prevention Conference in Atlanta, CDC director Koplan hailed HAART as a "tremendous public health accomplishment," and added, "I think you're hard-pressed not to say it's a public health triumph when people can live longer."

But there was a big difference between antibiotic treatments for, say, tuberculosis and HAART for HIV. The antibiotics were curative, when properly used, and thus decreased the size of the contagious TB population. HAART, in contrast, was *not* curative and had greatly increased the size of the population of Americans and Europeans living with HIV—living behind the leaky HAART dam.

There, they could transmit HIV to their sexual partners, in some cases passing on mutant, highly drug-resistant forms of the virus.

"Clearly HAART was a great boon for medicine," Thomas Jefferson University's HIV expert Roger Pomerantz said. "For public health, though, it's a challenge, maybe an obstacle."

In the early months of 2000 President Clinton seemingly settled the debate, declaring the global AIDS pandemic a U.S. national security threat.

And so the twentieth century ended on a confusing, ominous note for public health in the United States. Humanity's old nemesis, the microbial world, was creating so many new challenges that scientists and doctors were hard-pressed to keep track. Globalization opened America to fantastic new economic and cultural horizons, but left her vulnerable to a higher order of microbial threat. The aging population was increasingly going to fill oncology and cardiology wards, just as the nation's health care financing system was finding novel, creative ways to deny access to such care. Ever more Americans were outside the system, denied health insurance and access. Politically, many Americans decried anything that reeked of "government," thus undermining support for public health.

Horribly, hospitals had been transformed in a remarkably short period of time from esteemed bastions of medical bravado to financially managed hubs for transmission of drug-resistant, lethal microbes. Tough CDC infection-control standards, coupled with decreased use of catheters and other invasive devices, brought nosocomial infection rates down in the U.S. during 1999 in top hospitals, but spread of bacteria in medical facilities still cost America about forty-four thousand to ninety-eight thousand lives and up to $29 billion that year.[747]

The sheer complexity of treatment for previously simple bacterial infections had become mind-boggling. Hospitals, physicians, and public health leaders made valiant attempts at limiting emergence and spread of antibiotic-resistant, ubiquitous bacteria, discovering by 2000 that despite fifty years of the drugs' use they had barely an inkling of how to perpetuate their efficacy in such complicated American ecologies as intensive care units, child care centers, and prisons.[748] Not surprisingly, novel staph and strep strains capable of resisting the last-ditch drug, vancomycin, continued to crop up across America.[749]

Though many of America's major health threats by 2000 came from outside the country, the nation's public health infrastructure was not at all prepared to deal with such external menaces. Agencies that traditionally had ignored public health, such as the CIA[750] and the Center for Strategic and International Studies,[751] were by 2000 addressing concerns about globalized infectious diseases far more vigorously and anxiously than were most public health agencies.

U.S. public health at the end of the twentieth century had also been stymied in its meager attempts at addressing racial gaps in life expectancy and other basic indicators of well-being. An average white baby boy born in America in 1980 had a life expectancy that was seven years longer than that of an African-American infant born the same year. By 1990 that life expectancy gap was slightly wider: 7.3 years. And in 1996 that gap was eight full years.[752] Public health's abysmal track record in minority communities had not, despite greater prominence of Hispanic and African-American leaders in relevant government leadership positions, much improved during the 1990s.

In New York City, for example, the African-American neighborhood of central Harlem had Gotham's highest overall death rate in 1998 and led the metropolis not only for most infectious diseases mortality rates but also for cancer and heart disease. The death gap between Harlem and whiter, wealthier parts of the city was on the order of 30 percent.[753]

Prevention of chronic killers—cancers, heart diseases—continued to stump American public health leaders in 2000, partly because of contradictory scientific findings regarding diet and behavioral issues. But even where the science of both prevention and treatment seemed clear there were terrible failures. Topping the list were hypertension and obesity, both of which rose dramatically among Americans during the 1990s. In a 1999 survey in Minnesota, for example, more than half of all tested adults were hypertensive (39 percent of whom didn't know it, and only 16.6 percent of whom were in treatment of any kind.)[754]

Though health care was not synonymous with public health, by 2000 it was glaringly obvious in the United States that lack of access to medical treatment, and insurance company limitations on such care, were affecting life expectancies. The National Coalition on Health Care announced that lethal false diagnosis rates soared during the 1990s, approaching 35 percent of all 1997 deaths. And an estimated 180,000 Americans died annually during the late 1990s because of nontreatment or improper medical care.[755] A University of Wisconsin study found that some managed care–dictated early hospital discharge policies during the 1990s *tripled* infant death rates.[756]

At the close of 1999 a team of Harvard and University of North Carolina researchers surveyed the status of the United States public health system. The analysts gave detailed questionnaires to every local public health leader in the country, asking them to rate the performance of their own departments and services. On average, those polled gave themselves a 35 percent rating out of a possible 100 percent.

In other words, by the end of the century, public health leaders themselves said that they were only achieving one-third of the functions essential to protecting the health of the population of the United States.[757]

What would ancient Greece's Asklepio have thought of America's great bastions of health in 2000, her prestigious teaching hospitals? Strolling along hallways resonating with the sounds of beeping heart monitors and emergency audio pages, Asklepio might turn to daughters Panakeia and Hygeia.

"Where is the solution to this mess?" Asklepio might ask.

Panakeia would cast her eyes upon the plethora of high-technology devices to which patients were attached and the long lists of drugs they were receiving. She would note the spread of diseases inside the hallowed chambers of panacea. And she would be at a loss.

"Sister," Panakeia would say in desperation, "have you an answer?"

And Hygeia would shake her head sadly, whispering, "Most of these suffering souls should never have been here in the first place."

CHAPTER FIVE

BIOWAR

Threatening biological terrorism
and public health.

Could it not be contrived to Send the Small Pox among those Disaffected Tribes of Indians?

—Sir Jeffrey Amherst, British commander-in-chief, American colonies, July 1763, writing in reference to an uprising among the Pontiac. Two weeks previously, smallpox-infested blankets had been distributed to the Shawnee and Delaware peoples.[1]

Above 700 Negroes are come down the River in the Smallpox. I shall distribute them about the Rebel Plantations.

—British General Alexander Leslie, July 13, 1781, writing of his plans to use smallpox against supporters of General George Washington, during the American Revolution.

The bright sunlight and glare off freshly falling, sparkling snow belied the danger of the day. The wind chill factor on this January morning in Minneapolis was 50°F—cold enough to quickly kill any ill-prepared fool who ventured far from shelter.

Through the glass panel of his tiny, drab government office Mike Osterholm eyed his heavily clad employees as they tromped toward their respective cubicles, peeling off layers of down, Gore-Tex, and wool as they went. Peering through heat-steamed glasses one waved a good-morning greeting to Osterholm who, as befits a classic Minnesotan, cheerfully waved back and shouted, "Cold enough for you?"

"Yup. Gonna be good ice fishing this weekend," the young state health worker joked. They both knew he'd be about as likely to spend a day off in a tent on one of Minnesota's hundreds of frozen lakes as he would dance with the Rockettes at Radio City Music Hall.

Two eighteen-inch-wide slits of glass afforded Osterholm a few rays of winter sunlight and a glimpse of snow drifting down onto leafless trees. On the white Sheetrock walls were ominous old State Health Department signs, one reading: SMALLPOX EXISTS ON THESE PREMISES. Osterholm was in unusually good spirits, as he'd just received a remarkable telephone call.

Mike Osterholm, an epidemiologist in America's Siberia, was preparing to play an historic role in the politics of a Middle Eastern nation about which he knew next to nothing. He had just been summoned by the king of Jordan to brief the monarch about a subject that had caused Osterholm many sleepless nights: biological terrorism.

While his staff of exceptionally astute disease-detectives on that January 5, 1999, icy day were busy tracking the trail of a new outbreak of listeria food poisonings Osterholm spoke from his office with Washington, getting details of the planned meeting from the State Department and National Security Council.

King Hussein, leader of the Hashemite Kingdom of Jordan, held a position of strategic global import that far outweighed the size and economic clout of his tiny desert nation. He was the longest-ruling head of state in the latter twentieth century, having acceded to the throne at the age of seventeen. But his continued survival was in jeopardy. Just five days earlier Hussein had hastily left his six-month-long cancer care at the nearby Mayo Clinic, having not yet completed a final round of bone marrow transplant procedures. His sudden, unexpected departure, accompanied by American-born Queen Noor and eighteen-year-old Prince Hamzah, had caused consternation at the Mayo and sparked rumors of political intrigue. Now, with cancer cells coursing throughout his body, the sixty-three-year-old monarch had an apparently sudden interest in biological terrorism. It seemed to have been sparked shortly before Christmas when Osterholm, on a visit to the Mayo Clinic, met teenaged Prince Hamzah and struck up a conversation not about deadly tumor cells but about lethal microbes. The young prince, who was enrolled at Britain's prestigious Sandhurst military school, was impressed by the energetic Swedish-American.

Shortly after that chance meeting, the king and his family had made their hasty departure, stopping first in London, where the royal family owned a taste-fully appointed home not far from Buckingham Palace. Even Osterholm was unaware that the king was in London, and in preparation for meeting with the monarch he was boning up on information about Amman, a desert city he could barely imagine from the vantage point of his American Siberia. Yet if the place seemed unfathomable the subject did not, as bioterrorism had obsessed Osterholm for nearly six years.

As he prepared to meet Hussein, he explained to a visitor that the interest began on May 11, 1993, in the CDC's Auditorium A, at precisely 1:00 P.M. He remembered such details because the moment was for the state epidemiologist an epiphany the likes of which he had never previously experienced. The topic on the agenda was possible destruction of remaining laboratory stocks of otherwise eradicated smallpox virus. During the debate information was revealed regarding former Soviet scientists who had defected to the United States and United Kingdom, giving Westerners information on a previously secret Soviet biowarfare program. The classified word was that Soviet scientists had developed a weapon of mass destruction, made of smallpox viruses.

"And I thought to myself, 'Jeez! In this century alone, 500 million people died of smallpox, and all of the wars combined were only 320 million,' " Osterholm recalled.

Like most American biologists and physicians Osterholm had always considered talk of bioweapons the stuff of silly science fiction, paranoid conspiracy fantasies, or old-fashioned red-baiting. He had never previously imagined that someone might actually use germs as weapons. And the meeting was shattering if for no other reason than it made terribly real a concept he had for his entire life comfortably dismissed as, to be frank, silliness.

After that fateful CDC meeting Osterholm had drinks with General Philip Russell, the military's highest-ranking biologist, who revealed still more alarming details: it wasn't just smallpox; it wasn't just the Russians; it wasn't even just belligerent countries that had bioweapons. Russell told Osterholm that such horrors had found their ways into the hands of groups of political zealots, armed terrorists, religious cults, and American ultraright-wing militiamen.

"And it started me on a journey," Osterholm said. For the next three years Osterholm sat as a civilian advisor on military and foreign affairs secret committees that were focused in Washington on biological warfare and terrorism issues. He racked up a lot of frequent-flier miles jetting back and forth to the nation's capital, growing more anxious with every new secret revelation. He could tell his colleagues in the Minneapolis office nothing—even the names of his Washington committees were classified.

It was driving him crazy, Osterholm said, because the further he got into the issue, "the more I realized we really didn't know what was going on."[2]

Osterholm recognized by 1996 that the only effective response against a bioterrorism event would come from public health, "and meanwhile I'm watching the infrastructure for public health in this country deteriorate."

Never one to mince words, he soon spoke his mind in these meetings. And in Washington an emboldened Osterholm came under attack. The more he cried at secret meetings that no one was prepared, the more he was accused of grandstanding, trying to wave his ego around the capital. One New York City official privately charged that Osterholm was out for personal glory, rather than public protection.

Osterholm had retaliated, saying that he saw "two enemies. The perpetrator. And the ones who are supposed to respond to it, who instead have blindfolded themselves. . . . Right now we are missing enough rods in public health we could not stop that [metaphoric] nuclear reaction of bioterrorism."

By the close of 1996, having patiently sat on FBI committees, briefed Vice President Al Gore, and been through innumerable classified gatherings, Osterholm was convinced it was time to go public. He turned to Dr. D. A. Henderson, one of public health's most venerable spokespersons. He urged the smallpox expert to speak out. Henderson, he knew, had the greatest credibility. The senior scientist ran a unique program at Johns Hopkins University's School of Public Health, called the Center for Civilian Biodefense Studies. And Henderson had been in even more classified meetings than Osterholm.

Thinking back on these events that January morning prompted Osterholm to put a call through to Henderson, who served as a sort of mentor on the bioterrorism issue. Osterholm turned to him for advice on what to tell the king of Jordan.

A week later the Minnesotan found himself seated across from the royal family of Jordan in their opulent home. Queen Noor, her son Hamzah, and the king's security chief listened and energetically partook in the hours-long discussion. Osterholm was impressed with King Hussein's vigor and keen intellect. He decided that rumors of King Hussein's imminent death were greatly exaggerated. And there was no doubt whatsoever in Osterholm's mind as he left the royal family that King Hussein, for reasons unstated, had cause for acute concern about the possible use of biological weapons inside his kingdom, or regionally in the volatile Middle East.

The king told Osterholm that he wanted to host an international meeting of world leaders to discuss bioterrorism. And Osterholm was, in turn, in awe of the Jordanian leader.

Jordan was defended against hostile neighbors on every side by an armed force of 82,250 men and 35,000 reserves. It was a tiny military force compared to those amassed around it. To the north Syria spent more than $3 billion a year building an armed force of more than 306,000 men, 392,000 reservists, and strategic missile, tank, and aircraft capability, all of it well tested in battles against Israel and in Lebanon's long civil war. To the south was the Hashemite's ancient tribal nemesis, the House of Saud, protected by a Saudi Arabian highly trained military force of some 50,000 men, including twenty air bases stocked with the most expensive high-technology aircraft, missile, and reconnaissance equipment available in the global marketplace. To Jordan's west was Israel, the only country in the region with which the Hashemite Kingdom had in recent decades waged war. With military spending that topped $8 billion annually, a standing army of 140,000 men and women, including seasoned combatants and highly sophisticated air and land strategic capacity, Israel was the Middle East's most significant tactical force.

Most troubling for King Hussein, however, were two things: the forces massed on his eastern flank and domestic insurgents. On the east was Saddam Hussein's Iraq, with a standing army of some 450,000 men, combat-seasoned fighter pilots, an ambitious SCUD missile program, and military spending well in excess of $5 billion annually.

Domestically, King Hussein had always been plagued by would-be assassins, terrorists, attempted coups, and religious fanatics, who readily gained political and financial support from Jordan's belligerent regional enemies. Even within his own army was a 1,200-man Palestinian subdivision that swore allegiance not to the king, but to PLO leader Yasir Arafat. The majority of Jordan's population was Palestinians, most of whom considered themselves refugees from Israeli-occupied Palestine. On innumerable occasions during his reign the PLO and other Palestinian organizations had used Jordan as a staging ground for unauthorized attacks on Israel, carried out violent demonstrations within the kingdom, and even attempted to overthrow the king. It was rumored King Hussein had survived more than fifty assassination attempts: publicly thirty were acknowledged by the Hashemite government.

The king did not discuss these matters with Osterholm in their London meeting, but they surely formed a backdrop to his avid interest in bioterrorism. At the close of their meeting the king, queen, and prince cordially thanked Osterholm and withdrew to their private chambers. The following day King Hussein piloted his own jet home to Amman.

Seven days later, on January 26, the king stunned the entire world by announcing that his brother, Prince Hassam, would not inherit the throne, which for thirty-four years had been his promise. Rather, the comparatively obscure Prince Abdullah, a thirty-seven-year-old Jordanian military leader and son of the king, would take control of the nation. Amid rumors of court intrigue that were described in scales of Shakespearean drama a lengthy letter from the king to Prince Hassam explained the radical change. Among the issues discussed at length in the fourteen-page missive was germ warfare. The king warned Hassam—and the Jordanian people—of the grave dangers of deliberately fomented epidemics. Echoing lessons learned in his hours with Osterholm, Hussein described bioweapons as a terrible new resource for the stateless terrorist or rogue nation. Realizing his letter would be published in Jordanian newspapers and resonate across the Arab world King Hussein pointedly warned that there could be no winners in a world of man-made epidemics.

A few hours after completing the letter the dying king boarded his jet and under U.S. Air Force escort winged his way back to the Mayo Clinic. Prince Abdullah was sworn in the following day.

And then the king died.

Osterholm would never know what role—if any—his discussion with the royal family had on the king's shocking twelfth-hour decisions. He recognized some of his remarks in the king's letter and knew from the questions the royal family had posed in London that a few of his themes had gotten through: that new scientific technology made genetic manipulation and creation of superbugs fairly simple feats. And systems of civilian defense against bioweapons were virtually nonexistent. The Minnesotan's brief moment in the world of international intrigue served, however, to confirm Osterholm's belief that he had been right a year earlier when he insisted that the bioterrorism issue be placed on the agenda for public concern.

For months he had bugged Henderson about it, pressing the older scientist to reveal to the press what they both had heard in all those secret Washington meetings. Henderson first gingerly tested the waters at the September 1997 meeting of the Infectious Diseases Society of America.[3] He carefully restricted his comments to published information, but made reference to larger concerns he had picked up in the secret Washington meetings. Henderson stuck to historical ground, outlining the destruction and terror produced by outbreaks of smallpox and anthrax during the latter half of the twentieth century. He kept the academic litany remarkably dry, given the horror he was describing. And he concluded his remarks with an observation that stood in stark contrast to the almost nonchalant tone of his previous comments: "The specter of biological weapons is every bit as grim as that of nuclear winter," a reference to the theory that use of nuclear weapons would sink the world into an ice age that would obliterate nearly every life-form on earth.

Osterholm wasn't satisfied. He pushed his mentor for more. And he got it six months later at an enormous public meeting in Atlanta.

D. A. Henderson decided that the time had come to speak his mind in the manner Osterholm had urged. It was, frankly, hard to imagine the tall, barrel-chested baritone ever doing otherwise. His presence dominated any conversation, filled any room.

Seas of colleagues parted when Henderson entered a room, in deference to his leadership role in probably the most dramatic public health victory of the twentieth century, the elimination of smallpox. By his own admission Henderson, then an officer of the World Health Organization, had broken every rule in the UN bureaucratic book by the time the various strains of human smallpox viruses were vanquished in 1977. It was necessary, he insisted. After all, they were fighting to defeat a virus responsible for killing more human beings in the twentieth century than all wars combined.

Henderson had, for example, rationalized open cooperation between military and public health personnel and collaboration across 1970s Cold War boundaries. After all, the global campaign to eliminate smallpox was originally a Soviet idea, announced in Moscow in 1958. And the Soviets had a profound—perhaps unnerving—knowledge of the two species of viruses capable of causing smallpox. So at a time when virtually all other communication between Moscow and the capitals of the capitalist West were tightly shut, Henderson encouraged public health alliances with hands outstretched across the Berlin Wall.

When all traces of wild human smallpox had been eradicated, Henderson had to go along with WHO's diplomatic plan for dealing with the fate of remaining laboratory samples of the virus. One set went into the deep freezers of the maximum security laboratory at the Centers for Disease Control and Prevention in Atlanta, Georgia. The other was placed in frozen isolation in a Moscow laboratory that, Henderson knew, was physically less secure. He didn't much like the Moscow setting but compromised: after all, with all other known lab samples of smallpox scheduled for immediate destruction the WHO scheme limited global concern and security to just two sites. In 1977 that had seemed reasonable.

Henderson didn't then know, of course, that Soviet Premier Leonid Brezhnev had other plans for those viruses—indeed, for hundreds of different lethal pathogens. Twenty years later military and intelligence experts in the West would confess that they hadn't a clue about the program Brezhnev dubbed Biopreparat until at least ten years after the smallpox bilateral accord was reached. They'd known nothing of Brezhnev's great scheme for offsetting American nuclear deterrence, nor of his absolute resolve to violate the Biological Weapons Convention signed with U.S. President Richard Nixon in 1973.

They had no idea that by 1977 the Soviet Union was well along in construction of what eventually would be forty-seven biologic weapons laboratories and testing sites, employing upward of fifty thousand scientists, technicians, and support staff in facilities spanning at least ten time zones. Most crucially, they knew nothing about the secret laboratories in Siberia.

By 1998, seven years after the collapse of the Soviet Union, though, Henderson was aware of at least some of the facts about Biopreparat. He confessed that it was "damned hard" to sift fact from fiction, to know which former Biopreparat scientists could be trusted. They could all be exaggerating the hell out of the situation. Or they could be hiding enormous information that was vital—

Henderson felt with no sense of overstatement—to the survival of the human race.

The horrible possibility that a politically—even pathologically—crazed group or individual could get their hands on the Moscow viruses hit home when Henderson watched televised reports of the 1993 standoff between Boris Yeltsin's government and a loose coalition of armed dissidents, ranging politically from relatively moderate members of the Duma to angry Afghan war veterans shooting guns on behalf of a return to power of the Communist Party. Like most non-Russians Henderson had no sense of what was to come when American TV networks quipped on September 21 that Boris Yeltsin had issued a decree on reform that was found objectionable to most of the Duma. But as days passed, the standoff escalated, and Henderson's fear for the safety of Moscow's stash of smallpox grew.[4]

"I learned that they dispatched soldiers to guard the Virology Institute and at that point it seemed logical to get [the smallpox] out of there," Henderson later recalled. But when the protectors of Russia's smallpox stash were questioned closely it appeared "that they moved it before that," secretly, to the former Biopreparat facility located about an hour's drive from Novosibirsk, in central Siberia. Henderson was stunned, as the Russians had never told WHO that the tubes of lethal microbes had been relocated, and no international representative had seen the new repository or could vouch for the safety of the smallpox storage.

When U.S. intelligence officials discovered that the Russian smallpox supplies were moved, Henderson recalled, "They asked, 'Why didn't they get permission to move it?' and I said, 'We never gave them a mandate to request permission from WHO.' So they moved it."

Now, four years after Yeltsin's White House confrontation Henderson remained unsure about where all of Russia's lethal smallpox supplies were located. Had they all gone into the Biopreparat freezers in Novosibirsk? Or had they secretly been dispersed, a test tube at a time, over the years to other Biopreparat laboratories? Was it even right to think in terms of Russian test tubes of the terrible virus, or might the old Soviets have cloned and mass-produced gallons of the viruses? Such uncertainty, coupled with classified intelligence reports he'd heard, made Henderson very, very nervous.

"Until recently the subject of biological terrorism has been little discussed or written about in the medical literature or, for that matter, in the public press," Henderson began, addressing a tense March 1998 gathering of some six thousand professionals in Atlanta for the first International Conference on Emerging and Infectious Diseases.[5] The moment Henderson, dressed in a black-and-white check jacket, starched white button-down shirt, tie, suspenders, and black pants, stepped to the podium a hush came over the audience—unusual in its makeup as military personnel, academics, researchers, U.S. government scientists, investigators from all over the world, and the media commingled. Henderson casually ran his fingers through his white hair, adjusted his steel-rimmed bifocals, and continued.

"Until recently, I personally had doubts about publicizing the subject because of concern that it might entice some to undertake dangerous, perhaps catastrophic experiments,"[6] Henderson said. "However, events of the past twelve to eighteen months have made it clear that likely perpetrators already envisage every agenda one could possibly imagine."

Among recent events that had escalated U.S., European, and United Nations concerns about biological weapons were UN inspectors' findings in Iraq, recent innovations in biotechnology that streamlined genetic manipulation of microbes, elucidation of the scope of Russia's Biopreparat program, and evidence that some of its former scientists may have moved their expertise and products onto the international arms market. Though most of these elements for concern had been known to experts before, it was only in 1997 that the full picture—the sense of threat—coalesced in Western military, intelligence, and some scientific circles.

Until the late 1990s few experts in any field considered biological weapons a viable threat. Lederberg, like Henderson, was part of that scientific fraternity of advisors on the subject, said there were several mistaken assumptions that previously steered world leaders away from concern about weaponized viruses, bacteria, and biological toxins. Paramount, Lederberg felt, was the thankful fact that no one had yet committed the biological equivalent of Hiroshima.

In the absence of a bio-Hiroshima, Lederberg argued, it was all too easy to dismiss concerns about biological weapons on other grounds: biobombs, if you will, were more likely to kill a protagonist's own colleagues or troops than its opponents; it was impossible to weaponize biologicals, making them deliverable to enemies via missiles or a localized dispersion device; it was assumed there were sufficient vaccines and medicines invented and available to counter the effects of such weapons, should they be deployed; any nation or organization that used such weapons would be greeted with disgust and moral repugnance from the rest of the world, therefore bioweapons represented a poor choice, even for outlaws.[7]

"Each of these arguments is without validity," Henderson insisted. "We now know that there are nations and dissident groups who have both the motivation and access to skills to selectively cultivate some of the most dangerous pathogens and to deploy them as agents in acts of terrorism or war."

Henderson dangled the prospect of germ terrorism before the assembled public health experts, beckoning them to get on board for a journey previously taken only in secret, largely by military and law enforcement personnel. The invitation carried risks, he knew. Military and police cultures rarely mixed well with that of public health.

But the CDC's Dr. Scott Lillibridge had no such reservations, and made it clear that biological weapons were a public health issue: "My extreme concern . . . is that these events will exploit vulnerabilities in our public health system. The lack of capacity at the local level means [biological] isolates may not be confirmed in a timely manner. Preparedness must include the public health community as a full partner."[8]

The event that set off the first apprehension in public health, military, and intelligence circles occurred in Tokyo on March 20, 1995.

It was rush hour. Tens of thousands of Japanese office workers were boarding Tokyo's vast subway system. Three of the key, extremely crowded subway lines came from the residential districts to the west and north of Tokyo, particularly Asakusa and Aoyama, converging in the Kasumigaseki government center of the city. At 8:00 A.M. these trains were particularly mobbed as hordes of civil servants headed for their workday, which commenced at 8:30 A.M.[9]

At 8:09 A.M. a small bomb detonated in Kasumigaseki station as the Eidan, Marunouchi, Chiyoda, and Hibiya subway lines converged, releasing a deadly nerve gas called sarin.[10]

Four minutes later another bomb detonated inside busy Kasumigaseki station. At least three individuals carried additional plastic bags of nerve gas on the subways, which they poked open at the same time. The simple bombs released an invisible chemical, 1-Methylethyl methylphosphonate, bringing hundreds of passengers to their knees, overcome with nausea, bleeding from their noses and mouths, and suffering headaches, a profound sense of chemically induced anxiety, coughs, and, in three cases, pulmonary edema. The Tokyo Fire Department rushed to the scene, responding to word of bomb blasts. Many were, themselves, overcome by the gas.

Hundreds of commuters staggered out of Kasumigaseki station and made their ways to local hospitals.

In the end, 5,510 people were harmed in the sarin attack, about 100 of whom required hospitalization. Twelve died.

Japanese police soon discovered the culprits were members of a bizarre religious cult called Aum Shinrikyo, or Buddhist "Om" and Supreme Truth.[11] Led by a forty-year-old Rolls-Royce–driving, long-haired, bearded guru named Shoko Asahara, Aum Shinrikyo was on a mission to bring about the end of the world, placing themselves in dominion over the survivors. While religious cults in many cultures have long forecast Armageddon, Aum Shinrikyo was determined to hasten its arrival.

Subsequent years of police investigation and court proceedings revealed that Aum Shinrikyo was an enormous organization with minimally forty thousand devotees in Japan, Russia, Europe, and the United States. Japanese police swiftly discovered that the Kasumigaseki subway attack was just a trial run: the organization had stockpiled enough sarin to, in a future attack, kill 4.2 million people. Further, the March 1995 sarin attack followed at least two prior gassings, several botulism toxin assaults, endeavors to kill Japan's leaders with anthrax, and attempts to acquire and develop Q fever bacteria and Africa's dread Ebola virus.[12]

With a donated and earned $2 billion treasury at its disposal thanks to a computer software company it ran, the cult bought the best expertise, including former KGB agents and Russian military advisors. In 1991 cult members even solicited advice from Russia's Minister of Defense Grachov and Oleg Lobov, a member of President Yeltsin's advisory council. The cult was negotiating purchase of nuclear weapons materials, using Ukrainian and Russian mobsters as go-betweens with ex-Soviet military personnel. Even the isolationist and vehemently anti-Japanese North Korean government provided the cult with arms and advice.

Aum Shinrikyo's activities proved to a once-skeptical national security community that weapons of mass destruction, and in particular bioweapons, could and were being developed by groups well outside of traditional government control.[13]

A few days after the Tokyo attack a classified national security forum convened at the White House, attended by President Bill Clinton, Vice President Al Gore, several cabinet members, and a select group of scientists, defense, and emergency officials. Kenneth Adelman, vice president of the Institute for Contemporary Studies in Washington, asked Joshua Lederberg at the meeting whether there weren't technological "fixes" that could prevent biological and chemical attacks in the United States. As an example of what he was getting at, Adelman cited the positive role metal detectors were playing in virtually eliminating terrorist attacks at airports and on commercial planes.

Lederberg responded carefully by comparing prevention approaches for nuclear, chemical, and biological attacks:

"Well, for the most part, it is not detection and prevention but deterrence which is the keystone of our security in the nuclear area. . . . That breaks down when you have a kamikaze—when you have people willing to commit suicide as part of the game. Deterrence is not a feature there."

Lederberg discussed options for detecting nuclear devices that had fallen into terrorist or rogue nation hands, noting that "in the nuclear field there is some room for detection."

But, he added ominously, "It is much more difficult in the chemical and biological area—it is next to impossible."

Were an Aum Shinrikyo–type of attack to occur in America one of the key responding agencies would be the federal Office of Emergency Preparedness and National Disaster Medical System. Its director, Dr. Frank Young, listened as Lederberg speculated that an effective bioattack on the New York City subway system posed the possibility of "6,000 dead, 100,000 in perilous condition. Your local authorities cannot begin to cope with events of that kind."

"That is absolutely correct," Young responded soberly.

It was the sort of nightmarish vision the congressional Office of Technology Assessment had conjured in 1993 in a now-classic scenario: a crop duster plane, loaded with one hundred kilograms of anthrax spores, flies over the White House, Capitol Hill, the Pentagon, and much of Washington, D.C., in a criss-cross pattern before being detecting and forced to land.[14] Over the next days and weeks three million people die.

The Aum Shinrikyo attack served as one wake-up call, alerting officials that the once-unthinkable was not only possible, it might even be probable. This was no longer science fiction.

President Clinton promised the gathering that he would seek ways to strengthen the anemic 1972 Biological Toxins and Weapons Convention, but there was little immediate satisfaction on that score—no one knew how to make violations of the treaty verifiable.[15]

The first genuinely tough attempt to enforce the treaty targeted Saddam Hussein's regime in Iraq. It demonstrated clearly that controlling a government's use, or threatened use, of biological weapons was difficult if not impossible with available technical and diplomatic tools.

On August 2, 1990, an estimated force of 545,000 Iraq troops and tanks marched on neighboring Kuwait, seizing Kuwaiti oil reserves and instituting martial law.[16] Seven months later an allied force of some 690,000 combatants, led by the U.S. administration of President George Bush, carried out an air and land war against Iraq's then million-man army, taking 175,000 Iraqi soldiers prisoner and inflicting some 85,000 casualties. The vanquished Iraqi leadership was compelled to sign a treaty that, among other things, guaranteed all of Iraq's chemical and biological weapons and stockpiles would immediately be destroyed. This allowed United Nations inspectors, at least technically, the greatest investigational access to Iraq's war machine ever afforded under the Biological Toxins and Weapons Convention.

But the following year, on July 5, 1992, Iraq denied UN inspectors entry to a suspected bioweapons storage site. International tension rose, U.S. sanctions of Iraqi trade were put in place, and three weeks later Baghdad yielded, allowing UN inspection of the contested site. No suspected materials were found; some inspectors claimed Iraq was playing a shell game, moving the weapons from one place to another, hiding the incriminating evidence.

The rationale for UN suspicion appeared strong. In 1989 the Iraqi Air Force had successfully launched its first orbital three-stage rocket, and appeared to have ballistic missile capability. With its $5 billion annual military budget Iraq spent heavily on acquisition of high-technology equipment. And in April 1990 Saddam Hussein had grandiosely announced that his forces had developed missile-loaded binary chemical weapons, mounted on modified long-range SCUD missiles. "I swear to God that we will let our fire eat half of Israel if it tries to wage anything against Iraq," Hussein declared in 1990.[17]

Saddam Hussein had rarely leveled a political or military threat without following through: in the 1980s Hussein obliterated every Iranian town and village he threatened.[18] The ensuing Iran/Iraq war lasted eight bloody years and claimed an estimated 240,000 Iranian civilian and military lives.[19]

Some of those casualties had been victims of Iraqi chemical weapons, inflicted from the first days of the war. Iran claimed, and UN inspectors had at least partially verified on site in 1984, 1986, and 1987, that mustard gas and a nerve gas called tabun were dispersed by airplanes and rockets. A UN team determined that Iraq was in violation of the Geneva Protocol.[20] It is estimated that 5 percent of all Iranians who were exposed to these chemicals during the war died, but exact numbers of dead are not known.[21]

Shortly after Iraq signed a cease-fire in 1988 Saddam Hussein refocused his attention on his country's Kurdish minority. On March 19, 1988, the Iraqi Air Force attacked the Kurdish village of Hallabja, killing nearly all its inhabitants. Though international observers didn't learn of the attack or reach the site for several days, Western intelligence experts concluded that the Kurds were victims of cyanide and mustard gas.[22]

Thereafter, Iraq began, by its own admission, an unprecedented chemical weapons buildup. And in 1996 Saddam Hussein's government conceded that biological weapons production had also commenced at that time.[23]

In the late 1980s Hussein had gone full bore on acquisition and development of chemical and biological weapons, with the complicity of U.S., Japanese, Austrian, British, Swiss, Dutch, and German commercial suppliers and technicians. Enormous chemical plants were built in Samarra, Falliyah, Al Muthanna, and just outside Baghdad. And, in collaboration with Argentina and Egypt, Iraq developed Condor missiles capable of delivering CBW to distant targets. Further, Iraq modified several SCUD missiles to give them very long-range capacity—capable of reaching targets in Israel.

After the Operation Desert Storm war's end, Iraq for several years employed a cat-and-mouse game with UN inspectors, hiding as much chemical and biological evidence as possible.

In 1994 Germany's BND intelligence unit (Bundenachrichtendienst, or Federal Intelligence Service) discovered a complex acquisitions trail used by Iraq to obtain weapons and biowar materials, largely from Western European sources. Among the mountains of supplies obtained illegally by Iraq, despite international sanctions, were thirty-nine *tons* of bacterial growth medium, purchased mostly from Oxoid, a British subsidiary of Unilever.[24]

"It is absolutely inconceivable that Iraq could have had legitimate medical uses for that much growth medium," Henderson insisted. "Claiming legitimate use defies all boundaries of credibility."

All of Iraq's medical and scientific laboratories previously consumed less than 441 pounds of medium annually, or 0.5 percent of the tons that were imported. Iraq was never able to account for the use or whereabouts of seventeen tons of that imported medium.[25]

Iraq's original seed sample of anthrax had been purchased aboveboard from American Type Culture Collection, then based in Rockville, Maryland, during the mid-1980s. The purchase was cleared by the U.S. Department of Commerce during the Reagan Administration.

United Nations inspectors eventually concluded that Iraq had built an impressive biological weapons armamentarium before the Desert Storm war,[26] including about eight thousand pounds of anthrax, eight kilograms of concentrated botulinum toxin, and at least four other types of bacteria, five of viruses, and three other biotoxins. Just before the war broke out, the UN team concluded, Iraq had grown 340 liters of *Clostridium* for botulism toxin production. At numerous sites—particularly the Al Hakam Single-Cell Protein Plant, located a few miles south of Baghdad—stainless steel fermenters capable of holding 1,450 liters of biologicals were found.

Though the Iraqi government eventually admitted to some of those findings, no one outside the Iraqi military leadership knew how much of the material had actually been weaponized. Growing bacteria or viruses was one thing; figuring out how to keep it alive aboard a flaming missile or bomb was quite another.

The Americans knew a fair amount about that problem.[27] U.S. secret agents discovered during World War I that German laboratories were developing weaponized ricin toxin designed to be inflicted as a one-on-one weapon. (The protein ricin, found in castor beans, was a highly toxic neurological poison that would kill a human being who ingested as little as 180 micrograms of the compound. Though it was three hundred times less potent than botulism toxin, ricin was thirty times more potent than Aum Shinrikyo's sarin gas.) As far as is known these early weapons were never used. And at the war's end the League of Nations concluded that biological weapons were impractical and therefore did not pose a serious threat.

Twenty-seven years later in World War II, the U.S. Army maintained that biologicals remained impractical because they could never be weaponized. But

France, the United Kingdom, and Japan didn't agree: all three had substantial bioweapons programs during World War II. And Japan developed and used its bioweapons in Manchuria from 1933 to 1940. Using biobombs, it successfully caused outbreaks of typhus, cholera, and plague in China.[28] In addition, Allied investigations after the war revealed Japan's use of bioweapons for dysentery and paratyphoid.

A U.S. biological weapons program commenced in 1943 but was unable to weaponize any agents before the war's end.

With the Cold War came an escalation in American efforts to weaponize biology. In the 1950s special yellow fever–carrying mosquitoes were developed and tested. And unique bombs for release of pathogens were invented, as well as large-scale aerosolizers and submarine mines. Experiments were conducted, releasing microbes in New York, San Francisco, South Dakota, Minnesota, and, unintentionally, Canada.[29] A 1950 army experiment spraying bacteria from a boat sickened several San Franciscans, allegedly killing one.[30]

The most aggressive American biowarfare effort was conducted during the Korean War (1951–1953), and involved development and use of a variety of bacteria and disease-carrying mosquitoes. Though the U.S. Joint Chiefs of Staff gave the military's scientists a green light to develop and use whatever bioweapons they could, the entire effort was hidden from the American people, even Congress. The military brass was all too aware that their deliberate creation of epidemics in Korea would be viewed as morally repugnant by U.S. citizens.[31]

The offensive biological warfare program continued, still shrouded in secrecy, for fifteen more years in the United States.

By 1966 the United States was spending $38 million a year on development of biological weapons, having weaponized anthrax, *Pasteurella tularensis, Bacillus globigii*, and agricultural microbes such as stem rust, a fungus deadly to wheat. The weapons were stockpiled on a fifteen-thousand-acre spread outside Pine Bluff, Arkansas—thousands of gallons of death, nestled inside rusting metal canisters. Like their nuclear counterparts that were mounted atop missiles inside silos all over America the biobombs were Cold War weapons that few scientists or military leaders hoped to ever actually use. But the mentality of the capitalist-versus-Communist era dictated a sort of historic suspension of rationality in favor of paranoia-driven technological development. If there were rumors of bioweapons developments in Communist Korea, according to the mentality of the day, then surely capitalist America had better race toward technical superiority—even if the weapons of choice conjured nightmares of mass civilian death, perhaps genocide.

But the 1960s were a bad time for the United States to be in the bioweapons game (if there ever was a "good" time for such efforts): widespread antiwar demonstrations and public uncertainty about the veracity of American military statements put activities at Fort Detrick, Fort McClellan, and the Edgewood Arsenal under harsh political scrutiny.[32]

So in November 1969, President Richard M. Nixon announced that "the United States of America will renounce the use of any form of deadly biological weapons that either kill or incapacitate. Our bacteriological programs in the future will be confined to research in biological defense . . . and on measures of controlling and preventing the spread of disease."[33]

U.S. stockpiles were destroyed over the following five years, and U.S. offensive bioweapons programs abruptly stopped. The experience, however, taught the Americans that it was one thing to grow trillions of deadly bacteria or viruses; it was quite another to create a way to deliver those pathogens, alive and lethal, effectively sickening enemy soldiers.[34]

Similarly, British and French military researchers abandoned bioweapons research not simply for moral reasons, but also because it proved so difficult to truly weaponize living microorganisms.

So as United Nations inspectors struggled in the 1990s to discern exactly what Iraq had developed, they paid closest attention to sorting out what may have been weaponized. By 1994 the inspectors concluded that Iraq had, indeed, weaponized botulinum toxins, but, as Dr. Raymond A. Zilinskas put it: "Though in possession of several hundred biological weapons, Iraq's tactical biological warfare capability during the Persian Gulf War actually was quite limited . . . [and] had Iraq's biological warfare munitions actually been used, their effect would have been limited to contaminating a relatively small area of ground surrounding the point of impact and exposing nearby individuals to aerosolized pathogens or toxins."[35]

The Iraqis, it seemed, were technological klutzes. They had loads of nasty germs, but little capability of delivering biobombs to designated targets. Further, Iraq's SCUD attacks in Israel were wildly off target due, the inspectors later determined, to an almost complete lack of inertial guidance systems. Iraq in 1992 could no more have tactically biobombed Tel Aviv than it could drop an A-bomb on Paris.

But subsequent years of investigation convinced UNSCOM—the United Nations special commission responsible for CBW inspections—that the Iraqi government was clandestinely continuing to develop and weaponize biological agents throughout the 1990s. And Iraq had research and development collaborators, particularly in Libya. Zilinskas felt certain that Iraq could, within a matter of months, be capable of having, "remotely piloted vehicles, long-range fighter-bombers or cruise missiles equipped with tanks and sprayers and programmed to avoid detection by flying low and, following ground contours, could reach

populations located within one thousand kilometers of Iraq's borders and disperse agents under conditions favorable for carrying out a successful biological
attack."

In the summer of 1995, Saddam's son-in-law who was in charge of Iraq's
CBW effort, Lieutenant General Hussein Kamal al-Majid, defected to Jordan and
was closely grilled by the CIA, UNSCOM, and European intelligence experts.
Kamal told his interrogators that Iraq possessed vast stores of biological agents.
Confronted by the truth, Iraq was compelled to destroy much of its postwar
reserves, and Saddam admitted to having produced, among other things, a half
a million liters of anthrax and botulinum toxin. Further, boxes of damning documents were turned over to UNSCOM. Based on these papers, UNSCOM concluded that Iraq had imported *more* than the thirty-nine tons of bacterial growth
media originally estimated and experts were left to ponder the countless possibilities of its use.

Kamal, meanwhile, was lured back to Baghdad, along with another of Saddam's sons-in-law—both were soon assassinated.

UNSCOM director Richard Butler said Iraq admitted that in 1992 it had
seventy-five SCUD missiles loaded with either biological or chemical weapons.
UNSCOM managed to destroy thirty of them but did not believe Iraq had, as
claimed, eliminated the other forty-five, Butler said. And increasingly in 1997
Iraq blocked UNSCOM activities. By November of that year President Bill Clinton
was publicly prepared to once again wage a U.S./Iraq war over the matter—
which would have constituted the first war in world history fought over the lack
of transparency[36] in bioweapons matters.

The U.S. House of Representatives released a Task Force on Terrorism and
Unconventional Warfare report on February 10, 1998. The report claimed that
Iraq still then possessed forty-eight SCUD missile launchers and forty-five mis-
siles, "the majority" of which were loaded with bioweapons. Further, there were
minimally 8,400 liters of anthrax and tons of chemical weapons in Iraq. The
congressional report further charged that Iraq possessed ship-mounted drones
capable of dropping biobombs on Europe and select spots in the Middle East.
Biobombs and missiles were hidden from UNSCOM in Sudan and Libya. In Wau,
Sudan, Iraqi scientists were once again manufacturing chemical weapons in the
German-made Yarmook facility. And, the report also claimed, in Libya, Iraqi-
made biological and chemical weapons were mounted on medium-range ballistic missiles capable of hitting targets up to 3,000 kilometers from Tripoli. About
a dozen Iraqi scientists were making anthrax and botulinum in the General
Health Laboratories, located in Tripoli.[37]

Though many experts felt that much of the report could not be substan-
tiated, it set a mood in Washington, and among U.S. allies.[38]

Frustrated by an endless cat-and-mouse game between UN inspectors and

Iraqi authorities the United States waged two crucial attacks in 1998. The first targeted Khartoum, Sudan, hitting a site the United States claimed was used by Iraqi-trained Sudanese to manufacture biological weapons. This alleged weapons factory was, according to the United States, used by the same terrorists who weeks earlier bombed U.S. embassies in Nairobi, Kenya, and Dar es Salaam, Tanzania. The Sudanese government insisted that the targeted factory was a legitimate pharmaceuticals plant.

As the House of Representatives debated impeachment of President Bill Clinton the U.S. Air Force, on December 16, 1998, launched the second military assault: a series of bombing sorties aimed at alleged CBW manufacturing and storage sites in Iraq.

"Saddam Hussein must not be allowed to threaten his neighbors or the world with nuclear weapons, poison gas, or biological weapons," Clinton said in a televised speech that day. "I have no doubt today that, left unchecked, Saddam Hussein will use these terrible weapons again."[39]

What did Iraq, Libya, and Sudan actually have? No one outside those countries really knew; Iraq denied everything, and nobody in Khartoum or Tripoli was saying anything about the matter.[40] By mid-2000 renewed allegations surfaced, claiming Iraq was developing a new viral weapon, and doing so right under the noses of UN inspectors.[41]

The Iraqi situation made all too apparent the absurd weaknesses of the Biological Toxins and Weapons Convention of 1972. It was a toothless wonder, full of good intentions but utterly lacking in the key components of effective arms treaties: transparency, power of inspection, verification, and enforcement. For several years biologists from all over the world had been gathering in Geneva for meetings aimed at finding ways to strengthen the Convention. But none could deny that bioweapons treaty enforcement was, as Joshua Lederberg had told the White House, infinitely more complicated and difficult than nuclear arms control. It was too easy to make biobombs, and too hard to find them.

Opposition to inspection was by no means restricted to so-called rogue nations, such as Iraq. Worldwide the pharmaceutical industry protested provisions that would allow outsiders unannounced entry into drug manufacturing plants for purposes of inspection. Yet without such investigative power no one could ever enforce the Convention, as bioweapons production sites and pharmaceutical plants use the same sorts of equipment and personnel.[42] Gillian Woollett, spokesperson for the Pharmaceutical Research and Manufacturers of America, said such provisions would discriminate against legitimate businesses, yet fail to find anything because, "a treaty is only for those who play cricket."

Matters were only worsened by evidence that bioweapons production was, indeed, proliferating.

"Biological weapons may emerge as the principal proliferation concern of the next decade," wrote analyst Brad Roberts.[43] "Reports indicate that eleven countries are pursuing offensive-oriented biological warfare programs, up from just four in the 1960s."

Henderson only touched on such diplomatic issues when he addressed his colleagues in Atlanta. Nor did he say publicly what he had secretly told government officials: someone will inevitably cause a deliberate epidemic within a decade's time. His primary mission, at Osterholm's insistence, was to reveal details of possible bioterrorism, in hopes that he would inspire the public health community, spurring them to action. So Henderson turned to Iraq's admitted anthrax program—one that made more than enough of the bacteria to kill every man, woman, and child living in the Middle East.

"Iraq acknowledges making 8,000 liters [of anthrax]," Henderson said in his speech. "The ramifications of even a modest release in a city are profound."

He spun a tale of public health horror, by once again turning his Atlanta audience's attention to history: a Soviet Ministry of Defense anthrax experiment that went tragically awry on April 2, 1979, in a facility outside the city of Yekaterinburg.[44] An accident occurred in the weapons production facility, causing the release of an unknown quantity of dry anthrax spores. Some seventy-seven residents of the zone immediately south of the plant came down with the classic symptoms of inhaled anthrax: illness within one to six days of exposure, marked by muscle pains, fatigue, malaise, fever, and a nonproductive cough. Sixty-six of those individuals, or 83 percent of them, got much, much sicker, developing infections in their brains or nervous systems, leading to meningitis and seizures; or getting huge colonies of bacteria in their lungs that produced local hemorrhages and slowly caused them to suffocate; they usually died in shock. The Ministry of Defense realized the organisms had escaped their containment and distributed prophylactic antibiotics and vaccines. The local fire department was ordered to wash down the entire city. Hospitals, schools, and restaurants were scrubbed clean with disinfectants.[45] As days wore on, more succumbed, leaving a trail of death along the path of prevailing winds. Livestock found as much as fifty kilometers southeast of the military plant also perished. In some human cases symptoms didn't strike until six weeks after exposure.

The town nearest the bioweapons laboratory, Chkalovsky, was particularly hard hit, with perhaps one thousand deaths—all covered up by the Soviet government, only coming to international attention at the behest of environmental officer Sergei Volkov nineteen years later.[46] The U.S. Los Alamos National Laboratory would analyze lung biopsy material from several of those victims in 1997, concluding that at least four different strains were in the lethal mist that spewed out of the laboratory, and the concoction was resistant both to available vaccines and antibiotics. Thus, the Ministry of Defense's actions following the accident were useless, and it is possible that nearly every person who was exposed to the anthrax mixture succumbed.[47]

After the incident—which Soviet authorities originally denied was related to man-made anthrax—local medical experts tried to publish autopsy reports on forty-two victims, demonstrating that the massive internal hemorrhaging and lymphatic activity in the lungs was due to *inhaled* anthrax, not bacteria accidentally eaten from ailing sheep (as was claimed by the Soviet authorities). The report was suppressed until 1993.[48]

Finally, in 1992, the new Russian President Boris Yeltsin acknowledged that the accident had been part of a vast Soviet biological weapons program. "There will be no more lies—ever," Yeltsin declared in a 1992 speech to the U.S. Congress. Denouncing Soviet deceptions and the Communist beliefs behind them, Yeltsin swore "that we will not let it rise again in our land."

Harvard's Matthew Meselson calculated that Russia's lethal accident involved less than one gram of anthrax spores, an amount that could easily be hidden from inspectors, airport security guards, or police.

"So along comes [Yekaterinburg] and there you are with cases coming down what—forty-two days," Henderson recalled. "So I talked to [anthrax] experts and said, 'What's the probability this is resuspended particles in the air?' And they were adamant that couldn't happen. Since that time Friedlander at USAMRIID[49] has exposed monkeys to low-dose anthrax. One monkey came down at fifty-nine days postexposure. And the more awesome thing: is it possible we don't have an endpoint for exposure?"[50]

So, Henderson reasoned, "Suppose that somebody throws a little bit of anthrax into the subway. When do we decide that it's safe to go back into the subway?" How long might lethal spores drift about in the air, or nestle into nooks and crannies from where, under proper conditions, they might emerge years later, be resuspended in the air, and kill unsuspecting victims?

Henderson was convinced that even a minuscule, barely detectable quantity of anthrax spores would have a profound public health impact on a North American, Japanese, or European city. Though the spores could not be spread from person to person, those microbes could circulate in the air for days, perhaps months.

"Emergency rooms would begin seeing a few patients with high fever and some difficulty breathing perhaps three to four days following exposure," Henderson told his public health colleagues. "By the time they were seen, it is almost certain that it would be too late for antibiotic therapy. Essentially all would be dead within twenty-four to forty-eight hours. No emergency room physicians or infectious disease specialists have ever seen a case of inhalation anthrax; medical laboratories have virtually no experience in diagnosis. Thus, it is probable that a delay of at least three to five days would elapse before a definitive diagnosis.

"Once the diagnosis was made, one would be faced with the prospect of what to do over the succeeding six weeks. Should vaccine be administered to those who might have been exposed? Unfortunately, there is at present little [anthrax] vaccine available. . . . Should antibiotics be administered prophylactically? If so, which antibiotics and what should be the criteria for exposure? What quantity would be required to treat an exposed population of perhaps 500,000 persons over a six-week period? Should one be concerned about additional infections occurring as a result of anthrax spores being subsequently resuspended and inhaled by others? Does one request everyone who has been anywhere near the city to report to his or her local physician for treatment at the first occurrence of fever or cough, however mild? Undoubtedly, there would be many persons with such symptoms, especially in winter. How does one distinguish these from the premonitory symptoms of anthrax, which may precede death within twenty-four to forty-eight hours? Can one imagine the reaction of a large population confronted with this array of problems?"

A year later officials from the Pentagon, several other federal agencies, and the New York City government would role-play an anthrax terrorism event. In their scenario somebody placed aerosolizers inside Grand Central Station at rush hour, releasing anthrax spores. Two weeks later in this scenario Gotham was a ghost town because millions had fled in panic, antibiotic supplies were long since depleted, more than a million people were dead or ailing, the New York Stock Exchange had collapsed, and law and order had broken down. It was, as one participant would put it, "a highly unprobable event, but one with such horrible, catastrophic probable outcome that it simply had to be taken seriously."

Botulinum toxin posed fewer uncertainties; its lethal power in minuscule doses was well understood. As was its ease of manufacture. The toxin was derived from a common bacteria, *Clostridium botulinum*, which is an anaerobic microbe that grows readily on fruits and vegetables stored at room temperature in airtight containers. The precise pathogenicity of the toxin could vary from one *Clostridium* strain to another, but botulinum toxin generally killed any untreated individual who ingested 10 ng of the substance: an invisible microfraction of a minuscule droplet. The same dose, multiplied by the number of kilograms an individual weighed, was lethal when inhaled. Guaranteed.

Antibiotics were useless if an individual was exposed to pure toxin. All medicines were worthless. Only the rarely available sera of botulinum toxin could prevent death due to botulism.

The toxin, a protein, directly attached itself to receptors on the surface of nerve cells, gaining entry to the neurons. Once inside, the toxin interfered in the biochemical processes essential to production of chemicals that transmitted signals among nerve cells. Unable to communicate, the neuronal system would break down. The medical result was an illness that initially looked a bit like the flu but increased in severity within twenty-four to forty-eight hours to include dizziness, slurred speech, difficulty walking, dulled and incoherent thinking, severe muscle weakness, uncontrollable drooling and nasal drips, difficulty breathing, inability to swallow, and loss of appetite. Eventually—in two to four days—the lack of signals in the brain and nervous system shut down one or more key body functions and the individual died.

Because the toxin was not a living thing, but a protein, it was easy to store and aerosolize. A very small amount went a long way. About seventeen pounds of a concentrated liquid suspension of the toxin would be enough to kill about half of all people living in a 27,710-acre area, assuming they were exposed. That wouldn't be many people if the target was the desert region of the Persion Gulf. But if it were Hong Kong, Tokyo, Los Angeles, New York City, or London, millions of lives could be lost.

Horrible as the impacts of anthrax or botulinum might be, D. A. Henderson's chief concern, he told the visibly agitated Atlanta audience, was the microbe he had defeated two decades earlier: smallpox. Smallpox, Henderson thought, was the ultimate weapon of mass destruction or, in military-speak, WMD. The possibility that samples of smallpox might fall into nefarious hands—indeed, might already have found their way onto the international arms market—was Henderson's obsession.

"You cannot really be sure," Henderson said, that all the former Soviet samples of smallpox were accounted for and safely stashed inside Siberian freezers. Even assuming goodwill all-around, "Virologists are such squirrels. A lot of this stuff goes in deep freezes . . . at no time could you ever say, no matter what you did, that there was no [smallpox] virus anywhere."

Henderson asserted that he considered evil use of the virus a grave potential as long as any sample of smallpox remained in a freezer anywhere in the world. Yet elimination of all remnants of a biological species—even a lethal pathogen—was repugnant to many scientists, so by WHO agreement the American and Russian samples remained alive, in frozen limbo.

"I have no question I'd like to see it destroyed tomorrow," Henderson insisted.[51]

Despite such fears, in April 1999 President Clinton revoked U.S. support for destruction of the smallpox stocks.

The smallpox virus was highly contagious, both by contact and, under close conditions, through the air. Unvaccinated people were thought to have one-in-three odds of dying of the disease, and most survivors of the dreaded virus were physically scarred for life.

In truth few people in 1999 were particularly knowledgeable about humanity's former nemesis. Even Henderson conceded that such death toll estimates were matters of conjecture on his part. When he wanted hard facts Henderson called Australia and spoke to an eighty-six-year-old college professor named Frank Fenner.

Despite his age Fenner was a remarkably prolific author and advisor to numerous government committees, both in Australia and all over the world. His modest office in the University of Canberra was covered with stacks of unfinished manuscripts, photocopied research papers, laboratory data, and the texts of speeches he'd recently delivered. The walls were lined with arguably the best smallpox library in the world. And as he spoke with a visitor the spry Fenner often leapt to his feet, sprinting across the room to grab the perfect reference book or article to bolster a given statement. Ignoring shocks of white hair that fell across his face as he peered through manuscripts Fenner would periodically shout, "Ah! There it is. Come look! Here are the bloody facts."

He nonchalantly guided his visitor through the factoids of the fearful virus—offering some of the same details he had given President Clinton and Australia's Prime Minister John Howard when he in 1998 argued in favor of destroying the smallpox viruses. Though Fenner was one of the world's top virologists in his youth, and had devoted decades to the study of smallpox, he had no delusions about the danger that his pet research subject's continued existence posed.

"In the absence of the vaccine in London about 10 percent of all deaths in any given year were due to smallpox," Fenner began, referring to eighteenth-century documents. "The death rate among those who got infected was 25 percent for adults and 40 to 50 percent in children. There was a time when they wouldn't give names to children unless they had survived smallpox."

After vaccination became commonplace in Europe the 1870 Franco-Prussian War answered the question of how long immunity might last, because the Prussian Army revaccinated all its troops, but the French did not. The French suffered 125,000 smallpox casualties, 18.7 percent of which were fatal. The Germans, in contrast, had only 8,463 cases with a mere 5.4 percent fatality rate.

Fenner stared from behind clear blue eyes, shrugged, and said, "That tells you that immunity cannot be expected to last very long. You cannot expect that many people in the world today are still immune, given all vaccination ceased in 1980."

When he had spoken to President Clinton in early 1998 Fenner told the American leader that he ought to support destruction of all smallpox viruses: "Why don't you come out in the open and say you're scared of bioterrorism," Fenner asked, arguing that would be the most honest rationale for destruction of the microbes.

"The president said, 'But you can never be sure it's eradicated,' " Fenner recalled. And unless every single virus were truly destroyed some stocks ought to be saved as research tools, Clinton had continued, in the event of a catastrophe—of a deliberate release.

Fenner lost the argument.

And in the summer of 1999 the U.S. Congress released a report claiming that both Iraq and North Korea were in possesson of secret smallpox stockpiles.[52] The congressional public pronouncement drew from intelligence documents submitted a year previously to President Clinton.[53]

Fenner had not known of the report when he spoke with President Clinton. But it would not have swayed him: the Australian remained convinced that every single smallpox virus on earth had to be destroyed. Having seen firsthand what the virus could do to the human body, and knowing how rapidly it could spread, Fenner was adamant.

The disease process itself was the stuff of which nightmares were made. When enemies in old England cursed, "A pox on you!" they knew whereof they spoke. So great were the early-twentieth-century death tolls that in 1995 it was estimated that vaccination programs administered a generation previously were in the 1990s saving *$1 million a day* in the United States due to elimination of smallpox illnesses and deaths.[54]

The virus entered the cells lining human lungs and made its way from there to the lymph nodes all over the body. This usually took one to three weeks, during which the infected human felt fine, had no limits on his or her physical activity, and may have come in contact with dozens—even hundreds—of other people, possibly passing on the lethal virus.

Once billions of viruses were made and dispersed all over the infected body through the bloodstream, then fever, muscle pains, vomiting, headaches, and back pain set in. Two days later a rash appeared, spreading from the face and forearms down the trunk to the genitals and legs. After forty-two to seventy-two hours the rash would erupt into large, obvious poxes, some of which could have been hemorrhagic, bleeding out viruses. Two weeks into the illness scabs appeared over the poxes, which shed at week three, leaving acnelike scars all over the body and often grossly disfiguring the victim's face.[55]

No one in the world had been vaccinated since 1980, Fenner again reminded his visitor; some countries ceased smallpox immunization in the early 1970s. In the United States vaccinations stopped in 1972, rendering two generations of children and young adults at the turn of the century vulnerable to the virus. "It is doubtful," Henderson concluded, "that more than 10 to 15 percent of the population today have significant residual smallpox immunity."

Until September 1997 Henderson had limited his discussions of biological weapons to classified arenas, fearing that such information was likely to provoke panic in some, and evil ideas in others.

"I was concerned, worried about copycats," Henderson explained. But then Osterholm had persuaded him to rethink his position. "What I think persuaded me was I found people in the defense community who could not get their superiors to look on this with more seriousness."

A newfound sobriety on the issue first hit Western intelligence communities—especially in London and Washington—in the early 1990s, as news of the true scale and scope of the Soviet Biopreparat program became known. Nobody in the West had previously realized the gargantuan scale of the Soviet biodeath program.

Americans got their first chilling glimpses of Biopreparat in 1996, and this reporter was the first U.S. journalist to gain entry to their facilities.

A gray pallor hangs over Siberia's largest city, Novosibirsk. In winter's twilighted sun a stern city yields on its outskirts to vistas of belching smokestacks and decaying concrete apartment complexes. Farther on the visitor encounters forests of white birch and pine trees. Stark and largely leafless in the winter chill, the trees beckoned viewers into a natural environment that was at once awesome and threatening. Even a late-winter chill was enough to remind visitors that wandering about in Siberia's version of nature was dangerous business, indeed.

About an hour outside the city, near a top secret town called Koltsovo, the forest yielded to an enormous complex of a hundred large concrete-and-steel buildings, surrounded by an eight-foot-tall concrete wall. Three rows of electric wires topped the wall. A bird landed on one and remained perched, harmlessly, on wires that once electrocuted unwanted guests.

A Russian Army guard, shivering inside a glass booth, acknowledged visitors, welcomed to VECTOR if they possessed proper credentials.[56]

Six years after the fall of the Soviet Union VECTOR, the USSR's premier virus weapons facility, had a seedy, has-been look to it. Weeds sprouted from long-neglected cracks in the sidewalks and streets. The roads had potholes big enough to challenge even 4×4 sports utility vehicles. Most exposed steel was covered in rust, and large cracks in the concrete facades of several buildings appeared to be more than mere eyesores. Some of the laboratories and offices seemed in danger of collapsing.

Broken windows went unrepaired, the bitter Siberian wind left to sweep into the now ghostly halls of research. Once a bustling minimetropolis dedicated to the scientific pursuit of perfect vectors of man-made disease, by the end of the 1990s VECTOR lay nearly silent; only the sound of the cold wind's relentless pummeling of the deteriorating buildings resonated in the otherwise empty air.

Scattered about, dressed in tattered uniforms, Russian soldiers idled away the long, cold, boring hours, guarding microscopic charges. In Building Number 1, for example, row upon row of industrial freezers housed Ebola, Lassa, smallpox, monkeypox, tick-borne encephalitis, killer influenza strains, Marburg, HIV, hepatitis A,B,C, and E, Japanese encephalitis, and dozens of other human killer viruses. And there were dozens of different strains of smallpox viruses—140 of them were natural, wild strains. Some were handcrafted by the bioengineers of VECTOR, giving them greater powers of infectivity, virulence, transmissibility.

The Russian Army guards didn't fully understand what was in Building Number 1. They called them "superbugs." But they did know that the bugs were terribly valuable—worth their weights exponentially in incalculable amounts of gold. These young men, and tens of thousands of their counterparts, were guarding more than three hundred once-secret cities, factories, and laboratory complexes in Russia—former places of plutonium production, nerve gas manufacture, uranium mining, and biological weapons development.

By 1996 the two million Russian soldiers, most of them conscripts, represented a disorganized, underpaid (or unpaid), demoralized horde, armed with military skills and weapons in a country rife with economic hardship. While its colonels and generals loudly lamented the grand days of Soviet global military power, Russia's young soldiers were simply killing time, staying off the country's swelling unemployment lists, and waiting for opportunities—other than combat—to present themselves. Meanwhile, corruption was rampant in all tiers of the military. The enlisted men smuggled drugs and guns, while high-level officers ordered their troops to build dachas for their mistresses, sold Soviet arms on the world armaments market, and siphoned off millions of rubles for personal use. Yeltsin's government made arrests—even jailed a deputy minister of defense and the leader of Russian ground troops. But the pillage continued.

Russia policy experts Daniel Yergin and Thane Gustafson note that Yeltsin's attempts to downsize the country's army resulted in an incredibly top-heavy military force: of 1.5 million personnel 690,000 were officers, 2,200 of them generals.

"In many respects the Russian military and the security police remain states within a state," Yergin and Gustafson wrote in 1995.[57] "The military and the security forces still command large blocks of property in the form of parks, sanatoria, dachas, housing, clubs, bases, schools, and institutes. There have been many charges recently that senior officers have been selling these properties back into private hands—or their own. But Yeltsin has so far refused to open an investigation that would embarrass his senior officers. Both the military and the security forces have resisted internal reform, as time goes on this resistance is likely to grow."

Russia's most popular military leader, General Lev Rokhlin, was murdered mysteriously in his vacation dacha in early July 1998, prompting rising discontent in army ranks. A host of other former generals, including General Alexander Lebed, quit the military for the world of politics.[58] In the summer of 1998 the Russian stock market collapsed, and for the sixth time since he came to power,

Yeltsin watched his economy spiral into a tailspin, and his approval rating drop to just 2 percent. By the summer of 1998 Russian soldiers were literally eating dog food: one thousand tons of processed animal parts originally manufactured for canine consumption. All heat and electricity was shut off at most barracks, and the streets of Moscow were lined with panhandling uniformed soldiers. One mentally ill sailor, driven over the edge by the Russian Navy's poverty, hijacked a nuclear submarine in September 1998.

In such an atmosphere of humiliation, economic chaos, and political instability, it would be no wonder if a handful of soldiers decided to smuggle one or two test tubes of hellish power—undetectable, as they would be—to whatever group offered an appropriate political agenda or large amounts of cash. With each passing day of chaotic activity in Russia, American and European analysts grew more anxious, openly worrying that the former USSR stockpiles might become sources of leverage—or worse—fall into the hands of political renegades or dissident soldiers.[59]

However, the job of transferring bioweapons technology from a Siberian laboratory to freezers in some other belligerent nation—or to the control of a rebel faction within Russia—could best be handled not by a soldier but by a scientist. Indeed, biological weapons were almost unique in the 1990s in that the substance was perhaps of less value than the intellect behind it. A scientist who genuinely knew how to genetically enhance and weaponize a lethal virus need not risk his life smuggling frozen test tubes, however minuscule they might be: all his buyers needed was the knowledge of molecular biology stored in his brain. At the onset of the Cold War nuclear physicists were in that position. But by the early 1980s biology had replaced physics as the intellectual property of greatest global value. And though Russia's civilian scientific enterprise was in shambles, no nation had more men and women with the intellectual knowledge of how to turn microbes into weapons.

In a 1992 meeting U.S. President George Bush told Russia's Boris Yeltsin that the American government had learned of Biopreparat and wanted the program stopped, its stockpiles destroyed. Yeltsin professed ignorance of all but the bare bones of the program. He asked retired General Anatoly Kuntsevich to prepare a report on the Soviet Union's bioweapons program. Kuntsevich reported later that year that the USSR's efforts were breathtaking in scope. Dozens of killers had been weaponized for missile, rocket, and aerial bomb delivery, including anthrax, Q fever, tularemia, and a host of viruses. And these weapons were tested over the years on Vozrozhdeniya Island, located in the middle of the rapidly receding Aral Sea.[60]

The Kuntsevich report described a complex web of bioweapons programs, including Biopreparat and separate labs and test sites run by the Ministry of Defense. In addition to forty-seven Biopreparat sites, the Ministry of Defense had several bioweapons factories, labs—even in heavily populated Moscow—and missile test locations. Biopreparat, the Soviet government claimed, was merely a civilian pharmaceutics program. And the Ministry of Defense's bioweapons program did not, officially, even exist. Estimates are, however, that some seventy thousand scientists and technicians were employed in these efforts before 1992. But by 1997 most were no longer to be found toiling in the laboratories, bioweapons factories, or test sites. Where did they go?

"Nobody knows," Dr. Kanatjan Alibekov said.[61] In 1992 Alibekov defected to the West, moved to Virginia, and Americanized his name, becoming Ken Alibek. The Kazakhstani biologist started doing bioweapons research in 1975, rising through the ranks of Biopreparat to become deputy chief of the Soviet program in 1987 when he was just thirty-six years old.[62]

"Nobody can answer" the question of where all those bioweaponeers went, Alibek continued. "Some, like me, are in the United States. Some are in Europe. But, you know, there is a very high probability that some are in the Middle East. When you are suggested to make one thousand dollars a month—for them this is a huge amount of money."

Alibek said that Biopreparat employed thirty-two thousand civilians and scientists in his day, and the bioweapons program of the Ministry of Defense involved another ten thousand military scientists. In addition, thousands of test site personnel released sample biobombs at Yekaterinburg (where the 1979 anthrax accident occurred), Kirov, Sergiyev Posad, and Strizhi. Among the achievements Alibek claimed this program made were the weaponizations described above, and: antibiotic-resistant (incurable) plague, missile-mounted smallpox, mass scale production of the hemorrhagic fever viruses Ebola, Marburg, and Machupo, and antibiotic-resistant anthrax.

In their top secret Sergiyev Posad laboratory the Biopreparat scientists figured out how to mass-produce smallpox viruses, cultivating tons every year. At VECTOR in 1990—just one year before the collapse of the Soviet Union—Alibek led a team that figured out how to weaponize smallpox, dispersing the deadly microbes in aerosols. And under orders from President Mikhail Gorbachev, Alibek insists, they manufactured eighty to a hundred tons of the horrible stuff yearly.

Ghastly as their work was, the Biopreparat scientists—including Alibek—were convinced that the United States had a comparable biological arsenal, and that a major Cold War confrontation was inevitable. Fed paranoid and often false "intelligence" by the KGB, the Soviet scientists felt certain that Americans would soon unleash equally abominable epidemic weapons, slaying innocent civilians from Vladivostok to Leningrad.

Alibek was one of the last Biopreparat defectors to reach the West—but the first to publicly reveal the program's secrets. Alibek's claims received a lot of attention in Washington and came under attack in some circles for being exaggerations. But Henderson found Alibek "quite impressive," and Osterholm said the Kazakhstani's information gave him nightmares.

In London's intelligence circles Alibek's assertions didn't appear too far off the mark. British intelligence debriefed Alibek's boss, Vladimir Pasechnik, in 1989 when he defected to the United Kingdom. From Pasechnik they learned that many apparently legitimate enterprises, such as plasma clinics and vaccine plants, were actually parts of the Biopreparat nightmare. And the Russian revealed that he had personally supervised modification of cruise missiles, making them bioweapons delivery systems.[63]

Alibek's defection a decade later and the information he provided disabused Western authorities of any hope that the Soviets had abandoned bioweapons development. President George Bush, in a report to Congress in 1993, decried Biopreparat, saying: "The Russian offensive biological warfare program, inherited from the Soviet Union, violated the Biological Weapons Convention through at least March 1992. The Soviet offensive bioweapons program was massive, and included production, weaponization, and stockpiling."

Why did tens of thousands of biologists eagerly participate in creating weapons of mass destruction out of life, itself? There was the paranoia—including KGB misinformation, of course. But there also were the perks, both personal and scientific. Biopreparat scientists ate tomatoes in January in Siberia, traveled widely, had decent apartments where such things were reserved for Communist Party bosses, got their children in the best colleges, and—perhaps most significantly for the biologists—had open, remarkably free access to Western scientific literature, even conferences. At a time when it was forbidden for physicians to read American, Western European, or Japanese medical journals and texts, Biopreparat researchers studied whatever they liked. While Soviet geneticists, molecular biologists, and agronomists struggled to recuperate from the tremendous damage wrought by Lysenkoism, the bioweapons scientists blithely rejected all of Lysenko's idiocy, devoured the writings of Watson, Crick, Monod, Berg, Bishop, Baltimore, and Varmus, and eagerly learned to manipulate DNA.

"There were two different worlds of science," Alibek later explained. "In 1973 the Soviet Union signed a decree to increase work in genetic engineering. A lot of money was put into development of this program. A lot of work was secret. The final objective was to develop these weapons. And there was *no* contact between civilian and military scientists. We started from scratch, but we used all knowledge obtained by the West. A huge analytical system existed just to analyze the work of the West."

When the Ebola epidemic broke out in Kikwit, Zaire, in 1995 a group of VECTOR scientists sent word that they had long-since developed a vaccine, and tested its use on human volunteers during the heyday of Biopreparat. VECTOR's deputy director Sergei Netesov didn't know, or wouldn't say, from whence the Russians originally obtained their Ebola samples, nor how they had been aware of unpublished findings in Western laboratories, but clearly he and his VECTOR colleagues were up to speed on Ebola when they attended the 1996 Antwerp meeting on the virus.[64] Stored in Russia, Netesov said, were supplies of Ebola antisera made by infecting sheep and goats in the BL-4 lab at VECTOR. Ten volunteers got the antisera, with no ill effects, Netesov claimed. And when one of his colleagues was bitten by an Ebola-infected monkey at VECTOR repeated injections with the antisera saved the scientist's life.

Even more ambitious than Biopreparat's efforts were those of the Soviet military's Ebola program, which also mysteriously obtained samples of the virus and of unpublished American laboratory findings. In military facilities Ebola antiserum was made in horses and tested repeatedly on human beings.[65]

While top physicians in the Soviet Union scrubbed their OR walls, ignorant of all modern infection control practices, the scientists in Biopreparat approached molecular biology as if it were another Cold War race to the moon. For a bright young biologist in the 1970s, Biopreparat offered enormous intellectual advantages over just about any other Soviet options. As further enticement the USSR threw in chauffeured cars, priority A access to food supplies, state-of-the-art laboratories, almost unlimited supplies of experimental animals, and marvelous intellectual puzzles to solve. It was, by Soviet standards, an almost irresistible offer.

And it all went away in 1992. Poof! No more privileged status. No more research money. No more large Soviet salaries. With the stroke of a pen in late 1992, Yeltsin eliminated nearly all funding for bioweapons research. Or tried to.[66]

Suddenly there were in the world thousands of unemployed, humiliated bioweapons scientists. That worried Chris Howson, Colonel Dennis Duplantier, Alexis Shelokov, and their British counterparts enough that they hatched an unprecedented trilateral scheme to put some of the Biopreparat personnel on the U.S. payroll. Beginning in 1997 the U.S. Department of Defense and National Academy of Sciences, working in a trilateral arrangement with their counterparts in Russia and the United Kingdom, began, as Shelokov put it, "trying to get [the Russian bioweapons labs] converted to peacetime work."

Shelokov and Howson sat on a National Academy of Sciences committee that hatched the plan and helped run it. Howson explained that his interest in the effort was "to get my hands on that wonderful expertise and put it to work on improving global health, not harming it."

Handfuls of Russian scientists at VECTOR and other Biopreparat facilities were funded by the Pentagon to work on developing vaccines against the terrible microbes they had created. They collaborated directly with USAMRIID and the CDC. Under the scheme, some of the Russian scientists would get a chance to work in public health labs in the United States, and Americans would get inside Biopreparat.

American scientists who visited the Biopreparat facilities during the late 1990s got quite a shock. The crude quality of the laboratories—even, in some cases, primitive nature—demonstrated that very, very dangerous work and sophisticated molecular biology could be done in just about any facility, provided adequate intelligence was at the helm.

For example, in its heyday, VECTOR boasted more than four thousand scientists and thousands more support personnel, all laboring in relatively new facilities (built in 1974). It was a state-of-the-art showcase for Russian talent during the 1970s. But by 1997 more than half the VECTOR scientists and workers were gone. And those that remained were a dispirited lot, toiling for little or no money inside a rapidly decaying infrastructure.

Deputy Director Sergey Netesov got a peptic ulcer trying to run the virtually unfunded VECTOR complex in 1997. It was hard to raise interest in VECTOR and her scientists. No one had heard of the facility, of Netesov, or of their work until 1992 when its existence was declassified. While recovering from surgery Netesov continued efforts to find funds for the faltering facility.

"We are trying to use any opportunity to make money for our institution," Netesov said, his face drawn and pale. "We tried to make vodka but we couldn't make money because the taxes were too high."

To put Netesov's position in perspective, having VECTOR forced to consider vodka production as a last-resort means of financing was roughly equivalent to saying the Los Alamos National Laboratory in New Mexico should cease receiving funds from Congress and go into the manufacturing of robot toys to subsidize its scientific research program.

Netesov, who was VECTOR's expert on the Ebola and smallpox viruses, was nearly leveled by simple garden-variety bacteria following his ulcer surgery. The widespread antibiotic resistance in Novasiask forced his doctors to prescribe expensive drugs, which Netesov had to purchase on his own.

Some distance away from Netesov's office, past several weed-choked lawns and fissured sidewalks, loomed Building Number 5: Molecular Biology. No guards blocked its entry. Yet on the eleventh floor Sergei Shchelkunov toiled away, searching for the gene responsible for virulence—in monkeypox. Shchelkunov, a recipient of the U.S. Department of Defense funding, was sequencing smallpox, cowpox, and monkeypox viruses, he said, "to get a picture of evolutionary interrelatedness of these viruses."

At the request of the CDC and World Health Organization, Shchelkunov was working out the genetics of the strain of monkeypox that broke out in Congo in 1997.

The entry to nearby Buildings Number 6 bore a forbidding sign in Cyrillic:

ATTENTION. THIS BUILDING OPERATES UNDER RESTRICTED CONDITIONS. ONLY THOSE IMMUNIZED FOR SMALLPOX MAY ENTER. But no security guards were present in 1997 to enforce the stricture. Down long, dark hallways, unlit with expensive electricity, were unoccupied laboratories, seemingly caught in time somewhere around 1975. Like a scene out of the *Twilight Zone* it appeared that work in most labs simply stopped one day, midway in experiments. Dusty lab benches were loaded with out-of-date equipment.

Upstairs Alexander Guskov worked by muted winter sunlight. His task, also funded by the CDC, was to preserve VECTOR's hundreds of smallpox samples, periodically venturing into the maximum containment facility to verify the vitality of the twenty- to fifty-year-old frozen viruses.

Biologist Valery Loktov was also a participant in the collaborative program put together by the U.S. National Academy of Science. He was heading studies of a river fluke that had contaminated all the fish in local Siberian rivers and was increasingly found in Japanese and North American fish.

"Eighteen to nineteen percent of the local [human] population is infected," as a result of eating those contaminated fish caught in Novosibirsk's rivers, Loktov said. And in hamster studies the fluke caused liver cancer 100 percent of the time.

While Loktov's work could be done in minimal security facilities, VECTOR was designed for study of Biohazard Level-4 microbes—those that could kill humans more than 50 percent of the time and are both incurable and, so far, not affected by any known vaccine. Until 1996 VECTOR's BL-4 labs were filled with activity, including research on Ebola and several other hemorrhagic fever viruses, encephalitis viruses, and some unusual forms of hepatitis.

A year later, however, the BL-4 labs were silent, and the cages of the maximum containment animal colony were empty. Though it brought financial hardship into the lives of VECTOR scientists, the disuse of their BL-4 facilities was probably a good thing.

"We need to modernize the facility if we want to attain U.S. BL-4 standards," Loktov admitted, pointing out the ominous lack of proper exhaust air treatment filters to prevent escape of dangerous microbes. U.S. scientists said that even more troubling was the fundamental design of the place—a sort of huge, hulking industrial mass that bore many of the same flaws seen in Soviet designs of factories and nuclear power plants. For example, enormous ducts crisscrossed the ceilings, and exposed heating and ventilation pipes wended around them. The net effect was a ceiling spaghetti of exposed iron and steel that would be impossible to decontaminate in the event of a microbial leak.

Close inspection revealed that most of the antimicrobe filters in the lab were installed in 1981 and were originally designed not for biological control but as nuclear radiation barriers. Washed latex gloves, ready for reuse, hung on a pipe in one lab. Most of the airlock and pressure doors were heavy iron portals first made for Soviet nuclear submarines.

The space suits Russian scientists toiled in while working with lethal microbes were terribly uncomfortable and heavy, grumbled one of Loktov's colleagues as he reluctantly climbed into one, demonstrating safety procedures. It was difficult to move around in the heavy rubber and steel suit, much less manipulate tiny syringes and test tubes full of deadly viruses.

"We've had no incidents of infection of our personnel who worked with such equipment," Loktov insisted. "But it is old equipment. Very old equipment. And now we have no funds for new equipment. It's very dangerous work."

In Building Number 1 of the enormous VECTOR facility were row upon row of freezers, all on triply redundant electrical systems that supposedly ensured that even if the primary electricity grid for Novosibirsk Oblast went down, the freezers would remain colder than ice. Which was a good thing because inside of them were trillions of living viruses and bacteria, the mere names of which conjured fear in medical circles. Were they to escape their iced test tube environs, sneaking past old leaky seals and poorly maintenanced freezer insulations, many of the microbes could flood into the air, possibly infecting VECTOR personnel and starting an epidemic.

This extraordinary reservoir of human predators was comparable to the CDC's deadly warehouse in Atlanta. But the multilayered, intense security that protected the CDC cache was not mirrored in Novosibirsk.

"You can't preclude the fact that anyone can walk out with biological samples," bioweapons expert Anthony Cordesman, of the Center for Strategic and International Studies in Washington, said. Had someone already done so, taking microbes away from VECTOR to another, undisclosed location? In classic Washington-speak, Cordesman said, "If people in government were free to confirm or deny [the rumors] they probably would not confirm. But that does not imply that there is no evidence for concern."

In a statement released by the U.S. secretary of defense on November 25, 1997, William S. Cohen underscored this fear: "The United States remains concerned at the threat of proliferation, both of biological warfare expertise and related hardware, from Russia. Russian scientists, many of whom are unemployed or have not been paid for an extended period, may be vulnerable to recruitment by states trying to establish biological warfare programs. The availability of worldwide information exchange via the Internet or electronic mail facilitates this process."

Even beyond such sinister causes, microbial leaks could have occurred if the facilities and staff morale were not upgraded. That was because those viruses and bacteria could not simply sit forever in Building Number 1 freezers. To remain viable they must occasionally be removed, thawed, and injected into animals or cells. Such passaging, as the process was called, had not been done for most of the samples for years—eventually Netesov and his staff would have to choose between allowing the samples to deteriorate beyond use, or risking their health and the safety of others by climbing into those old rubber space suits and going back inside the antiquated BL-4 labs.

Should something go wrong the scientists could have turned to their thirty-year-old rotary telephones, dialed through an old-fashioned manually manipulated Siberian switchboard, and called Novosibirsk for help. It would probably have been faster, however, to turn to their computers and send an E-mail to Washington.

When Colonel Duplantier and the National Academy of Sciences (NAS) group first in 1996 envisioned their cooperation effort it seemed that funding for about twenty researchers would be enough. But, Duplantier said later, "When we went to visit, the magnitude overwhelmed us."

At a workshop in Kirov in July 1997, Duplantier was stunned by the numbers for Biopreparat alone: "Forty-seven institutes, forty thousand employees,[67] nine thousand scientists, eleven full-scale research institutes with two thousand people with special expertise in pathogens. That's how big it was!"

Clearly, then, the U.S./U.K. effort to make work for Biopreparat scientists was inadequate. Funding twenty could hardly halt the activities of forty thousand.

Bottom line: there weren't forty thousand people toiling inside Biopreparat by 1997. Where did they all go?

"It's very difficult to discuss this topic. It's a very sensitive discussion," Alibek said nervously. "I know what kind of weapon could be developed just using regular rooms. For me, I need to have just a very simple lab, equipment. Even without any agent developed by any cell culture house. I can go outside, take just soil samples. I can manufacture weapons."

Back in the summer of 1995 Western intelligence sources had accused the Russian military of continuing its bioweapons effort, and of assisting Iran in mounting a similar program.[68] Amid allegations of misconduct—including continued bioweapons production and sale of expertise to other governments—among Russians funded by the U.S. program the congressional General Accounting Office attacked the effort in early 1999, and its future appeared precarious.[69] The White House, however, seemed committed to the program, as signaled in President Clinton's 1999 State of the Union address, which pointedly referred to the importance of U.S./Russian cooperation to prevent spread of biological weapons.

Though Biopreparat opened its labs to the United Kingdom and United States, the Ministry of Defense did not. Henderson, for one, was thoroughly convinced that tremendous danger lurked in those MOD labs. So was Alibek.

In the spring of 1997, *Jane's Weekly*, a prominent British military publication, published a claim—based on information from sources in Britain's spy center, MI6—that Russian scientists had developed a genetically modified strain of anthrax that was resistant to all vaccines and antibiotics. On the face of it the claim appeared preposterous to biologists acquainted with the bacteria.

But weeks later Chris Howson made one of several site visits to Biopreparat facilities and asked about the alleged anthrax superbug. He was told, "Well, we do have strains here that are resistant to vaccines and antibiotics." As rumors of that encounter spread around Washington, Henderson and Osterholm, as well as the army scientists working at the Fort Detrick biodefense laboratory, grew increasingly anxious. They all hoped that Howson had heard braggadocio, not truth.

With the opening of 1998, however, came British publication of work by A. P. Pomerantsev and his colleagues at the State Research Center for Applied Microbiology, a Biopreparat facility in Obolensk.[70] Using sophisticated genetic engineering techniques the Obolensk team inserted virulence genes from a humanly harmless species, *Bacillus cereus*, into *Bacillus anthracis*, the organism that causes anthrax. In addition, the *anthracis* strain upon which these feats were performed was bred for complete antibiotic resistance. The result, it appeared, was an entirely new form of anthrax that was, indeed, resistant to penicillin and vaccines, and was capable of residing dangerously inside human cells in ways never previously seen with anthrax.[71]

Lederberg was stunned.

"This, as far as I know, is the first example of an artificially contrived new pathogen," the elder statesman of biology told his colleagues. "The kind of obvious cat is out of the bag. . . . It's the thought of this kind of work going on sub rosa that is really the black cloud hanging over us."

USAMRIID's Colonel Arthur Friedlander issued a statement saying that the American military felt that the Russians had developed "a new potential biological warfare agent.

"This new organism is based on anthrax and is reported to be resistant to the Russian vaccine," Friedlander continued. "It likely causes disease by a different mechanism than that used by naturally occurring anthrax strains. The development of genetically engineered new organisms using anthrax and other BW agents is a potential threat which must be carefully evaluated."[72]

Pomerantsev's group had obtained all that they needed from Western sources simply by exploiting the candid atmosphere of basic biology and public health research. The technique that they used to modify *B. anthracis* was borrowed from work published by cell biologist Daniel Portnoy out of the University of California, Berkeley. Portnoy worked with a different organism—*Bacillus subtilis*. In 1990 he succeeded in forcing *B. subtilis* to express genes from another bacterial species—*Listeria monocytogenes*—resulting in new capacities for the organism. In particular, Portnoy crafted *Listeria* genes for destruction of red blood cells into *B. subtilis,* making a new bacteria that could punch holes in red blood cells and survive outside of the sort of soil milieu in which such organisms were usually confined. It was an innocent sort of study, of the type academic researchers in the West were most inclined to perform. Call it a "proof of principle," the Portnoy effort simply showed that the more primitive bacterial organism possessed the necessary machinery for sophisticated activity, provided it got the right genetic blueprints.[73]

Pomerantsev's group paid homage to the Portnoy work: "The cloning of the structural gene for the *L. monocytogenes* hemolysin into an asperogenic mutant of *Bacillus subtilus* resulted in conversion of a common soil bacterium into a parasite that can grow in the cytoplasm of a mammalian cell. According to this model an acquisition of hemolytic properties by *B. anthracis* strains can allow them to escape host immunity by means of penetrating host cells. The data presented in this study confirm the statement that 'the evolutionary leap from an extracellular existence to an intracellular lifestyle may only require the acquisition of a limited number of genes.' "

In other words, a literal garden-variety bug could be transformed into one that could thrive inside the human bloodstream.

Portnoy was aghast. It had never occurred to him that the work he did converting the *B. subtilis* soil bacteria into one that could live inside mouse cells could also apply to other soil organisms—including anthrax. When he first learned of the Russian experiment Portnoy tried to throw skeptical water on it, casting doubt on the veracity of Pomerantsev's publication. But as he pored over the paper Portnoy realized with horror what had been done: his work had been perverted: "Now I'm getting scared," he said.

Portnoy wasn't the only scientist whose work was used by the Obolensk group. In order to accomplish their anthrax conversion the Russians needed special *Bacillus cereus* genes—for insertion into the anthracis genome. Once again, they exploited the uniquely open atmosphere of basic biology research. In the days of active Biopreparat effort they turned to Dr. Werner Goebel, a prominent biologist in Biozenthrun, located in Wurzburg, Germany. When Goebel was told of the use his genes were put to he was flabbergasted.

"I don't have any direct contacts to the Pomerantsev group," Goebel E-mailed. "I don't even know him personally. It is of course possible that I sent him (or more probably) a related person the genes which we cloned many years ago from *Bacillus cereus* as I did to many other people after its publication. He (or the other person) certainly did not mention that he wanted to put it into *B. anthracis.*"

Former Biopreparat leader Alibek chuckled at Western science's naïveté.

"We started from scratch, but we used all knowledge obtained by the West," Alibek explained. "And Western scientists are very, very open people—it's not a problem to write a letter and get all you need."

The need to share biologic samples had led decades previously to creation of special repositories of organisms, cells, and other biological material. As it was expensive to store such things in individual laboratories, these repositories maintained massive biological inventories and shipped requested samples to researchers all over the world.

Members of the U.S. Congress expressed outrage in the late 1990s when it was learned that one such repository, American Type Culture Collection (ATCC) of Virginia, in 1995 shipped anthrax samples to a lab in Iraq and plague to right-wing Ohio zealot Larry Wayne Harris—who was arrested outside Las Vegas in early 1998 with a supply of anthrax.

But in his defense to enquiring journalists ATCC Director Dr. Raymond Cypress insisted that there was "a tradition of exchange of materials in science, and we have no documentation of almost any of it."

For example, twenty-seven research laboratories in America in 1997 published work on *Yersinia pestis*, which caused plague, "but only four got cultures from us. So where did the rest come from?"

Well, there were 453 such repositories worldwide, according to the *World Directory of Collections of Cultures and Microorganisms*, 54 of which sold or shipped anthrax, 64 sold the organism that caused typhoid fever, and 34 offered the bacteria that produced botulism toxin. And 18 repositories, located in fifteen countries, traded in plague bacteria. These repositories were located not only in the United States and Europe, but also in China, Bulgaria, Iran, Turkey, Argentina, and sixty other nations. Some such repositories did business over the Internet, offering overnight shipment of microbes for nothing more than a credit card number—no proof of scientific credentials was required.[74] Like the open atmosphere of scientific exchange that allowed Pomerantsev access to Portnoy's and Goebel's work, the exchange of microorganisms had traditionally been fettered by little more than the prices dealers charged for their bugs. And such openness was thought to help public health, giving scientists speedy access to strains of bacteria and viruses for research use.

By Cypress's estimations 99.9 percent of all research uses of such organisms were, indeed, in the interests of public health, basic science, or pharmaceutics development. And that underscored the key problem with biological weapons verification and enforcement: dual use. While there could be no legitimate civilian use for discovered VX gas supplies or pellets of weapons-grade enriched plutonium, both the equipment needed to produce bioweapons and, by and large, the biological agents themselves could be put to honest medical and research aims.

Unlike nuclear, conventional, or chemical weapons production, bioweapons required no dedicated facilities. Any pharmaceutical or medical laboratory and production site could be the source of manufacture. And bioweapons could be dispersed using standard agricultural equipment: pesticide sprayers or crop dusters.

Every step, then, in production of bioweapons involved materials and equipment that could be put to legitimate exploits: thus it was all, in national security parlance, "dual use." And the dual use dilemma lay at the heart of weapons inspection obstacles.

Some members of the intelligence community believed that the Biopreparat anthrax had made its way to Iraq—an allegation that could never be proven, even if samples of a vaccine and antibiotic-resistant strain of *B. anthracis* were found. The Iraqis could always assert that the bacterial strain arose naturally—on Iraqi, not Russian, soil. And whatever criminal proof the intelligence operatives claimed to possess implicating a Russian scientist or two was never made public—indeed, it probably never could be without compromising sources. These uncertainties made it possible to use the act of accusation as a diplomatic weapon, tarnishing the reputation of a nation without offering a shred of proof. It seemed almost as bad as the state of diplomatic affairs during the Cold War.

Allegations concerning an illness dubbed Gulf War Syndrome further underscored the tremendous difficulties in diagnosing an ailment and determining its cause in the context of war. Did thousands of Allied soldiers suffer a unique ailment caused by exposure to a chemical or biological substance during the Persian Gulf War? Several veterans groups and their physicians said yes, pointing to a long list of symptoms shared by many returning soldiers. A host of causes were suggested: pesticides, U.S. Army vaccines, fumes from burning military vehicles, smoke from a bombed Iraqi chemical weapons depot, chronic fatigue syndrome, mass hysteria. Years after the war's end debate still raged in the United States, Canada, and the United Kingdom over every conceivable aspect of Gulf War Syndrome. The inability to resolve the public quarrel—even to reach consensus on whether Gulf War Syndrome existed—illustrated how difficult it would be to sort fact from fiction in any conflict if an unusual or subtle organism were inflicted on combat troops.

The Gulf War, coupled with news of Pomerantsev's superbug anthrax invention, prompted U.S. Defense Secretary William Cohen in May 1998 to allocate $130 million for anthrax vaccination of 2.4 million active duty military personnel. Almost immediately resistance surfaced as recipients of the vaccine claimed the immunization had caused severe health problems, and more than a hundred servicemen and women faced summary courts-martial rather than be vaccinated. As protest spread among U.S. soldiers, sailors, and airmen it became disturbingly obvious that Americans could no longer be counted upon to willingly undergo mass immunizations—even in the face of possible bioterror threats.

The anthrax vaccine was only one of many immunizations U.S. military personnel were required to receive. The lengthy list included vaccines against cholera, Japanese encephalitis, plague, typhoid, and yellow fever. No soldiers risked courts-martial over those vaccines, even though some of them posed significantly greater health hazards or were of a far lower efficacy. For example, the cholera vaccine was no longer recommended by WHO or the CDC because it could actually cause cholera in some people and offered only marginal immunological protection. The CDC had abandoned the plague vaccine, finding that cheap, low-risk prophylactic doses of tetracycline offered fine protection for individuals in *Yersinia*-infested areas. And the Japanese encephalitis vaccine produced severe allergic reactions in a fair percentage of recipients. Yet no protests were raised against those vaccines.

Between May 1998 and March 1999 more than 630,000 U.S. military personnel received the anthrax vaccine: forty-two of them, or 0.007 percent, suffered adverse reactions, seven of which were severe enough to require hospitalization. All recovered fully.[75]

Yet the antimilitarist peace organization Citizen Soldier waged strong protest against the anthrax vaccination campaign. The group's attorney Todd Ensign said that there was "good faith concern" about anthrax vaccination, boiling down to, "what is the hurry here? Is there some other agenda? I think it's, Number One, this has connotations of warfare, so that concentrates the mind. Cholera, diphtheria—they're just not dramatic in the same way. It raises the question, 'Wait, does this mean I'll be exposed to anthrax?' "[76]

Via the Internet, Citizen Soldier spread the gospel of anthrax vaccine protest. The group's perspective was decidedly from the left. But there were plenty of other groups on the political right who used the Internet to raise concern about the vaccine. Human Life International, an antiabortion group, alleged that the vaccine was laced with human chorionic gonadotrophin—a female pregnancy hormone—as part of a massive, top secret campaign to sterilize U.S. soldiers. Behind the effort, the group claimed, were WHO, the World Bank, and the Rockefeller and Ford Foundations. At a Gulf War veterans Web site soldiers were advised that human fetuses were destroyed, and their body fluids used in the anthrax vaccines. In darker conspiratorial tones various fundamentalist Christian and far-right groups warned of a NATO plan to take over America by weakening U.S. troops, giving them an anthrax vaccine that was filled with chemicals that would spark an autoimmune response, thereby turning the vaccinee's immune system against his own body. Similarly fantastic theories were espoused by Canadian opponents of that country's military anthrax vaccine program.

Some members of the U.S. Congress and its General Accounting Office were inclined to accept the notion that autoimmunity-inducing compounds were in the anthrax vaccine. And though there was absolutely no evidence to support the claims, GAO insisted that a chemical called squalene had been incorporated into the vaccine as an adjuvant. Further, GAO insisted that squalene sparked autoimmune responses.[77]

Social historian David Rothman of Columbia University saw a larger lesson in the suspicions and protests among active duty soldiers and veterans—one that he suspected would cloud all civilian and military vaccine campaigns aimed at offsetting bioterrorism. During World War II, he said, Americans had been very enthusiastic about the marriage of military and medicine, a union that produced mass penicillin use for bacterial diseases, refined blood transfusion procedures, and chloroquine prophylaxis for malaria.

With the advent of the Cold War after 1945, however, Americans began to feel uneasy about Pentagon medical efforts, particularly amid rumors of cover-ups regarding radiation dangers.

"Fear of the mad, dangerous scientist is something ancient in American culture. We also have long had anxieties about our government, about the idea of government. And the military has evoked its share of anxieties," Rothman explained.[78] "Until recently, however, all of these were separate suspicions. What you have now is something new."

To accept that the anthrax vaccine was inherently more dangerous than, for example, the almost universally condemned cholera immunization, Americans had to reject the repeated, contrary assertions of the White House, an assortment of federal agencies, the Department of Defense, and the nation's medical science establishment.[79] It constituted a constellation of doubt never previously expressed by Americans, Rothman insisted.

At Johns Hopkins University D. A. Henderson's Working Group on Civilian Biodefense carefully analyzed all available information on anthrax, concluding that any plan to protect American citizens against terrorist use of the bacteria had to include vaccination.[80] Without either immunization or immediate prophylactic antibiotic use inhalation of anthrax spores, the Group concluded, would be fatal to 80 percent of those who were exposed. The Group strongly recommended vaccination of emergency response personnel.

But the antivaccination movement inside the military revealed how hard it might be to gain compliance with immunization from average Americans. This, despite mounting evidence that anthrax and other bioweapons were finding their ways into the hands of more rogue nations.

As the twenty-first century approached, the following nations possessed biological weapons, developed for missile or large-scale aerosol delivery to enemy targets: Iraq, Iran, Syria, Libya, China, North Korea, Russia, Israel, Taiwan, and possibly Sudan, India, Pakistan, and Kazakhstan.[81]

The list cut across power blocs, ideology, political organization, and geography.[82]

In addition to these countries many nongovernmental international political organizations were thought to be developing or seeking to purchase bioterrorist weapons. Intelligence sources in Europe and the United States, including retired Central Intelligence Agency Director John Deutch, insisted this was the case, though for security reasons details were not provided.[83]

Beyond advances in delivery capacities, the sophistication of the bioweaponry itself was expected to improve by leaps and bounds. Until 1985, all of the world's bioweaponeers were stuck with the same limited list of agents that could be assured of killing thousands of enemies and were deliverable with missiles or other systems. Each nation knew the list and stockpiled antidotes and vaccines. It was a standoff.

But as the Pomerantsev case illustrated, biology was intellectually to the 1990s what physics was in the 1940s and 1950s: a field of exponential discovery. What seemed impossible in 1980 was done by 1990 and ho-hum fodder for high school biology classes in 1995. In 1993, the U.S. congressional Office of Technology Assessment (OTA) predicted that:

Genetic engineering is unlikely to result in "supergerms" significantly more lethal than the wide variety of potentially effective biological agents that already exist, nor is it likely to eliminate the fundamental uncertainties associated with the use of microbial pathogens in warfare. However, gene-splicing techniques might facilitate weaponization by rendering microorganisms more stabile during dissemination (e.g., resistant to high temperatures and ultraviolet radiation). Biological agents might also be genetically modified to make them more difficult to detect by immunological means and insusceptible to standard vaccines or antibiotics.[84]

Biology moved along far more rapidly than even the OTA anticipated. A multinational effort in the 1990s to determine the sequence and identify all of the genes of the human genome charged ahead at a pace far exceeding expectations. And it inspired efforts to sequence the DNA or RNA of microbes. With that came unwitting identification of unique targets in humans, and weapons in microbes.

In a 1996 editorial the British medical weekly *Lancet* noted that "a concern has slowly surfaced about biological weapons with selective ethnic targets. Anyone voicing such concerns at a meeting of molecular biologists or infectious disease specialists risks scorn. 'That's the stuff of science fiction.' But is it?"

Determining the genetic sequence of a virus, such as Ebola, was no longer much of a feat. John Mekalanos at Harvard Medical School figured out how to quickly find genes in bacteria that were responsible for virulence.[85] At Stanford University Stanley Falkow developed a way to see which genes in the organism that caused typhoid fever were switched on first, after the pathogen infected human cells.[86] This quick and dirty technique singled out virulence genes. Influenza researchers, in hopes of spotting a naturally emerging superflu before it caused a 1918-type pandemic, sequenced that virus and identified some of its key pathogenesis genes.[87] In 1998 scientists at the Frederick Cancer Research Center in Bethesda determined, genetically, exactly how anthrax kills human cells.[88]

By the late 1990s the tools were in hand. There was a massive pool of bioengineers.[89] They had genetic blueprints to guide their efforts.[90] There were precedents. And there were stockpiles. Western militaries hardened their biodefenses, vaccinating troops, stockpiling antitoxins, storing appropriate antibiotics, purchasing bioprotection suits and masks, carrying out war games drills involving biologic weapons, and supporting research on potential biodetection devices.

But protection of innocent men, women, and children was another matter.

"There's just been *no* looking at this on the civilian side," Henderson lamented.

In his speech that spring morning in Atlanta, Henderson warned that no one had a master plan for dealing with the collateral impact of bioweapons on civilians located around a combat zone—or the deliberate impact of bioterrorist damage inflicted on an unsuspecting community.

"To date, the focus of concern with respect to countering civilian terrorism has been almost wholly on chemical and explosive weapons and a response which is, at most, a modest extension of existing protocols to deal with a hazardous materials incident," Henderson intoned. "A chemical release or a major explosion is far more manageable than the biological challenges posed by smallpox or anthrax."[91] Following an explosion or a chemical attack, the worst effects are quickly over; the dimensions of a catastrophe can be defined; the tolls of injuries and deaths can be ascertained; and efforts can be directed to stabilization and recovery. Not so following the use of smallpox or anthrax. Day after relentless day, additional cases could be expected—and in new areas.

Comparisons to the impact of nuclear weapons, once considered ridiculous, arose in every 1990s policy discussion of biological warfare. The key similarities were their lasting effects long after an initial explosion or release and the likelihood that nearly all of the dead would be civilians. For example, national security analyst Brad Roberts felt that biological weapons constituted the "poor man's answer to the nuclear bomb," creating the possibility of asymmetric strategies of conflict.

"In such strategies," Roberts wrote, "weaker states seek to pit their strengths against the weaknesses of stronger ones in order to deter intervention or prevent the stronger state from bringing to bear its full military potential."[92]

The strategic superiority of biobombs over nuclear weapons, under such circumstances, would be greatly enhanced, Roberts argued, by creation of what might be termed "designer bugs," genetically engineered for such strategic advantages as racial targeting. With nuclear weapons there was always the risk that winds would carry radioactive fallout toward the bomber's own troops, and no living creature was immune to the mutational impact of ionizing radiation. But bioweapons designed to exploit a specific genetic vulnerability might be harmless to the inflictor's troops while devastating not only opposing armies, but also entire civilian populations.

As writer Robert Wright put it, "If someone asks you to guess which technology will be the first to kill 100,000 Americans in a terrorist incident, you shouldn't hesitate; bet on biotechnology."[93]

When U.S. Navy Commander James K. Campbell contemplated preparedness for biological weapons attacks he spoke of "the postmodern terrorist," who did not hesitate to target civilians. Campbell said that "of increasing occurrence is the ultraviolent terrorist act followed by silence," such as the bombing at the 1996 Olympics in Atlanta. Or the 1998 bombing of the U.S. embassies in Dar es Salaam and Nairobi. Such events, he argued, "suggest a 'shift' in terms of the message the terrorist was supposedly sending. Where traditional terrorists used the event to gain access to a 'bully-pulpit' to air their grievances, these silent terrorists send a silent message creating a superordering sense of overwhelming fear and vulnerability."

An action that seemed unimaginably ghastly to most people, Campbell said, was precisely the kind of step the new "postmodern terrorist" was likely to take. Unfettered by governmental restraints—indeed, unconnected to any government—this novel terrorist, Campbell argued, was likely to be so strongly motivated by religion or political issues that the damage inflicted by his or her actions could far exceed that caused in more traditional conflicts. The reason: the postmodern terrorist was often willing to take measures that were so dangerous as to be suicidal, as well as homicidal.

In the United States, Senator Sam Nunn was the politician in the 1990s who appeared most knowledgeable about defense and national security issues. Following the Aum Shinrikyo attack in Tokyo, Nunn, echoing concern about postmodern terrorism, said: "The number one security challenge in the United

States now and probably for years ahead is to prevent these weapons of mass destruction, whether chemical, biological or nuclear, and the scientific knowledge of how to make them, from going all over the world to rogue groups, to terrorist groups, to rogue nations."[94]

"As we enter the twenty-first century, we may well be facing weapons of mass destruction used not on the battlefield by warriors," wrote U.S. Air Force Lieutenant Colonel Terry Mayer, "but among dense population centers by deranged nonnation states—a sobering perspective."[95]

In May 1993, President Clinton echoed those sentiments in a key speech to the Annapolis Naval Academy, saying: "Rather than invading our beaches or launching bombers, these adversaries may attempt cyber-attacks against our critical military systems and our economic base . . . or they may deploy compact and relatively cheap weapons of mass destruction."

Preparing to meet the challenges posed by the use of biological weapons at the hands of such groups or individuals was an enormous task that was only beginning to be tackled in Europe and the United States at the turn of the century.

Just ask retired Atlanta fire chief Don Hiett. In 1996 he was in charge of all emergency responses for the Olympics, and in preparation he saw FBI files on attempted and successful terrorist events never made public. When it came to bioweapons, Hiett said, "We are far, far short of where we need to be. We're far, far short in detection. And as first responders we don't think in the big picture."

For example, when a bomb exploded during an Olympic rock festival Hiett was one of the first responders on the scene.

"Honey, let me tell you," Hiett said in a Georgia drawl, "nobody had the mind-set to think of biological or chemical. And nobody will think of it until we start seeing the canaries dropping in the coal mine. . . . There was some forethought, and it was mainly a chemical thing. Biologicals—first off, most people don't even think bombings happen in America. Well, let me tell you, there's twenty a day!" And increasingly, Hiett continued, terrorist threats and actions involve biological weapons. "The potential is here, there's no doubt about it."

Though twenty-seven American cities participated during the late 1990s Department of Defense–run training exercises, all of the nation's municipalities remained ill-prepared for such an eventuality. Henderson insisted that the focus of training was wrong: there needed to be a sustained, long-term effort to prepare emergency room and public health personnel, firefighters, or police.[96]

Were a terrorist to release what Henderson considered the ultimate weapon—smallpox—the once universally vaccinated population would be horribly vulnerable. The U.S. government had, two decades earlier, stockpiled enough vaccine for about 15.4 million people,[97] and the World Health Organization had warehoused 500,000 doses in the Netherlands. Various additional national stockpiles totaled about sixty million more doses, of varying quality and potency. Clearly, were smallpox released the majority of the world's population would be vulnerable and, given smallpox's 30 percent kill rate, nearly two billion people could die.

Two *billion* human beings.

In 1999 the picture actually worsened, amid discovery that the U.S. smallpox vaccines had severely deteriorated. Originally made in the 1970s by the Wyeth pharmaceutical company, the vaccines were stored at the CDC facilities in Atlanta, in the form of freeze-dried crystals, parceled out in 100-dose quantities inside vacuum-sealed glass tubes. The tubes were further sealed with rubber stoppers held tight by metal clamps. To their dismay CDC investigators discovered that condensation had built up inside many of the glass tubes, indicating that the rubber stoppers had decayed and vacuum pressure had been lost.

The Food and Drug Administration said that the nation's smallpox vaccine supply "failed quality assurance." And that was only the first of several problems shocked government and private scientists would discover as they scrutinized America's smallpox vaccine stockpile. The scrutiny only occurred because the White House, anxious about evidence that samples of the deadly virus might have been distributed beyond the two WHO-designated repositories, called for production of additional vaccine supplies for the U.S. armed forces. Investigators thought it wise to first check the status of the original stockpile—one that six presidents had, apparently mistakenly, assumed would protect the citizenry if ever needed. It was a good thing such eventuality hadn't arisen.

The condensation, it turned out, was simply problem number one. The second concerned a fluid, or diluent, that was supposed to be mixed with the freeze-dried crystals just before vaccination. The diluent had what was called a "brilliant green" indicator in it that was supposed to help the vaccinators see the droplets passing out of the needle onto the recipient's arm.

But the "brilliant green" had changed color, and appeared to be deteriorating rapidly.

And there was another problem: the needles. Smallpox vaccination is unlike other immunizations in that it cannot be administered as a simple shot. Rather, the droplets of vaccine must be scratched into the skin using a special instrument called a bifurcated needle. It turned out that the U.S. stockpile contained fewer than one million such needles, and nobody in the world still manufactured them.

But the largest problem was what scientists called VIG, or variola immunoglobulin. Whenever a large number of people were, back in the 1960s, vaccinated against smallpox a handful of them—less than 1 percent of all vaccinees—suffered severe adverse reactions. For them a quick shot of VIG was a lifesaver. CDC investigators became aware in 1999, however, that there were only enough stockpiled VIG doses to handle 675 adverse reactions, or the number of such events that would typically occur if three million people were immunized. And even those few doses of VIG seemed compromised as they had taken on a pink hue, rather than the acceptable colorless status of freshly made supplies.

Were an emergency to occur, the U.S. population would be completely vulnerable to smallpox. And though the other European and South African vaccine stockpiles hadn't undergone similar scrutiny there was little confidence in those, either. The last time a mass emergency vaccination had taken place in the United States was 1947, when a traveler from Mexico spread smallpox in New York City. Vaccines were then readily available, and 6.35 million New Yorkers were immunized in less than four weeks—a feat that a half century later U.S. authorities would not, were it necessary, be able to repeat. In 1961 a similar mass vaccination campaign was executed following appearance of smallpox cases in England: 5.5 million people were immunized in a month's time. A decade later the recognition of cases in Yugoslavia prompted rapid vaccination of 20 million people in that country. Were a smallpox crisis to emerge, in 2000, neither of these efforts could be repeated.

At the urging of the White House the Department of Defense had in 1997 awarded the small biotechnology company Dynport a $30 million contract to make 300,000 doses of smallpox vaccine for military personnel. It was as a result of queries from Dynport that the CDC and FDA had investigated the status of the old vaccine stockpiles. And upon learning of the sorry state of that supply the White House asked Dynport to look into the feasibility of making another forty million doses for civilian use.

Dynport looked into the question and came back with an offer—forty million doses for $1 billion.

"Outrageous," hollered Henderson. "I looked at what we paid at WHO in 1974 for vaccines we got from Switzerland, the U.S., the U.K. and Canada. It was between a half cent and 1.7 cents per dose. Now, allowing for inflation to, say, 10 cents, or heck, let's even say to $1 a dose, okay? You should only be talking about $300,000 to meet the DOD contract and, at most, $40 million for the civilian side."

While the haggling continued between Dynport and federal officials the Wyeth company quietly set to work making fresh vaccine diluent. But no company stepped forward to manufacture the needed forty to fifty million bifurcated needles. And the Baxter pharmaceutical company was having a tough time figuring out just what happened to the VIG supplies it had made twenty years earlier.[98]

Large-scale stockpiling of smallpox vaccines in key civilian zones of the United States and Western Europe might, after all, be of limited value for two reasons: only several days after exposure would individuals develop symptoms diagnosable as smallpox, by which time thousands—even millions—would have been exposed; and only several days or weeks after vaccination would individuals have developed sufficient antibodies to stave off infection.[99]

For other vaccine-preventable microbes, such as anthrax, the lag time between inoculation and development of powerful antibodies could be far longer—up to a year, even with boosters. And of course vaccines would be of no value whatsoever if the culprits created vaccine-resistant killer germs. Further, a determined enemy could simply try a succession of microbial weapons—or use a cocktail at the outset—defying even the best organized population vaccine defenses.

In the United States the federal model for civilian protection was essentially patterned after that of the military. Based on recommendations made in the spring of 1998 by a White House panel of scientific experts, President Clinton ordered hundreds of millions of dollars worth of vaccine stockpiles, advanced biodefense training for National Guard troops, and accelerated urban preparedness based on a military response model.[100]

The strategy almost immediately came under fire from public health advocates.

"I look at it this way," Henderson said following a 1998 U.S. Senate hearing on bioterrorism. "This is our main defense: state and local public health, local doctors. Here we are investing $300 million for fifty-plus twenty-two-man National Guard units, and what possible relevance are they to the problem? Why aren't we putting a billion dollars into strengthening what is actually our frontline response. Hell, we haven't even got a strategy!"

At the same Senate hearing,[101] Minnesota's Osterholm grew indignant when asked what it would take to get America's cities prepared to respond to bioterrorism: "There is simply nothing that scares me like this issue. . . . Today you hit a major building in this country with an aerosolizing device with smallpox, it could quickly be all over the country. The orientation here in Washington, D.C., is on chemical terror. But giving the National Guard $300 million does nothing for bioterrorism. The key is local public health."

"What I'm trying to determine is how much money you need to spend on the three Ps: planning, preparedness, and prophylaxis," CDC economist Martin Meltzer explained.

To figure that out, Zimbabwe-born Meltzer imagined a small city of 100,000 people, a calm warm evening, and a crop duster. That plane was loaded with one of three deadly bacteria: anthrax, brucella, or tularemia. A cloud of microbes enveloped the city, exposing everyone to its deadly contents. What would happen?

Meltzer discovered that in the case of such treatable bacterial diseases the severity of the attack, both in terms of lives lost and cost to the community, would depend on how quickly authorities recognized what had occurred and how rapidly they distributed prophylactic antibiotics to the population to prevent individual illnesses.

"The cost of delay—the cost of not being prepared, in the case of anthrax," Meltzer explained, "if you wait to day six [after the attack] before starting your prophylaxis program the difference in deaths is five thousand if you start on day one versus thirty-five thousand on day six."

The assumptions built into Meltzer's model were, if anything, overly optimistic. Doctors correctly diagnosed the exotic diseases, ideal treatments were administered, hospital costs were low, and if local authorities decided to administer prophylactic antibiotics to the population they, in their wisdom, selected the perfect drugs and had ready supplies on hand. Such assumptions were, Meltzer admitted, "a bit on the rosy side." Nevertheless, they revealed clearly that the costs of delay, and the numbers of lives saved with rapid response, were profound.

For example, if local officials in Meltzer's mythological city of 100,000 picked the correct antibiotic and administered it in the proper dose within twenty-four hours of an attack, about 5,000 people would die and the total cost of medical care for the community would be $128 million. If, in contrast, it took six days for authorities to realize what had happened, correctly diagnose the microbial culprit as anthrax, and commence mass antibiotic prophylaxis with the appropriate drug, nearly 35,000 people would perish and treatment costs for the dead and ailing would total $26.2 billion.

In terms of fiscal costs the difference was exponential. If an anthrax attack were recognized within twenty-four hours and widespread doxycycline prophylaxis was administered to the entire exposed population the costs for treatment, hospitalization, and lost productivity due to illness or death would be $3.7 billion. If the prophylaxis didn't commence until day six, the attack would cost the community nearly $25 billion—just a billion less than what no response at all might cost.

When asked what such an attack might cost a large metropolitan area such as New York and its neighboring suburbs, Meltzer thought out loud: "How much more difficult is it to aerosolize an agent to infect a population of fourteen million? Is it impossible? No. But there is some difficulty. If time isn't a factor, no problem. . . . Let's see, if 100,000 people were exposed would you have to prophylaxe fourteen million?"

Meltzer stopped his mental computation, concluding that a clever terrorist wouldn't even try to infect everyone. In a large, dense city, "How much do they actually have to disperse in order to create an all-out panic?"

In a larger urban center, then, the true costs of a bioterrorist event might be secondary factors associated with panic, such as the collapse of the stock market in New York or commodities market in Chicago.

So, from Meltzer's point of view, cities large and small would be well advised to get ready, stockpiling supplies of relevant antibiotics, vaccines, and general medical supplies.[102] Of these three, Meltzer concluded antibiotics were the most crucial. Of slightly less importance was preparing local police and military responders to contain order and forestall mass hysteria.

"Do you want to be so scared that you paralyze yourself," asked Meltzer rhetorically. "Or do you want to become alerted, informed, and prepared? . . . You have to be prepared to deliver postexposure prophylaxis to a large number of people. That is the challenge that bioterrorism represents."

Meltzer was, of course, the first to admit that his scenario didn't speak to the potentials of either drug-resistant bacteria or viruses. Such agents, Meltzer asserted, were too fearsome for even he to contemplate, as few potentially lethal viral illnesses were treatable or preventable with available vaccines.

The Meltzer study was one of the key influences on the Clinton administration's decision to develop antibiotic stockpiles for use in defense of civilians. Former New York City Commissioner of Health Dr. Margaret Hamburg was placed in charge, working inside the U.S. Department of Health and Human Services. Her tasks were to determine which antibiotics could actually save lives in the event various bacterial agents were released in a U.S. city, what the shelf lives of those drugs were, how they ought to be stored, and how in a crisis they could be equitably and rapidly distributed. It was, Hamburg said, "an almost overwhelming challenge."

Henderson asserted that, were a highly infectious virus released, the primary protection would be air-filtered quarantine units. But few hospitals had such facilities, as New York City discovered earlier in the decade when the superdrug-resistant group W strain of tuberculosis appeared on AIDS wards in several facilities.

Recognition that a bioterrorist event has occurred was the key, regardless of whether the agent was bacterial or viral. And if Navy Commander Campbell was correct, the modern bioterrorist wasn't likely to issue warnings, claim credit, or in any way acknowledge the event.[103]

It would be a surprise.

Local authorities "probably aren't going to be able to recognize it has happened . . . until the incubation period is over," Clark Staten, executive director of the Emergency Response and Research Institute in Chicago, insisted.[104] "And by then you've got it spread over a wide area. And it may take longer to recognize there's a pattern going on."

It will begin, the experts say, with a couple of cases of "flu" in one hospital, three in another, and so on. Hours or days may pass before health care workers start wondering why there is so much "flu"—and most of these diseases do begin with flulike symptoms—flooding into the hospitals. Eventually someone would call the local public health department, alerting officials that some sort of epidemic is occurring, or so authorities hope. Of course when an unusual encephalitis outbreak struck New York City during the summer of 1999 only one physician took note and made such a call to Department of Health authorities. Retrospective investigation revealed that New Yorkers had been taking ill and dying of encephalitis for weeks before the city realized what was going on. And once the existence of such an outbreak was known federal CDC scientists incorrectly diagnosed the cause as St. Louis encephalitis. Weeks passed before academic researcher Dr. Ian Lipkin of the University of California in Irvine correctly determined that the deceased patients were victims of, instead, West Nile virus, a North African microbe never previously seen in the Americas.

As the clock ticks away in an outbreak an epidemiologist would be dispatched to determine the cause of the cases. If the bioagent were a fairly common bacterium, such as *Clostridium botulinum*, local hospital laboratories should be able to identify the culprit.

But if a microbe not usually seen by local physicians, such as anthrax, Q fever, Ebola, smallpox, or plague appeared, local facilities probably would not be able to diagnose the problem. With precious time passing, people dying, and disease possibly spreading, local officials would then await word from the diagnostic labs at the CDC in Atlanta. And if any truly dangerous organism were the suspected culprit—such as smallpox—all CDC analysis would be handled in the Special Pathogens BL-4 laboratory.

During the summer of 1994 Dr. Marcelle Layton started her job as New York City's chief of infectious disease control, learning that "by the way, part of your job description is planning for biological warfare," Layton said in a 1998 speech to her colleagues.[105]

"It is easy to be overwhelmed by the more than sixty agents that the DOD says have the capacity to be weaponized," Layton continued, noting that "for many of these agents there are very limited supplies of treatments . . . and capacity to do specimen analysis and autopsies. Panic and terror could be expected, even among the health care providers, themselves."

By order of New York City Mayor Rudolph Giuliani municipal employees like Layton were generally forbidden to publicly discuss any details of the city's response plan. When Office of Emergency Management Director Jerry Hauer did address the topic he deliberately spoke in dry, even boring, tones. The concern was that individuals with evil intent would spot fears and weaknesses, which they would exploit in a terrorist attack.

But Layton summarized the city's situation by saying, "Most of us . . . have grave concerns about whether or not our current public health system has the capacity to respond. Are we prepared? No."

And New York City had actually undergone DOD training, staged 1997 and 2000 bioterrorism citywide drills, and put some serious thinking into the problem. In 1996 Mayor Rudolph Giuliani created the Office of Emergency Management, placing at its helm Hauer, a professional emergency manager and firefighter with ten years experience in corporate and government preparation. Hauer traveled to Israel to learn how that country planned to respond should microbes be released by terrorists in Tel Aviv. He studied Pentagon plans. He conducted drills involving forty-one New York City hospitals. And to most public queries he either declined to comment or told the public that the city was ready for the worst.[106] But in public meetings Hauer acknowledged that a bioattack involving a human-to-human transmissible agent would quickly overwhelm the city's hospital emergency rooms, require hasty construction of alternative care facilities, and if not handled excruciatingly carefully, provoke widespread panic that could not be controlled by the New York Police Department.[107] In a 1999 role-playing anthrax scenario Hauer's staff and the New York City Police Department quickly lost control of the populace and Gotham descended swiftly into an hysteric, nightmarish scene unlike any seen in North America since the 1918 flu pandemic.

Osterholm scoffed at Hauer's confidence, and there was no love lost between the two government officials. Osterholm insisted that New York, or any other city, couldn't consider itself "prepared" for a bioattack unless it had stockpiles of millions of doses of vaccines and antibiotics—which no city did. And he wasn't sure that Hamburg's antibiotic stockpiles could ever reach New York or any other city and be distributed rapidly enough to stave off disaster.

"Look, suppose the president is coming to New York to speak at the UN," Osterholm suggested. "He gets out of the car. A plane flies down the East River. You know, the president and the bum on the street are breathing the same air. So that plane spews out anthrax. Are you going to tell me New York is ready for that?"

Could any city be ready for such an evil act? Perhaps not, Osterholm conceded. But the degree to which any municipality was prepared for such an abomination would depend not on emergency personnel such as police, but on the strength of the city's basic public health infrastructure.

Osterholm insisted that Hauer, and all other city emergency planners, were grossly underestimating the amount of panic such an event would provoke: "I can tell you, a single case of meningitis in a local high school causes enough fear and panic to bring down a whole community. . . . Now imagine you're telling people, 'This is going to unfold for eight weeks, and I can't tell you if you're going to die.' And with every symptom people in the public feel, real or imagined, they're going to think, 'I've got it! I'm gonna die!'

"You don't think that's panic? Think again," Osterholm continued. "Part of my message has been sharpened because of a lack of response by these people who want to say, 'We're prepared.' Heck, it's like stealing candy from a baby. Just ask, 'So where are your vaccines?' "

If New York City wasn't prepared, how could its neighboring towns and villages, from Newark to East Hampton, possibly be expected to know how to respond to such an attack?

Colonel David Franz, deputy commander of the U.S. Army Medical Materiel Command, devoted years of his life to readying the military for bioweapons. He insisted that this tremendous American vulnerability "underscores the need for a strong technical base that we cannot get away from in this nation. We need far forward capabilities. . . . The timelines are critical, even for a hoax. We've got to know what we're dealing with to treat people properly and to prevent panic."

Though Congress directed the military to develop that technical base, the Department of Defense was shorthanded. Until 1997, for example, Franz ran USAMRIID, located inside Fort Detrick. USAMRIID was the military's only BL-4 top security facility in which such superlethal microbes as Ebola and smallpox could be safely studied. And USAMRIID had responsibility for developing and testing treatments and vaccines for potential biological weapons.

Between 1991 and 1998, due to budget cuts, USAMRIID lost 30 percent of its scientists and technicians, and across the board they could no longer promote junior scientists.

"We're eating our seed stock," said USAMRIID scientist Peter Jahrling. The budget situation froze all of the agency's scientists and physicians in tiers they had occupied for years. No one advanced, and no young, fresh scientists entered at the bottom level, training to one day take over the nation's vital laboratory. USAMRIID became a laboratory full of aging, demoralized men and women who collectively possessed most of the West's knowledge of biodefense.

If an emergency developed due to biological weapons use, Franz said, "We would have . . . to pull people in from all other divisions."

So many federal, state, and local agencies were supposed to respond if a bioweapons event occurred in the United States that it was doubtful anyone would know precisely who was supposed to be first notified and which group would be in charge.

"We need a 'wiring diagram' of how federal assets are requested," Charlotte, North Carolina, Fire Chief Luther Fincher Jr. declared.[108] "What is the federal 911 number? How is it activated? Who determines what assets will be spent? What are the defined roles for each federal agency dispatched? Do they understand that they will report to the local incident commander for assignment? . . . There can be no hesitation or confusion about any of this after an incident occurs."[109]

Interestingly, the one federal agency that was *not* supposed to be in charge was the Department of Health and Human Services—public health. In most scenarios it was law enforcement that called the shots, despite the near certainty that federal and local police forces would know next to nothing about viruses, biotoxins, or bacteria. Law enforcement tended to be slow to recognize such threats, and then to respond in classic police fashion, throwing every available weapon or tactic at the situation regardless of the scientific wisdom of its use.

On April 24, 1997, for example, events in Washington, D.C., proceeded precisely by the book according to the FBI. But public health terrorism experts say what happened at the B'nai B'rith national headquarters that Passover day offered terrible evidence of the flaws and vulnerabilities in America's prepared- ness—or lack thereof—for a biological attack.

It was the third day of Passover and the Jewish human rights organization was closed, save its security guards. Amid the April 23 mail was an eight-by-ten- inch padded envelope that sat twenty-four hours in the B'nai B'rith mail room.

On Friday morning one of the mail room employees noticed that the pack- age was leaking a red sticky substance—blood, perhaps. And written on the package—which had passed through the U.S. mail—were the words *Yersinia* and *anthrachs*. The first referred to *Yersinia pestis*, the bacterium that cause plague. The second was a misspelling of *anthrax*.

For the following nine hours the B'nai B'rith building was surrounded by the Washington, D.C., fire department, police, FBI, and District of Columbia emergency management personnel. The air-conditioning system was shut down, and the mail room was designated a "hot zone," D.C. Fire Department Battalion Chief Alvin Carter recalled.

"The area was cordoned off. There's a hot zone, a warm zone, and a cold zone. Each zone required different protective equipment," Carter explained. "All civilians are in the cold zone."

All of the people who were in the "hot zone" mail room were required to remain there until, Carter said, "the area was decontaminated." The suspect bioterrorist package was placed in an airtight HAZMAT, or Hazardous Materials Team, container and transported by car to the Naval Medical Research Institute in Bethesda, Maryland.

The sample was brought to G. W. Long's lab where, Long said, "within minutes we were able to say it was negative for plague and anthrax," the two agents the envelope claimed were enclosed.

While navy scientists worked to determine the actual contents of the pack- age, D.C. authorities and the FBI took the following measures: the entire B'nai

B'rith building and neighboring structures were quarantined; fire department personnel dressed in Level A, fully encapsulated suits hosed down the "hot zone" with chlorine; and a set of sheets were strung out in the Washington, D.C., street and potentially exposed individuals were ordered to strip and submit to a spraying with a chlorinated water pounded at them by high-powered fire hoses.

"That's how you decontaminate," Carter explained.

An FBI supervising Special Agent who asked that he not be identified said that the emergency response "went slowly, but everybody wanted to be careful. . . . There's a federal disaster response plan that kicks in and you follow certain protocols." And key to the federal protocols were local HAZMAT teams: such fire department HAZMATs would, he said, play the lead role in any bioterrorist event.

"Pretty much any good metro fire department has materials for chemical hazards—same thing."

As it turned out, thankfully, the package contained a broken petri dish full of nothing but strawberry Jell-O, along with a note from the would-be assailant, Counter Holocaust Lobbyists of Hillel, an Orthodox Jewish group that stridently opposes liberal Judaism.[110]

Contrary to the FBI's view public health experts say responses to chemical versus biological hazards should *not* be the same.[111] They argue that several mistakes were made at B'nai B'rith that could have spread disease had the package contained anthrax or plague.

First, by orders of the local HAZMAT, which was trained to handle chemicals or explosives, the air-conditioning system at B'nai B'rith was shut down. But this didn't occur until emergency services was notified of the suspicious package—twenty-four hours after it arrived in the building. That means that potential microbes could have circulated throughout the building, making the entire complex a "hot zone," not just the mail room.

The second concern was for the decontamination procedure used on one mail room employee, a B'nai B'rith security guard, and two emergency personnel—the sprayed fire hoses. The FBI insisted that chlorine in the water "kills everything. If it's biological, it will kill it. That's all you have to do."

But biologists said that some organisms—such as anthrax spores—could well resist droplets of chlorine. And high-powered hoses could actually spread the organisms into an aerosolized mist that could rain down over the area.

Further, D.C. HAZMAT and the FBI benefited from their proximity to the navy's top—indeed, *only*—bioterrorism laboratory—Bethesda. When asked what would happen elsewhere were such an incident to occur, the navy's Long shrugged and said, "I'm not aware of anything for the rest of the country. If somebody put up the money some of this could be used elsewhere. But I'm not willing to go testing all over the country."

In other words, the rest of America would be on its own, unable to rapidly determine the contents of suspicious terror packages.

In 1997 to 1999 the FBI had the lead role in training local firefighters—HAZMATs—in first response to biological weapons attacks. Nearly seventy thousand firefighters were trained in WMD (Weapons of Mass Destruction), operating in manners that equated chemical and biological attack responses.[112] It was, Osterholm insisted, *the* fundamental flaw in all American plans for defending the nation's citizenry against bioweapons attacks. Osterholm said that "biological weapons cause diseases that exist in nature and may occur spontaneously in human populations. . . . The investigative steps for detection and identification of the agent would be the same as that for a naturally occurring agent. Therefore, the first and most fundamental strategy for dealing with bioterrorism was to develop effective means for combating all infectious diseases. . . . improving the public health infrastructure and biomedical research capacity."

Long, long before it became chic in America to point out the possibility of a bioattack on U.S. citizens, a religious cult did, indeed, wage bioterrorism. And, underscoring Osterholm's point, it was local public health that recognized what had happened and responded. It took place on September 17, 1984, in a remote corner of northern Oregon. Four days later patients contracted acute stomach pains, fever, chills, headaches, bloody stools, and vomiting; by September 24 more than 150 people in rural Wasco County, Oregon, were violently ill. In the sparsely populated county of 21,000 people such a sharp increase in gastrointestinal cases drew attention from Oregon state authorities.

By the end of September, 751 cases of acute gastroenteritis had occurred in the county, representing 9 percent of the total population. And lab tests showed that all the victims were infected with *Salmonella typhirium*.

"Usually the county sees less than five cases of salmonellosis a year," Dr. Michael Skeels, chief epidemiologist for Oregon's state health department, said.[113] The incident sparked a large public health investigation because, "it was the largest food-related outbreak in the U.S. in 1984," he added.

It took a year of intense study for Skeels's team, working with CDC and FBI experts, to figure out what happened. And it took another twelve years for the Oregonians to gain permission from state and federal investigators to publish the details in the *Journal of the American Medical Association*. Federal authorities feared that merely describing the incident would spark copycat crimes nationwide.

It all traced back to Big Muddy Ranch, located near the town of Antelope in Wasco county. A religious cult there planned to take over the county's political apparatus.

In the early 1980s Bagwan Shree Rajneesh was an Indian guru who claimed enormous numbers of followers in the United States, most of whom wore red, orange, or fuchsia clothing because the Bagwan said he loved the colors of sunrise. The cult bought Big Muddy Ranch and quickly outnumbered the local residents. In 1984 the Rajneesh group, having many grievances with county officials, pushed for a special election, which might have given them control of the county's affairs.

As the election approached, the Rajneesh group, led in these efforts by an American nurse who had taken the Indian name Puja, built a biology laboratory at Big Muddy and ordered samples of several microbes, including *Salmonella typhirium*, from American Tissue Type Culture, then located in Maryland. The laboratory, called Pythagoras Clinic, had actually been licensed by the Oregon State Health Department.

"I licensed it," Skeels said with a shrug. "The irony of that did not escape me."

Following a variety of books and medical articles readily available in libraries and bookstores, Puja's lab grew large supplies of *Salmonella*.

And on the eve of the county election, hoping to make hostile voters too ill to go to their polling booths, the Rajneesh followers put the bacteria in dressings at salad bars in the county's ten most popular restaurants.

Fortunately the religious cult lacked sufficient biological sophistication to breed drug-resistant strains of the bacteria, and all the illnesses responded swiftly to antibiotic treatment.

When Skeels and the FBI raided Big Muddy Ranch a year later, however, they discovered "a bacteriological freezer-dryer for large-scale production" of microbes, Skeels said. They also found a library of such things as *The Anarchists Cookbook*, literature on manufacture and use of explosives, and military biowarfare articles.

"We lost our innocence over this," Skeels said. "We really learned to be more suspicious. . . . Obviously these pathogens are too easy to purchase.

"These cases were first picked up by the Wasco County health department," Skeels concluded, adding that "the first significant biological attack on a U.S. community was not carried out by foreign terrorists smuggled into New York, but by legal residents of a U.S. community. The next time it happens it could be with more lethal agents. . . . We in public health are really not ready to deal with that."

If Wasco County hadn't had an alert disease surveillance system, the sudden increase in salmonellosis would have gone unnoticed. The Rajneesh cult would have gotten away with it. And perhaps, emboldened by its success, the religious cult might—as Aum Shinrikyo would years later—have escalated their efforts. If the agent they used the next time were more toxic even Skeels's alert group would be at a loss to prevent large-scale homicide.

"I'm concerned with, how are we going to make the diagnosis? Fire departments aren't going to play a role in this thing unless it's a hoax," Osterholm insisted. "For most of these illnesses what's going to get picked up is an undiagnosed illness that suddenly overwhelms doctors' offices, emergency rooms, and ambulances."

In two chilling role-playing scenarios public health and law enforcement officials staged responses to bioterror events, revealing critical flaws in the nation's safety net. At a December 1998 Biological and Chemical Weapons Conference at Stanford University public health officials failed in their role-playing scenario to mount an effective response to deliberate release of a superflu virus: in a few months one million Americans would have been dead, had their scenario been real.

A more elaborate scenario was enacted in February 1999 in Crystal City, Virginia, by the Johns Hopkins Center for Civilian Biodefense Studies. The details played out over an eight-hour period in a packed, tense room full of public health, military, and law enforcement personnel. Under the scenario the vice president of the United States visits a prestigious university located in a mythological town dubbed Northeast. It's April 1. Eleven days later a twenty-year-old student who heard the vice president shows up in the university hospital's emergency room with flulike symptoms: high fever, muscle aches, fatigue, headache. She is sent home with aspirin and the old maxim: get plenty of rest and drink lots of fluids.

Two days later the young woman returns to the hospital, now fighting for her life. And a university janitor who cleaned up after the vice president's speech turns up with the same symptoms. By six o'clock that night, April 13, the hospital infectious diseases expert is ready to gingerly voice an outrageous conclusion: both patients have smallpox.

Since smallpox was officially eradicated from the face of the earth in 1977 and samples of remaining viruses are supposed to be under lock and key only in Atlanta and Siberia there can be but one conclusion: someone has stolen laboratory samples of the virus, and deliberately released them in a bioterrorist attack aimed at the United States vice president.

Under this scenario, within two months more than fifteen thousand people have died of smallpox worldwide and epidemics are out of control in fourteen nations. All global supplies of vaccine are depleted and it will take years to manufacture enough to save humanity. The global economy teeters on the brink of collapse as nations close their borders and sink into nationalistic isolation, barring all Americans from entering their countries. In the city of Northeast utter chaos reigns, and the National Guard has imposed martial law over the two million residents.

Similarly, government authority has either broken down or reverted to military-style control in cities all over the world as smallpox claims lives and pits terrified citizens against one another.

A top smallpox expert scribbles projections on the back of an envelope and gently slides it in front of the governor of his state: within twelve months eighty million people worldwide will be dead.

"We blew it," declared California's top state public health laboratory expert Dr. Michael Ascher. "It clearly got out of control. Whatever planning we had . . . it didn't work. I think this is the harsh reality, what would happen."

While most of the public in North America and Europe remained ignorant of the sorts of issues raised in the scenarios, handfuls of Internet-hooked extremists, right-wing militiamen, psychiatrically imbalanced men of anger, and postmodern fascists were cognizant of the fine points of bioterrorism. Recipes for botulinum and anthrax production were on the Internet. Books describing biotoxin assassination techniques were readily available. Some private militia groups trained in the use of bioweapons.

For example, Uncle Fester, as he called himself, was a Green Bay, Wisconsin, devoted father of two. He was also the author of *Silent Death*,[114] a book adorned with a skull and crossbones that purported to teach readers hundreds of ways to kill using chemical and biological poisons. While his youngest cried for attention, forty-year-old "Fester," who declined to reveal his real name, bragged on the phone to a reporter[115] that the book "sells a couple thousand copies per year," to people he imagined were "holed up in their bunkers waiting for Armageddon to come. And then they will come out of their bunkers and use these skills."

Fester's book told readers how to be a "crafty executioner" by poisoning individuals with botulinum toxin, noting that "once these symptoms of botulism appear, the antitoxins that medical science has developed are completely useless."

Fester, who said he had degrees in both biology and chemistry, told his readers how to manufacture and use several of the world's deadliest microbes, suggesting that they ship them through the U.S. mail. One should "have no contact with any delivery service," Fester said, pointing out dozens of ways to ensure that no evidence would turn up in victims' autopsies.

"Look around the world," Uncle Fester challenged. "There are multiple places in the world where the skills in this book could be used to good purpose. In the United States? Not as long as we have free speech. But there are rat holes all over the world."

Asked if he had ever tested his "recipes," the Wisconsin assassination guide hedged. After all, under congressional law that had recently been enacted such activity would be illegal.

"Let's just say I know they work," Uncle Fester said with a chuckle. And then he recommended his Web site on the Internet, where further "cooking" details were available.

Ex-biker and former Klan member Kurt Saxon, age sixty-six, also had a Web site that was full of the same sorts of things one could read in his books, *The Poor Man's James Bond*, Volumes 1–4.[116] The books were chockablock full of ways to maim, kill, and torture victims, including with biological weapons. In the introduction of the first volume, Saxon told his readers that "this book is power," and praised right-wing "militants" who, he wrote, would be transformed by his book. Yet, he insisted, most would-be American terrorists were "a bunch of hate-filled losers."

When asked about Larry Wayne Harris, who had twice been arrested with plague and anthrax, Saxon chortled, "The guy who was caught with anthrax in Vegas? Well, he was a member of Identity. And that means he's clinically insane." But Harris had his mind straight enough in 1997 to be able to write a book: *Bacteriological Warfare: A Major Threat to North America*. In it, Harris cleverly avoids violating federal laws, telling readers how to make biobombs by describing actions he claims outsiders plan to execute against the U.S.

Thus, the information was readily available to those who wanted it, and apparently many Americans did. In its 1998 annual report, the Southern Poverty Law Center identified 474 so-called hate groups in America, representing a 20 percent increase over the previous year. The largest, Identity, had fifty thousand members in 1998.[117] It is estimated by some observers that there were eight hundred right-wing militia groups in the United States in 1999, some of which advocated the overthrow of the U.S. government and conducted tight Green Beret–style training of their members, who carried sophisticated weaponry.[118]

A Washington, D.C., FBI Special Agent, who spoke on condition he not be named, said the numbers of terrorist threats called into the nation's capital every year had increased steadily, by 1998 topping five per day.

An unreleased White House 1995 report on terrorism predicted that a terrorist could kill millions of residents of the nation's capital by dropping a hundred kilograms of a biological agent out of the back of a crop duster flown on a windless day over Washington, D.C. The authors of the White House report predicted that a virtual amateur could develop bioweapons which, if dispersed in the New York subway system, would claim tens of thousands of lives.

But were America's militants and fanatics ready to try biological terrorism? Law enforcement leaders claimed that religious cults and militant political groups were the *most* likely to try bioweapons. After all, they argued, the first domestic mass biological poisoning was carried out in 1984 by members of the Rajneesh religious cult. And the first bombing of a fully occupied government office building was in 1995 in Oklahoma City—executed by American political extremists.

It was, perhaps, the tone of their rhetoric that sparked the most concern. In *The Poisoner's Handbook*, for example, author Maxwell Hutchkinson told readers that they could poison or kill IRS workers by filling out phony 1040 tax return forms, lacing the forms with a mixture of ricin toxin and DMSO—a concoction the author claimed was 100 percent lethal.[119]

"The purpose of all this is to disrupt the operations of the Internal Revenue Service," Hutchkinson wrote. "If done on a large enough scale, it would serve two purposes—it would make it more difficult for the IRS to operate efficiently, thus helping tax cheats and tax protestors. It might also awaken the politicians to the depth of resentment felt by the taxpaying public."

Fortunately, Hutchkinson was a lousy chemist: DMSO only serves as a solvent, passing substances through the skin into the bloodstream, if a simple chemical is involved. Proteins, such as ricin, couldn't dissolve in DMSO.

But the depth of Hutchkinson's antagonism was unmistakable. He suggested his readers kill Catholics by soaking their rosary beads in *Phytotoxin abrin*, a toxin derived from precatorious beans; he wrote that "botulism is fun and easy to make"; and he urged survivalists worldwide to hone their skills, readying themselves for biological defenses in the Armageddon.

In light of all this, the U.S. Congress passed a number of laws aimed at making it harder for anyone—citizen or overseas agent—to attack America with bioweapons. In 1991 it passed an export controls law, soon put in force against Iraq, that barred U.S. companies from trading with countries believed to be developing bioweapons. In 1989 it passed the Biological Weapons Act, which made it illegal for any American to possess, trade, sell, or manufacture a biological substance "for use as a weapon."

After the Oklahoma City bombing, Congress passed the Anti-Terrorism Act of 1996, which allowed federal authorities to arrest anyone who even "threatens" to develop or use biological weapons. And the following year, by order of Congress, the CDC named twenty-four infectious organisms and twelve toxins as "restricted agents," use or possession of which required a federal permit.

Congress sought technological solutions as well, allocating money for Department of Defense research on devices that might sniff out bugs and sanitize contaminated areas. First on line was the navy's TagMan, a three-hundred pound sophisticated gene scanner that could in less than half an hour identify whether a liquid sample contained any of several known agents. But the system had significant limitations: at three hundred pounds it was hardly portable. And it could not be used for serious Biohazard Level-3 or BL-4 agents—precisely the most worrisome microbes. Most significantly, it couldn't analyze air samples.

The DOD's Defense Advanced Research Projects Agency, or DARPA, had $2 billion to fund wild and crazy science ideas—notions so far-out that standard civilian funding sources would not consider them. Among DARPA's many projects were $61.6 million of bioweapons defense efforts. The primary DARPA hope was that someone would develop a fast, cheap, safe, and portable way to sample air for the presence of nasty biologicals. Most of the research under way focused on unique genetic attributes of bacteria and viruses.

One project involved trying to grow human nerve cells on microscopic chips that would change color or light up if the nerves detected some sort of neurotoxic agent. Such a device—were it ever practicably developed—could be a sort of early warning system that would sense the presence of such nerve-damaging agents as botulinum.

Several laboratories—notably Argonne National Laboratory in Chicago—were trying to develop chips that were lined with thousands of pieces of DNA from bacteria, to serve as probes. Argonne's goal was to have an air detection device that was small enough that it could be handheld, akin to a police radar gun. But research director Eli Huberman said such a thing "is years away from mass production or for widespread use."

Furthermore, neither the Argonne device nor any others in development envisioned sampling the air for viruses. Even the DARPA wild thinkers hadn't imagined how that could be done.

Even the simplest technological approach to bioweapons proved to be too much for DOD contractors. In the spring of 2000, Defense Department officials revealed that protective space suits U.S. troops had relied upon in the Persian Gulf, and that still formed the basis of soldiers' defense against deadly microbes, were defective. At least 5 percent of the 900,000 suits DOD had purchased during the 1990s were useless, and the reliability of the entire inventory was suspect.[120]

It seemed unlikely, then, that a technological quick fix would soon be found.[121]

Thus, the three immediate Western responses to bioterrorism appeared to be seriously flawed: military defense, HAZMAT reactions, and high-technology sensors.

If the Red Army had succeeded in releasing, let us hypothesize, drug-resistant anthrax spores in the Bourse Station of the Paris metro at 8:00 A.M. on a warm Wednesday in June, what would be the role of the French military, Sûreté, Paris police, or any number of high-tech sensor devices? None. The most important responders wouldn't be from the military or law enforcement branches of the French government. They would be the doctors, epidemiologists, ambulance drivers, nurses, and bureaucrats of the Paris public health system. It is they who would note—days after the event—that large numbers of Parisians appeared to be ill, suffering similar symptoms. And with questioning they might realize that all the ailing individuals routinely took the same metro train, or stopped at the same station.

And regardless of whether or not anyone ever realized that the lethal biological mist was dispersed in the Bourse metro station—or caught the terrorists responsible—it is the public health system that would track down and treat the patients, determine who should receive prophylactic antibiotics and dispense the drug, conduct epidemiology that could determine whether the new anthrax outbreak was spreading from person to person, and analyze the organism to see what special attributes it might have.

Yet it was a militarylike response that dominated government thinking. Legally the Department of Defense was on shaky constitutional ground in asserting its right to seize command in the event of a domestic bioterrorist event. Defense Secretary William S. Cohen announced on February 1, 1999, creation of a special command within DOD, designed to coordinate responses to domestic biological attacks.[122] A popular 1995 movie, *Outbreak*, had depicted such a scenario, in which the U.S. Army declared martial law and took full control of an American city in order to limit spread of an air-borne transmissible form of the Ebola virus. Such a clear violation of the United States Constitution might be okay for Hollywood, civil libertarians cried, but not for the real world.

In his January 22, 1998, speech to the National Academy of Sciences President Clinton said that "we will be aggressive. At the same time I want you to know that we will remain committed to uphold privacy rights and other constitutional protections, as well as the proprietary rights of American businesses. It is essential that we do not undermine liberty in the name of liberty."[123]

That day Clinton requested congressional approval for a $10 billion antiterrorism program, including $86 million for improving public health surveillance, $43 million for research on vaccines for anthrax, smallpox, and other potential BW agents, and $300 million for stockpiles of essential drugs and vaccines. The proposed expenditures marked a doubling in the previous year's bioterrorism budget.[124]

In an interview the previous day with the *New York Times* President Clinton acknowledged that he had "spent some late nights thinking a lot about this and reading a lot about it . . . For example, we know that if all of us went to a rally on the Mall tomorrow with ten thousand people, and somebody flew a low-flying crop duster and sprayed us all with biological agents from, let's say, two hundred feet, that, no matter how toxic it were, half of us would walk away for reasons no one quite understands. You know, either we wouldn't breathe it, or we'd have some miraculous resistance to it. And the other half of us, somebody would have to diagnose in a hurry and then contain and treat."[125]

The job of building the nation's drug and vaccine stockpile fell to Hamburg. In her new capacity as assistant secretary of health for the U.S. Department of Health and Human Services, she was racing to catch up with the Department of Defense and the FBI. Public health was a late entrant into the bioterrorism field, she said, and significant dangers lurked in the developing antiterrorist infrastructure. Beyond the already voiced civil liberties issues Hamburg worried that "the danger is we don't want public health identified with the CIA and FBI activities. Particularly in terms of global infectious disease surveillance. We in public health need to have public trust and confidence."

Already local public health departments were having a hard time striking that balance in responding to fake bioterrorism events. It seemed that claiming to have placed or shipped an anthrax-containing device had suddenly become chic. Jessica Stern of the Council on Foreign Relations had counted forty-seven such hoaxes in the United States since 1992.[126] In all forty-seven cases local fire and police authorities had reacted seriously, decontaminating two thousand people in these incidents and appearing on the scenes dressed in full body protection suits. And Stern's list was by no means comprehensive.[127]

Secretary of the Navy Richard Danzig warned that panic, in and of itself, was becoming the new terrorist tool, adding that "only through a new union of our public health, police, and military resources can we hope to deal with this dangerous threat."[128]

But Hamburg was worried that the hoaxes were occurring precisely *because* the police and FBI were responding. It seemed bioterror hoaxes attracted some of the same sick individuals as enjoyed watching fire departments douse buildings that they had set afire.

"When an envelope comes in saying 'This is anthrax,' we don't need the fire department in full protective gear on site," Hamburg insisted. "What we need is to discreetly move the envelope to a public health laboratory for proper analysis. Mass decontamination and quarantine only added fuel to the fire of the hoax perpetrators and it's totally unnecessary in terms of public health."

It was obvious that public health, law enforcement, and defense had very different priorities. For public health the paramount concerns were limiting spread of disease, identifying the causative agent, and, if possible, treating and vaccinating the populace. Law enforcement, however, was in the business of stopping and solving crimes, and the scene of any bioterrorist incident was, first and foremost, a source of evidence.[129] Managing an outbreak response would, for the FBI and police, constitute a conflict of interest, as they would by mandate be focused on detaining witnesses and obtaining evidence even if their efforts ran counter to public health.[130]

The primary mission of the Department of Defense is to protect the United States against military foes. Secondary to that is defending the health of its troops. How that squared with intervening—indeed, *commanding*—responses to domestic bioterror incidents wasn't at all clear.

When public health needed to intrude upon individuals' lives in order to protect the larger community it did so in limited ways and under the usually hard-and-fast promise of confidentiality. For example, during an epidemic individuals may be asked to submit to blood tests and medical exams, and their medical charts may be scrutinized.

On a more long-term basis public health protects the community by monitoring disease trends, logging who is suffering or dying from what diseases. Again, the information is generally stored in confidential or anonymous form.

Globally the World Health Organization and a variety of other groups kept similar count of nations' diseases, monitoring for emergence of new epidemics. After the 1995 Kikwit Ebola epidemic WHO sought to create a more rigorous surveillance system and pushed countries to be more open about epidemics in their populations.

All these functions, in all tiers of public health from villages to global levels, required maintenance of a crucial social contract: the individual or country agrees to openly disclose information for the sake of the health of the larger community. And in return public health authorities promise never to abuse their trust, maintaining discretion and protecting patient privacy.

But the fear of bioterrorism threatened to destroy that vital social contract, as it was not one shared by law enforcement or defense. The closer public health drew to the other two, the greater the danger that it would lose all trust and credibility in the eyes of the public it served.[131]

Some public health advocates were frankly convinced that no marriage between their profession and law enforcement could ever work, and denounced all efforts to heighten bioterrorism concerns. One prestigious group argued that "bioterrorist initiative programs are strongly reminiscent of the civil defense programs promoted by the U.S. government during the Cold War . . . fostering the delusion that nuclear war was survivable."[132]

For many older public health leaders the bioterrorism issue at the turn of the century brought up nasty memories of Cold War cover-ups and suppression of science. By adopting the issue, they warned, public health was buying into a framework of paranoid thinking. And, indeed, in 1999 biologists for the first time found their work facing censorship in federal laboratories in the wake of allegations of Chinese espionage at the Los Alamos National Laboratory. The Department of Energy, which ran the national labs, clamped down so hard in 1999 that the National Academy of Sciences warned that the future of the U.S. scientific enterprise could be imperiled. Though the DOE's primary concern was computer and nuclear secrecy, the threat of bioterrorism prompted the agency to broaden its new security restrictions to embrace basic biology research as well.

"This is a truly pernicious list," declared Nobel laureate Burton Richter, director of the Stanford Linear Accelerator center in Palo Alto, addressing the National Academy of Sciences.[133]

Overall, many advocates argued, public health's role in the bioterrorism issue could only be a comfortable one if it were an equal partner with the military and law enforcement. Or, perhaps, better than equal.

In his historic speech in Atlanta during the winter of 1998 D. A. Henderson had beckoned public health to jump on board a train already in motion, conducted by the defense, intelligence, and law enforcement communities. Less than a year later public health was on board the train, but clearly not in the conductor's seat. Some public health advocates gleefully confided that concern about bioterrorism might be the political trigger that restored funding for their collapsing infrastructures. But the wiser among them recognized that dollars earmarked for bioterrorism issues would never be applicable to such essential programs as syphilis monitoring, well baby programs, HIV counseling, immigrant TB screening, or cardiovascular disease surveillance.

Osterholm knew that he had instigated the public airing of previously secret biological weapons fears. And he took no satisfaction in that—not so long as the essential role of public health remained unresolved.

"I use this analogy," Osterholm explained. "It's like riding giant waves in Maui. You can't be an inch farther out than the data. But you can't wait to act, either. For three years I was almost the lone voice on biological terrorism."

He rode his Maui big wave, Osterholm said, dreaming of surfing while Arctic winds blasted the walls of his office. Now the trick would be to keep public health from being wiped out. Hunched over his phone the Minnesota State epidemiologist was watched over by a sign on the wall behind him.

It read THE BUG STOPS HERE.

CHAPTER SIX

EPILOGUE

The changing face of public health and future global prophylaxis.

Responsibility requires *freedom.*

—Amartya Sen, 1999[1]

The poor, we're told, will always be with us. If this is so, then infectious diseases will be, too—the plagues that the rich, in vain, attempt to keep at bay."

—Dr. Paul Farmer, 1999[2]

There is *a chain that runs from the behaviour of cells and molecules to the health of populations, and back again, a chain in which the past and the present social environments of individuals, and their perceptions of those environments, constitute a key set of links. No one would pretend that the chain is fully understood, or is likely to be for a considerable time to come. But the research evidence currently available no longer permits anyone to deny its existence.*

—*Why Are Some People Healthy and Others Not?* Robert Evans, Morris Barrer, and Theodore Marmor 1994[3]

In 1346 a particular set of circumstances occurred, in a peculiar sequence, resulting in what may have been the first true global epidemic. Perhaps only the Americas and Antarctica were spared humanity's globalized Black Death.

The event involved no dark, conspiratorial forces concocting evil means of deliberate spread. It simply entailed the right mix of human social evolution, weather, and ecology occurring simultaneously with a force that was devastating to *Homo sapiens* of Europe, Central Asia, the Indian subcontinent, Indochina, the South Seas, the Middle East, northern Africa, and the Arctic.

With epidemics, timing is everything.

Yersinia pestis had undoubtedly been infecting fleas and rodents for centuries, occasionally happening upon a human victim who fell mysteriously to the bacterium's lethal force. But by the 1300s the human race had millions of its members scattered across the globe, many of them—perhaps a fifth of the population—living in cities and trading posts. Caravans loaded with goods were making their ways across the most forbidding terrains, from the Gobi Desert to the Sahara. Sailing ships carried goods from port to port, continent to continent. It was an era of profound globalization in which cooks in Venice were discovering the wonders of pepper and cinnamon, London's tailors were sewing wondrous silk garments, and the emperors of China witnessed the chemicals they used for fireworks exploited effectively in the West as gunpowder.

In that earlier epoch globalization brought riches and wonders to some, sparked an intermingling of cultures and languages with sprinklings of ideas from faraway places, and forever changed the nature of economics, politics, and warfare.

It also created new opportunities for *Yersinia pestis*. At some point in 1345 to 1346, weather conditions favored large flea and rat populations in Mongolia, giving *Yersinia* ample opportunities to reproduce and spread between the insects and rodents. The weather must also have been favorable for the horses and camelback caravans that wended their ways from Mongolia, through China, and along the Silk Route of Asia.

Stowaways made the journey: fleas, rats, and *Yersinia*. And within eighteen months the Black Death was claiming millions of lives all over the Old World.

In the fourteenth century, as a response to the Black Death, some of the basic tools and laws of public health were created: quarantine, ship inspections, leprosariums, mass burials during epidemics. These were applied crudely, without any understanding of the causes of the scourges sweeping through the fourteenth and fifteenth centuries. All too often such methods of epidemic control were accompanied by ruthless, brutal repressions of the populations thought to be responsible for given diseases, such as the Jews of Europe and Infidels of the Ottoman Empire.

Wherever globalized trade went, disease hitchhikers cotraveled, taking their tolls on Incas, Aztecs, Maoris, Polynesians, Russians, Laotians, French, and Moroccans. A price, it seemed, had to be paid for the first internetting of human beings, connecting Iroquois via English ships indirectly to Hawaiians, and Irish via the Dutch armada to Papua New Guineans. Even such slow-motion fourteenth-century globalization came at a cost.

In the twentieth century global economics and power were the causes of three world wars, two fought on battlefields, and one "cold" one, involving the constant threat of thermonuclear weapons. (Only a handful of people realized that the world also lived under the peril of biowarfare catastrophe at the time.) In the final decade of the century the global power struggle was settled: there were winners, and there were losers. The United States won largely because it outspent the USSR. And when the world awoke to a post–Cold War hangover— after a brief period of *Pax Europa* euphoria—the true cost of the clash between communism and capitalism was clear.

With the 1989 fall of the Berlin Wall and 1991 collapse of the Soviet Union the nations and populaces of the world suddenly faced three unshakable new realities. First, the capitalist market system was the basis for all trade and economics, and Marxist approaches to economic equity or distribution were dead.[4] Second, the old alliances were no longer meaningful, and superpower protection of corrupt, dictatorial proxy state leaders was over. And third, the price hundreds of millions of people had paid for the Cold War and its subsequent global structural readjustments was their health and well-being.

It may seem paradoxical to hear that there are voices of discontent— including my own—decrying the global state of public health, claiming that the triumphs of our time are transient, under siege, even doomed. At the close of the twentieth century, life expectancies are soaring, not just in wealthy industrialized nations, but in many of the world's poor countries, as well. The World Health Organization forecast in 1999 that average life expectancy globally in 2025 will be seventy-three years—up from just forty-eight in 1955. In 1955, some twenty-one million children died before their fifth birthdays; in 1995, only eleven million did.[5]

Yet these promising overall trends disguised local and regional reversals that were profoundly disturbing to health experts. The double epidemics of TB and AIDS set sub-Saharan Africa's hard-fought health advances spiraling backward toward the nineteenth century: life expectancies shot downward regionally in the 1990s, and infant mortality rates jumped upward. By 1998, for example, Malawi's average life expectancy rate had fallen below its pre–World War II levels, thanks almost entirely to the human immunodeficiency virus.[6] So dire was the situation by 2000 that the World Bank declared the AIDS pandemic its "number one priority," and Bank president James Wolfensohn vowed that "no sensible AIDS program would be stopped for lack of money." Never before had a public health issue been given such prominence in the Bank's portfolio.

Advances made in poor countries proved frighteningly fragile. They were easily reversed by wars, corruption, global economic shifts, new epidemics, or refugee movements.

In the former Communist world—particularly in the nations that once made up the Soviet Union—life expectancies have reversed course with such rapidity and drama as to exceed anything seen in the absence of war over five previous centuries. Indeed, some regional downturns were proportionally greater than anything witnessed during peacetime since the pneumonic plague reached Moscow in the fourteenth century.

In 1955 the world was deeply divided: Communist bloc versus capitalist West. The roughly 2.5 billion people living on earth in 1955 grew up in an explosively prosperous economy. In 1973, however, the world's economy fell into a twenty-year-long sluggish recession that was most strongly felt in developing countries. By 1994, when global economic recovery began, there were 5.8 billion mouths to feed, most of them left malnourished.

In the wealthy world the artificial trade and currency alliances in the capitalist market economies—united by their opposition to communism during most of the twentieth century—turned competitive with a vengeance after the fall of the Berlin Wall. There was no longer any need for concern that European workforces would embrace socialism or communism, so government handouts didn't have to be used as lures to an obedient proletariat. Western European economies, long taxed by national and cultural commitments to social welfare, found their national health systems were baggage too weighty to carry during the competitive sprint for global economic power. As health care costs inflated, physicians throughout Europe reduced the numbers of procedures, medications, and therapies they administered to their patients. Nevertheless, national health systems sank into debt, physicians failed to get full reimbursement for their services, and government calls for managed care resonated from Lisbon to Oslo. With the twenty-first century approaching, Europe prepared to merge into a single economy, lean and strong, ready for fiscal showdowns with American, Japan, China, even the new Russia.

Russia staggered, however, seemingly unable to transform itself into a viable, first world market economy without succumbing to the tragedies of the developing world: corruption, political instability, capital centralization, and the complete collapse of social service infrastructures.

Some of the same frailties, long masked by stupendous capital growth and productivity, brought the economic powerhouses of Asia to their knees just two years before the millennium. In rural Japan and South Korea the crash of 1998 signaled the greatest fiscal and public health hardships since World War II.

And in the poorest countries of the world the already difficult became impossible. As former Tanzanian President Julius Nyerere put it: "When the world sneezes we catch pneumonia." The economic gap between the world's richest, versus her poorest, nations widened from 1961 to 1997 from about a twelvefold difference to a thirtyfold one. The sharpest widening took place between 1994 and 2000—at the same time as the inequalities in life expectancies and infant mortality rates grew most disparate. By then Nobel laureate Amartya Sen was no longer a lonely voice: his was echoed by a chorus of economists and public health experts who showed that the wealth of nations, and the degree of fairness with which that wealth was distributed within nations, determined countries' infant mortality rates. Poverty, they declared, killed babies.[7]

In contrast, at the eve of the twenty-first century Americans enjoyed a phenomenal boom; their economy was the strongest on the planet. Though artificialities also plagued the U.S. economy—notably the investment character of its stock exchanges—Americans had so much cheap food that more than half of the population was medically obese. They were literally living high off the hog.

But beneath the veneer of America's political and economic world domination problems lurked. By 1997 some 43.4 million Americans—more than 15 percent of the population—had no health insurance.[8] In 1998 that figure jumped to 44.3 million, or 16.3 percent of the population. Since 1993, when the Clinton administration first initiated the U.S. health care reform debate, the uninsured population had grown by 4.5 million,[9] among them one out of every four children in the country. An additional 71.5 million Americans lacked health care insurance for at least part of 1997, with a disproportionate percentage of the uncovered drawn from Hispanic, African-American, and poor white populations. The government's safety net—Medicaid and Medicare—didn't reach to protect a third of all Americans living below the poverty line. And many who were insured had coverage under plans that put a straitjacket on their care, limiting patients to the medical practices deemed cost-effective within a profit-making paradigm.

"Two-thirds of all deaths under the age of sixty-five are now postponable, if not preventable," American Public Health Association President Dr. Joyce Lashoff declared in 1991.[10] Yet, with each passing day more and more Americans put off vital health care needs, clogged public hospital emergency rooms, or went bankrupt trying to pay their medical bills.[11]

America had reached a critical health juncture, the seriousness of which was written in the numbers. Studies in 1997 showed that 56 percent of the uninsured put off treatments due to lack of funds, and 47 percent found it difficult or impossible to obtain medical care when needed.[12]

Most insured Americans had coverage through their employers, a victory that had been won decades earlier through labor union collective bargaining. But the end of the twentieth century brought significant changes in the American workplace resulting in millions of fully employed Americans having no health insurance. And millions more had coverage, the costs of which were docked from their pay: in other words, they were paying some or all of their medical coverage themselves.[13]

By the end of 1998 fully a third of all Americans favored some form of radical reconstruction of their health care system, registering the highest level of dissatisfaction seen in any major industrialized society.[14] They were spending twice as much annually on their out-of-pocket health needs as Canadians, and more than triple the $1,347 annual per person payments made by citizens of the United Kingdom.[15] The average American in 1997 spent $4,090 on personal health care, compared to $2,339 for a typical German.

Americans were, by the late 1990s, nearly matching out-of-pocket every uninsured dollar spent on medical care with another dollar for treatments delivered outside of the system. From use of acupuncture to herbal remedies, quartz bedtime crystals to magnet therapy, Americans lacked faith that mainstream medicine could adequately meet their needs, and spent billions of dollars on alternative health remedies, to the tune of more than $2,000 per capita annually.

Despite spending more on their health than any other peoples, citizens of the United States had the slowest rate of improvement in life expectancy of any industrialized nation. Americans born in 1960 had a life expectancy of 69.7 years, and in 1996 of 76.1 years, for a gain of 6.4 years. In contrast, Japanese born in 1996 could expect to live 80.3 years, with a gain of 12.6 years since 1960.[16] The Japanese paradox directly challenged U.S. health assumptions, as that country's populace had experienced the most rapid increase in life expectancy seen anywhere in the world during the second half of the twentieth century. Yet Japanese per capita spending on health ranked the lowest of any industrialized nation. The biggest health spender—the United States—ranked far behind Japan on every significant health index.[17]

Another crucial public health indicator—maternal deaths—was on the rise in America, after a fifty-year decline. In 1987 the rate of maternal deaths associated with pregnancy was 7.2 per 100,000 women in the United States. Three years later it was 10 per 100,000, according to the Centers for Disease Control and Prevention.[18] On a global scale, young children in the United States were certainly better off than their counterparts in Central Africa, India, or the former Soviet nations, but they fell well behind twenty-nine other nations when ranked by UNICEF for under-five mortality. Among the countries whose children had better 1996 survival rates were Slovenia (just four years after its war of secession from Yugoslavia), the Czech Republic, South Korea, and all of Western Europe.[19] The Children's Defense Fund argued that most of the comparatively poor health of America's youngsters was a function of poverty and lack of health insurance, noting that half of the country's children lived in single-parent homes, a quarter were poor, and one out of twenty-four was born to a mother who lacked any prenatal care.[20]

The twenty-first century opened on a new age of market globalization, joyfully embraced by some, dreaded by others. Massive, rapid change could irrefutably be forecast.

It posed interesting and troubling questions for public health.

At a time when the former Soviet public health infrastructure was moribund, when HIV was devastating sub-Saharan Africa, when impoverished India was spending a fortune on nuclear weapons development at the expense of its populace's health, and when long-antagonistic groups were taking advantage of the end of Cold War policing to slaughter ethnic enemies, public health was in a shambles. It could not meet its basic twentieth century core duties, that is, to ensure the public's safety at the community level, much less handle the new challenges posed by twenty-first century globalization. The safety of individual communities was eroding amid dwindling commitments to protection of the air, water, food supply, and hygiene systems. The drugs and pesticides that had insured miraculous improvements for the Northern Hemisphere during the sixth and seventh decades of the twentieth century were losing effectiveness by the final decade.

Risk increased. Though HIV surfaced in 1981 it might better be considered the first great pandemic of the twenty-first century. It spread swiftly from country to country, continent to continent in a retrovirus form that used human DNA as its vehicle and hideaway. Globalized sex and drug trades ensured HIV's ubiquity. And HIV, in turn, facilitated the circumnavigation of new, mutant forms of tuberculosis, the one taking advantage of the weakened human state caused by the other.

In the fourteenth century global travelers were few and slow. By the seventeenth century European nations were amassing wealth through global conquest and trade, conducted at the behest of kings, queens, and royally sanctioned companies. No European nation could hope to have power without spreading its tentacles to the south, east, and Americas.

The nineteenth and early twentieth century saw shifts in power and the end of colonialism, but trade remained encumbered by Cold War restrictions and the great costs of maintaining those far-flung corporate tentacles. Telecomputerization and the fall of communism erased such barriers, for the first time making the world a potential oyster for hundreds of millions of vacationers, immigrants, entrepreneurs, speculators, and home television viewers. Cars were assembled from parts made in a dozen different countries; Indians made software that was programmed into computers made in South Korea, Sri Lanka, California, and Mexico; air travel grew so commonplace and popular that few of the world's major airports in 2000 could handle the traffic.

Once the world was globalized for kings and queens, then for wealthy industrialists. In the twenty-first century globalization would be ordinary, accessible not just to the patricians but also to plebeians.

Millions on the move.

Billions of humans on earth.

Shipping trillions of tons of cargo, crops, and animals.

And, by doing so, increasing everybody's risks, from Guadalajara to Guang-zhou.

And ahead lurked new global risks that could exact painful prices from the public's health.

The world's population was aging, most significantly in North America, Western Europe, Japan, Korea, and China. This would have two key impacts on public health: first, on economics, and then on infectious diseases. In financial terms the wealthy West and Asia were approaching crisis points as their national tax and productivity bases were soon to shrink considerably, placing enormous burdens on their smaller, young adult populations. For the West this would be the result of the retirement of its Baby Boom generation, leaving behind two much smaller adult generations to carry the societies' fiscal burdens. In Japan, Korea, and China a combination of shrinking birth rates and phenomenal lon-gevity meant that many Asians would live well into their nineties but be financial burdens to their families or states.

Part of the "problem" was that these peoples had embraced concerns about a population explosion and come to understand that smaller families were healthier and financially more stable households. Instead of having six children and hoping two would be males who survived into their thirties, taking care of their aging parents, the late twentieth century saw these societies recognize a new concept: have two children, both of whom survive, and the parents try to make enough money so that they can care for themselves in retirement.

By 1999 the United Nations Population Fund proudly announced that, yes, the global population had grown from one to six billion during the twentieth century. But its swelling was slowing, and it would only hit 7.5 billion by 2040, then actually begin to decline.[21] If true, that would mean that wise government and careful management of Planet Earth's resources could allow humanity and nature to coexist without horrendous damage to the globe's biodiversity and ecological integrity. It just *might* be possible.[22]

But the generation born between World War II and 1970 would pay a price in their old age for not leaving a large tax base in their wake. In the United States, for example, the over-sixty-five-year-old population grew from 26 million elders to 38.6 million between 1977 and 1997, and their health costs to the federal government climbed from $21.5 billion to $214.6 billion. By 2020 the individual medical costs per elder were expected to have risen from $9,200 on average in 1995,[23] to more than $25,000. And there would be 69.3 million elders in the United States requiring Medicare coverage: simple math forecasts to a cost of $1.7 trillion for elder care.[24]

Globally in 1998 there were 580 million over-sixty-year-olds, 355 million of whom lived in the world's poorest countries. By 2020, predicted the World

Health Organization,[25] there would be a billion elders on earth with 700 million of them residing in developing countries.[26]

And the World Bank forecast that the number of elders living in developing countries by the mid-twenty-first century could, for the first time in human history, exceed the numbers of children under fifteen years of age.[27]

Beyond economics, this radical restructuring of the global population, from an overwhelmingly youth-dominated demography in the mid-twentieth century to an aging one less than eighty years later, posed an interesting and potentially dangerous herd immunity issue.

As people age their immune systems erode, replacing white blood cells and lymphatic tissue at a slower pace and in a less diverse repertoire over time. As a result, elderly bodies are simply more vulnerable to disease than youthful ones. Their immune systems are less able to scavenge for aberrant cells, thereby blocking tumor development. Regulatory mechanisms break down with age so that elders suffer more autoimmunity as their antibodies attack bone (arthritis), glands (Graves' disease), and vital organs. And the aging defenses fail more frequently when confronted with microbial diseases. That is why influenza and pneumonia, for example, are often lethal infections in elders, while the identical microbes may produce little more than a few days discomfort in young adults.

Herd immunity was a well-known, but remarkably poorly understood, concept in the twentieth century. Vaccinologists had long realized that unless a crucial threshold of immunization was crossed—say, 90 percent of a given community was vaccinated—the disease-causing microbes would continue to lurk and kill vulnerable individuals. Few scientists could predict what would occur when the percentage of societal pools with weakened immune systems increased and the efficacy of their childhood vaccinations waned. HIV offered some clues, albeit in the context of young adults and children. Wherever the percentage of HIV-positive adults exceeded 10 percent of a given society waves of opportunistic secondary epidemics followed, notably of tuberculosis.

But HIV depletion of youthful immune systems wasn't a clear mirror of what transpired in the aging process; like all body functions, the immune system decayed over time at different rates in every individual, usually unpredictably. What would happen with epidemic disease in the twenty-first century? Would moderately virulent influenza strains claim millions of lives, spreading among the elderly? Would drug-resistant bacteria emerge at an accelerated pace, transmitted readily with nursing homes and centers of elder populations? Nobody could predict empirically what might occur when a given society's elder population exceeded 30 percent in wealthy countries or 10 percent in poor ones. There simply weren't any precedents from which to derive reckonings.

For twenty-first-century public health leaders, the prospect of diminished herd immunity due to societal aging posed significant challenges. To reduce the threat of contagion, microbe surveillance both locally and globally would need to be significantly better than it was at the close of the twentieth century; it needed to be more widespread, based on far more sophisticated laboratory capabilities, and far more vigilant. Public health scientists would also need to learn more about how aging bodies responded to vaccines, perhaps designing immunizations tailored to elders much as nearly all twentieth-century vaccines were designed specifically for children under twelve years. Only in the 1990s were influenza vaccines created especially with elders in mind. Would it be necessary after 2010 to design special elder vaccines for measles, diphtheria, polio, pertussis, and the other ancient child killers in order to stave off waves of ancient microbial pandemics?

Water supplies, too, would pose a particular public health challenge in the twenty-first century because such microbes as *Cryptosporidium* and *Legionella* were most dangerous to elders. As the sheer numbers of elders in global communities rose the need for ever purer water would also increase.

And the forecast called for more pain.

At the close of 1998 the U.S. Health Care Financing Administration projected a doubling in health care costs, jumping from $1 *trillion* in 1996—already a staggering figure—to $2.1 trillion in 2007. Per capita the world's highest spending on health—13.6 percent of personal income—would soar to 16.6 percent by 2007, and annually costs would rise by 6.5 percent.[28] According to government projections, the burden of those increased costs would fall directly on the shoulders of average Americans, as federal and state expenditures were expected to shrink.

How in the world could Americans pay for their personal and collective health?[29] By 1990 one out of every six Americans, or 13 percent, lived below the poverty line. In 1999 the U.S. Census Bureau redefined poverty, pushing the line from the roughly $16,000 income annually for a family of four to $19,500. With that definition fully 17 percent of the U.S. population was impoverished.[30]

And a worrisome wealth gap was swelling in the United States. From 1989 to 1998 the poorest fifth of American society lost an average of $587 in real annual income while the richest 5 percent of the country gained $29,533. During the 1990s median American family income increased by $600, and thanks to personal real estate and investment values net family worth jumped $11,900. But debt also rose during the decade, driving more families to the edge.[31] The number of families classified as "very poor"—those living on less than $8,018 per year—increased, and as the Children's Defense Fund put it, "We have five times more billionaires but four million more poor children."[32]

The net effect was increasing poverty, decreasing expenditures on social and health services, and rising housing costs. History clearly demonstrated the critical importance of a strong middle class to the maintenance of public health.

Yet most of America was witnessing both a shrinkage of its middle class and greater financial pressure on the strata of society between the expanding ranks of the poor and the enlarging bank portfolios of the superrich.

If America was so rich in 2000 where was all the money going? The top 5 percent of the society saw its wealth, compared to poorest Americans, expand from a ten-fold differential in 1970 to a twenty-fold one in 1996. In 1998 elite business executives earned 419 times more than their office and factory workers, compared to a forty-two-fold difference in 1980.[33]

A key study executed by Fordham University found that despite overall U.S. economic growth the American social-health index had fallen steadily since its peak in 1973.[34] The index annually evaluated sixteen social factors (such as numbers of impoverished children, adults lacking health insurance, and average weekly earnings in real income terms), rating them on a scale of 0 to 100. In 1973 the U.S. index topped at 77.5. By 1993 it was down to 40.6. And it kept falling thereafter.

In 1999 the World Bank concluded that there were more people living in dire poverty at the close of the twentieth century than at any time since World War II. Of course, overall there were more human beings; but a greater percentage of them were surviving in 1999 on less than one dollar a day than had since the 1950s: 1.5 billion in all. The surge in global poverty was largely credited to the collapse of the "Asian Miracle," an economic calamity for much of South Asia and the western Pacific region.[35] In some Asian countries the percentage of the population living on less than one dollar a day doubled in a single year (1997 to 1998). And within nations the wealth gap had caused the middle class to shrink or disappear.[36]

With the very notable exceptions of Singapore and the United States, the wealthiest nations in the world, all of them democracies, had large middle classes, and their richest citizens controlled less than 30 percent of the country's wealth. In most—notably the northern European states—the wealthiest fifth of the societies controlled less than 23 percent of the national wealth.

The reverse was the case in the poorer nations of the world, where more than a third of national wealth was concentrated in the hands of a small societal elite. In most cases these figures underestimated the true proportions of the developing and post-Communist nations' wealth gaps, as they reflected only disparities in the official economies. If corruption and black market economies were factored into these estimates then the concentrations of wealth in such countries were even more severely skewed toward the elite, often just to a handful of families or clans.

In 1996 just 358 superrich individuals controlled as much personal wealth as the combined income and assets of the 2.3 billion poorest people in the world.[37] Three men—Bill Gates, Warren Buffett, and Paul Allen—had a combined 1999 wealth of $156 billion, or $20 billion *more* than the combined GNPs of the forty-three poorest nations.[38] Global critics charged that this signaled a sort of capital lawlessness; globalization, they said, was really about an effort to concentrate the planet's wealth in the hands of perhaps one-hundredth of a percent of its population.[39] Less radical critics pointed to the need for stronger national governments and rules of law to protect the integrity of the marketplace and ensure free access to trade for entrepreneurs and small businesses. Limiting lawlessness and monopolies, they argued, was the key to more equitable distribution of wealth in the twenty-first century globalized community.[40]

Regardless of the macroeconomic finger-pointing it was clear in 2000 that the gap between rich and poor nations was widening.[41]

The United Nations Development Program decried what it called this "dangerous polarization," insisting that it was being driven by the telecomputer age.[42] And finance giant J. P. Morgan said that by the close of 1999 only $119 billion worth of capital would have flowed from the richer nations to the poorer ones—less than half the sum that moved from rich to poor in 1997.[43]

A comparison of key nations worldwide at the close of the twentieth century demonstrated the factors most responsible for the health of citizens.[44] If the observer began with the small Central American nation of Costa Rica it seemed that a rather poor nation, with average per capita shares of GDP (gross domestic product) at just $2,640 a year, could achieve remarkable health for its people, even though its climate was tropical and environment rife with parasitic and mosquito-born disease potential. On a scale of 1 to 188, with 188 being best, little Costa Rica ranked an impressive 144 for child mortality rates, its infant mortality was a low 12 per 1,000 live births, and average life expectancy was seventy-seven years.

In contrast, Russia, with almost equal per capita GDP earnings, ranked only 115 in child mortality, had an infant mortality rate of 20 per 1,000 births, and life expectancy of just sixty-five years. And the United States, with an impressive per capita GDP of over $28,000 a year, ranked 159 in child mortality, had an infant mortality rate of 7 per 1,000, and life expectancy of seventy-seven years—equal to Costa Rica.

What did that mean? Why would the wealthy United States and poor Costa Rica have roughly equal public health indicators, while nearly fiscally equal Costa Rica and Russia had markedly variant health statuses? The answers lay in other telltale figures, such as the percentage of GNP spent on health (8.5 percent in Costa Rica versus 4.8 percent in Russia), though after a point excessive spending (such as 14 percent of U.S. GNP) offered no added benefit. Classic public health mainstays were also crucial, such as access to safe drinking water—nearly every Costa Rican could trust the safety of water coming from his or her tap, but fewer than half of all Russians could be so confident.

A careful reading of the data also demonstrated that adult literacy rates correlated more closely with life expectancy and infant mortality than did GDP per capita.[45]

Zambia and Zimbabwe offered striking evidence of the complexities of public health. Once called Northern and Southern Rhodesia, the nations shared much common culture, were divided by the Zambezi River along a lengthy common border, and both ranked as nations with greater than 20 percent adult HIV rates. Yet Zambia, which provided safe water to only a third of its people and spent only 3.3 percent of its GNP on health, had an infant mortality rate more than double Zimbabwe's, an average life expectancy of forty-three years, and ranked horribly as 12 in the world for child mortality.

Next door, Zimbabwe was hardly a picture of perfect health, with life expectancy a mere forty-nine years. But it offered safe drinking water to 79 percent of its population, spent 6.2 percent of GNP on health, and ranked 58 for child mortality. It was AIDS that brought Zimbabwe's life expectancy down to forty-nine—the nation's chief premature death toll was among its young adults, not, as was the case in neighboring Zambia, its babies and infants.[46]

In the 1950s famed public health advocate René Dubos admonished his colleagues to "think globally, act locally." Fifty years later the reverse was also wise: global efforts were needed to protect local public health. The 1977 eradication of smallpox signaled worldwide recognition that a grave global threat could *never* be eliminated locally unless it was knocked out of every nook and ecological cranny of the planet. The world rallied then but failed to follow through afterward, by mixing global and local public health action across the board.

Global public health action on an ongoing basis would, if it truly existed, constitute disease prophylaxis for every locality, from rich nation to poor. New York City need not worry about its inability to stop plague at JFK Airport if India's infrastructure can do the job in Surat, preventing spread beyond that Gujarati city. And Tokyo need not fear Ebola if Congo's hospitals are sterile environs in which the virus cannot spread. Safety, then, is as much a local as international issue. In public health terms every city is a "sister city" with every other metropolis on earth.

But for such an international system of health to exist every nation needed demonstrable political and economic will. The World Bank, under the leadership in 1999 of James Wolfensohn, and World Health Organization under Dr. Gro Harlem Brundtland scolded national leaders, telling them that the age of handouts from the rich was over. If a national government failed to make good faith efforts to improve the health of its people it could not expect assistance from the United Nations agencies or the wealthy West.

Public health infrastructures were remarkably delicate entities. The instant crash of public health in the former USSR nations offered striking proof of their fragility. And the hospital-acquired and hospital-spread epidemics of Ebola in Kikwit, MRSA in Manhattan, and multidrug-resistant tuberculosis in Russian institutions proved that a poorly maintained medical infrastructure could in some ways be worse than no system at all, undermining public health.

Public health is a bond—a trust—between a government and its people. The society at large entrusts its government to oversee and protect the collective good health. And in return individuals agree to cooperate by providing tax monies, accepting vaccines, and abiding by the rules and guidelines laid out by government public health leaders. If either side betrays that trust the system collapses like a house of cards.

Many factors contributed to the diminution of the public health trust worldwide at the close of the twentieth century: some were related to the erosion of old systems of protection; others signaled a failure to address the new paradigms of health for the globalized twenty-first century.

In terms of the classic, older systems in 1990, the U.S. Department of Health and Human Services released its 675-page *Healthy People 2000*, a manifesto of public health goals for the millennium. At the time, the report stated, Americans were spending annually $65 billion on smoking-related illnesses, $4.3 billion on AIDS treatment, and $16 billion on drug- and alcohol-associated ailments.[47] The 1990 report was an update of the original one, released in 1979, and reflected failure to meet most of the timetable of health improvement then laid out, during the Carter administration.[48] Noting that health care spending had jumped from 5 percent of GNP in 1960 to 12 percent in 1990, and lost productivity due to death and illness had risen, the official report estimated that "injury alone now costs the nation well over $100 billion annually, cancer over $70 billion, and cardiovascular disease $135 billion."

The report detailed a very, very long list of health goals for America, most of which were to be achieved not through expenditures of dollars on government regulation and services, but on "health promotion," a catchall phrase for public education efforts aimed at convincing the nation that it should eat less and more healthfully, exercise more, stop smoking, have fewer (but healthier) children, avoid violent behavior, and cease abusing alcohol and recreational drugs.[49]

The report recognized that none of its goals could be reached unless the then thirty-one million uninsured Americans got access to primary care, and it stipulated that *Healthy People 2000* goals wouldn't be attainable until all Americans could afford to see doctors regularly.

Sadly, the draft *Healthy People 2010 Objectives*[50] noted little improvement in basic health indicators, such as life expectancy. It reflected utter defeat in improving access to health care for Americans. The disparity between white and non-white American health widened during the 1990s. And the numbers of

Americans who were losing work and leisure time due to illness rose, from 18.9 percent in 1988 to 21.4 percent in 1995. The report noted a startling series of deficiencies in basic public health information, and chart after chart was filled with "not available" in place of numbers for such things as percentages of diabetics receiving primary care, oral cancer death rates by race, and blood cholesterol levels in poor Americans. This dearth of data reflected what the report labeled America's primary problem: its declining public health infrastructure:

> This report made clear that the infrastructure upon which the national public health system functions requires definition, coordination, and strength to realize the universal public health mission. [The report] documents continued deterioration of the national public health system: health departments are closing; technology and information systems are outmoded; emerging and drug-resistant diseases threaten to overwhelm resources; and serious training inadequacies threaten the capacity of the public health workforce to address new threats and adapt to changes in the health care market.

While the federal government worried about the nation's weakening public health infrastructure academic public health veered into new territory, far removed from its traditional role: based on large epidemiological surveys—some of which were of shoddy design—academicians issued strong recommendations regarding personal behavior and health.

If health could not be purchased by individuals, some argued, society as a whole could improve its status through nonmedical interventions. And certainly there were American public health victories during the last quarter of the twentieth century, all of which contributed to the country's rising life expectancy. Antismoking campaigns and litigation could be credited with a tremendous decline in tobacco use, which, in turn, prompted annual 1 percent decreases in cancer deaths from 1970 to 1995 and was the key factor in heart disease downturns. Another contributor to America's healthier hearts was the nation's changing diet, away from saturated fats. Seat belts and drunk driving campaigns lowered the car accident death rates. And an enormous national campaign during the 1990s brought teen pregnancy rates down from the highest in the industrialized world in the mid-1980s to about the OECD median by 1998.

Some of these successes came at credibility cost, however. As academic researchers sought to refine their recommendations, particularly regarding diet and lifestyle, contradictions surfaced.[51] Confused Americans worried, for example, about heart disease and lowered their consumption of fatty foods but increased their overall caloric intake, increasing the national rate of obesity— also a contributor to heart disease.

The credibility of the public health message was further undermined by racial stigma, as those diseases most prevalent in minority communities were commonly linked to African-American, Native American, or Hispanic diets and behaviors. When the messenger was perceived as the "white government" the message was viewed with suspicion, even hostility. The Tuskegee legacy haunted absolutely every public health effort aimed at black Americans during the 1990s.

During the 1980s and 1990s public health seemed to be in a "blame the victim" mode: if diseases were personally preventable through proper diet, exercise, and lifestyle, it was axiomatic that the presence of cancer, atherosclerosis, and other potential killers was indicative of poor personal behaviors. Some insurance companies took the logical step of financially penalizing individuals who defied such public health messages as "stop smoking" and "lower your cholesterol count."

This did not endear public health to its public.

In March 1999 the Centers for Disease Control and Prevention conducted a public opinion poll, finding that 57 percent of questioned Americans could not define public health properly, even when given clear descriptions from which to select. Most said that they had "negative evaluations" of the public health system. And, in order of their ranking, the survey group said contaminated drinking water, toxic waste, air pollution, bacterially contaminated food and pesticides represented their greatest health fears.[52]

For many Americans the "blame the victim" perspective of the last decade of the twentieth century flowed from the same science that throughout the 1970s had issued nearly daily warnings about cancer-causing substances in the nation's food, water, environment, and workplaces. Many of the chemicals viewed with panic and trepidation in the 1970s proved to be only marginally hazardous in environmental doses a decade later. Nevertheless, fear of environmental carcinogens had driven creation of a tough and expanded federal regulatory apparatus involving the Environmental Protection Agency, Food and Drug Administration, Occupational Safety and Health Administration, and continued to dominate public concern three decades later.[53]

In this environment of restrictions, amid strong business antipathy to public health regulatory programs, Ronald Reagan swept into the presidency in 1980. His two terms in that office were marked by the dismantling of public health's regulatory powers. Within eight years the Reagan administration had so thoroughly defeated its regulatory adversaries that public health was forced into defeat, even on issues of bona fide community health threats, its most outspoken voices of environmental concern sidelined along the margins of academia and political activism.[54]

As the twenty-first century approached, the combined impact of mounting numbers of uninsured Americans, slashed public health budgets, and widespread antigovernment sentiment could be felt in the rundown county health offices, clogged public hospital emergency rooms, and mounting squabbles over which diseases were most deserving of federal research dollars.

It made the job of public health an increasingly political one, forcing its advocates to defend not only their policies but also the role of government itself. To be fair, public health always was a very political pursuit. After all, its budgets were politically controlled, and implementation of public health principles invariably came up against one interest or another. But now public health in much of the richest country in the world was fighting for its life.

Medicine, too, was struggling. In 1999 the always conservative American Medical Association voted to support unionization of doctors—a move so radically different from the organization's historic stances as to prompt jaw-dropping gasps from the health industry. The AMA's vote reflected rising anxiety among doctors in the United States, who feared their profession was losing not only income but also dignity, power, and respect. American physicians were not, at the close of the twentieth century, a happy lot.[55] Physician dissatisfaction was topped only by the angst among American nurses, and by health consumers.[56]

In response to this collective anxiety, optimists within the health care industry referred to the turn of the century as a transition period that, like so many times of change, might be a bit rocky before the envisioned Nirvana was reached. But the future, they insisted, would usher in a glorious age of New Medicine, drawing from the tools of New Biology. Just as antibiotics had vanquished the bacterial scourges that had plagued humanity for centuries, so New Biology would conquer the chronic killers—cancer and heart disease—as well as mental disorders and addictions.

Would cancer still be a major killer of Americans in the twenty-first century? Probably not, forecast the director of the National Cancer Institute, Dr. Richard Klausner,[57] because Science was entering an era of "dramatic, unimaginable change," in which cancerous cells, and even cancerous genes, would be spotted and controlled or eliminated long before tumors even developed.[58]

"I think that's the scenario," a clearly excited Klausner exclaimed. Revolutionary breakthroughs made in biology over the previous twenty years opened up the possibility of developing an actual strategic plan for elimination of cancer in the United States, Klausner said, and "we've decided on a path and we're already heading down it."

For heart disease, too, a light shone brightly at the end of a treatment innovation tunnel, predicted pharmaceutical industry insider Randall Tobias, and the millennium offered "truly miraculous possibilities" that would, he insisted, include "an end to surgery."

An end to open-heart surgery and invasive oncology? Had the former

CEO of Eli Lilly pharmaceutical company morphed into a hopeless Pollyanna? No, insisted Tobias, because "in the not-so-distant future . . . the life sciences will have accomplished the biological equivalent of putting a man on the moon."

At the root of Klausner's and Tobias's grand optimism were three key areas of basic science innovation: human genetics, protein chemistry, and nanotechnology. The National Institutes of Health's Human Genome Project was racing to the finish line, having nearly completed the delineation of the entire code contained within the DNA of all twenty-three human chromosomes. Hundreds of private and public laboratories were hard at work deciphering the newly discovered code sequences, figuring out what genes actually coded for, how to turn them on and off, and what sorts of mutations led to particular diseases.

The Holy Grail of medicine (and, by inference, public health) in the next millennium was prevention of chronic diseases—cancer, strokes, Alzheimer's, schizophrenia, diabetes, and hundreds of others—through intervention either at the genetic or protein levels. Since all life functions and malfunctions usually boiled down to protein interactions, "nothing is too *Star Trek*kie," Klausner insisted.

For example, cancer cells usually bore proteins on their surfaces that were different from those found on normal cells, and resulted from expression of certain genes. In the future, scientists planned to inject microscopic detectors into outwardly healthy people, and these nanoprobes would "seek out cancers. It's absolutely possible." Klausner continued, "We're working on it with NASA. It's really exciting. If we can think of stellar probes where the signal-to-noise ratio is much, much greater, we're going to be able to find a cancer cell in the human body."

And the next step, Klausner predicted, was "why not arm those little molecular machines? Send them into the body to seek and destroy cancer cells. So I can actually envision treating cancer before it happens," long before anybody has tumors, when cellular change is still in the "precancerous pseudodiseases" phase, as Klausner put it.[59] And that, in Klausner's vision, constituted high-tech public health, focusing prevention not on the carcinogenic environment and diets of the community, but on the appearance of aberrant cells in individuals. It moved the very concept of public health from outside of the human body deeply inward.

Similarly, a number of genetic factors appeared to play roles in the buildup of cholesterol and other physical sources of vulnerability to heart disease and stroke. Researchers had already by 1998 manipulated the cells and DNA of mice to make them skinnier versus fat, smart versus Alzheimer's-like, and cancer-free for a variety of malignancies. There were genetically manipulated mice that had human immune systems, were drug addicts (or not), and suffered a range of human diseases. Cloned cells could grow into tissues, perhaps in the future into whole replacement parts. Need a new heart? Clone it. Or better yet, inject seed cells into the damaged heart to grow replacement tissue and strengthen the organ.[60]

As the secret code of human DNA was deciphered the next step was translation. Having the alphabet soup was one thing: knowing what signals and proteins it encoded was quite another. There were two basic ways to get at that mystery: through the front door or the back. Using massive high-speed computers "front door" analysts took random sequences of DNA and scanned all available protein databases in search of matches. Once a match was found, the position of that particular protein's DNA code within human chromosomes might reveal something about how production of that compound was regulated—switched on or off. And neighboring DNA sequences might contain other vital proteins that carried out related functions in the human body.

The back door approach started with cells and vital hormones, receptors or activators (such as chemokines or neurotransmitters). Scientists used superpowerful magnets or X rays to tease out the three-dimensional structures of these vital proteins and manipulated those shapes to guess what might be the nature of a compound that normally fit into the bends, folds, and pockets of the targeted protein. Those clues would lead to construction of chemicals designed to block or stimulate crucial proteins in the body. In such a way it might be possible to switch on or off hormones, enhance vitamin effectiveness, block addiction-triggering nerve cell receptors in the brain, or turn off cancer-promoting chemicals.[61]

"In thirty to fifty years we'll have it *all* done," predicted Nobel laureate Dr. David Baltimore, president of Caltech.[62] "And we will have the value of that research in terms of drugs in a continual pipeline of discovery. Chemistry is the key to all of this—computorial and structural chemistry is just so powerful. . . . The number of protein structures we'll get a year will be measured in the thousands."

The twentieth century began with a revolution sparked by the microscope, which opened humanity's eyes upon the world of gyrating, fiercely active germs. The Germ Theory was the engine that drove biology for half a century of published health discovery and triumph. With the 1953 discovery of DNA and, perhaps more critically, the early 1970s inventions of genetic engineering techniques, biology entered the Genome Era.

As the new century dawned, the Genome Era was passing its baton to the Age of Proteomics, promising an upheaval in pharmaceutics and medicine that proponents argued would be every bit as dramatic as had been Pasteur's and

Koch's discovery of microbes, Fleming's finding penicillin, and Salk's and Sabin's polio vaccines. Surgeons would be on the unemployment lines, along with psychologists and drug rehab workers. Doctors of the twenty-first century, proponents opined, would practice an elegant new protein-based preventive medicine.[63]

A sort of "public health, if you will." That's what industry leader Tobias called it: public health. And Glaxo Wellcome's Vice President Dr. Allen Roses agreed.[64]

"People are going to come in to their doctors with computerized medical records, genetic blueprints" embedded on small plastic strips, like credit cards," Roses predicted. Those cards would represent a new marriage of sorts, between public health and medicine. Each card would carry the individual's entire genetic blueprint, and "medicine will shift to true family medicine, based on a family's genes."

In the twenty-first century, predicted the National Institutes of Health's Mark Boguski, physicians' textbooks "will be our genes."

But long before such fantasies could be fulfilled a few serious, sobering public health realities need to be faced.[65] The paramount one for the United States was a question of race and, perhaps, class. African-Americans consistently since the Civil War had lagged at least a decade behind whites of all economic brackets in achievement of such public health milestones as life expectancy, infant and maternal mortalities, and adult premature deaths. It was not that they had been more likely to get sick—although in some cases that was the case. Rather, they were more apt to die of their illnesses. And there was little evidence, U.S. Surgeon General David Satcher argued, that African-Americans' DNA was to blame. Rather, a complex set of social and behavioral factors, combined with a lack of access to care on a par with that provided for whites, were the roots of the chasm that separated black and white health.

Similar disparities in health existed between whites and Asian-Americans on the one side, versus African-Americans, Native Americans' and Hispanics on the other, insisted Dr. Phil Lee, former undersecretary of the U.S. Department of Health and Human Services.[66]

"For example, American Indians who come into contact with a different culture—what's the impact? Diabetes," Lee said. "That's not because their genes changed. Their diet changed. And the answer isn't to change their genes—it's change the lifestyle."

Nobody could argue with the desirability of discovering means—genomic or otherwise—of intervening to prevent dreadful disabilities and chronic disease, even death. But would such high-technology approaches as genomic and proteomic drugs get at the core of global public health? If Russia's drinking water was still heavily contaminated in 2020 would proteomic nanoprobes constitute wise public health interventions? At the core of the biotechnology industry's use of the term "public health" in reference to their genomic innovations was the word *prevention*. Public health leaders, unable to reach a consensus on the definition of their field during the 1990s, were ill-prepared at the millennium to debate New Biology's usurpation of their nomenclature. Was prevention, on an *individual* basis, equivalent to public health?

There was certainly plenty of money invested in genomic medicine, both by wealthy nations' governments and by the pharmaceutical industry. Even "small" biotechnology companies had more than $1 billion in research and development of genomic and proteomic products on the line by 2000.[67] For the larger pharmaceutic giants billions of dollars spent on research and development in the genomic arena was an annual routine expenditure.[68]

The excitement was at fever pitch in the industry. Investors commonly claimed that biotechnology would be in 2010 what cyberspace, the Internet, and computers were for the 1990s. The global economy, they argued, would go from the silicon age to the DNA era. Former Eli Lilly CEO Tobias grinned as he pronounced, "Something truly amazing is happening in medicine."[69]

In anticipation of these radical changes mammoth chemical, drug, and foods companies merged or formed partnerships during the 1990s, creating behemoth companies that controlled chemical, drug, and food manufacture on scales exceeding $100 billion.[70] For example, two New Jersey corporations—Warner-Lambert and American Home Products—prepared to merge in late 1999. In the previous year each had revenues exceeding $10 billion and combined market capital of $150 billion. United, the companies were major pharmaceutical and veterinary product manufacturers, controlled numerous vaccine and biotechnology spin-off companies, and manufactured some of the biggest-selling over-the-counter drug and hygiene products in the United States.[71]

In the mid-1990s, the U.S. Congress changed laws that previously regulated the boundaries among medicine, food, and dietary supplements. The lines were so blurred by the close of the decade that more Americans were already taking "preventive medicine" in the forms of vitamin pills and modified foods than were taking prescribed prophylactic drugs. Between 1990 and 2000 the dietary supplement market for everything from orange juice enhanced with echinacea, vitamin C, and zinc to vitamin D plus calcium–enriched milks soared from $3.3 billion in the United States to more than $14 billion.[72] In an odd state of affairs, companies could almost without regulation add a long list of physiologically active chemicals to foods but would be required to undergo extensive FDA approval tests in order to be permitted to sell the same blend of chemicals in pill form.

"For the first time in the 1990s you got a food product where you say, 'If you eat this you live longer,' and that's fiber for your heart," Harvard University's

Juan Enriquez explained.[73] "We're beginning to understand the biochemistry of foods. . . . It's not that you're going to pay $20,000 for surgery at the end of your life. In the future you'll pay $20,000 for nutraceuticals over twenty years."

Long life wasn't, of itself, the goal of residents of the wealthy world: they wanted those many decades to find them sexually adept, slim, in possession of a full head of hair, and, overall, youthful. In the early sixteenth century Juan Ponce de Léon risked a fortune and the lives of himself and a crew of men to sail from Spain to Florida in search of an elixir of youth. Youth-seekers of the twenty-first century will travel inward, to their genes, in pursuit of elusive im-mortality. As the global population aged, so did collective vanity. No price—or profit margin—seemed too high to preserve the vanities of youth. Thus by the late 1990s the biggest-selling drugs were those that promised the individual a cheery personality (e.g., Prozac), plenty of hair on their head (e.g., Propecia), and staying power during sexual intercourse (Viagra). Each of these drugs when released proved wildly popular, were sold at enormous profit margins (Viagra at a 98 percent annual profit),[74] and pushed up stock market values for the relevant manufacturers. Indeed, the same Baby Boomers of the West who were the targets of these so-called lifestyle drugs were also betting their pensions and retirement years on stocks and mutual funds, with pharmaceutical companies ranking among the most popular in which to bank their futures.[75]

In 1998 the pharmaceutical industry earned $99.5 billion in profits in the United States, alone: an 11 percent increase over 1997. In 1999 drug sales profits rose another 16.6 percent. Expenditures on pharmaceutical drugs nearly dou-bled in the United States between 1993 and 1998, rising from $50.6 billion in 1993 to $93.4 billion in 1998.[76]

Global sales were also up, rising 7 percent in just a single year (1997 to 1998) and making pharmaceuticals the fastest-growing and highest-profit legit-imate industry in the world.[77]

Skyrocketing gross sales mirrored astounding net profit growths industry-wide as well. During a time in 1997 to 2000 when typical Fortune 500 corpora-tions had annual profit growths of 4 to 7 percent the average pharmaceutical company's profits grew by 14 to 18 percent annually, and such expansion was expected to continue, if not quicken in pace, after 2000.[78]

The result was fantastic price upgrowth for medicines, making pharma-ceutics the new engine of health care inflation at the dawn of the twenty-first century. Just a decade previously it had been hospitals that drove inflation: by 1999 the real question facing policy makers was no longer whether insurance companies, governments, and individuals could afford the costs of hospitaliza-tions, but whether they would be able to afford to buy the drugs intended to prevent these hospitalizations. Drug companies not only increased the average price tags of newly released drugs, claiming such high costs were necessary to reimburse their research and development investments, but also boosted prices on older and generic drugs. And they were getting away with it, charging as much as $15 *per pill* for some medications.[79]

Consumers searched frantically for sources of cheaper drugs, often by-passing doctors and pharmacies in favor of purchasing off the Internet or their local black market. The result was a deterioration of physician control, a rise in side effects and drug-associated deaths, and a potential public health calamity due to antimicrobial self-medication and consequent promotion of drug resistance.[80]

The drug industry responded to rising criticism of its high profits and prices by saying, as Enriquez had put it, that the future would witness *not* a net increase in health costs, but a shifting of those costs from hospitalizations and treatments to preventive medications. And this would shift expenditures from the late-twentieth-century norm of predominantly the last decade of an individual's life to a trend more evenly distributed throughout life.

At Boston University attorney and ethicist George Annas found any notion of such cost shifting "hilarious," noting that "the major ethical pitfall is going to be how are we going to pay for this? What's the point? They say all expense will be at the front end—that's ridiculous! There's no way to get rid of the back end," Annas insisted. "Short of suicide or euthanasia there's no way to get rid of those last years of really compromised life."

Everybody will die someday, of something. And few, Annas argued, were fortunate enough to feel terrific for decades and then one day simply fall down dead. Most people—even in the brave new world of genomic medicine—would slowly deteriorate and suffer an eventual degeneration and costly hospitalization.

Boguski of the National Institutes of Health said that in the future every single far-out idea was possible, and the only limits "were social and economic."

Most problematic was the world outside the United States. Assuming, for example, that the great breakthroughs forecast for mental illness were realized for the 400 to 500 million residents of North America and Western Europe, what would be available to the six to seven billion other human beings on planet Earth? Christopher Murray, chief epidemiologist for the World Health Organization, calculated that by 2020 depression would jump ten notches to rank as the second-most common debilitating illness in the world, driven by an aging and increasingly frustrated human population.[81]

While Americans in the 1990s obsessed over their neuroses and flights of blues the United States ranked comparatively low on the depression scale, with just 5 percent of the population at some time in their lives being so diagnosed.

And there were already medicines available that dramatically improved the lives of depressed Americans. The annual bill for treatment of depression and lost national productivity due to time away from work or suicide topped $44 billion.[82]

But in France a staggering 16.4 percent of the population was clinically depressed at some point in their lives, 19 percent in Lebanon. And in many countries, notably China and India, millions suffered undiagnosed depressions that WHO's Murray predicted would draw both attention and demand for treatment by 2020. But how could countries such as Lebanon, China, and India afford to spend their equivalents of $44 billion a year on the disease? And assuming the predicted fruits of New Biology appeared in the coming decades, would they be affordable for mental patients in Brazil, Egypt, South Africa, and Thailand?

Even in the wealthy world the burden of depression hit hardest among the poor—precisely those least likely to be able to afford mood elevators and antidepressants. For the most part, it wasn't rich depressed or psychotic Americans who wandered the streets of New York City, homeless and babbling to unseen voices. If the poor of America couldn't afford access to the innovations of psychiatric medicine, certainly the even poorer populaces of the rest of the world could not.

Drug research and development was moving at a feverish pace at the close of the twentieth century. In the United States alone, the drug industry spent $17 billion on research and development in 1998, and some of the National Institutes of Health's $13.6 billion budget went toward pursuit of new medicines.[83] Between 1975 and 1996 nearly 1,240 new drugs were licensed—a very promising figure.

Except that of those 1,240 drugs only 379 were for therapeutic interventions—for treatment of disease states. And just thirteen were for diseases that were the world's leading killers, primarily afflicting residents of tropical and poor countries.[84] Dr. Patrice Trouiller of the Centre Hospitalier Universitaire de Grenoble, argued that "pharmaceutical firms operate like any private industry, they have no specific social welfare mission and respond to economic rather than social or human imperatives. All things considered, drug development for tropical diseases may not have a promising future in the current context. The profit-driven system is not responding to tropical medicine needs."[85]

It was a position with which Dr. Harvey Bale Jr., head of the International Federation of the International Pharmaceutical Association, had little disagreement. He asserted that there was no marketplace to speak of in the poor world. And where any glimmerings of a market—purchasing power—existed, the World Trade Organization's Trade-Related Aspects of Intellectual Property Rights, or TRIPS, was routinely violated by local patent-busting drug companies. Only strong patent protections, coupled with improved local purchasing powers, could serve as true incentives for research, development, and distribution of drugs aimed at the health needs of the developing world, he argued.[86]

Trevor Jones, director of the Association of the British Pharmaceutical Industry, insisted that it cost, on average, $500 million to research and develop a new drug, and a drug company expected to earn back that investment within the first three to five years of sales, thereafter making a profit. Estimates of drug research and development costs per licensed product varied wildly, from that $500 million figure[87] to an incredulously lowball figure of $16 million.[88] Regardless of how much a company invested in research and development of a new drug, Jones insisted, the manufacturer and its stockholders had a right to expect a full return on that investment within three to five years. Bale and Jones neatly sidestepped the question of how much pharmaceutic research was actually funded by American and European taxpayers, both through government support of basic science and tax exemptions granted to the drug industry. When such subsidies were factored into the R&D equation industry claims of justifiable profit margins withered. Even more challenging to the industry's economic calculus was mounting evidence that drugs were deliberately marketed in the U.S. at prices significantly higher than those demanded of medical consumers in Europe and Canada. By 2000 American taxpayers and politicians were questioning why, if the U.S. paid the lion's share of tax-supported global medical research, should its consumers also be paying the most exorbitant prices for the fruits of that scientific mission.

But the drug access problem extended well beyond new products just emerging out of the R and D pipeline. Some 150 nations had drawn up essential drugs lists, naming products considered to constitute their bottom line pharmacological needs. About 90 percent of the drugs on such lists were no longer covered by TRIPS or any form of patent protection—and the original manufacturers had long since earned back their R and D investments. Nevertheless, these drugs remained unattainable in much of the world because of global distribution problems, local corruption that funneled such purchases directly to black markets, and still-high costs. The lowest-priced drugs were often unavailable, as no manufacturer found reason to continue producing such things as the valuable antibiotic streptomycin to combat tuberculosis; five drugs used against African sleeping sickness; aminosidine for the parasitic disease leishmaniasis; uninterrupted supplies of cheap insulin for diabetes treatment; even the great post–World War II public health innovation, the polio vaccine.[89]

The push for record-breaking profits "leaves you focused on 300 to 400 million people in rich countries. But on a human rights level, of course, this is unacceptable," Dr. Bernard Pécoul of the Nobel Prize–winning Médecins Sans Frontières insisted.[90]

"Our role is to organize a fight against this effort to reduce the pharmaceutical market to a very small population. We cannot accept . . . that for most of the world the essential drugs list is things from the 1950s and 1960s, many of which cause [drug] resistance."

Among the many examples cited by Pécoul and his Médecins Sans Frontières colleagues was the deadly diarrheal disease shigellosis, which claimed hundreds of lives in Rwanda following that country's 1994 civil war. The *Shigella* bacteria developed resistance to all but one drug, ciprofloxacin, which cost more than Médecins Sans Frontières or other humanitarian organizations could afford. Médecins Sans Frontières negotiated a price break with the manufacturer, Bayer, ultimately saving thousands of lives. But Bayer's willingness to cut costs in order to stop an African epidemic was not, Pécoul insisted, typical. More commonly people simply died for lack of affordable medicine.

Further exacerbating the problem was poor, even fraudulent local production of drugs, usually in violation of TRIPS international patent laws. In some cases locally produced products were as good as the patented American-made ones, and simply cost local consumers 50 to 90 percent less. But in all too many cases, Pécoul said, the results were substandard, even dangerous. The most egregious example cited in their study occurred in Nigeria during a massive West African meningitis epidemic in 1996 to 1998. A Nigerian company counterfeited vaccine labels for Pasteur Merieux and SmithKline Beecham products and sold sixty thousand doses of nothing but contaminated water. Injected into sixty thousand Nigerians, the dummy vaccines constituted a public health catastrophe that perpetuated the country's epidemic and cost thousands of lives, Pécoul charged.

What was to be done? The Médecins Sans Frontières group offered a list of recommendations, beginning with changes in global treaties that protected patents and pharmaceutical trade and allowing "realistic pricing of potential drugs" sold in developing countries in exchange for local patent enforcement.

The group also called for a far more activist role in these issues on the part of the World Health Organization.[91] And insisted that strong financial incentives would be needed to propel the otherwise dismal state of research and development on tropical diseases. The Médecins Sans Frontières group concluded that access to lifesaving medicine was a human right.

When the World Trade Organization met in Seattle in November 1999 riots broke out, pitting an array of protestors from around the world against the gathering political and corporate leaders. Among the dissidents were public health advocates enraged over pharmaceutic pricing and health care access inequities.[92] Five weeks later President Bill Clinton addressed the elite Trade Forum in Davos, Switzerland, promising tax benefits to pharmaceutical companies that manufactured drugs for poor countries, and calling for reduced pricing on essential drugs. And when the World Bank convened its annual meeting in Washington, D.C., in April 2000, protestors again rioted, many of them denouncing pharmaceutic pricing and inequity. Inside the Bank meeting, as well, the gross disparities between life-and-death drug needs versus availability for most of the world's population were the subjects of lengthy, often heated, discussion.

While the drug companies applauded Clinton's promised tax breaks, they were loath to accept any responsibility for lack of equitable medication access worldwide.

Glaxo's Roses said that "it's not the drug companies that are inhibiting getting the right drugs to the right patients. For a fraction of the cost of peace-keeping in those countries[93] we could get people all the drugs they need."

Consider, Tobias and Roses said, the example of antibiotics. These drugs were widely available and sold in every country in the world, yet the infectious diseases they targeted remained rampant. That was not because of the costs of drugs, they argued, but due to lack of proper health delivery infrastructures: doctors, nurses, hospitals, and clinics.[94]

Not so, countered Pécoul. He argued that drug-resistant microbes were arising in the wealthy world, where the problem was usually handled by simply switching to secondary or tertiary newer drugs—all of which were more expensive, in some cases more than ten times costlier. And at the bottom end of the market drug companies had stopped making such stalwarts of infectious diseases control as penicillin, streptomycin, and chloroquine. Thus, the world's poor faced a squeeze play in which their old drugs were no longer available, the midpriced 1960s and 1970s drugs were losing utility due to drug resistance, and the super new drugs were completely unaffordable.[95]

At stake, Pécoul insisted, was "a time bomb" that would explode not just in the world's poorest countries, but in Europe and America as well. A time bomb of resurging infectious diseases, most of which would acquire phenomenal drug resistance capacities due to improper use and insufficient availability of anti-microbial agents.

A University of California, San Francisco, forecast predicted that by 2070 the world would have exhausted all antimicrobial drug options, as the viruses, bacteria, parasites, and fungi would have evolved complete resistance to the human pharmaceutic arsenal. That apocalyptic nightmare was, remarkably, shared by many of the world's top microbiologists and infectious diseases experts.

Although several laboratories were working on novel ways to kill bacteria and viruses, most do not anticipate that fundamentally new approaches will emerge within the next ten years.[96] Even if such drugs did eventually reach the marketplace, they would undoubtedly follow the financial pattern set with antibiotics: each newer drug cost far more than its predecessor. And the newer agents were usually more toxic, fraught with fiercer side effects.

"The biggest concern is staphylococcus, where only one drug is left," Stanford's Stanley Falknow said, referring to vancomycin. "If that were incurable it would be devastating."

Dr. Anthony Fauci, director of the U.S. National Institute of Allergy and Infectious Diseases, warned that mutated microbes, resistant to hosts of drugs, were the real crisis looming for the twenty-first century. "There is more of a chance of a virulent influenza A wiping out whole populations than you and I getting a gene card," he declared, dismissing the genomic future vision.

Examples of such lurking microbial threats, and humanity's apparent impotence to deal with them, abounded at the millennium, the three most potentially catastrophic being HIV, malaria, and tuberculosis. Combined in 1998 the three microbes claimed five million lives, according to the World Health Organization.[97]

HIV was, by the close of 1999, a lightning rod for protest against pharmaceutical companies, TRIPS, and global inequities in public health. The forecast for the future of the global pandemic was very, very grim. Already, according to the UNAIDS Programme, the virus's impact on Africa was "catastrophic, and the scenario will only worsen unless global leaders work together to invest more—much more—in prevention efforts and programmes to address the multitude of social and economic problems that AIDS has wrought."[98]

Experts envisioned nations obliterated by the world's newest plague, held out little (if any) hope of a cure for the viral disease, and differed significantly at the end of the century only on one point: how many more decades would pass before an effective, affordable HIV vaccine could be used worldwide.

The National Institutes of Health reached the conclusion that an HIV vaccine was the only thing that could slow the virus's seemingly relentless expansion around the world. By 1999 half of the agency's $1.5 billion HIV budget was aimed directly, or indirectly, at the search for a vaccine, offered Office of AIDS Research director Neal Nathanson. "We're in it for the long haul," he said with a sigh. But he argued that the private sector lacked similar long-term commitment to the vaccine problem, and "none of the big players are seriously involved in developing a vaccine because they don't see the profit in it."

When AIDS first surfaced in 1981 the global response was a medical, not public health, one: resources were skewed to the search for a cure. Fifteen years later Science offered up HAART, or highly active antiretroviral therapy. But in the long run HAART clearly was not the answer. Its price tag—$10,000 to $60,000 a year for the drugs alone—rendered HAART unusable for more than 90 percent of the word's HIV population, estimated in 1999 by the United Nations AIDS Programme to number forty million people.

And in North America and Western Europe, where hundreds of thousands of people were on HAART in 1999, trouble was brewing. Many patients—about 50 percent, depending on which studies were cited—had failed their initial rounds of HAART either because they could not tolerate the drugs' toxic side effects or they had difficulty adhering to the rigorous daily schedules of medicine ingestion that HAART necessitated.

With the bloom clearly off the HAART rose AIDS advocates were calling for rapid development of drugs that hit novel targets on HIV, possibly outwitting the virus's awesome mutation capacities. But Merck's vice president, Emilio Emini, said that there wasn't much in the drug development pipeline and it was "impossible to answer" when such novel agents might be ready: "It's the temporal zone of chaos."

"Where will we be in ten, twenty years?" Dr. Peter Piot, Director of UNAIDS, asked.[99] "It's really, really hard to say. We haven't done [forecasts] going out more than to 2005. We've learned that projections turn out to be awfully wrong."

Wrong, in that the epidemic had consistently outpaced worst case scenarios, particularly in Africa and Asia.

The key question for forecasters was the proverbial bell-shaped curve. Most, if not all, epidemics started at a low level, rose rapidly claiming large numbers of human victims, and then naturally slid back down the bell-shaped curve, ending up permanently at a modest, endemic level in the population. The reasons for that downward curve were multitudinous, and they varied from epidemic to epidemic. But the curve was always there.

Was there evidence of a bell-shaped curve for HIV, or would the epidemic continue to claim even more lives, ascending its death toll year after year well into the twenty-first century?

Piot believed that HIV might by 2005 hit the top of its bell in some hard-hit African countries, such as Uganda, Tanzania, Zambia, and Zimbabwe. But what a bell it was! The peak was only reached when upward of a third of all adults under fifty years of age were infected in most parts of those societies, meaning a third of each generation would perish.

"What you have is a kind of modern conflagration. It's the modern equivalent of the great Plague," said Larry Gostin, professor of law at Georgetown and expert on AIDS human rights. "And that's what you're going to get in all of the developing world. It's going to be losses of whole generations. We're on the verge of the twenty-first century with all this modern technology and yet we're as vulnerable to pathogens as we were decades ago.

"The critical difference," Gostin continued, "is that at those times we as a world community sat by and cried because we couldn't do anything. And now we stand by and watch, expressionless, because we choose not to do anything.

And that's a clear measure of how far we as a species have moved, from compassion to disinterest, or self-interest."

Piot said that reaching what appeared to be the top of the bell in some African societies had meant national bankruptcy, "pushing households into poverty and starvation, people ending up on the streets. And then we'll be giving food aid, instead of investing in [HIV] prevention."

The first community to reach an HIV bell curve was San Francisco's gay population, where the bell peaked in the mid-1980s when the infection rate exceeded 50 percent. Since that time, due largely to the gay community's own education campaigns, the HIV rate had declined steadily, yet it still claimed a terrible 20 percent of the remaining San Francisco gay population in 1998.

For more than a decade epidemiologist Jim Chin, retired in 1999 and living in California, executed HIV forecasts for the World Health Organization and UNAIDS. He believed that "there will continue to be from twenty-five to thirty million persons with HIV alive each year for the next twenty-five years, and hopefully by then (or before) the African countries can get their act together and begin to significantly reduce their annual incidence of new infections so that from twenty-five to fifty years from now, when my grandchildren become parents and then grandparents, the global prevalence of HIV infections will begin to drop to about ten to twenty million."[100]

Grim as that scenario was, Chin conceded that India, with a population of one billion people, was the "wild card" that could throw off all his forecasts. It was one thing for Botswana, for example, with a population of 1.4 million people, to have a 32 percent infection rate among its young adults, or about 200,000 HIV cases. It was quite another for 32 percent of all young adult Indians, or about 200 *million* people, to be infected. Piot said that Asia, particularly China and India, where two out of every five human beings living in 1999 resided, was the key to the future of the planet's HIV bell curve.

A 1998 joint publication of the World Health Organization, Harvard School of Public Health, and the World Bank entitled, "Health Dimensions of Sex and Reproduction," sought to forecast HIV bell curves region by region for the world. The team predicted that much of Africa wouldn't see its HIV epidemic peak until 2005 to 2010. Asia's epidemics, they said, wouldn't peak until a decade later.

If true—and if an adult infection rate of more than 30 percent was fated to constitute societies' HIV bell peak, by 2020 the world could have nearly half a billion people living with HIV and AIDS.

Some studies suggested the elusive bell curve might be unimaginably high. A U.S. national security analysis of African armed forces found 1999 prevalence rates among soldiers ran as high as 60 percent—a staggering figure unmatched by any other infectious disease of the twentieth century except, perhaps, the 1918 swine influenza.[101] Well surpassing any flu toll were HIV levels seen in the

South African armed forces—infection rates as high as 90 percent, according to a March 2000 United Nations survey.

Given such a dire backdrop it came as a surprise to no one that the arrival of HAART for wealthy countries sparked rage in poor, HIV-plagued nations. They could not afford the drugs, even when pharmaceutical companies reduced the prices. And various donor schemes for providing HIV drugs to poor nations, particularly in Africa, floundered on the rocky shores of long-neglected public health. If, after all, doctors in the United States were finding it extremely difficult to administer HAART to patients without prompting hard-to-treat side effects and drug resistance, how in the world could impoverished clinics such as Kikwit's General Hospital do the job? The HAART dilemma proved the cases of both Pécoul and Roses: for poor countries the wrong sorts of drugs had been developed; and even free drugs could not be used properly in countries lacking viable public health infrastructures.[102]

In most of the world the only viable solutions to HIV in the long run were a safe, 100 percent effective vaccine; a cheap pill that in one or a very few doses completely eliminated infection; or a vaginal and rectal microbicide that was very cheap (less than 10 cents per use), nontoxic, and highly effective in blocking HIV sexual transmission. In 2000 none of these solutions were at hand. And, more importantly, none were in the R and D pipelines of major pharmaceutical companies, primarily because of a lack of perceived future profitability.

The HAART model opened a set of profitable doors for the pharmaceutical industry. First, it allowed an acute infection to be treated as a chronic disease, dragging out treatment (and drug sales) for decades. Second, it escalated the level of socially acceptable public health disparity in the world, finding the companies and wealthy world governments facing remarkably little criticism for sparing the lives of European and North American citizens while witnessing obliteration of populations elsewhere. Third, the treatment was based on a class of drugs, called protease inhibitors, that were very costly and difficult to produce; patent violation was minimized by the sheer scale of production obstacles. And fourth, even an extraordinarily expensive set of drugs could prove profitable within targeted wealthy nations if the sense of urgency was high enough to commit governments to their subsidized purchase. That Brazil, a developing country, committed to purchasing HAART drugs and dispensing them for free to its entire HIV population testified to the scale of acceptable pricing in a perceived national crisis.

Finally—most important—the HIV/HAART model showed that a public health problem could be "acceptably" medicalized: even public health authorities bowed before the HAART model though, in truth, it offered more obstacles than solutions for HIV prevention and control.

Malaria was medicalized decades earlier, when chloroquine was invented. As the parasites acquired drug resistance new drugs were used. But resistance emerged to those, too. By the late 1990s some three thousand children were dying daily of malaria, 90 percent of them in the same African countries that were struggling against HIV. The parasites had acquired tremendous powers of drug resistance, rendering prophylactic therapy useless in much of the tropical world and treatment perilous. And global climate change brought warming trends that made higher elevation regions of Africa, Asia, and Latin America newly hospitable to malaria-carrying mosquitoes.[103]

In 1998 the World Health Organization launched the Roll Back Malaria campaign, working with UNICEF and the World Bank to find incentives for development of new antimalarial drugs. Though there were promising potential drugs in the research pipeline, no pharmaceutical company in 1999 had an internal malaria research program.[104]

Tuberculosis offered the most startling case of the failure of the medicalized model of public health. The catastrophic TB epidemic of Russia and neighboring formerly Soviet nations was out of control by 2000, despite considerable efforts to rein it in through the use of antibiotics. In 1997 and 1998 the World Health Organization stuck to its DOTS mantra, repeating over and over that the region's governments should adopt the directly observed short course therapy approach to TB control.

But it didn't work.

Drug-resistant TB swept over the Russian region, even in areas where authorities obediently followed WHO's protocols.[105]

Far away in the Andes Mountains of Peru Dr. Paul Farmer and his colleagues were working with residents of Carabayallo, the poorest neighborhood of Lima. They discovered in 1997 that many of these Peruvians were suffering from tuberculosis, despite having received DOTS at local clinics. The Harvard group collected sputum samples from the TB patients and submitted them for analysis at a Massachusetts laboratory. In an urgent 1997 letter to colleagues and financial backers, Farmer and his partners described the situation:

> A number of these patients we have identified have been found to have strains with resistance patterns more alarming than those documented in any other setting. None of these patients has been receiving appropriate treatment, since the medications necessary to cure their resistant disease are not available through the public health program. This restrictive policy is in sharp contrast to the provision of free "first-line" medicines for patients with the more usual, drug-susceptible strain of TB.
>
> It became evident to us that these impoverished patients were neglected and at about the same time infecting a large number of individuals,

including family members, coworkers, neighbors, and even casual contacts. Through in-depth interviews with these patients, we have been able to identify the processes by which poor Peruvians become sick with drug-resistant TB: inequalities in access to effective treatment are producing a vicious cycle which permits the emergence and transmission of this deadly disease.[106]

Farmer and other DOTS critics were increasingly uneasy. They argued that multidrug-resistant strains of TB had by 1999 emerged in more than one hundred countries, as the microbes stubbornly defied WHO's prescribed treatment. Further, most developing countries lacked a public health infrastructure that could effectively distribute the WHO-recommended drugs, especially to their poorest citizens.[107]

In 1998 the World Health Organization brought together top pharmaceutical leaders, hoping to gain their support for development of some form of pill that, taken alone, would have the impact of the complicated schedule of multiple drugs that formed the basis of DOTS. If a sufficiently inexpensive formulation could be found, combining several drugs that were then made by competing companies, TB control would be far easier. But the meeting was a disappointment. The companies told WHO that their targets were $1 billion "big hitters" in the United States, not drugs that might sell for pennies in poor countries. There was no TB drug in the research pipelines of any major pharmaceutical or biotechnology company, anywhere in the world. The reason: no drug company was interested in pursuing *any* project that could realistically yield profits of less than $350 million a year, for five or more years. Even if all of the roughly estimated eight million TB sufferers worldwide went on the new superpill, each taking the medication for six months at an average total cost of eleven dollars per patient, the profit numbers simply wouldn't add up, the companies said.[108]

Though WHO continued its optimistic DOTS chanting, its own dire reports forecast that 200 million people alive in 1998 would eventually develop tuberculosis, which far exceeded the total estimated number of worldwide tuberculosis cases that occurred over the course of the entire nineteenth century.[109]

It was time to take stock: what was an appropriate strategy for TB control? Could catastrophe—globalization of completely drug-resistant, incurable tuberculosis—be averted without new drugs? Or an effective vaccine? In late 1999 the Centers for Disease Control and Prevention issued its recommendations, which boiled down to elimination of the one-size-fits-all WHO/DOTS approach, in favor of tailor-made strategies on a country-by-country basis. No strategy would work, the CDC warned, in the absence of a strong public health infrastructure.

Thus, the U.S. federal agency concluded, the only way residents of Los Angeles, Minneapolis, Paris, Tokyo, and London could truly be sure that their children wouldn't grow up in a world of threatening, incurable tuberculosis was by joining in a global commitment to basic public health.[110]

The most condemning, most sobering report of all came from the auspices of billionaire George Soros in October 1999.[111] Harvard's Farmer, the scientists in New York City's Public Health Research Institute, Soros's Open Society Institute, and researchers from all over the world collaborated on the massive report. They concluded that multidrug-resistant TB *already had globalized*, with strains having surfaced in at least one hundred nations. In horrifying detail the 258-page report documented failure after failure to control TB, and promotion of emergence of resistance as a result of inappropriate use of antibiotics. The worst examples were in Russia and the former Soviet Union nations, but the scientists documented terrifying death tolls due to antibiotic-resistant microbes all over the world.

"The best way to work toward elimination of TB is to provide effective treatment to all patients with active disease," the report argued. "Had DOTS been established before the emergence of resistance to antituberculosis drugs, DOTS alone might have been sufficient for TB control. But MDR-TB 'hot-spots' have been identified on four continents, and the transmission of *M. tuberculosis* continues apace, as yet unchallenged by any coherent strategy."

The report called for "DOTS-Plus," a strategic approach that involved use of still more drugs for longer periods of time, coupled with laboratory monitoring for resistance and strict supervision of patients to ensure compliance. It estimated a price tag of $1 billion a year to bring the global cataclysm under control. Soros had personally committed millions of dollars for such efforts in Russia, but far more was needed.

"If new money isn't made available immediately the epidemic may become virtually impossible to contain," Farmer warned.

Malaria, tuberculosis, and the new scourges of hospitals (MRSA, VRE, VISA, and the like[112]) shared one critical feature: all had at some point been treatable or preventable with medicines that ultimately were failing due to microbial evolution and inadequate public health. Would the list lengthen in coming years? Definitely, biologists warned. Would industry supply alternative drugs? Probably not—certainly not within an urgent time frame.

The drug companies were banking on vaccines. They said innovative products, such as vaccines made from the DNA of viruses or bacteria, would be available for tuberculosis, malaria, schistosomiasis, and other killers within twenty years. And, they promised, these vaccines would be affordable.

Affordable to societies such as those in sub-Saharan Africa, that spent less than ten dollars per citizen per year on all health care needs?

"Here we are, one hundred years after Pasteur identified the cause of rabies and Koch the cause of tuberculosis," former Health and Human Services Assistant Secretary Lee said. "Yet we did more to control TB by social factors," in Koch's day than through antibiotics a century later.

"Here we are," Lee continued,[113] "one hundred years out and we still don't have a vaccine for tuberculosis or malaria."

Meanwhile the opportunities for emergence and spread of such microbes would increase in coming years as the density, mobility, and relative poverty of the human population grew.

In the end, he argued, humanity was left with a disturbing, contradictory picture of the New Medicine. On the one hand, true miracles were ahead. On the other, a grim global social context challenged all optimism.

In Gostin's nightmarish vision of 2040, "you'll have a population with virtual absence of disease and disability. And another overwhelmed by disease and disability."

At the dawn of the twentieth century the Western world fused the ideas of civic duty and public health. Conquering disease was viewed as a collective enterprise for the common good.

"And now we end the century really rejecting the right of the health of societies in favor of the individual," Gostin said sighing.

Where did we go wrong? Why had the sense of collective good disappeared? On a microscale, it seemed neighbors were less willing at the dawn of the twenty-first century to take minute risks or pay taxes on behalf of the health of the overall community. And on a macroscale, the wealthy world seemed in 2000 to be less willing than they in some cases had been during the days of colonialism a century earlier to come to the aid of African, South Asian, Eastern European, and Latin American populations. Why?

One obvious answer—perhaps *the* answer—was the very success of the medicalized approach to public health. Antibiotics, vaccines, antivirals, pesticides, antiparasitic drugs—these had been triumphs when first introduced. And they had worked, pushing the microbes into retreat and allowing whole societies to relieve themselves of the collective burden of plagues and childhood deaths. For societies that had full access to these boons—these genuine scientific miracles—it was possible for individuals to shift their entire mind-sets from concern for the collective well-being to personal concerns about cancer, heart disease, diabetes, and countless other noncommunicable chronic ailments and killers.

It would be unfair to characterize such thinking as selfish. True, microbial death and disabilities continued to stalk the poor throughout the twentieth century, despite these great advances. But for those fortunate enough to grow up without such threats in their environs, pure practicality dictated a shift in focus.

It is hard to fear that which doesn't visibly threaten when other worries and killers are lurking.

But the individualized and medicalized approaches no longer made sense by the close of the twentieth century, amid global travel, international economic trade, rising drug resistance, and a widening wealth gap.

What did? The World Health Organization was in the late 1990s accused of having no strategy or sense of mission for global public health.[114] It had for decades focused on provision of medicines—on the medicalized model of public health—leaving such basics as clean drinking water, decent primary health care, and safe, abundant foods up to local governments. And governments displayed a remarkable range in senses of responsibility for their populaces, from the Scandinavian cradle-to-grave all-inclusive health model down to the level of gross negligence, such as existed in Mobutu's Zaire.

In 1999 WHO Director-General Brundtland set out a new strategy for the global health organization, focused on those governments that seemed to shirk responsibility for their people.[115] Under the scheme government and business leaders were presented evidence of the deleterious economic consequences of having a population that was in poor health. It was, in short, an appeal to the venal nature of such leaders, arguing that ignoring their people's public health needs would eventually hurt their financial balance sheets.

But as Lenin would no doubt have noted, this was not a strategy, but a tactic. And though it might constitute a clever approach toward raising concerns and dollars from the world's powerful, it did not supply a strategic plan for the expenditure of those resources.

More challenging was the task of forecasting, providing policy makers with a glimpse of humanity's medical future that might help make tough decisions about whether, for example, to build two new neonatal intensive care units, a few dozen rural clinics, or one large geriatrics center with scarce government funds.

The amazing thing, Harvard public health expert Christopher Murray argued, was that no one really knew how many people in the world died or suffered from *any* disease or injury.

"If you go to WHO offices and ask, 'How many young adults die of your respective diseases?' TB, or HIV, or cancer, whatever, the total when you add them all up exceeds the number of human beings who die annually by two- to three-fold," Murray said.[116]

About fifty million people died on earth every year in the late 1990s: only fourteen million deaths were ascribed to any cause in formal death certificates. An additional unknown number of people—probably a quarter of the world's six billion living human beings—suffered some form of illness, injury, or disability every year that was serious enough to warrant a day or more off from work or school. If the cause of humanity's deaths remained obscure, Murray said, its nonlethal illness burden was an utter black hole, largely because "problems are brought to the attention of the world through the lenses of advocates. And despite everyone's best intentions you get distortion as a result. As much as possible we have to separate epidemiology assessment from advocacy."

Diseases common to well-educated, well-heeled Westerners had their constituency groups that lobbied hard for medical research and treatment dollars. Key to that political effort was demonstration of need—and need equaled a death toll. So cancer advocacy groups, for example, rounded their numbers upward to claim the maximum percent of the world's annual death toll as theirs.

Lost in the numbers game was the most obvious fact: most deaths and illnesses in the world occurred among the poorest citizens of the planet, and their biggest killers simply didn't have powerful advocacy groups in Geneva, Washington, London, or Moscow. Malaria, tuberculosis, malnutrition—these were not ailments with formidable lobbies.

Murray headed a team of 150 scientists and physicians from throughout the world aimed at filling in the vast data gap and, as he put it, separate advocacy from epidemiology. The effort began under the direction of the World Bank in 1992 and had expanded to include the involvement of World Health Organization and the Harvard School of Public Health. By the time the effort would be completed early in the twenty-first century ten volumes of information on the burden of human disease and several policy implication documents would have been published.

And they would be quite controversial.[117] The World Health Organization's reports painted grim pictures of humanity's efforts to stave off infectious diseases such as HIV, tuberculosis, and malaria. They forecast a resurgence of old scourges, including those that were then vaccine-preventable.

The Harvard group's *Investing in Health*, in contrast, viewed the future as one rife with chronic disease, mental illness, cancer, and heart disease. By 2020, the report argued, microbes would be responsible for only 40 percent of the burden of disease. The majority of all illness and death would be due to cancer, heart disease, stroke, clinical depression, and automobile accidents.

As a result, the report stated, research and development spending should shift toward the search for cheap ways to treat then-costly ailments such as myocardial infarction, breast cancer, acute depression, trauma, and stroke.

Murray's group concluded that the single biggest force pushing health priorities of the future was the aging of the world's population. In Japan, Europe, and North America the majority of the population would by 2020 be over sixty-five years old.[118]

Forecasting was a dangerous business, of course. Health planners in the United States had been absolutely certain in the late 1960s that more than 85 percent of all deaths in America by the close of the century would be due to such chronic diseases as cancer and heart disease. In 1900 nearly 800 Americans out of every 100,000 died annually of infectious diseases. By 1980 that number was down to 36 per 100,000. That certainly seemed to bear out the forecasts. But then infectious diseases deaths started rising again in the United States, hitting 63 per 100,00 in 1995.[119]

In an extensive, largely classified study the U.S. Central Intelligence Agency scrutinized the Harvard and WHO forecasts, deciding that both captured "some real trends" but "overstate the progress achievable, while underestimating the risks."[120]

The intelligence group concluded that the most likely scenario was one of future deterioration in global health, followed in the mid-twenty-first century by limited improvement. Key to the CIA's pessimism were "persistent poverty in much of the developing world, growing microbial resistance and a dearth of new replacement drugs, inadequate disease surveillance and control capacity, and the high prevalence and continued spread of major killers such as HIV/AIDS, TB, and malaria."

In 1999 the World Health Organization settled for the following breakdown of global deaths: 53.9 million people died in 1998; 31 percent suffered cardiovascular diseases, 25 percent infectious diseases, 13 percent cancer, and the remainder was comprised of deaths due to accidents, respiratory and digestive diseases, maternal childbirth fatalities, and 6 percent "other."[121]

Better data for policy makers would result from vastly improved disease surveillance systems, vital statistics reporting, and primary health infrastructure.

It was hard to escape that word—*infrastructure.* Such a deceptively banal-sounding term failed utterly to convey the millions of lives that might be long and healthy, or short and tragic, based on whether or not infrastructure existed.

During the Great Depression Paul de Kruif, who had been a true believer in the medicalized strategy of public health, witnessed the dreadful death toll that preventable and treatable diseases were taking on America's poor children. Embittered, prone to sarcasm, he asked in 1936:

When you think that this science is really the right of all humanity, should be owned by humanity, by the living, by all who, half-dead, have a chance for life—

Then what, fundamentally, could be more hopeful?

Because when they understand that all their own babies can be brought to this strong and beautiful life, the people of the world will at last rise up and ask: Are or are not all of our children really going to live?

And if not, then in the name of misery, why keep them alive.[122]

Nearly seventy years later the question remained germane. Science had, indeed, offered humanity a treasure trove of discoveries of public health significance. But at the close of the century everything seemed up for patent grabs, even the genomes of killer microbes that, once deciphered, were placed under corporate locks and keys, away from the utility of public health advocates.[123]

Yet de Kruif's question contained a glimmer of an idea: democracy.

It's impossible as an individual to believe in a future if you don't believe in your power to influence the present. Making choices and taking actions to prevent theoretical future catastrophes or better the lives of your children, or grandchildren, are formidable steps to take for those who feel impotent in their day-to-day lives.

Public health in the twenty-first century will rise or fall, then, with the ultimate course of globalization. If the passage of time finds ever-widening wealth gaps, disappearing middle classes, international financial lawlessness, and still-rising individualism, the essential elements of public health will be imperiled, perhaps nonexistent, all over the world. Capital will be skewed away from social service infrastructures in such a scenario, particularly those that meet the needs of the poor. Few public health barriers will be in place to prevent global spread of disease, and ever more drugs will be rendered useless by microbial resistance. United Nations agencies, including the World Health Organization, will witness further deterioration in their funding and influence. And political instability will foster increasingly irrational nation-state and rogue activities including, perhaps, bioterrorism.

There was another potential for the future. It didn't cast the world in a bed of aromatic roses, but neither did it forecast hell on earth.

The people of the world were coming to know a great deal about one another at the millennium, thanks to worldwide distribution of movies, the Internet, television, and twenty-four-hour-a-day broadcast news. In the short term the global population witnessed one another's miseries with powerful impact in the 1990s. Earthquakes, carnage, ethnic cleansing, hurricanes, famines—these once-remote events filled living room TV screens and blared headlines from Cape Town to Moscow.

In the longer run, perhaps on a more subtle level, humanity also began to see the scale of planetary inequities. The writer was reminded of an experience in Harare, Zimbabwe, watching the film *Ruthless People* in a neighborhood theater. Bette Midler and Danny DeVito's amusing performances, curiously, drew no laughter from the audience, though the Zimbabweans did enjoy the film immensely. Rather than guffaw at Midler's slapstick virtuosity the crowd loudly sighed, "oohed" and "ahed" over the cars, stereos, houses, clothing, jewelry, electronic devices, and lifestyles displayed on the silver screen. They reveled in a sort of jealous fantasy state, gasping at the amazing and wonderful lives that they imagined all Americans enjoyed.

In American movies and internationally distributed television shows no modern characters ever fretted over their diphtheria-slain child or malarial toddler. Life was free of such care, filled instead with gun-toting Clint Eastwood cops, glamorous Julia Roberts love affairs, and madcap Robin Williams adventures.

In the future was it not possible that, faced with such glaring evidence of the shortcomings in their own existences, more and more of the world's poor would demand accountability from their governments? Was it Pollyannaish to imagine that in coming years politicians and government leaders who denied clean drinking water, safe foods, ample medicines, and basic public health to their constituencies would pay a price for such negligence and arrogance?

And one could hope that in the future violations of that trust would be punished.

That was the essence of U.S. foreign policy in the post–Cold War period. The Agency for International Development, for example, devoted most of its resources to what it called "democracy building."

Perhaps, such proponents argued, the day would come when Indians would demand that their government spend 5 percent of its GDP on noncorrupt public health activities. Perhaps the Zairois would one day cease their civil war and ethnic battles, face their national leaders, and cry out for health for their children. Perhaps African leaders who failed to place HIV prevention on their top priority lists would be drummed out of office by millions of grown-up AIDS orphans. Perhaps Russian voters would one twenty-first-century day come to believe in the power of the ballot and opt for candidates that espoused not tired ideological and nationalistic rhetoric but concrete programs for provision of social services.

And perhaps—indeed, probably—Americans would grow fed up with their irrational public health and medical systems, demanding the long overdue, bold reappraisal of the nation's priorities for the health of its people. By 2000 there were already organizations forming all over the United States, as well as internationally, demanding that the pharmaceutical and health insurance industries shift their priorities away, at least incrementally, from profits toward humanity's most urgent public health needs.[124]

Health, broadly defined, may not qualify as a right for every human being. But the essentials of public health most assuredly were human rights. Every government in the world knew by 2000—irrefutably—that an unfiltered, unclean drinking water system could kill children. Every government knew that black market sales of antibiotics fueled emergence of deadly drug-resistant microbes. No political leader could believably deny knowledge that allowing unfettered tobacco advertising and sales in his or her country would destroy the lungs, hearts, and other vital organs of the smoking citizenry. Leaders could no longer deny that an HIV-loaded syringe, passed from one person to another, was every bit as dangerous as a loaded gun. Ignorance might have protected world leaders in the mid-twentieth century, but after the millennium it would be difficult to dodge a charge of negligent homicide against a national leader who deliberately shunned provision of safe drinking water in favor of military or grandiose development expenditures. Trust and accountability: above all else, these were the pillars of public health.

After the Persian Gulf War the U.S. government demanded global accountability regarding biological weapons. Together with its European allies the United States called for complete transparency in the manufacture and distribution of agricultural chemicals, pharmaceuticals, and petrochemicals. Only in an atmosphere of openness and accountability, the Clinton administration argued, could there be truth.

But *no* drug or chemical company, whether located in Baghdad or Baltimore, wanted outsiders inspecting its plants and operations. Trade secrecy, alone, necessitated barriers and blocked transparency. Resorting to typical law enforcement solutions in confronting such obstinance, the United States funded research on high-tech solutions, such as devices that could "sniff out" nasty microbes in the air or detect them in the water supply.

It was just another example of a public health threat confronted with technological solutions. There was not demonstrable justification for placing public trust in such options.

Were a biological attack to occur, or a naturally arising epidemic, the public would only have one viable direction in which to place its trust: with its local, national, and global public health infrastructure. If such an interlaced system did not exist at a time of grave need it would constitute an egregious betrayal of trust.

To build trust there must be a sense of community. And the community must collectively believe in its own future. At the millennium much of humanity hungered for connectedness and community but lived isolated, even hostile, existences. Trust evaporated when Tutsis met Hutus, Serbs confronted Kosovars, African-Americans worked with white Americans or Estonians argued with Russians.

The new globalization pushed communities against one another, opening old wounds and historic hatreds, often with genocidal results. It would be up to public health to find ways to bridge the hatreds, bringing the world toward a sense of singular community in which the health of each one member rises or falls with the health of all others.

NOTES

INTRODUCTION

1. Published in 1994 by Farrar, Straus & Giroux, New York, and in 1995 in paperback by Viking Penguin, New York.

2. Decosas, J. Plenary address to the 11th International Conference on AIDS, Vancouver, July 1996.

3. "World hunger." *The Economist* (November 6, 1999): 108.

4. Food and Agriculture Organization. *The State of Food Insecurity in the World.* Food and Agriculture Organization, Rome, 1999.

5. "Risky economies." *The Economist* (November 13, 1999): 114.

6. Indeed, by 1998 violent crime rates in most American cities had fallen to their lowest levels in more than three decades, yet politicians continued to garner public support and votes by increasing police spending and building more jails.

7. Committee for the Study of the Future of Public Health. "The future of public health." Washington, D.C.: National Academy Press, 1988.

8. Ibid, page 3.

9. In addition to overall government cutbacks, this reflected a change in the sources of funds. As part of the anti-"Big Government" effort of the Reagan era control of public health shifted from the federal to state levels. In 1980 states received their public health funds as follows: 45 percent from state taxes, 28 percent from the federal government, and 20 percent from local (city and county) taxes. Just four years later state taxes accounted for 54 percent of the public health budgets, federal revenue for 37 percent, and local just 2 percent.

In 1966 the United States Congress had passed the Partnership in Health Act, the goal of which was to provide funds to poor states. In 1982 the program was amended, becoming a block grant allocation to each state, to be used in key areas of public health as the states saw fit. As time and the 1980s recession wore on, the states increasingly used those federal block grant funds to retire debts, raise long-stagnant salaries, and save programs in counties that were devastated by lost tax revenues. Federal monies were like an addictive drug for the states, particularly in those that suffered local tax revolts and stagnation in municipal revenues.

10. Numbers of Uninsured Americans (in millions) (Based on data from the U.S. Department of Health and Human Services.)

11. Callahan, D. *False Hopes: Why America's Quest for Perfect Health Is a Recipe for Failure.* New York: Simon & Schuster, 1998.

12. "Support for some public health programs increased in appropriations for FY 1997." *The Nation's Health* (November 1996): 5–6; and "Appropriations process tough on public health." *The Nation's Health* (August 1995): 1.

13. Editorial. "WHO: Where there is no vision, the people perish." *The Lancet* 1350 (1997): 749.

14. Al-Mazrou, Y., Berkley, S., Bloom, B., et al. "A vital opportunity for global health." *The Lancet* 350 (1997): 750–51.

15. McKeown, T. *The Origins of Human Disease*. Oxford, U.K.: Basil Blackwell, 1988.

16. McKinley, J. B. and McKinley, S. M. "The questionable contribution of medical measures to the decline of mortality in the United States in the twentieth century." In *Health and Society. The Milbank Memorial Fund Quarterly* 1977, 55: 405–28.

CHAPTER ONE

1. I was in Surat, as well as much of the rest of India, during the plague outbreak of 1994. See: Garrett, L. "Plague triggers a panic in India." *Newsday* (September 23, 1994): Al; Garrett, L. "Surge to flee plague in India." *Newsday* (September 24, 1994): A12; Garrett, L. "Plague spreads across India." *Newsday* (September 29, 1994): A6; Garrett, L. "India plague under control." *Newsday* (October 3, 1994): A12; and Garrett, L. "Anatomy of a plague." *Newsday* (October 9, 1994): A26.

2. Sardesai, R. "Black death." *The Telegraph* (September 25, 1994).

3. Chakravartty, N. "The rats will play . . ." *Economic Times* (Bombay) (October 4, 1994).

4. Dixit, J. N. "Controlling crisis." *Indian Express* (Bombay) (October 4, 1994): 8.

5. "Reaping a grim harvest." *India Today* (October 15, 1994): 4.

6. For earthquake details and photos, see Nayar, R. "Latur revisited: One year later." *Sunday* (September 25, 1994): 23–38; and Unhale, S. "Unending tragedy: A year after the Marathwada quake." *Frontline* (October 21, 1994): 28–30.

7. Hinnebusch, B. J., Perry, R. D., and Schwan, T. G. "Role of the *Yersinia pestis* hemin storage (hms) locus in the transmission of plague by fleas." *Science* 273 (1996): 367–70.

8. Brown, R. "Is behavioral thermoregulation a factor in flea-to-human transmission of *Yersinia pestis*?" *Lancet* 345 (1995): 931.

9. An excellent summary of the type III secretion can be found in Barinaga, M. "A shared strategy for virulence." *Science* 272 (1996): 1261–63.

10. World Bank. *World Development Report 1994: Infrastructure for Development*. New York: Oxford University Press, 1994.

11. In the same year China garnered nearly $35 billion in foreign investment.

12. From 1995 to 1997 India's growth increased to 6 percent a year, but the Asian crash of '98 put brakes on Indian growth. See: "Time to let go: A survey of India." *The Economist* (February 22, 1997), Special Supplement; and "When China and India go down together." *The Economist* (November 22, 1997): 41–44.

13. Modi, K. "Surat textile and diamond industries grind to a halt." *Business Standard* (New Delhi) (September 26, 1994): 1.

14. "The plague within." *Business Standard* (Bombay) (September 27, 1994): 11.

15. World Health Organization. *The World Health Report 1996*. Geneva, WHO, 1996.

16. Robboy, R. "IDA extends record health sector credit to India." *World Bank News* (March 28, 1996): 1–2.

17. Kumar, S. "Non-governmental report spells out failings in India's health care." *Lancet* 352 (1998): 380.

18. The number of deaths broke down as follows:

YEAR	PLAGUE DEATHS
1896–1906	6,032,693
1907–1918	4,221,528
1919–1928	1,702,718
1929–1938	422,880
1939–1948	217,970

YEAR	PLAGUE DEATHS
1949–1958	59,056
1959–1968	678

19. "Surat 'fever' claims 45." *Mid-Day* (September 22, 1994): 1.

20. Express News Service. "Shankaranand issue hots up." *Indian Express* (October 6, 1994): 1; and Press Trust of India. "Plague under check, says Shankaranand." *Times of India* (September 22, 1994): 1.

21. For example, Dr. Musunuri Suresh of Vijayawada insisted that a homeopathic compound called Pyrogenium 200 was superior to antibiotics in treatment of plague.

22. Express News Service. "Plague rages on; a death every hour in Surat." *Indian Express* (September 24, 1994): 1.

23. In 1995 a strain of multidrug-resistant *Yersinia pestis* did surface in a fifteen-year-old boy in Madagascar. The strain was resistant not only to tetracycline, but also to all anti-*Yersinia* antibiotics, save, fortunately, trimethoprim. The case may have been related to a small Mozambican bubonic plague outbreak that occurred in September 1994—at the same time as India's outbreak. Or it could be part of Madagascar's July–October 1995 bubonic plague outbreak, which involved 348 cases, five deaths. Because there are many Indians living in both Madagascar and Mozambique and trade and travel between the countries is frequent, there is no way to know where this boy's ominous drug-resistant *Yersinia* originated. See: Rasolomaharo, M., Rasoamanana, B., Andrianirina, Z., et al. "Plague in Majunga, Madagascar." *Lancet* 345 (1995): 983–84; and Bonn, D. "Multidrug-resistant plague case causes concern." *Lancet* 350 (1997): 788.

24. For a flavor of this, see the front page of Calcutta's *The Telegraph* for September 27, 1994, and Pfizer ads such as "Don't Get Plagued with Fear," appearing on page 19 of the *Sunday Times of India*, October 2, 1994.

25. *Times of India* News Service. "Rajasthan tourism affected by plague." *Sunday Times of India* (October 2, 1994): 29.

26. Mary, J. "Plague hits Kerala economy hard." *Indian Express* (September 30, 1994): 10.

27. All travelers bound for the United Kingdom from India were given a leaflet, which stated: "Advice to Passengers Arriving in the UK by Air from India.

"An outbreak of plague has recently been reported from Gujarat and Maharashtra states of India.

"If you have traveled in these states, or to other areas where plague cases are known to have occurred, there is a remote risk that you may have caught the infection.

"If during the next *week* you become unwell with any of the following:

1. A fever
2. Cough or breathing problems
3. Tender swellings in the neck, armpits or groin

Please seek medical advice from a doctor immediately and take this note with you to show the doctor."

The note then detailed information for physicians, calling for immediate tetracycline therapy, lab work, and notification of the UK's Communicable Disease Control Office.

28. Press Trust of India. "Indian harassed at Heathrow." *Times of India* (October 3, 1994): 1; and Agencies. "U.K.-bound passengers found plague-free." *Times of India* (October 4, 1994): 13. For samples of other detentions of Indian travelers, see: Agencies. "China bars

entry of Indian travelers." *Times of India* (October 5, 1994): 13. The same page has briefs detailing detentions in Russia and Ukraine.

29. Sources for this section include interviews with and presentations by the key players, and: Mojica, B., Heffernan, R., Lowe, C., et al. "Detection of notifiable diseases through surveillance for imported plague—New York, September–October 1994." *Morbidity and Mortality Weekly Report* 43 (1994): 805–07; and Advisory Committee on Immunization Practices (ACIP). "Prevention of Plague." *Morbidity and Mortality Weekly Report* 45 (1996): ii–15; Campbell, G. L., and Hughes, J. M. "Plague in India: A new warning from an old nemesis." *Annals of Internal Medicine* 122 (1995): 151–53; and Fritz, C. L., Dennis, D. T., Tipple, M. A., et al. "Surveillance for pneumonic plague in the United States during an international emergency: A model for control of imported emerging diseases." *Emerging Infectious Diseases* 2 (October 2, 1997): 1–9.

30. A CDC assessment two years after the plague outbreak in India would find that "it is unrealistic to expect any system to effectively screen all travelers returning from areas of recognized disease outbreaks. It is impossible to assess the sensitivity of the described surveillance system since no cases of pneumonic plague were identified either within or outside the system. In retrospect, the risk for an imported plague case was quite small, since the epidemic in India was limited in time and space and had far fewer cases than originally suspected. The WHO investigative team found no evidence of transmission in metropolitan areas other than Surat. Most of the patients with suspected plague in Surat came from poor neighborhoods, residents of which would be unlikely to travel internationally. In addition, the short incubation period and severe symptoms of pneumonic plague and the rapid deterioration of the patient's condition substantially limited the contagious period and the opportunity for secondary transmission." Fritz, C. L., Dennis, D. T., Tipple, M., et al., op cit.

31. Adhikari, G. "A plague upon us." *Times of India* (October 1, 1994): 16.

32. For details related to lab efforts and controversies see: Assorted letters and authors. "Plague in India." *Lancet* 345 (1995): 258–59; Altman, L. K. "Was there or wasn't there a pneumonic plague epidemic?" *New York Times* (November 15, 1994): C3; Bharadwaj, R., Kagal, A., Deshpandey, S. K., et al. "*Burkholderia pseudomallei* and Indian plague-like illness." *Lancet* 346 (1995): 975; Bharadwaj, R., Kagal, A., Deshpandey, S. K., et al. "Outbreak of plague-like illness caused by *Pseudomonas pseudomallei* in Maharashtra, India." *Lancet* 344 (1994: 1574; Chand, V. K. "Plague in India." *Lancet* 344 (1994): 1298; Dance, D. A. B., Sanders, D., Pitt, T. L., et al. "*Burkholderia pseudomallei* and Indian plague-like illness." *Lancet* 346 (1995): 904–5; Desai, D. "Now doctors say it is *melioidosis.*" *Indian Express Bombay* (October 4, 1994): 7; Editors. "Plague in India: Time to forget the symptoms and tackle the disease." *Lancet* 344 (1994): 1033–35; Express News Service. "NICD, AIIMS lock horns over blood samples." *Indian Express New Delhi* (October 6, 1994): 3; Holden, C. "Plague in India confirmed." *Science* 267 (1995): 1268; John, J. T. "Final thoughts on India's 1994 plague outbreaks." *Lancet* 346 (1995): 765; John, J. T. "IAMM inauguration, President's speech." Pune, India, November 12, 1994; John, J. T. "India: Is it plague?" *Lancet* 344 (1994): 1359–60; John, J. T. "Learning from plague in India." *Lancet* 344 (1994): 972; Kumar, S. "Confirmation of Indian plague outbreak?" *Lancet* 345 (1995): 443; Kumar, S. "Plague in India." *Lancet* 344 (1994): 941–42; Kumar, S. "Surat plague caused by a novel strain." *Lancet* 345 (1995): 626; Jain, K. "60 employees of AIIMS down with viral hepatitis." *Times of India* (October 8, 1994): 1; Lalit, D., Thakur, R., and Dar, V. S. "India: Is it plague?" *Lancet* 344 (1994): 1359; Prasannan, R. "Military microbe." *The Week* (July 23, 1995); and The Times News Service. "Not plague, but *melioidosis.*" *Times of India, Bombay* (October 4, 1994): 5.

33. Dr. Jacob John, president of the Indian Association of Medical Microbiology, fa-

vored the notion that another bacterial disease, tularemia, was the culprit. "I am not declaring that the epidemic was tularemia without laboratory evidence," John said. "But I am stating that the epidemic has not yet been aetiologically diagnosed. It is by no means confirmed to be plague. In all probability it is not plague. Alternate diagnosis must be considered, for example tularemia." John went on to attack the lack of epidemiological detective work executed by authorities in Surat, Maharashtra's Beed District, or anywhere else in the country, concluding: "Has anyone heard about the case definition, we cannot accept that there was an epidemic."

34. Kimball, A. M. Speech to the Center for International Studies, University of Toronto, October 30, 1998.

35. "Was it the plague?" *The Economist* (November 19, 1994): 38–40.

36. On October 10 the Indian Ministry of Health issued this breakdown of cases:

| | SUSPECTED CASES | | CONFIRMED CASES | |
| | Cumulative to Oct. 9 | | Cumulative | New on |
State/District	*Cases*	*Deaths*	*to Oct. 8*	*Oct. 9*
Andhra Pradesh	0	0	0	0
Delhi	1,003	3	54	6
Surat	944	52	118	0
Rest of Gujarat	605	0	4	3
Haryana	17	0	1	0
Madhya Pradesh	112	0	8	1
Bombay	383	0	0	0
Beed District	449	0	46	0
Rest of Maharashtra	2,341	0	33	2
Rajasthan	245	0	0	0
Uttar Pradesh	59	0	8	2
West Bengal	118	0	0	0
Bihar	3	0	0	0
Karnataka	43	0	0	2
Punjab	22	0	0	0
TOTAL	6,344	55	272	16

37. "Were Ultras responsible for Surat plague?" *Hindustan Times* (July 9, 1995): A1.

38. It first assumed that any unusual features in Surat's *Yersinia* could not possibly have arisen naturally. The last Indian *Yersinia* strain available for comparison was from Karnataka in 1963, and it did not possess this novel genetic sequence. Several scientists—notably a biotechnologist from AIIMS and a virologist from Pune—claimed that it was "categorically impossible" for such change to occur as a result of natural evolution. One went so far as to assert that there were no known examples of evolution adding, versus deleting, genes.

39. John, J. T. "IAMM inauguration, president's speech," op cit.

40. Chand, V. K., 1994, op cit.

41. UNICEF, Information Statistics/India. UNICEF Web site: www.unicef.org/statis/country_1page81.htmlfil, 1998.

42. Kumar, S. "India has the largest number of people infected with HIV." *Lancet* 353 (1999): 48.

43. "Plague in India: Time to forget the symptoms and tackle the disease," op cit.

44. Krishnan, E. Letter to *Lancet* 344 (1994): 1298.

CHAPTER TWO

1. Translated from "Le virus ebola à Kikwit: mythe, mystère ou réalité." Editions Baobob, Kinshasa, Democratic Republic of Congo, 1998.

2. Translated from N. Kibari and M. Lungazi, ibid.

3. For descriptions of the Kikwit people's perception of the events during the 1995 Ebola epidemic I have relied on a combination of my own observations on site at the time, numerous local interviews conducted in May 1995 and March 1998, and on the seminal work of University of Bandundu professors Kibari N'sanga and Lungazi Mulala, 1998, ibid.

4. Garret, L. "Yambuku." In *The Coming Plague. Newly Emerging Diseases in a World Out of Balance.* New York: Farrar, Straus & Giroux, 1994.

5. UNICEF.*The State of the World's Children 1998.* New York: Oxford Press, 1998. The eleven worse-ranked nations were, in order of greatest child mortality rates, Niger, Angola, Sierra Leone, Afghanistan, Liberia, Guinea-Bissau, Mali, Malawi, Mozambique, Somalia, and Guinea. All but three of the thirty-two highest child mortality nations were in 1995 in Africa. Those three exceptions were Afghanistan, Pakistan, and Cambodia.

6. Estimates of maternal death rates are hard to come by, as coroner records typically list other causes of mothers' demises in Africa. A survey of autopsies in Brazzaville, Congo, found rates so high as to mean that one out of every twenty-five women in that city died prematurely due to complications in pregnancy. Given that Brazzaville is the capital, where medical services are concentrated, this certainly indicates rural mortality rates are far higher. See LeCoeur, S., Pictet, G., M'Pelé, P., and Lallemont, M. "Direct estimation of maternal mortality in Africa." *Lancet* 352 (1998): 1525–26.

UNICEF estimates that across the Congo river in Zaire maternal mortality was higher, still, in the late 1990s. They say 870 mothers annually of every 100,000 pregnant women died, which is 14 percent higher than the LeCoeur estimate for the Congo.

7. Muyembe, T. Speech to the International Colloquium on Ebola Virus Research, Antwerp, September 4–7, 1996.

8. The sorry history of Lumumba's assassination and Mobutu's rise to power is well documented. I refer readers to several sources, including: Kalb, M. G. *The Congo Cables: The Cold War in Africa—From Eisenhower to Kennedy.* New York: Macmillan, 1982; Fanon, F. *Toward the African Revolution.* New York: Grove Press, 1967; Nkrumah, K. *Africa Must Unite.* New York: International Publishers, 1963; Western Massachusetts Association of Concerned African Scholars. *U.S. Military Involvement in Southern Africa.* Boston: South End Press, 1978; and Winternitz, H. *East Along the Equator.* New York: Atlantic Monthly Press, 1987.

9. American, French, Belgian, and South African troops, as well as mercenaries, fought on behalf of the Mobutu regime, quashing rebellions against the dictator's brutal government. Occasionally these interventions were financed by Saudi and Israeli sub-rosa government funds. From his first days in office, Mobutu was unable to fully control Shaba and Katanga provinces, even his eastern flank bordering Rwanda, Burundi, and Zambia, which were always hospitable to rebel troops. When Cuba sent soldiers in support of the MPLA in Angola and the government of Ethiopia the Carter administration widened its backing for Mobutu. The French government's position, particularly during the François Mitterand years, was even more adamantly in support of Mobutu. In 1978 alone, fifteen thousand French troops fought in Zaire, defending the Mobutu regime in a *corps d'intervention.*

10. To get an idea of the scale of wealth lying beneath Zaire's soil consider these points, gleaned from the 1997 annual stockholders report for the Canadian mining company Melkior Resources, Inc.: "2,800 square kilometres of the World's richest known Copper-Cobalt deposits, in an area that has already produced over 14 million tonnes of copper and

560,000 tonnes of cobalt since the beginning of the century and is poised to be the World's biggest supplier of these minerals. The region has also yielded uranium and gold."

This statement refers to a single mining site in Zaire, and even with its obvious bravado cannot come close to expressing the scale of gem, mineral, and petroleum reserves nationwide.

11. Garrett, L. "Plague Warriors." *Vanity Fair* (August 1995): 85–161.

12. For details in this and the following section of this chapter I refer the reader to my many reports at the time, appearing in *Newsday* between March–September 1995. In addition, see: "Ebola: The beginning of the end?" *African Medical News*, Nairobi (June 1995): 1; "Return of a killer virus." *U.S. News and World Report* (April 17, 1995): 20; Altman, L. K. "New skin test will help track Ebola infection in remote areas." *New York Times* (September 19, 1995): C1; Ambassade des Etats-Unis. "U.S. government donates $25,000 in emergency disaster assistance for virus outbreak in Kikwit, Zaire." Press Release, Kinshasa, May 11, 1995; Banea, M., Tylleskär, T., and Rosling, H. "Konzo and Ebola in Bandundu Region of Zaire." *Lancet* 349 (1997): 621; Benini, A. A. and Bradford, J. K. "Ebola virus—From medical emergency to complex disaster?" Thesis, Social Sciences Department, California Polytechnic State University, 1995; Bonnet, M., Akamituna, P., and Mazaya, A. "Unrecognized Ebola hemorrhagic fever at Mosango Hospital during the 1995 epidemic in Kikwit, Democratic Republic of the Congo." *Emerging Infectious Diseases* 4 (1998): 508–10; Bray, M., Davis, K., Geisbert, T., et al. "A mouse model for evaluation of prophylaxis and therapy of Ebola Hemorrhagic Fever" *Journal of Infectious Diseases* 178 (1998): 651–61; Breman, J. B., van der Groen, G., Peters, C. J., et al. "International Colloquium on Ebola Virus Research: Summary Report." *Journal of Infectious Diseases* 176 (1997): 1058–63; Centers for Disease Control. "Outbreak of Ebola Viral Hemorrhagic Fever—Zaire, 1995."*MMWR* 44 (1995): 381–82; Centers for Disease Control. "Update: Outbreak of Ebola Viral Hemorrhagic Fever—Zaire, 1995." *MMWR* 44 (1995): 468–69; French, H. "Fear stalks the quick and the dead in Zaire." *New York Times* (May 28, 1995): A1; Garrett, L. *Vanity Fair*, op cit; International Colloquium on Ebola Virus Research. Proceedings (various papers and authors), September 4–7, 1996, Antwerp, Belgium; International Commission. "Ebola haemorrhagic fever in Zaire, 1976." *Bulletin of the WHO* 56 (1978): 271–93; Jaax, N., Jahrling, P., Geisbert, T., et al. "Transmission of Ebola virus (Zaire strain) to uninfected control monkeys in a bio-containment laboratory." *Lancet* 346 (1995): 1669–71; Johnson, E., Jaax, N., White, J., et al. "Lethal experimental infections of rhesus monkeys by aerosolized Ebola virus." *International Journal experimental Pathology* 76 (1995): 227–36; Kelley, M. J. "Research on Ebola virus." *Lancet* 347 (1996): 691; Swanepoel, R., Leman, P. A., Burt, F. J., et al. "Experimental inoculation of plants and animals with Ebola virus." *Emerging Infectious Diseases* 2 (1996): 321–25; Walker, P. V. "In search of . . . Ebola and other deadly agents help scientists on the move." *Army Times* (July 24, 1995): 1; Wickelgren, I. "A method in Ebola's madness." *Science* 279 (1998): 983–84; Wool-Lewis, R. "Understanding how Ebola virus gets into cells." First International Conference on Emerging Infectious Diseases, Atlanta, March 10, 1998; World Health Organization. "WHO team investigates fatal outbreak of Haemorrhagic fever in Zaire." Press Release (May 10, 1995); World Health Organization. "WHO teams further efforts to control Ebola virus outbreak in Zaire." Press Release WHA/13 (May 12, 1995); World Health Organization. "The Ebola epidemic in Zaire: The acute phase is over." Press Release 40 (May 26, 1995); World Health Organization. "The Ebola epidemic in Zaire: International aid increases." Press Release WHO/39 (May 27, 1995); World Health Organization. "Combatting the Ebola epidemic in Zaire: A model of international collaboration." Press Release WHO/45 (June 12, 1995); World Health Organization. "Ebola Fever epidemic: WHO Director-General visits Kikwit." Press Release WHO/50 (June 29, 1995);

World Health Organization. "Ebola epidemic in Zaire could be over by September, says WHO Director-General." Press Release WHO/52 (July 4, 1995); World Health Organization. "Report of WHO meeting to review epidemic preparedness, epidemic control and research in outbreak situations." WHO/EMC/95.4, 1995; and Yang, Z., Delgado, R., Xu, L., et al. "Distinct cellular interactions of secreted and transmembrane Ebola virus glycoproteins." *Science* 279 (1998): 1034–37.

13. "Quatre-vingt" is *Eurapatorium odoratum*, a weed found in the tropics of Africa, Asia, and even Latin America. Where it originated is unclear. It was noted well to the north of Congo, in Nigeria, in 1963. (See Adams, C. D. *Flora of West Tropical Africa*. 2nd Edition, 1963.) It is, as local Kikwitians noted, a very aggressive weed, and a member of the daisy family. I thank Roy E. Gereau of the Missouri Botanical Garden and Clifford W. Smith of the University of Hawaii for assistance in determining the identity of "quatre-vingt."

14. The Latin name for "quatre-vingt" is *Eurapatorium odoratum*.

15. Charlotte Kilesa and Augustin Bisambu were Gaspard Menga's grandparents, or the parents of his father, Innocent Menga. When Gaspard elected to be a Jehovah's Witness his older brother, Philémon, changed his own surname to Nseke as a sign that he remained a Catholic. As had his wife, Marie-José, Philémon died of Ebola.

16. At the time there was concern that Ebola, Marburg, or other deadly hemorrhagic fever viruses might break out in Goma. See: Garrett, L. "Few drills—or skills—to foil a super plague." *Newsday* (July 31, 1994): A7; and Garrett, L. "Refugee crisis worsens as aid is sent to Goma." *Newsday* (July 24, 1994): A14.

17. Pécoul, B., Chirac, P., Trouiller, P., et al. "Access to essential drugs in poor countries: A lost battle?" *Journal of the American Medical Association* 281 (1999): 361–67; and Paquet, C. and Van Soest, M. "Mortality and malnutrition among Rwandan refugees in Zaire." *Lancet* 344 (1994): 823–24.

18. The use of patient names is a very serious matter. Obviously, all patients, regardless of their nationality, have a right to full confidentiality. I have chosen, however, to use Kimfumu's name, as well as those of other Ebola patients, for two reasons. First, most of these names were widely published all over the world during the epidemic, and appear fully listed in Zairois publications. And secondly it seems important to humanize the epidemic and conditions in the African country. I hope that by personalizing such things residents of wealthy countries can identify more closely with the conditions under which their African counterparts live—and die.

19. His leader, Pastor Eloi Mulengamungu, would later declare Kikwit to be a Sodom upon which God was levying revenge in the form of Ebola.

20. Muyembe was one of the first scientists in Yambuku in 1976, arriving when that Ebola epidemic was peaking and out of control. Since that time Ebola had been one of the primary foci of his professional life.

21. The army would later provide seven experienced BL-4 scientists on temporary loan to CDC, to supplement the exhausted Special Pathogens Lab staff.

22. For a good rendition of the CDC funding problems at that time see: Cimons, M. "Budgetcutting puts disease control lab at risk." *Los Angeles Times* (May 19, 1995): A10.

23. The U.S. Agency for International Development—itself a target for severe cuts, perhaps even dissolution, in FY 1996—agreed on June 1, 1995, to provide the CDC with $750,000 in Ebola-control assistance. And Senator Russell Feingold (D-Wis) held a press conference that week to specifically warn that further erosion in foreign-aid funding could lead to more outbreaks in poor countries of Ebola and similar diseases. Eventually the CDC would spend more than $1 million on Ebola control and lab work, most of which was ultimately reimbursed by USAID and Congress.

24. New York City Commissioner of Health Dr. Margaret Hamburg shared the concerns of her counterparts in other major U.S. ports of call that someone infected with Ebola might land on American soil. As she had done nine months earlier when pneumonic plague broke out in India, Hamburg set into motion in New York City an elaborate system of surveillance for Ebola. Doctors and hospitals were notified of the following: should a suspect Ebola case appear at JFK International Airport or under your care it will be sent to one of two designated isolation wards located in City hospitals.

But there were three serious flaws in the New York City plan, Hamburg acknowledged.

First, some of the hospital workers unions threatened to strike if their members were ordered to deal with Ebola cases. The CDC's Dr. Ruth Berkelman said similar threats were issued by hospital unions in other U.S. cities. None of the New York City unions acknowledged that they, individually, had made such threats, though representatives conceded that "other unions" might have issued such warnings.

The second problem concerned the handling of laboratory samples.

"If a suspect case came into a New York hospital we would obviously want to do routine tests to rule out other causes—malaria, other viruses—for the symptoms." Hamburg said, "But there was genuine concern that the hospital labs couldn't handle samples that might contain Ebola."

The city's public health lab, which has a BL-3 facility, was designated as the testing site.

Finally, Hamburg and her counterparts in Chicago, Los Angeles, and other major U.S. cities were assured that the U.S. Public Health Service was screening airline passengers arriving in the United States from Zaire. That screening—which was supposed to involve airline employee examinations of passengers during the flights followed by dispersal of health alert information to passengers as they passed through U.S. Customs—was the linchpin of all surveillance efforts.

Yet this reporter passed freely through U.S. Immigration and Customs, despite having flown directly from Kinshasa, without any examination, questioning, or provision of Health Alert Notice cards.

25. Benini, A. A. and Bradford, J. K., op. cit.

26. The reporters were Michael Skoler of National Public Radio, French photographer Patrick Robert, and *Time* magazine's Andrew Purvis.

27. There is a large question in the friction between public health personnel and representatives of other professions, whether they are journalists, soldiers, development workers, or humanitarian aid providers. In any epidemic occurring in a remote area the local populace generally lacks the financial resources to travel any significant distance and in only rare circumstances could be expected to jet their ways to London, Tokyo, or Omaha. But foreigners on site are another matter. United Nations employees, media, peacekeeping forces, humanitarian aid distributors—these people typically fly in and out of hot spots frequently, returning to their home bases within twenty-four to forty-eight hours of leaving the epidemic. If they were exposed to Ebola—or any contagion—these individuals would still be asymptomatically incubating their infections when they reached their home countries.

Yet as a practical matter—and as events in Zaire confirmed—it is impossible to keep determined foreigners out of such a hot spot, or to block their departures.

What is the answer? Ideally epidemic control teams should include liaison professionals who would allow other groups access to the situation on safe, reasonably monitored terms, careful never to use "safety" as a cover for access denial that is actually motivated by other interests. In Kikwit WHO or CDC should have had a press liaison on site from the beginning of team activities. In Goma during the Rwandan refugee crisis each major organization should have had press and humanitarian aid liaisons to coordinate activities.

In the Kikwit situation the lack of a media specialist was particularly heinous, as the town had no media of its own and could have benefited from daily publication of accurate reports, posted about town in French and KiCongo. For Kikwitians the single most reliable source of epidemic information was Radio France, broadcast from Paris and received on their battery-operated shortwave radios. It is ironic in the extreme that the French were, in turn, gleaning their information from David Heymann's group in Kikwit.

During periods of extreme stress participants in crisis intervention are most likely to vent pent-up frustrations upon targets that are of less consequence to them. In Kikwit, for example, it was essential that friction among team members be handled calmly, professionally. And certainly it would have been inappropriate for any team member to turn their rage or fear upon local Kikwitians. The media was a safe target, as few scientists hold the journalistic profession in high—or even middling—regard.

No matter how much professionals loathe or distrust one another, however, any action that potentially compromises infection control must be condemned in the strongest possible terms. If one of the reporters had become infected—either through the individual's carelessness or because of a belligerent action by a public health worker—the global repercussions would have been profound.

28. It's worth asking what would have happened in Brazzaville if one of these reporters had been carrying Ebola. In the context of the 1995 epidemic, given the very brief amount of time the journalists were in Kikwit and the rather superficial nature of their interaction with the epidemic it would seem a near impossibility. But at a time when the movements of Zairois people were so terribly restricted and when Zaire nationals were being detained at international airports out of fear of spreading the frightening virus, the apparent free mobility of the media seems inconsistent. Detaining reporters would make no sense either. What would be appropriate policy in future epidemics? Clearly it will depend on the organism, its mode of transmission, the nature of journalists' contact with the situation, and WHO policies.

All of this would be far easier to sort out, and policies of containment would make more scientific sense, if trained media liaisons were on the ground from day one of epidemics, carefully balancing reports' needs for access against the greater exigencies for epidemic control. Some journalists, convinced that they would ultimately be placed under quarantine, booked passage on local boats, crossed the wide, muddy Congo River, and made their ways to Brazzaville, capital of the Congo. Lacking appropriate visas they were stuck in Brazzaville for considerable amounts of time.

29. Former American presidential candidate Dr. Pat Robertson turned up in Kinshasa, offering medical supplies purchased, he said, with funds raised from television viewers of his conservative, Christian "700 Club" program. In an old brewery warehouse in Kinshasa Robertson's staff stacked supplies suitable for treatment of bacterial dysentery and malaria: oral rehydration kits, dextrose, saline, streptomycin, ampicillin, chloramphenicol, and the like.

On May 17 Robertson, dressed in a stifling business suit, quietly paced in front of the warehouse, awaiting an old friend. With the media in full attendance two black Mercedes limousines approached, loaded with automatic weapons–toting bodyguards. And the dictator, dressed in a French suit and silk tie, stepped out of a limo and embraced his comrade, Robertson. Obviously well acquainted, the duo explained their agendas to the media.

Robertson decried the Clinton administration's stance on the regime, which was one of condemnation.

"I think he [Mobutu] cannot understand why the United States has turned against him," Robertson said. "He wants to be a friend. And I want him to be a friend. I want America to come here and invest. And President [Mobutu] really cannot understand why America has turned against him. And neither can I."

Robertson's donated medical supplies were loaded onto an ancient Caribou cargo plane and flown by two Vietnam veteran Navy SEALs to Kikwit. When questioned about their familiarity with local flight paths the pilots explained that the old Caribou was part of a small fleet of planes owned by Robertson and used to haul goods to the 700 Club leader's diamond mining operations in Zaire and nearby Angola. Robertson said that he was trying to raise funds, via his television viewers, to rebuild railway lines that once connected diamond and mineral mines of Angola to that country's capital, Luanda. Robertson's holdings in the region were well known to competing diamond and mining operators. A top Canadian mining executive who had conducted numerous diamond and gold excavations in the region confirmed that Robertson had a longstanding interest in Central African mining. See Garrett, L., "Plague warriors," op cit; and Maier, T. "Robertson's ties with Zaire leader questioned." *Newsday* (May 21, 1995): A43.

30. While I was in Kikwit I followed, for the most part, the same hygienic precautions I observe throughout the poor, tropical world. I washed in liquid biodegradable soap and drank two to three liters daily of bottled water or water that I filtered myself. I followed the old maxim of tropical medicine: don't eat it unless you can boil it, peel it, shell it, uncan it, or burn it. I was careful not to shake hands with anyone. And when eating in villages, where food is drawn with bare hands from a collectively used bowl or pot, I distributed disposable latex gloves, instructing my hosts and fellow diners that during an epidemic this was a wise precaution for all of us. To my distress, however, after sharing meals with a man known to have been exposed to Ebola I realized that latex was not protective against the oils used locally in food preparation, and the gloves leaked.

31. Kelly, M. J. "Research on Ebola virus." *Lancet* 347 (1996): 691; Jaax, N. K. "Author's reply." *Lancet* 347 (1996): 691; Jaax, N., Jahrling, P., Geisbert, T., et al. "Transmission of Ebola virus (Zaire strain) to uninfected control monkeys in a biocontainment laboratory." *Lancet* 346 (1995):1669–71; and Johnson, E., Jaax, N., White, J., et al. "Lethal experimental infections of rhesus monkeys by aerosolized Ebola virus." *International Journal of Experimental Pathology* 76 (1995): 277–86.

The design of Jaax's experiment is important. Six rhesus monkeys were placed in separate cages about three meters apart. Two received sprayed doses of interferon, which here was a placebo. These were the controls. Four others got a moderate aerosolized dose of Ebola ($2.6 \log_{10}0$PFUs). The exposure was done on the animals while they were fully anesthetized and laid inside airtight boxes. The solutions were pumped into these boxes, and the monkeys breathed that contaminated air for ten minutes. All four Ebola-exposed animals got infected and died of the disease within twenty-two days. Critics challenged the experiment's applicability to human exposure, as few people might be expected to remain in an airtight room for ten minutes with a patient. And, more problematic, they charged, was the assumption that ailing patients exhale or cough up such high doses of viruses.

32. Zaki, S. R., Greer, P. W., Goldsmith, C. S., et al. "Ebola virus hemorrhagic fever: Immunopathological and ultrastructural study." International Colloquium on Ebola Virus Research, September 4–7, 1996, Antwerp, Belgium; and Garret, L. "Ebola gets under people's skin." *Newsday* (September 21, 1995): A17. According to the CDC's C. J. Peters, autopsies showed that colonies of viruses clustered in the alveoli of patients' lungs. Whether such lung-bound viruses could be exhaled to another person was unclear, Peters said, because "when you cough you cough from the bronchi, not the alveoli."

The skin exposure situation seemed more worrisome, as the CDC found large viral colonies in sweat glands, macrophages, and dendritic cells of the skin of Ebola patients.

33. "2d Ebola fever case suspected in Liberia." Reuters (December 11, 1995); Georges-Courbot, M. C., Lu, C. Y., Lansoud-Soukate, J., et al. "Isolation and partial molecular characterization of a strain of Ebola virus during a recent epidemic of viral hemorrhagic fever in Gabon." *Science* 349 (1997): 181; Koffi, M. "Foreign Ebola experts enter war-ravaged Liberia." (December 10, 1995); Koffi, M. "Foreign experts find Ebola suspects in Liberia." Reuters (December 11, 1995); Susman, T. "Four more suspected Ebola cases found in Liberia." Associated Press (December 11, 1995); Susman, T. "Medical workers search Liberia for possible Ebola." Associated Press (December 11, 1995); World Health Organization. "Ebola case confirmed in Côte d'Ivoire." Press Release WHO/89 (December 8, 1995); and World Health Organization. "WHO-led collaborative study in Côte d'Ivoire." Press Release WHO/93 (December 15, 1995).

34. Amblard, J., Obiang, P., Edzang, S., et al. "Identification of the Ebola virus in Gabon in 1994." *Science* 349 (1997): 181–82; Morell, V. "Chimpanzee outbreak heats up search for Ebola origin." *Science* 268 (1995): 974–76; and Stone, R. "Ebola virus re-emerges in West Africa." *Science* 268 (1995): 19.

35. "Neuf personnes décédés après avoir consommmé de la viande de chimpanzé." *Agence France Press* (February 10, 1996); "South African Ebola scare eases; case tied to Gabon." *New York Times* (November 19, 1996): A15; Choo, V. "Ebola fever outbreak confirmed in Gabon." *Science* 347 (1996): 528; French, H. "The hunt for the creature that Ebola calls home." *New York Times* (November 24, 1996): A3; Garrett, L. "Killer virus strikes Africa for the third time in a year." *Newsday* (February 17, 1996): A7; Garrett, L. "Ebola outbreak deepens mystery." *Newsday* (February 20, 1996): A16; Okamba, L. "Seven dead from deadly Ebola virus in Gabon." Associated Press (October 11, 1996); Purvis, A. "Where does Ebola hide?" *Time* (March 4, 1996); Sharp, G. and Dusé, A. "Ebola in South Africa." Proceedings, Infection Control Congress, Cape Town, South Africa, April 22–24, 1998; World Health Organization. "Medical team investigates outbreak of suspected Ebola Haemorrhagic Fever in Gabon." Press Release WHO/11 (Febuary 16, 1996); World Health Organization. "Ebola Haemorrhagic Fever in Gabon." Press Release WHO/12 (February 19, 1996); World Health Organization. "Rapid government response stems Ebola outbreak in Gabon." Press Release WHO/13 (February 23, 1996); World Health Organization. "Ebola virus strikes again in Gabon." Press Release WHO/69 (October 15, 1996); and World Health Organization. "Update: Ebola in Gabon." Press Release WHO/1 (January 10, 1997).

36. In South Africa concerns about Ebola and other rare but deadly viruses is far from abstract. South Africa has faced its own frightening outbreaks—including one of Ebola—and the new openness with her African neighbors means the continent's most prosperous and internationally connected nation could well face further microbial dangers.

"Our view is that it's not really a threat as such to us so long as we all abide by public health measures," Dr. Olive Shisana, director-general of the South African Ministry of Health, said in an interview in Cape Town. "We have drawn up guidelines. . . . Whenever there is an epidemic anywhere in the country the people call me immediately. We have a very qualified response team. And immediately when they hear of anything they are on the plane and into the fight. We are fortunate to have very qualified help in South Africa."

Prior to 1994 South Africa was cut off from its African neighbors, who opposed the nation's apartheid policies, which separated the races and gave the white minority population virtually absolute control over every facet of the society. But with the election of Nelson Mandela to the presidency and elimination of all apartheid policies South Africa has become the darling of the continent, and the number one destination for young fortune seekers from every corner of Africa.

"The old borders are colonial," Dr. Neil Cameron, secretary-general of communicable diseases for South Africa, explained. "A huge paranoia against immigrants exists here, and its advocates use communicable diseases as a barrier."

The position of the new government is that South Africa has plenty of its own diseases that might also travel northward. For example, some 160,000 people suffer from active tuberculosis, Shisana said, which kills 10,000 South Africans yearly. And the HIV/AIDS crisis has reached nightmarish proportions in the country, with some areas showing HIV-positive rates as high as 30 percent among young adults. A report from the National Assembly says 1,500 South Africans are newly infected with HIV every day.

37. International Colloquium on Ebola Virus Research, 1996, op. cit.

38. Heymann presented this data on the Ebola outbreaks:

Site	Date	Cause of Viral Amplification? Or Control?	Deaths
Yambuku	1976	Poor infection control measures; reused nonsterile syringes	280
Tandala	1977	Good infection control measures in hospital	1
Kikwit	1995	Poor infection control nursing	245
Mayibout	1996	Good infection control measures in hospital	21*

*None were hospital-acquired cases.

39. United Nations Childrens Fund. *The State of the World's Children*. New York: UNICEF, 1998.

40. The infectable bats were the insect-eating little free-tailed bat and Angola free-tailed bat. And the Wahlberg's epauleted fruit bat was readily infected. These animals made billions of Ebola viruses in their bodies.

41. Gonzalez presented this data at the Antwerp meeting in 1996. In detail he found:

Species	Year	% Positive for Anti-Ebola Antibodies
Human: Pygmies of the Central African Republic	1979	5.4
	1985	34.6
	1987	26.9
	1995	18.4
	1996	11.0
Human: Kikwit residents	1990	2.0
Human: Makokou, Gabon residents	1987	21.7
Human: Bantus of Central African Republic	1995	14.0
Cereopitheus aethiops (monkeys)	1996	1.0
Patas	1996	1.0
Human: Oubangin River residents	1996	11.3–24.6

42. For details see Garrett, L., *The Coming Plague*, op. cit., 371–80.

43. Phillips-Conroy, J. E., Jolly, C. J., Petros, B., et al. "Sexual transmission of SIV agm in wild grivet monkeys." *Journal of Medical Primatology* 23 (1994): 1–7; and Chen. Z., Telfer, P., Reed, P., et al. "First simian immunodeficiency virus from a free-ranging sooty mangabey is equidistant from SIV and HIV-2 suggesting a new subtype." *Ann. Symposium on Nonhuman Primate Models for AIDS* 10 (1994).

44. Gao, F., Bailes, E., Robertson, D. L., et al. "Origin of HIV-1 in the chimpanzee Pan

troglodytes troglodytes troglodytes troglodytes." *Nature* 397 (1998): 436–41; Garrett, L., "Save the Chimps." *Newsday* (February 1, 1999): 1; Golden, F. "The first chimpanzee." *Time* (February 8, 1999): 52–53; Gurtler, L. G., et al. "HIV-1 subtype O: Epidemiology, pathogenesis, diagnosis, and perspectives of the evolution of HIV." *Archives of Virology Supplement* 11 (1996): 195–202; Sharp, P. M., Robertson, D. L., Gao, F., et al. "Origin and diversity of human immunodeficiency viruses." *AIDS* 8 (1994): S27–S42; Simon, F., et al. "Identification of a new human immunodeficiency virus type 1 distinct from group M and group O." *Nature Med.* 4 (1998): 1032–37; and Weiss, R. A. and Wrangham, R. W. "From Pan to pandemic." *Nature* 397 (1998): 385.

45. Environmental groups estimate the Congo Basin/Tai Forest logging rate is eleven million cubic meters of wood per year. The equivalent for all of Asia is ninety-two million; for all of Latin America it's twenty-eight million. See: World Society for Protection of Animals. "Slaughter of the Apes." London: WSPA, 1995; and McRae, M. "Road kill in Cameroon." *Natural History* 2/1997: 36–75.

46. Studies of bushmeat consumption throughout the region show that ungulates, such as dykers, are the main targets for hunters and account for between 58 to 95 percent of all bushmeat consumed by people. Further, bushmeat accounts for upward of 75 percent of all protein consumed by people living in and around Africa's equatorial rain forests. See: Wilkie, D. S. and Carpenter, J. F. "Bushmeat hunting in the Congo Basin: An assessment of impacts and options for mitigation." *Biodiversity and Conservation* (1999), in press. This is a major, comprehensive review of the literature.

47. Sources on the overthrow of Mobutu and subsequent Kabila regime include: "A continent goes to war." *The Economist* (October 3, 1998): 47–49; "New Congo, same old ways." *The Economist* (May 2, 1998): 41–42; "War in the heart of Africa." *The Economist* (August 22, 1998): 35; Chiahemen, J. "Congo's Kabila sacks outspoken minister." Reuters (November 11, 1998); Duke, L. "Congolese seethe over Tutsi presence among Kabila forces." *Washington Post* (November 11, 1998): A1; Edwards, M. "Central Africa's cycle of violence." *National Geographic* (June 1997): 124–133; Fisher, I., and Onishi, N. "Congo's struggle may unleash broad strife to redraw Africa." *New York Times* (January 12, 1999): A1; French, H. W. "Congo leader losing luster." *New York Times* (May 21, 1998): Al; and McNeil, D. G. "A war turned free-for-all tears at Africa's center." *New York times* (December 6, 1998): WK5.

48. "Africa's economies." *The Economist* (September 19, 1998): 126.

49. Breman, J. G. and Henderson, D. A. "The authors' reply." *Lancet* 339 (1998): 2027; Centers for Disease Control and Prevention. "Human monkeypox—Kasai oriental, Zaire, 1996–97." *Morbidity and Mortality Weekly Report* 46 (1997): 304–7; Centers for Disease Control and Prevention. "Human monkeypox—Kasai oriental, Democratic Republic of Congo, February 1996–October 1997." *Morbidity and Mortality Weekly Report* 46 (1997): 1168–71; Cohen, J. "Searching for the ghost of smallpox." Unpublished, 1998, cited by permission of the author; Hooper, C. "To the Editor." *Lancet* 339 (1998): 2027; and World Health Organization. "Largest outbreak of suspected monkeypox reported in Democratic Republic of the Congo." Press Release WHO/86 (December 2, 1997).

50. The World Health Organization was deprived of its logical Nobel Prize for elimination of smallpox because of these protests. For more than a decade teams of scientists combed Central Africa in search of monkeypox epidemics. No evidence was found at that time of significant human-to-human transmission of the virus.

51. The allegation is not entirely fair. WHO did set up a surveillance communications network that would allow physicians in Kikwit to notify authorities swiftly, were Ebola or other microbes to resurface. It is, however, interrupted by local warfare.

As for the health infrastructure, itself, WHO does not, under its United Nations mandate, get involved. The construction of hospitals and provision of supplies is somebody else's problem—a bilateral donor, a humanitarian organization, the World Bank. Unfortunately, as of this writing no moneyed group anywhere in the world was, as a matter of priority, dedicated to health infrastructure development.

52. "The cost of Kabila." *The Economist* (October 2, 1998): 48–9.

CHAPTER THREE

1. Translation by Constance Garnett, Book of the Month Club edition, 1985.

2. Sinyavsky, A., *The Russian Intelligentsia*. New York: Columbia University Press, 1997.

3. See the table "Health Care Systems in the United States and Former Soviet States, 1989" on page 608.

4. See the table "Regional Basic Indicators" on page 610.

5. See the table "Russian Life Expectancy Changes, 1958–1995" on pages 613–615.

6. The Ukrainian government changed the official spelling of Kiev to Kyiv in 1993.

7. See table "Life Expectancy and Economic Indicators" on page 612.

8. Shkolnikov, V., and Meslé, F., "Health crisis in Russia, Parts I and II." *Population and Society* 8 (1996): 123–90.

9. Primary Russian demography sources include: "Russian mortality double that in West." Russia Today Online, November 13, 1998; Belaeyev, E., *Role of Sanitation and Epidemiology Service in Maintaining the Sanitation, Epidemiology and Well-being of the Russian Federal Population*. Perm: Tyniga Publishing House, 1996; Centers for Disease Control and Prevention. "Vital and health statistics: Russian Federation and United States, selected years 1980–93." U.S. Department of Health and Human Services, Washington, D.C., June 1995; DaVanzo, J., ed., *Russia's Demographic Crisis*. RAND Corporation, Santa Monica, 1996; Demick, B., "Communism gone, death rates climb." *Philadelphia Inquirer* (March 26, 1995): E1; Feshbach, M., "Comment on current and future Russian demographic and health problems." Georgetown University, Washington, D.C., June 9, 1997; Feshbach, M., "Dead souls." *The Atlantic* (January 8, 1999); Feshbach, M., "A different definition of national security: Environmental and health issues in Russia and its impact on the West." First Symposium in the 40th CERES Anniversary Series, September 11, 1998; Feshbach, M., ed., *Environmental and Health Atlas of Russia*. Moscow: PAIMAS Publishing House, 1995; Feshbach, M., *Russia in Transition: Ecological Disaster*. A Twentieth Century Fund Report, New York, 1995; Feshbach, M., "What a tangled web we weave: Child health in Russia and its future." Science Applications International Corp., Inc., Washington, D.C., July 1998; Garrett, L., "Crumbled empire: Shattered health." 28-part series of reports. *Newsday* (October and November 1997); Gerasimenko, N. F. "Report of the Chair of the State Duma Committee on Health Protection." Moscow, May 13, 1997; Ivanova, A., "Marriage and Russian women." *Population and Society* No. 12, Moscow, 1996; Komarov, Y. M., Kiselev, A. S., Romensky, A. A., et al., "Vital and health statistics: Russian Federation and United States, 1980–93." Research Public Health Institute, Ministry of Health of Russia, Moscow, 1995; McCarthy, M., "Adults die younger in former Soviet republics." *Lancet* 349 (1997): 1890; Meslé, F., Shkolnikov, V. M., Hertrich, V., et al., *Tendances récentes de la mortalité par cause en Russie 1965–1994*. Institut National d'Etudes Demographiques, Paris and Center for Demography and Human Ecology, Moscow, 1996; Notzon, F. C., Komarov, Y. M., Ermakov, S. P., et al. "Causes of declining life expectancy in Russia." *Journal of the American Medical Association* 279 (1998): 793–97; Onyschenko, G., Various reports and tables from the Ministry of Health, Moscow, 1997; Presidential Committee on Issues of Females, Family and Democracy. "On the contemporary mortality status of the population of the Russian Federation." Report to President Boris Yeltsin, Moscow,

HEALTH CARE SYSTEMS IN THE UNITED STATES AND FORMER SOVIET STATES, 1989

(Sources: Statistical abstract of the United States 1992. "Take a number: The USSR's Constituent Republics, past and present." *Population Today* [November, 1991]; and American International Health Alliance, Washington, D.C., 1997.)

1989 data	U.S.A.	Armenia	Belarus	Georgia	Kazakhstan	Kyrgyzstan	Moldova	Russia	Turkmenistan	Ukraine	Uzbekistan
Physicians per 10,000	26.1	42.7	40.6	58.5	40.9	36.6	40.1	47.3	35.5	43.9	35.8
Nurses per 10,000	67.5	62.6	61.0	71.5	74.1	69.8	67.1	65.5	66.9	65.6	72.4
Hospital beds per 10,000	49.0	90.2	135.4	110.0	135.6	119.3	126.9	138.7	110.6	134.7	123.1
Polyclinics per 10,000	n/a	137.7	177.9	240.1	179.4	124.9	191.0	213.8	112.7	167.6	130.8
Hospitalization rate per 100	14	14.7	26.9	16	25.5	24.4	24.9	24.9	21.5	26.1	25.2
Percentage (%) beds occupied per year	69.6	71	82.2	58.9	82.2	84.7	86.3	80.8	80.0	85.5	84.1
Average # days per hospital stay	6.5	15.5	15.1	14.9	16	15	16.1	16.2	15	16.1	14.9
Health expenditures as a percentage (%) of GDP	11.7	2.7	2.4	3.0	3.1	3.7	3.3	2.2	3.6	2.5	4.5
Health expenditures per person in U.S. dollars	$2,556	$13	$15	$13	$13	$22	$14	$14	$11	$12	$12

1997; Shkolnikov, V. and Meslé, F., 1996, op. cit.; Specter, M., "Plunging life expectancy puzzles Russia." *New York Times* (August 2, 1995): Al; Specter, M., "Russia's declining health: Rising illness, shorter lives." *New York Times* (February 19, 1995): A1; United Nations Children's Fund. *The Progress of Nations: 1997.* UNICEF, New York, 1997; United Nations Children's Fund. *Regional Monitoring Report: Central and Eastern Europe in Transition.* UNICEF, New York, reports for 1993, 1994, 1995, and 1997; United Nations Children's Fund. *The State of the World's Children.* UNICEF, New York, annual releases for 1995, 1996, 1997, and 1998; Vishnievsky, A. G., ed., *Population of Russia.* Institute of Prognostics and Center for Demography and Human Ecology, Moscow, 1997; The World Bank. *World Development Report.* New York: Oxford University Press, annual reports for 1993, 1994, 1995, 1996, 1997, and 1998; World Health Organization. *The World Health Report.* WHO, Geneva, annual reports for 1994, 1995, 1996, 1997, and 1998; and Ykogynikov, B., "Life expectancy and mortality in Russia." *Population and Society* No. 2, Moscow, 1994.

    10. Feshbach, M., personal communication, 2000.

    11. See table "Forecasts, Russia" below:

FORECASTS, RUSSIA

(Source: Presidential Committee on Issues of Females, Family and Democracy)

Year	Premature deaths per 1,000 people			Russian Total Population Size
	Total	*Urban*	*Rural*	
1996	15.1	14.6	16.5	147 million
1997	15.2	14.7	16.6	
1998	15.4	14.9	16.8	
1999	15.5	15.0	17.0	
2000	15.6	15.1	17.0	
2001	15.8	15.3	17.1	141.6 million (RAND Corporation)
2002	15.9	15.4	17.1	
2003	16.0	15.6	17.2	
2004	16.1	15.7	17.2	
2005	16.2	15.8	17.3	
2006	16.2	15.8	17.1	
2007	16.1	15.8	17.0	
2008	16.1	15.8	16.9	
2009	16.0	15.7	16.7	
2010	15.9	15.7	16.6	136 million (Murray Feshbach) 134 million (Yevgeniy Andreyev) 128 million (Gennady Onyschenko)

    12. See table "Basic Demographics" on page 616.

    13. Very few genuine photographs of Joseph Stalin exist. His face was always touched up, hiding the disfiguring poxes and giving him a far handsomer physiognomy than he ever

REGIONAL BASIC INDICATORS

(Sources: The World Bank, World Health Organization, UNICEF)

Country	Under 5-year-old mortality per 1,000, per year, 1996	Infant mortality per 1,000 babies per year	Per capita GNP (in US$)	Life expectancy at birth, 1996	Adult population literacy % in 1995	Under 5-year-old mortality rank (#1=highest)	% population with access to safe water, 1993	% of 1-year old children fully vaccinated for: (in 1995)				1995 Population (millions)
								TB	DDT	Polio	Measles	
Armenia	30	25	$ 730	71	100	108	–	82	86	97	89	3.76
Azerbaijan	44	34	480	71	100	85	–	90	95	97	99	7.42
Belarus	18	14	2,070	70	99	139	–	93	95	94	74	10.28
Bulgaria	19	16	1,330	71	98	136	–	98	100	94	93	8.40
Czech Rep.	7	6	3,870	73	100	164	–	96	97	98	97	10.33
Estonia	16	13	2,860	69	98	145	–	99	90	93	86	1.48
Georgia	29	23	440	73	99	113	–	30	58	82	63	5.37
Hungary	12	11	4,120	69	99	152	–	100	100	100	100	10.23
Kazakhstan	45	38	1,330	68	100	84	99	93	94	98	97	16.82
Kyrgyzstan	50	39	700	68	97	80	–	90	82	81	80	4.47
Latvia	20	16	2,270	68	100	133	–	100	64	77	82	3.72
Lithuania	18	14	1,900	70	99	139	–	98	91	93	96	2.52
Moldova	32	26	920	68	99	102	50	50	83	81	90	4.34
Poland	14	12	2,790	71	–	147	–	94	95	95	91	38.59
Romania	25	21	1,480	70	98	117	–	100	98	97	94	22.68
Russia	25	20	2,240	65	99	117	–	97	87	97	95	147.86

continued

Slovakia	11	10	2,950	71	—	154	—	98	98	98	99	5.36
Tajikistan	76	56	340	67	100	61	—	96	93	96	80	5.94
Turkmenistan	78	57	920	65	98	58	91	88	80	83	66	4.16
Ukraine	24	18	1,630	69	99	121	—	92	94	95	96	51.53
Uzbekistan	60	46	970	68	100	71	22	95	89	99	81	23.21
World norm	88	60	4,812	63	75	—	42	—	86	89	83	—
Norm for industrialized countries	7	6	25,926	77	98	—	—	89	80	81	79	—

LIFE EXPECTANCY AND ECONOMIC INDICATORS

Country	Male Life Expectancy at Birth (in Years) in:						Gross Domestic Product Growth Rates (annual percentage change)						The Economist Emerging Market Indicators (percentage change)				
	1989	1990	1992	1993	1994	1995	1989	1990	1992	1993	1994	1995	Sept. 7, 1996	May 3, 1997	Jan. 17, 1998	Nov. 21, 1998	Jan. 30, 1999
Czech Rep.	68.1	67.5	68.5	68.9	69.5	70.0	+2.4	−1.2	−6.4	−0.9	+2.6	+5.2	+4.3	+4.5	+0.8	−2.4	−2.9
Slovakia	66.9	66.6	66.8	68.4	68.3	68.4	+1.1	−2.5	−7.0	−4.1	+4.8	+7.4	—	+5.0	+2.0	—	—
Hungary	65.4	65.1	64.6	64.5	64.8	65.3	+0.4	−3.3	−3.0	−0.8	+2.9	+1.5	−1.0	+2.5	+5.1	+5.1	+5.6
Poland	66.8	66.5	66.7	67.4	67.5	67.6	−0.1	−11.9	+2.6	+3.8	+5.2	+7.0	+4.0	+5.5	+6.9	+5.3	+5.0
Bulgaria	68.6	68.4	67.8	67.7	67.2	67.2	−0.3	−9.1	−7.3	−1.5	+1.8	+2.5	—	−4.5	—	—	—
Romania	66.6	66.6	66.6	66.1	65.7	65.9	−5.8	−8.2	−8.8	+1.5	+3.9	+6.9	—	−3.8	—	—	—
Estonia	65.7	64.6	63.5	62.4	61.1	61.7	−1.1	−6.6	−14.1	−8.6	−2.7	+2.5	—	+4.8	—	—	—
Latvia	65.3	64.2	63.3	61.6	60.7	60.8	+6.8	+2.9	−34.9	−14.9	+0.6	−1.6	—	+5.0	—	—	—
Lithuania	66.9	66.6	64.9	63.3	62.8	63.6	+1.5	−5.0	−39.3	−30.4	+1.0	+2.3	—	+5.0	—	—	—
Belarus	66.8	66.3	64.9	63.8	63.5	62.9	+8.0	−3.0	−9.6	−10.6	−15.8	−10.0	—	—	—	—	—
Moldova	65.5	65.0	63.9	64.3	62.3	61.8	+9.8	−2.7	−29.1	−1.2	−31.2	−3.0	—	—	+1.0	—	—
Russia	64.2	63.8	62.0	58.9	57.6	58.3	+1.6	−2.0	−14.5	−8.7	−12.6	−4.0	−6.0	+1.0	+1.0	−9.9	−9.9
Ukraine	66.0	66.0	64.0	63.5	62.8	—	+5.0	−3.6	−13.7	−14.1	−23.0	−12.0	—	−2.0	+1.5	—	—
Armenia	69.0	68.4	68.9	67.9	68.1	—	+14.2	−7.4	−52.3	−14.6	+5.5	+5.2	—	—	—	—	—
Azerbaijan	66.0	67.0	65.4	65.2	65.2	63.4	−5.8	−12.7	−22.6	−23.1	−21.9	−17.2	—	—	—	—	—
Georgia	68.1	68.7	—	—	—	—	−4.8	−12.4	−40.3	−39.4	−30.0	+2.4	—	+10.0	—	—	—
Turkmenistan	—	—	—	—	—	—	—	—	—	—	—	—	—	—	−2.0	—	—
Uzbekistan	—	—	—	—	—	—	—	—	—	—	—	—	—	—	+1.0	—	—

RUSSIAN LIFE EXPECTANCY CHANGES, 1958–1995

(Source: Center for Demography and Human Ecology, Moscow)

Year of Birth	LIFE EXPECTANCY, ALL RUSSIANS			URBAN RUSSIANS			RURAL RUSSIANS			Net Change	Notes
	Both Genders	Males	Females	Both Genders	Males	Females	Both Genders	Males	Females		
1958–59	67.9	63	71.5	67.9	63	71.5	67.8	62.9	71.3	—	USSR-wide introduction of antibiotics and childhood vaccines as standards of medical practice
1959–60	68.2	63.3	71.8	—	—	—	—	—	—	⇐	
1960–61	68.5	63.5	72.1	—	—	—	—	—	—	⇐	
1961–62	68.8	63.8	72.4	68.7	63.9	72.4	68.6	63.4	72.3	⇐	
1962–63	68.9	63.9	72.5	68.8	64	72.4	68.7	63.4	72.5	⇐	
1963–64	69.4	64.4	73	69.2	64.5	72.7	69.3	63.9	73.1	⇐	Leonid Brezhnev takes power
1964–65	69.6	64.6	73.3	69.5	64.7	73	69.4	63.8	73.5	⇐	
1965–66	69.5	64.3	73.4	69.4	64.6	73.1	69.1	63.3	73.5	⇒	
1966–67	69.5	64.2	73.5	69.5	64.5	73.2	69	63.1	73.5	—	Overall decline commences
1967–68	69.3	63.9	73.5	59.4	64.3	73.3	68.9	62.8	73.6	⇒	
1968–69	69.1	63.5	73.3	69.1	64	73.2	68.5	62	73.6	⇒	
1969–70	68.8	63.1	73	69	63.5	73.3	68.1	62	73.1	⇒	
1970–71	68.9	63.2	73.6	68.5	63.8	73.5	68.1	61.8	73.4	⇐	
1971–72	69	63.2	73.6	69.3	63.9	73.7	67.9	61.4	73.3	⇐	
1972–73	68.9	63.2	73.6	69.3	64	73.6	67.6	61.1	73	⇒	
1973–74	68.9	63.2	73.6	69.4	64.1	73.7	67.4	60.6	73.1	—	

RUSSIAN LIFE EXPECTANCY CHANGES, 1958–1995
(Source: Center for Demography and Human Ecology, Moscow)

Year of Birth	LIFE EXPECTANCY, ALL RUSSIANS			URBAN RUSSIANS			RURAL RUSSIANS			Net Change	Notes
	Both Genders	Males	Females	Both Genders	Males	Females	Both Genders	Males	Females		
1974–75	68.6	62.8	73.4	69.2	63.8	73.6	66.8	59.7	72.8	⇒	
1975–76	68.1	62.3	73.0	68.8	63.4	73.2	66.1	58.9	72.4	⇒	
1976–77	68.0	62	73.1	68.5	63.1	73.2	65.8	58.2	72.4	⇒	
1977–78	67.9	61.8	73.2	68.5	63.1	73.3	65.5	57.7	72.5	⇒	
1978–79	67.7	61.7	73.1	68.2	62.5	73.2	66.3	59.6	72.6	⇒	
1979–80	67.5	61.5	73	68	62.3	73.1	66	59.3	72.4	⇒	
1980–81	67.6	61.5	73.1	68.1	62.4	73.2	66	59.3	72.5	⇑	
1981–82	68	62	73.5	68.5	62.8	73.5	66.3	59.7	72.8	⇑	
1982–83	68.3	62.3	73.6	68.7	63.1	73.7	66.5	59.8	73	⇑	Brezhnev dies; Andropov takes power
1983–84	67.9	62	73.3	68.4	62.9	73.4	66.1	59.4	72.7	⇒	Andropov dies; Chernenko takes power
1984–85	68.1	62.3	73.3	68.6	63.1	73.4	66.3	59.8	72.6	⇑	Chernenko dies; Gorbachev takes power
1985–86	69.3	63.8	74	69.6	64.5	74	67.9	61.8	73.6	⇑	Gorbachev declares a war on alcoholism
1986–87	70.1	64.9	74.6	70.3	65.4	74.4	69.1	63.2	74.4	⇑	Anti-alcohol campaigns continue; Chernobyl nuclear disaster in Ukraine
1987	70.2	65	74.6	70.4	65.4	74.5	69.1	63.2	74.5	⇑	Historic peak life expectancy
1988	69.9	64.8	74.4	70.1	65.4	74.2	68.7	62.7	74.4	⇒	
1989	69.6	64.2	74.5	69.9	64.8	74.5	68.5	62.6	74.2	⇒	

Year											
1990	69.2	63.8	74.2	69.6	64.4	74.4	67.9	62	73.9	⇒	Baltic states pull out of USSR
1991	69	63.5	74.3	69.4	64.1	74.3	67.7	61.7	73.9	⇒	Soviet Union collapses
1992	67.9	62	73.8	68.2	62.5	73.8	66.9	60.7	73.5	⇒	Reaches 1958 level
1993	65.1	58.9	71.9	65.4	59.3	72	64.3	57.9	71.5	⇒	
1994	64.1	57.4	71	64.3	57.7	71	63.4	56.9	70.9	⇒	War with Chechnya; high military mortality
1995	64.6	58.2	71.7	64.7	58.4	71.7	64.2	57.9	71.7	⇒	Chechnyan war ends
1996											Male life expectancy in Sweden is 76
1997		57.7	71.0							⇒	Male life expectancy in USA is 72
1998		56.0								⇒	
2010 projections		55	72								Source: Murray Feshbach

BASIC DEMOGRAPHICS
(Source: Population Reference Bureau, Washington, D.C., 1996)

Country	Population in millions	Births per 1000	Deaths per 1000	Population Growth	Infant Mortality	Life Expectancy Male	Life Expectancy Female	GNP p/c
USA	265.2	15	9	+0.6	7.5	72	79	$25,860
Belarus	10.3	10	13	−0.3	13.0	64	74	2,160
Bulgaria	8.4	9	13	−0.4	15.5	68	75	1,160
Czech Rep.	10.3	10	11	−0.1	7.9	70	77	3,210
Hungary	10.2	11	14	−0.3	11.5	65	74	3,840
Moldova	4.3	14	12	+0.3	23.0	64	71	870
Poland	38.6	12	10	+0.2	13.5	68	76	2,470
Romania	22.6	10	12	−0.2	23.9	66	73	1,230
Russia	147.7	9	15	−0.5	18.0	57	71	2,650
Slovakia	5.4	12	10	+0.3	11.2	68	77	2,230
Ukraine	51.1	10	15	−0.5	14.0	63	73	1,570
Latvia	2.5	9	16	−0.7	19.0	61	73	2,290
Lithuania	3.7	12	12	−0.1	14.0	63	75	1,350
Estonia	1.5	9	15	−0.5	15.0	64	75	2,820
Sweden	8.8	12	11	+0.1	4.4	76	81	23,630

truly possessed. For details of Soviet photo fakery see King, D., *The Commissar Vanishes.* New York: Metropolitan, 1997.

14. Gerasimenko, N. F., 1997, op. cit.

15. The Soviet Union invaded Afghanistan in 1979, and the war persisted until 1988. Russian tanks rolled into Chechnya in December 1994, and that war continued until November 1996. It is estimated that 80,000 people died in the Chechnyan conflict, one million lost their homes, and roughly 280,000 Soviets died in Afghanistan.

16. Gerasimenko, N. F., 1997, op. cit.

17. Notzon, F. C., Komarov, Y. M., Ermakov, S. P., 1998, op. cit.

18. Meslé, F., Shkolnikov, V. M., Hertrich, V., et al., 1996, op. cit.

19. For example, age-adjusted mortality is crucial to determining life expectancy. When life expectancies started declining, the Soviets used different age adjustments that yielded more positive answers. Thus, they buried the disturbing news in statistical trickery. The same was true for infant mortality data.

20. A very nice biography of Feshbach is Murphy, C., "Watching the Russians." *Atlantic Monthly* (February 1983): 33–51.

21. Feshbach, M., and Friendly, A., Jr., *Ecocide in the USSR: Health and Nature under Siege.* New York: Basic Books, 1992; Feshbach, M., *Russia in Transition: Ecological Disaster*, 1995, op. cit; and Feshbach, M., ed., *Environmental and Health Atlas of Russia*, 1995, op. cit.

22. UNICEF expresses this another way, comparing the trends in births versus deaths in terms of amount of rate increase or decrease compared to 1989. So, if a number 100 is assigned to 1989, a 1995 death rate of 140 would represent a 40-person per 1,000 increase in annual death rate between 1989 and 1995. Using this approach UNICEF found for 1996:

DEATH AND BIRTH RATES AND RATE CHANGES, 1995–1996

Country	Death Rate Change 1995	Death Rate Change 1996	Birth Rate Change 1995	Birth Rate Change 1996
Czech Republic	92.7	102.7	75.0	91.8
Slovakia	96.1	104.2	75.2	100.8
Hungary	102.9	112.4	93.2	98.1
Poland	99	107.6	75.2	101.9
Bulgaria	113.3	110.3	67.7	90.7
Romania	112.1	121.9	64.6	97.1
Estonia	119.5	119.5*	58.7	58.7*
Latvia	127	95.0	58.9	90.9
Lithuania	118.4	110	73.5	92.9
Belarus	128.7	112.8	65.3	91.8
Moldova	132.6	107.5	68.8	84.6
Russia	138.3	100.6	64.4	93.7
Ukraine	132.8	132.8*	72.2	72.2*
Armenia	111.9	100	59.9	89.2
Azerbaijan	101.6	101.6*	73.5	73.5*
Georgia	89.5	89.5*	66.5	66.5*

(* = a 1995 figure used in the absence of available 1996 data)

23. See table "Regional Life Expectancy at Birth" on page 618.

24. According to UNICEF the North American "Great Depression" was marked by even more severe economic changes than those felt between 1989 and 1993 in Russia and Ukraine, and the population of the United States then was larger than the 1989 Russian and

REGIONAL LIFE EXPECTANCY AT BIRTH

(Source: UNICEF)

(* = endpoint 1994 data)

Country	1980		1985		1989		1990		1991		1992		1993		1994		1995		Net Change* 1980-95 (in years)	
	Male	Female	M	F	M	F	M	F	M	F	M	F	M	F	M	F	M	F	Male	Female
Czech Republic	66.8	74	67.3	74.7	68.1	75.4	67.5	76	68.2	75.7	68.5	76.1	68.9	76.6	69.5	76.6	70	76.9	+3.2	+2.9
Slovakia	—	—	—	—	66.9	75.4	66.6	75.4	66.8	75.2	66.8	75.3	68.4	76.7	68.3	76.5	68.4	76.3	+1.5	+0.9
Hungary	65.5	72.7	65.1	73.1	65.4	73.8	65.1	73.7	65	73.8	64.6	73.7	64.5	73.8	64.8	74.2	65.3	74.2	−0.2	−1.5
Poland	66.9	75.4	66.9	75.3	66.8	75.5	66.5	75.5	66.1	75.3	66.7	75.7	67.4	76	67.5	76.1	67.6	76.4	+0.7	+1.0
Slovenia	67.4	75.2	67.9	75.9	68.8	76.7	69.4	77.3	69.5	77.4	69.4	77.3	69.4	77.3	69.6	77.4	70.3	76.8	+0.9	+1.6
Albania	67.7	72.2	68.5	73.9	69.6	75.5	69.3	75.4	—	—	68.5	74.3	68.5	74.3	69.5	75.6	—	—	+1.8*	+3.4*
Bulgaria	68.4	73.6	—	—	68.6	75.1	68.4	75.2	68	74.7	67.8	74.4	67.7	75.1	67.2	74.8	67.2	74.9	−1.2	+1.3
Romania	66.5	71.8	66.8	72.8	66.6	72.7	66.6	73.1	66.6	73.2	66.1	73.2	65.9	73.3	65.7	73.4	—	—	−0.8*	+1.6*
Estonia	64	74	65	75	65.7	74.7	64.6	74.6	64.4	74.8	63.5	74.7	62.4	73.8	61.1	73.1	61.7	74.3	−2.3	+0.3
Latvia	63.6	73.9	65.5	74.5	65.3	75.2	64.2	74.6	63.8	74.8	63.3	74.8	61.6	73.8	60.7	72.9	60.8	73.1	−2.8	−0.8
Lithuania	65	75	66	75	66.9	76.3	66.6	76.2	65.3	76.1	64.9	76	63.3	75	62.8	74.9	63.6	75.2	−1.4	−0.2
Belarus	65.9	75.6	66.7	75.5	66.8	76.4	66.3	75.6	65.5	75.5	64.9	75.4	63.8	74.4	63.5	75	62.9	74.3	−3.0	−1.3
Moldova	62.4	68.8	63.1	69.5	65.5	72.3	65	71.8	64.3	71	63.9	71.9	64.3	71.1	62.3	69.8	61.8	69.7	−0.6	−0.9
Russia	61.5	73	63.8	74	64.2	74.5	63.8	74.3	63.5	74.3	62	73.8	58.9	71.9	57.6	71.2	58.3	71.7	−3.2	−1.3
Ukraine	64.6	74	66	74	66	75	66	75	66	75	64	74	63.5	73	62.8	73.2	—	—	−1.8*	−0.8*
Armenia	69.5	75.7	70.5	75.7	69	74.7	68.4	75.2	68.9	75.6	68.7	75.5	67.9	74.4	68.1	74.9	—	—	−1.4*	−0.8*
Azerbaijan	64.2	71.8	65.3	73.1	66.6	74.2	67	74.8	66.3	74.5	65.4	73.9	65.2	73.9	65.2	73.9	63.4	73.5	−0.8	+1.7
Georgia	67.1	74.8	67.4	75.1	68.1	76.7	68.7	76.1	—	—	—	—	—	—	—	—	—	—	—	—

Ukraine combined populations. Yet the health impact seen in the 1990s in Russia and Ukraine out-stripped that of the "Great Depression." Two reasons are cited. First, Prohibition, which greatly reduced alcohol consumption during the "Great Depression," and second, the introduction of antibiotics reduced child death rates. Neither of these factors had any beneficial impact on death rates in Russia or Ukraine in the 1990s.

25. UNICEF continued: "In addition, recent changes in mortality, nuptiality, and fertility parallel or even surpass those normally observed in wartime conditions."

In Russia and Ukraine the "excess mortality" seen between 1992 and 1993, "was greater than the total number of war losses borne by the United States during World War Two and higher than the number of deaths recorded during the entire Afghanistan war."

26. Shkolnikov, V., Meslé, F., and Vallin, J., 1996, op. cit.

27. In 1940, having suffered Stalin's wrath and a complete ban on both his writings and entry into the power-hub Griboyedov House, dying Ukrainian Mikhail Bulgakov completed his masterpiece, *The Master and Margarita*, in which he lampooned the cowardly writers who had kowtowed to Stalin's admonishments:

Who will say anything in defense of envy? It is a nasty emotion. Nevertheless, one should consider the visitor's position too. For what had he seen upstairs was not yet all; it was, in fact, quite far from all. The entire lower floor of [Griboyedov] house was occupied by a restaurant, and what a restaurant! It was justly considered the best in Moscow. And not only because it was housed in two large rooms with vaulted ceilings, adorned by lilac horses with Assyrian manes; not only because on every table there was a lamp with a silk shawl draped around the shade; not only because it was impossible for the man in the street to gain admission to it; but also because, in the quality of its fare, Griboyedov's beat any restaurant in Moscow, and because this fare was served at the most moderate, most reasonable prices. [Bulgakov, M., *The Master and Margarita*. Translated by Mirra Ginsburg. New York: Grove Weidenfeld, 1967.]

28. Even in the 1990s the affordable condoms in the countries of the region were thick, cumbersome items that, men said, blocked all pleasurable sensation. Thus, they were rarely used.

29. Popov, A. A., "Family planning and induced abortion in post-Soviet Russia of the early 1990s: Unmet needs in information supply." Chapter 3 in DaVanzo, J., 1996, op. cit.

30. Vishnievsky, A. G., op. cit, 1996.

31. Ibid.

32. Eberstadt, N., "Russia: Too Sick to Matter?" *Foreign Affairs* (June 1999): 3–24.

33. Smith, H., *The Russians*. New York: New York Times Book Co., 1976.

34. A recent UNICEF report shows that the suicide rate for teen males has jumped from 11 per 100,000 in the Czech Republic in 1988 to 17.8 in 1995. During the same period, it doubled in Belarus from 14 to 28; and soared in Lithuania, from 22.3 in 1989 to 35. In 1995, the United States saw 17.4 suicides in the same age groups, according to the National Center for Health Statistics.

35. DaVanzo, J., 1996, op. cit.

36. A striking exception is the wine-growing nation of Georgia, where consumption of distilled spirits declined 100 percent between 1985 and 1990, and has leveled off since. Georgian health officials say this reflects the strong local preference for wine, which has a low alcohol content and is much less expensive because it is locally produced.

37. By comparison, the National Institute of Drug Abuse and Alcoholism in Bethesda,

Maryland, said that the consumption rate for American adults annually is 2.21 liters, and declining steadily since an apparent peak of 2.7 liters in 1981.

38. Feshbach, M., *Russia in Transition: Ecological Disaster*, 1995, op. cit.

39. Chernobyl authorities claim that the nuclear material inside that sarcophagus is no longer in danger of escape or explosion. They even dispute the need to fortify the hastily constructed concrete shroud.

But Ukraine's substantial, independent physics community, as well as foreign experts, disagree. They say that the material inside the shroud is still in danger of undergoing an uncontrollable chain reaction, setting off a catastrophic nuclear explosion that could rain radioactive fallout over an area larger than that originally affected in April 1986. There are 200 tons of radioactive fuel inside the sarcophagus, 135 tons of which have the consistency of molten lava. That's enough to create an explosion greater than the Hiroshima bomb blast.

The sarcophagus was showing signs of weakening under the building fuel pressure inside. And in the other reactors inexplicable auto-shutdowns and electronic problems were common. On the tenth anniversary of the disaster *Science* published several unsettling findings in its April 19, 1996, issue.

40. Sources on the environmental impact of the Chernobyl disaster include numerous interviewees, and: Zakharov, Y. M., and Krysanov, E. Y., eds. *Consequences of the Chernobyl Catastrophe: Environmental Health*. Center for Russian Environmental Policy, Moscow, 1996; and Feshbach, M., *Russia in Transition: Ecological Disaster*, 1995, op. cit.

41. According to Zakharov and Krysanov, 1996, op. cit., soil samples collected in 1991 in Bryansk Oblast, Russia, were as follows. Note: global PU^{238} fallout from 1960 A-tests was 1Bq/Kg.

Site	Pu^{238} Bq/Kg	$Pu^{239} + Pu^{240}$ Bq/Kg	Ci/Km² of all fission products
Zaborye	9.2	26.8	290
Yalovka	5.5	28.6	190
Svyatsk	6.6	80	700
Stary Vyshkov	6.3	22.6	320
St. Bobrovichi	22.8	89.4	910
Dobrodeyevka	19.6	24.5	360
Vyshkov	5.9	15.6	170
Barki	22.4	24.5	390
Uscherpye	8.9	17.2	210
Veprino	19	22.8	340

42. Ratushinskaya, I., "Leningrad Triptych." In *Irina Ratushinskaya Poems*. Ann Arbor, MI: International PEN Book, 1984.

43. Feshbach, M., *Russia in Transition: Ecological Disaster*, 1995, op. cit.

44. Feshbach, M., *Environmental and Health Atlas of Russia*, 1995, op. cit.

45. Ibid.

46. Adult 1998 cancer incidence in Irkutsk was 14.5 times more than in the United States.

47. Feshbach, M., *Environmental and Health Atlas of Russia*, 1995, op. cit.

48. World Health Organization. "Dramatic increase in thyroid cancer among children in Belarus and Ukraine after Chernobyl accident." Press Release WHO/84, October 19, 1993.

49. Mitchell, P., "Ukrainian thyroid-cancer rates greatly increased since Chernobyl." *Lancet* 354 (1999): 51.

50. Pacini, F., Vorontsova, T., Molinaro, E., et al., "Prevalence of thyroid autoantibodies in children and adolescents from Belarus exposed to the Chernobyl radioactive fallout." *Lancet* 352 (1998): 763–66.

51. Gluzman, D. F., "Leukemias and myclodysplastic syndromes following the Chernobyl accident." *Experimental Oncology* (Russian) 18 (1996): 120–27; Gluzman, D. F., Abramenko, I. V., Vasilenko, O. S., et al., "Aberrant lymphocytes and sensitivity to apoptosis at low dose radiation." Courtesy of Gluzman; Gluzman, D. F., Abramenko, I. V., Sklyarenko, L. M., et al., "Approaches to the diagnosis and studies of leukemias after the Chernobyl accident." *Hematology and Transfusion* (Russian) 41 (1996): 35–39; and Gluzman, D. F., Simonet, M. L., Moutet, A., Pinchouk, L. B., "Ionizing radiation induced leukemias." *Experimental Oncology* (Russian) 16 (1994): 83–95.

52. Michielis, J., Kaletsch, U., Burkart, W., et al., "Infant leukemia after the Chernobyl accident." *Nature* 387 (1997): 246.

53. Bard, D., Verger, P., and Hubert, P., "Chernobyl, 10 years after: Health consequences." *Epid. Reviews* 19 (1997): 187–204.

54. "Chernobyl, cancer and creeping paranoia." *The Economist* (March 9, 1996): 81–82.

55. Larisa Ignatyeva's findings were:

Source	TCDD (parts per trillion)	
Butter	62	ppt
Milk	15	ppt
Riverbank soil	0.133	ppt
Sewage water	38.5	ppt
Irkutsk drinking water	5.5	ppt

The United States had no allowable contamination standards for dioxins in food or dairy products. The Environmental Protection Agency allowed a maximum of 30 parts per quadrillion TCDDs in drinking water, so Irkutsk's water seems to be safe by U.S. standards. But the U.S. Food and Drug Administration allows no measurable dioxins in foods, so the contaminants found by Ignatyeva would be illegal in America.

56. Klebnikov, P., "A company built on bones." *Forbes* (November 6, 1995).

57. Revich, B., Gervich, E., et al., "Regional and local problems of chemical contamination of the environment and health of population." 1st edition. Eurasia, Moscow, 1995.

58. Revich, B. A., "Public health and ambient air pollution in Arctic and subarctic cities of Russia." *The Science of the Total Environment* 160 (1995): 585–92.

59. On July 1, 1935, the first 1,200 slaves arrived in Noril'sk and "lived" in tiny unheated shacks. Most perished during the 1935–36 winter, and for his service the first Noril'sk manager was executed at Lubyanka in 1935, charged with being a "People's Enemy."

The second Noril'sk manager fared a little better. A KGB man, he survived two years of Noril'sk and then was arrested on an old murder rap and, like his predecessor, executed.

By 1939, however, managers had figured out how to build in the frigid permafrost, and how to dig mile-deep mine shafts. The slaves perished, perhaps at a rate of 25 percent of them every winter, men, women, and children. The poet Anna Akhmatova, for example, perished in Noril'sk after her husband and child died. With her blood she wrote this final poem on the wall of her barracks:

My husband, in a grave.
My son, in jail.
Pray for me.

During World War II Noril'sk operations sped up to provide Soviet troops with metals for weapons production. At the war's peak in 1942–45, 27,000 slaves and 5,000 "free people" worked in Noril'sk.

The wartime slave force included citizens of twenty-two nations, even an American. And toward the end of the war a large complement of German POWs worked—and died— in Noril'sk.

After the war the Noril'sk slave force became a more formalized political prison population, dominated by Soviet poets, intellectuals, and alleged dissidents. In 1951 some 100,000 gulag slaves worked in Noril'sk. And upon learning of Stalin's death in 1953 the slaves—who outnumbered "free people" of Noril'sk—rebelled, sparking a violent Arctic conflict that lasted five months and ended with a series of KGB-run public executions.

By order of Nikita Khrushchev the slave camps of Noril'sk were closed in 1954, and the political prisoners were transferred to other Siberian locales. In 1957 Noril'sk was officially declared a "free city," and construction was completed by Komsomol volunteers recruited from all over the USSR.

No one knows how many slaves perished in the Noril'sk gulag, as the Communists—unlike the German Nazis—didn't keep reliable records. Russian orthodox crosses dot nearby Schmidt Mountain, which, according to the most reliable estimate, holds half a million bodies.

Among the dead, Dolgan native and teacher Elena Sotnikova said, were all of the shamans and tribal leaders of the Arctic native peoples. "Innocent people suffered," she explained. "Those who didn't even speak Russian. They died without knowing what they were accused of. They were just dying for things like having too many reindeer," or speaking their native languages, which Stalin banned.

60. A. Galich, 1977.

61. For an excellent flavor of this bizarre social scene, see McQueen, A., "Survivors." *Granta* 64 (1999): 38–53.

62. Revich, B. A., "Public health and ambient air pollution in Arctic and subarctic cities of Russia." *The Science of the Total Environment* 160 (1995): 585–92.

63. Klebnikov, P., 1995, op. cit.

64. For a disturbing picture of Aral Sea devastation see Ellis, W. S., "A Soviet sea lies dying." *National Geographic* (February 1990): 73–93.

65. Revich, B., "Child health level in Moscow as related to ambient air pollution." *The Science of the Total Environment* 148 (1994): 57–60.

66. Revich, B., "Exposure to lead and its effects on children's health—the results of two studies implemented in Belovo (Metallurgical Plant) and St. Petersburg (production of batteries)." Personal communication.

67. Revich, B. A., Dvoyrin, V., et al., "Dioxins in the environment of Chapaevsk (Russia), health of its population." *Organohalogen Compounds* 30 (1996): 350–54.

68. Šrám, R., Bens, I., Binková, B., et al., "Teplice Program—The impact of air pollution on human health." *Environmental Health Perspectives* 104 (1996): 699–714; and Šrám, R. "Future research directions to characterize environmental mutagens in highly polluted areas." *Environmental Health Perspectives* 104 (1996): 603–7.

69. Sinyavsky, A., 1997, op. cit.

70. United Nations Children's Fund. *Children at Risk in Central and Eastern Europe: Perils and Promises.* UNICEF, New York, 1997: 16.

71. For the bounce-backs in these countries, according to the World Bank and UNICEF, see chart, "The Global Picture: A Sampler," on pages 611–17.

72. "Russia's fear-worse factor." *The Economist* (June 1, 1996): 45–46.

73. In Russia the kingpins were Boris Berezovsky, Mikhail Khodorkovsky, Vladimir Goussinsky, Rem Vyakhirev, Vladimir Potanin, Alexander Smolensky, and Yuri Luzhkov. In Ukraine Sergei Tigipko and Paulo Lazarenko. In Belarus it was its dictator, Alexandr Lukashenko, who allegedly was lining his pockets. In Uzbekistan the new moguls were Islam Karimov, Kayim Khakulov, Alisher Azizkhojaev, Sharaf Rashidov, and Ismail Jurabekov. In Kazakhstan it was said President Nursultan Nazarbaev was the key robber baron. See Quinn-Judge, P., "Battle of the Bankers." *Time* (October 20, 1997): 66–68; and Blasi, J. R., Kroumava, M., and Kruse, D., *Kremlin Capitalism: The Privatization of the Russian Economy.* New York: Cornell University Press, 1997.

74. Specter, M., "Yeltsin's plan to cut military touches a nerve." *New York Times* (July 28, 1997): A1.

75. For examples, see: Slackman, M., "Fanning anti-Semitic flames." *Newsday* (February 23, 1999): A18; Bohlen, C., "Russia's stubborn strains of anti-Semitism." *New York Times* (March 2, 1999): A1; and Gordon, M. R., "Russian Jews turning edgy as the country's chaos creates an ugly mood." *New York Times* (March 9, 1999): A12.

76. Consider these figures drawn from the November 16, 1998, issue of *Forbes*: Russia's top ten publicly owned companies lost, on average, 80 percent of their stock market value between October 1997 and October 1998. Yuri Luzhkov, mayor of Moscow and much-favored candidate to succeed Yeltsin, openly favored defaulting on $12 billion worth of Russian T-bills, which would leave Western banks in a crisis the likes of which they hadn't seen since the Brazilian debacle of the early 1980s. Already by the autumn of 1998 Western investors had lost $50 billion gambling on Russia—money no one ever expected to see again.

In two weeks in August the ruble fell from trading at 6.5 rubles to the dollar to 9 to the dollar. Some estimates are that the Russian people, in that blink of an economic eye, lost 80 percent of their collective personal savings.

And those banking moguls? Well, eighteen of Russia's twenty largest banks went under during the summer of 1998.

77. Powell, B., "Russian roulette." *Newsweek* (September 7, 1998): 25–31.

78. Clifford Gaddy and Barry Ickes argue that even these numbers hide Russia's reality: a GDP of only $466 billion, or 6 percent of the U.S. GDP, and a rapid deterioration of all cash exchanges, in favor of a largely barter economy. See Gaddy, C. and Ickes, B., "Russia's virtual economy." *Foreign Affairs* 77 (1998): 53–67.

79. "Competitiveness." *The Economist*, (April 22, 2000): 98; and Soros, G., "Who Lost Russia?" *The New York Review of Books* (April 13, 2000): 10–16.

80. See Yergin, D. and Gustafson, T., *Russia 2010 and What It Means for the World.* New York: Vintage Books, 1995.

81. Agence-France Presse. "2 million orphans" (November 18, 1998); and Associated Press. "Younger workers in Russia found more likely to be poor" (November 18, 1998).

82. Wadhams, N., "Economic crisis sending more children onto streets in Russia." Associated Press (October 13, 1998); International Youth Foundation. "Policies, programs and philanthropy for children and youth in Russia." IYF, Baltimore 1998; and Basu, S. J., "The health of street children in Moscow and St. Petersburg." Honors Thesis, Program in Human Biology, Stanford University, May 23, 1998.

83. Kohlmeir, L., Mendez, M., Shalnova, S., et al., "Deficient dietary iron intake among women and children in Russia: Evidence from the Russian Longitudinal Monitoring Survey." *American Journal of Public Health* 88 (1998): 576–80.

THE GLOBAL PICTURE: A SAMPLER

Country	Ranking for under-5-year-old child mortality	% of pop. with access to safe water	GNP per capita (in 1996 $)	% of pop. below $1 per day income	Infant mortality rate (1997)	Adult literacy rate (%) (1995)	Life expectancy at birth (years) (1997)	Health expenditures total, as % of GDP (1995)	% children immunized against measles (1997)	% children under 5 who are growth-stunted due to malnutrition Males (1995)	Females (1995)
Afghanistan	4	12	250	—	165	32	45	—	58	54	49
Albania	89	—	820	—	34	—	71	—	95	—	—
Angola	3	31	270	—	170	42	47	—	82	27	23
Argentina	118	71	8,380	—	21	96	73	9.7	98	7	2
Armenia	103	—	630	—	25	100	71	7.8	92	—	—
Austria	181	—	28,110	—	5	—	77	8.0	90	—	—
Azerbaijan	81	—	480	—	34	100	71	6.1	—	24	20
Bangladesh	44	95	260	—	81	38	58	2.4	97	54	55
Belarus	138	—	2,070	2	14	99	70	6.4	98	—	—
Belgium	163	—	26,440	—	6	—	77	7.9	64	—	—
Bolivia	51	63	830	7	69	83	61	7.1	98	33	26
Bosnia	142	—	—	—	14	—	73	—	85	—	—
Botswana	78	90	3,210	33	39	70	51	2.9	79	—	—
Brazil	84	76	4,400	24	37	85	67	4.6	99	12	9
Bulgaria	136	—	1,190	3	16	98	71	6.9	93	—	—
Burundi	17	52	170	—	106	35	47	—	—	—	—
Cambodia	23	30	300	—	106	65	54	7.2	68	—	—

THE GLOBAL PICTURE: A SAMPLER

Country	Ranking for under-5-year-old child mortality	% of pop. with access to safe water	GNP per capita (in 1996 $)	% of pop. below $1 per day income	Infant mortality rate (1997)	Adult literacy rate (%) (1995)	Life expectancy at birth (years) (1997)	Health expenditures total, as % of GDP (1995)	% children immunized against measles (1997)	% children under 5 who are growth-stunted due to malnutrition Males (1995)	Females (1995)
Cameroon	50	50	610	—	64	63	56	1.4	43	27	25
Canada	163	—	19,020	—	6	97	79	9.2	—	—	—
C. Afric. Rep.	19	38	310	—	113	60	49	—	—	27	30
Chad	14	24	160	—	118	48	48	3.7	30	41	39
Chile	146	91	4,860	15	95	11	75	6.2	92	—	—
China	80	67	750	22	80	38	70	3.8	96	32	31
Colombia	103	85	2,140	7	91	25	71	7.4	89	16	14
Congo	45	34	670	—	81	75	51	6.3	18	—	—
Congo, Dem. Rep.	11	42	130	—	128	77	53	—	20	47	44
Costa Rica	144	96	2,640	19	12	95	77	8.5	99	6	7
Côte d'Ivoire	27	42	660	18	90	40	51	3.5	68	25	24
Croatia	157	—	3,800	—	8	98	72	10.1	93	—	—
Cuba	159	93	1,170	—	7	96	76	—	99	—	—
Czech Rep.	163	—	4,740	3	6	—	73	9.1	96	2	2
Denmark	171	—	32,100	—	6	99	76	6.4	84	—	—
Dominican Rep.	75	65	1,600	20	82	44	71	5.7	80	12	9
Ecuador	90	68	1,500	30	90	30	70	5.3	75	—	—

THE GLOBAL PICTURE: A SAMPLER

Country	Ranking for under-5-year-old child mortality	% of pop. with access to safe water	GNP per capita (in 1996 $)	% of pop. below $1 per day income	Infant mortality rate (1997)	Adult literacy rate (%) (1995)	Life expectancy at birth (years) (1997)	Health expenditures total, as % of GDP (1995)	% children immunized against measles (1997)	% children under 5 who are growth-stunted due to malnutrition Males (1995)	Females (1995)
Egypt	65	87	1,080	8	51	54	66	3.7	92	26	23
El Salvador	95	66	1,700	—	72	31	69	5.9	97	23	24
Eritrea	40	22	100	—	73	—	51	2.0	53	36	41
Estonia	144	—	3,080	6	13	98	69	—	88	—	—
Ethiopia	18	25	100	46	111	36	50	2.6	52	66	63
Finland	188	—	23,240	—	4	—	77	7.5	—	—	—
France	181	—	26,270	—	5	—	79	9.7	83	—	—
Gabon	29	67	3,950	—	85	63	55	—	—	—	—
Gambia	55	69	320	—	66	39	47	—	91	33	28
Georgia	109	—	850	—	23	99	73	—	95	—	—
Germany	181	—	28,870	—	5	—	77	10.5	—	—	—
Ghana	47	65	360	—	68	65	58	1.5	59	28	24
Greece	159	—	11,460	—	7	97	78	5.9	90	—	—
Guatemala	74	77	1,470	—	56	43	67	3.2	74	50	49
Guinea	13	46	560	53	36	36	46	—	56	—	—
Haiti	34	37	310	—	92	45	54	3.6	—	32	32
Honduras	81	76	660	47	36	73	70	5.6	89	39	40
Hungary	149	—	4,340	2	10	99	69	7.3	100	—	—
Iceland	181	—	26,580	—	5	—	79	8.0	—	—	—
India	45	81	380	53	71	52	62	5.6	81	52	52

Indonesia	68	75	1,080	12	45	84	65	1.8	92	43	41
Iran	96	90	1,033	—	32	69	69	4.8	96	20	18
Iraq	37	81	1,036	—	94	58	62	6.4	98	—	—
Ireland	163	—	17,110	—	6	—	77	4.1	—	—	—
Israel	171	—	15,870	—	6	96	78	7.6	94	—	—
Italy	171	86	19,880	4	5	98	78	4.9	75	—	—
Jamaica	149	—	1,600	—	10	85	75	7.2	88	—	—
Japan	171	93	40,940	2	4	—	80	—	—	—	—
Kazakhstan	84	53	1,350	50	37	100	68	2.6	97	18	14
Kenya	55	81	320	—	57	78	54	—	32	35	32
North Korea	103	93	970	—	23	—	72	5.4	94	—	—
South Korea	171	71	10,610	19	6	98	72	—	85	—	—
Kuwait	146	44	18,720	—	12	79	76	—	95	—	—
Kyrgystan	79	—	550	—	38	97	68	5.3	98	—	—
Latvia	132	94	2,300	—	16	100	68	—	97	13	12
Lebanon	93	62	2,970	49	30	92	70	—	89	46	41
Lesotho	31	46	660	—	95	71	59	—	53	—	—
Liberia	6	97	490	—	157	38	50	—	—	—	—
Libya	115	—	5,540	—	22	76	65	—	92	16	14
Lichtenstein	163	—	—	—	6	100	—	—	—	—	—
Lithuania	143	—	2,280	2	13	99	70	—	96	—	—

THE GLOBAL PICTURE: A SAMPLER

Country	Ranking for under-5-year-old child mortality	% of pop. with access to safe water	GNP per capita (in 1996 $)	% of pop. below $1 per day income	Infant mortality rate (1997)	Adult literacy rate (%) (1995)	Life expectancy at birth (years) (1997)	Health expenditures total, as % of GDP (1995)	% children immunized against measles (1997)	% children under 5 who are growth-stunted due to malnutrition Males (1995)	Females (1995)
Madagascar	25	26	250	72	96	46	58	—	27	51	48
Malawi	8	47	180	—	135	56	41	—	87	50	47
Malaysia	149	78	4,370	6	10	84	72	—	—	—	—
Mexico	96	85	3,670	15	29	90	72	4.2	97	23	23
Mongolia	27	40	360	—	105	83	66	—	—	—	—
Morocco	67	65	1,290	2	58	44	66	3.4	92	24	24
Mozambique	10	63	80	—	130	40	47	—	70	—	—
Nepal	48	71	210	50	75	28	57	5.0	85	47	50
Netherlands	171	—	25,940	—	5	—	78	8.6	96	—	—
New Zealand	163	97	15,720	—	7	—	77	—	—	—	—
Nicaragua	71	62	380	44	42	66	68	8.6	94	25	22
Norway	188	—	34,510	—	4	—	78	7.9	—	—	—
Oman	138	85	4,950	—	15	59	71	—	98	19	13
Pakistan	38	79	480	12	95	38	64	3.5	74	—	—
Panama	132	93	3,080	26	18	91	74	6.7	92	—	—
Papua New Guinea	43	32	1,150	—	79	72	58	—	—	—	—
Paraguay	99	60	1,850	—	27	92	70	5.1	61	14	14
Peru	72	67	2,420	49	44	89	68	3.7	94	26	25
Philippines	88	84	1,160	29	32	95	68	—	—	—	—

Poland	149	—	3,230	7	10	—	71	6.0	94	—	—
Portugal	159	—	10,160	—	7	90	75	8.2	81	—	—
Romania	114	—	1,600	18	22	98	70	—	97	8	8
Russia	115	—	2,410	2	20	99	65	4.8	92	12	13
Rwanda	21	—	190	46	105	61	40	—	66	50	47
Saudi Arabia	112	95	6,800	—	24	63	71	3.4	92	—	—
Senegal	36	63	570	54	72	33	51	—	65	24	22
Seychelles	138	—	6,850	—	14	84	71	—	100	—	—
Sierra Leone	2	34	200	—	182	31	37	3.6	28	—	—
Singapore	188	100	30,550	—	4	91	77	3.5	90	—	—
Somalia	9	26	110	—	125	24	49	—	—	—	—
South Africa	69	87	3,520	24	49	82	65	7.9	75	24	22
Spain	181	—	14,350	—	5	97	78	7.7	—	—	—
Sri Lanka	136	57	740	4	17	90	73	1.9	94	23	25
Sudan	41	73	320	—	73	46	55	0.3	92	34	34
Swaziland	52	50	1,210	—	66	77	60	—	57	—	—
Sweden	188	—	25,710	—	4	—	78	7.3	93	—	—
Switzerland	181	—	44,350	—	5	—	79	9.8	—	—	—
Syria	99	86	1,160	—	27	79	69	—	93	23	18
Tajikistan	61	60	340	—	56	100	67	—	95	—	—

THE GLOBAL PICTURE: A SAMPLER

Country	Ranking for under-5-year-old child mortality	% of pop. with access to safe water	GNP per capita (in 1996 $)	% of pop. below $1 per day income	Infant mortality rate (1997)	Adult literacy rate (%) (1995)	Life expectancy at birth (years) (1997)	Health expenditures total, as % of GDP (1995)	% children immunized against measles (1997)	% children under 5 who are growth-stunted due to malnutrition Males (1995)	Females (1995)
Tanzania	30	66	170	11	92	68	51	–	69	45	42
Thailand	92	81	2,960	2	31	52	50	5.3	–	–	–
Tunisia	99	98	1,930	4	27	67	69	5.9	92	22	23
Turkey	81	49	2,830	–	40	82	69	4.2	76	21	20
Turkmenistan	59	74	940	5	57	98	65	–	100	–	–
Uganda	31	46	300	69	86	62	41	3.9	60	40	37
Ukraine	118	–	1,200	–	18	99	69	–	–	–	–
United Arab Emirates	154	97	17,390	–	9	79	75	2.5	95	–	–
United Kingdom	163	–	19,600	–	6	–	77	6.9	95	–	–
USA	159	–	28,020	–	7	99	77	14.0	–	2	2
Uraguay	127	–	5,760	–	18	97	73	13.4	99	10	9
Uzbekistan	70	90	1,010	–	46	100	68	–	88	34	29
Venezuela	115	79	3,020	12	21	91	73	7.5	68	15	12
Vietnam	86	43	290	–	32	94	67	5.2	96	47	47
Yemen	49	61	380	–	76	39	58	2.5	51	36	47
Yugoslavia	127	76	–	–	18	98	72	8.3	98	–	–
Zambia	12	38	360	85	112	78	43	3.3	69	43	42
Zimbabwe	58	79	610	41	53	85	49	6.2	73	–	–

(Sources: The World Bank, UNICEF, and WHO, annual reports, 1998)

— = no data available

84. "Russia: How do they survive?" *The Economist* (October 3, 1998): 60–61; and Gordon, M. R., "Facing severe shortage of food, Russia seeks foreign relief aid." *New York Times* (October 10, 1998): A1.

Interestingly, a Czech study of nearly 3,000 families during that country's most severe economic downturn of 1993 found no correlation between socioeconomics and child health, as measured by growth rates between ages three and six years. The only factors that did strongly correlate with stunted growth were maternal smoking and poorly educated mother. See Bobák, M., Bohumír, K., Leon, D. A., et al., "Socioeconomic factors and height of pre-school children in the Czech Republic." *American Journal of Public Health* 84 (1994): 1167–70.

85. Slackman, M., "Desperate Times." *Newsday* (September 5, 1999): A5.

86. See Gerasimov, G., "An overview of IDD status, control programmes, and salt supplementation in countries of Central and Eastern Europe (CEE), Commonwealth of Independent States (CIS) and Baltic States (BS)," Moscow, 1997; International Council for Control of Iodine Deficiency Disorders. "IDD in the former USSR." *IDD Newsletter* 8 (1992): 1; Ministry of Health of the Russian Federation. "Reference materials: On the problem of micronutrients malnutrition of the population of Russia for the U.S.-Russia Health Committee" (November 12, 1996); Program Against Micronutrient Malnutrition. "Elimination of iodine deficiency disorders in the Republic of Georgia." Rollins School of Public Health, Emory University, Atlanta, undated; and U.S. Agency for International Development. "The problem of micronutrient malnutrition in the Russian Federation." Trip report, June 24–July 2, 1997, Moscow.

87. Drakulić, S., *Café Europa: Life After Communism.* New York: W. W. Norton, 1997.

88. These were statements made in a June 18, 1995, press conference at WHO, in Geneva. To put those numbers in perspective, over the sixteen-year period 1980 to 1994 in the United States there were forty-one diphtheria cases, none of which spread to a second person. All of the cases involved inadequately vaccinated children. See Bisgard, K. M., Hardy, I. R. B., Popovic, T., et al., "Respiratory diphtheria in the United States, 1980 through 1995." *American Journal of Public Health* 88 (1998): 787–91.

89. Centers for Disease Control and Prevention. "Diphtheria epidemic—New Independent States of the former Soviet Union, 1990–1994." *Morbidity and Mortality Weekly Report* 44 (1995): 177–81; Efron, S., "Epidemic rages despite plea to other nations." *Los Angeles Times* (November 13, 1995): A11; Vitek, C. R. and Wharton, M., "Diphtheria in the former Soviet Union: Reemergence of a pandemic disease." *Emerging Infectious Diseases* 4 (1998): 1–12; Vitek, C. R., Brennan, M. B., Gotway, C. A., et al., "Risk of diphtheria among school-children in the Russian Federation in relation to time since last vaccination." *Lancet* 353 (1999): 355–58; and World Health Organization. *World Health Report 1996.* WHO, Geneva (1996): 26–27.

90. Umnov, B., "Who would think a shot? From childhood we are brought up thinking vaccines are safe. But is this always true?" *Komsomolskaya Pravda* (September 15, 1988).

91. For more on the Chervonskaya story see: "We don't want to 'Run with the herd'—More on vaccinations." *Meditsinskii Vestnik* 8 (1994); "Experiments on 'state' children." *Rossiskaya Gazetta* (April 8, 1994); "Debilitation of the country." *Stolitsa* 17 (1993); "Universal vaccination of Russians contradicts the declaration on human rights." *Sevodnya* (February 23, 1993); Chervonskaya, G., "Medical workers don't know their figures." *Nezavisimaya Gazetta* (December 15, 1990); and Chervonskaya, G., "Vaccination not the only defense against disease." *Moscow News* (September 15–21, 1995).

92. I thank Robert Steinglass for this translation.

93. Tatochenko, V. K., "Reasons for negative attitudes of physicians to vaccination

in Russia." Novgorod Seminar, September 1996; Steinglass, R., "Challenges in immunization: Issues related to service delivery." Russia-USA Joint Conference on Public Health Communication, October 2–4, 1995, Moscow; and Tatochenko, V. K., "Prophylactic vaccination of children in Russia and the USA." *Meditsinskii Gazetta* (December 4, 1996).

94. Stark, K., Barg, J., Molz, B., et al., "Immunity against diphtheria in blood donors in East Berlin and West Berlin." *Lancet* 350 (1997): 932.

95. That may account for the high rates of congenital birth defects seen in the region, Murray Feshbach argues, because maternal rubella virus infection during pregnancy is extremely dangerous to growing fetuses.

Between 1980 and 1991, when the Soviet Union dissolved, child immunization rates fell precipitously regionwide, to the point where nearly 40 percent of Russian children were still unvaccinated for polio by age two, and 29 percent lacked diphtheria, pertussis, and tetanus (DPT) shots or measles vaccinations, both of which are commonly required for school registration in the United States.

In Ukraine, the situation is even worse, UNICEF has reported, with barely a third of the nation's infants vaccinated at all. In Georgia in 1992, only 0.5 percent of the country's infants were given shots for DPT and only 9 percent got measles vaccines.

Gennady Onyschenko, Russia's first deputy health minister, reported that during the first seven months of 1997, the number of whooping cough cases had jumped two times the figure reported for all of 1996. And incidence of childhood mumps had risen 30 percent over two years.

96. Hardy, I. R. B., Dittman, S., and Sutter, R. W., "Current situation and control strategies for resurgence of diphtheria in newly independent states of the former Soviet Union." *Lancet* 347 (1996): 1739–44. And Vitek, C. R. and Wharton, M., "Diphtheria in the Former Soviet Union: Reemergence of a Pandemic Disease." *Emerging Infectious Diseases* 4 (1998): 539–49.

97. Because most vaccines are made of living bacteria or viruses, the principle says, they must be scrupulously maintained in a refrigerated state during every step in the chain of production, transport, and delivery. If allowed to warm up the vaccines will lose their potency or be destroyed.

98. Hardy, I. R. B., Dittman, S., and Sutter, R. W., 1996, op. cit.

99. For polio details see Oblapenko, G. and Sutter, R. W., "Status of poliomyelitis eradication in Europe and the Central Asian Republics of the former Soviet Union." *Journal of Infectious Diseases* 175 (1997): S76–S81; and Sutter, R. W., Chudaiberdiev, Y. K., Vaphakulov, S. H., et al., "A large outbreak of poliomyelitis following temporary cessation of vaccination in Samarkand, Uzbekistan, 1993–94." *Journal of Infectious Diseases* 175 (1997): S82–S85.

100. Sutter and his Uzbek colleagues concluded that: "Failure to vaccinate, rather than vaccine failure, appears to be primarily responsible for the outbreak of poliomyelitis in Samarkand. . . . The outbreak in Samarkand is also an example of how a disease controlled well for many years (low endemicity) can suddenly cause an explosive outbreak (epidemic)." From Sutter, R. W., Chudaiberdiev, Y. K., Vaphakulov, S. H., 1997, op. cit.).

101. There is no way to know whether Irakli survived the chilly Georgian spring. The impoverished Sherodzle family is not accessible by phone, fax, or mail.

102. December 1995, influenza: Though flu that year was mild for the United States and Europe, Russia and Ukraine suffered the worst epidemic in decades. At peak, days before Christmas, more than 200,000 people per day fell ill in Russia, and estimates are that more than a million Muscovites were sick with the flu on Christmas Day. The epidemic was so

large in Ukraine that the government shut down, as did most schools and companies, due to illness. Why was the epidemic so severe? One reason: all vaccination campaigns have collapsed. Another: more people were homeless or lived in crowded, nonhygienic settings.

103. For malaria details see Sharipov, A., "Malaria in Tajikistan." International Conference on Emerging Infectious Diseases, Atlanta, March 8–11, 1998.

104. Under the old Soviet system all production of goods was coordinated out of Moscow with specific components made in one territory and assembled elsewhere, often thousands of miles away. When the Soviet Union collapsed, production of raw products and goods was dispersed to different, new countries. In the case of disinfectants, such as chlorine products for water purification, 1991 brought a crisis: the raw chlorine had long been produced in Armenia but processed into appropriate chemical formulations in central Russia and bottled in numerous sites scattered around Russia. The Armenian chlorine site fell apart for lack of its old Soviet subsidies from Moscow and every step up the line closed down, unable to obtain the resources to manufacture saleable products.

105. Gerasimenko, N. F., 1997, op. cit.

106. According to the nongovernmental Moscow Center for Prison Reform the escalation of both crime and the jail populations began in the Soviet 1960s; crime rates grew by 2.2 percent annually throughout the 1970s. In the 1980s the pace of crime picked up, swelling by nearly 9 percent a year. And by the mid-1980s crime—nonpolitical criminal activity—was growing at a rate of 23.9 percent annually. The Center offers these startling figures for the post-Communist years:

CRIMINAL JUSTICE ACTIVITY: POST-COMMUNIST RUSSIA

Category	1991	1992	1993	1994	% Change 1991–1994
Number of people arrested	251,200	332,600	392,300	404,300	+16.9%
Number sentenced					
by courts	593,800	661,400	792,400	924,600	+55
to imprisonment	207,500	225,900	292,900	332,700	+60.3
to death	147	159	157	160	+108.9
Number of criminal reports filed with the police	2,978,000	3,617,000	3,669,000	3,394,000	+114
Number of criminal cases solved	1,023,000	1,217,000	1,395,000	1,578,000	+54.2
Number of persons brought to trial	654,800	782,500	967,100	1,117,200	+70.6
Percentage of those brought to trial needlessly	2.8	3.7	5.6	7.9	+282
Number of cases returned by courts for further investigation	109,700	66,000	119,800	115,000	+53.3
Number of penitentiary prisoners	680,000	745,000	772,000	876,000	1995 = 910,000 1996 = 1,017,000

Source: Moscow Center for Prison Reform, *In Search of a Solution*, Human Rights Publishers, Moscow, 1996.

According to the Moscow Center, Mirian's recall of the overcrowding at Matrosskaya Tishina jail actually understated the problem: in 1995 there were 460 inmates in a holding cell designed for 110 prisoners.

107. Data on prison populations in Europe are as follows:

NUMBER OF PRISONERS
per 100,000 citizens

Country	Pre-1950 Average	Post-1990 Average
Russia	60	740
Austria	53	100
England	72	53
Belgium	35	167
Denmark	47	67
Netherlands	31	70
Norway	47	49
France	47	78
Switzerland	47	120
United States of America	55	580

108. Wares, D. F. and Clowes, C. J., "Tuberculosis in Russia." *Lancet* 350 (1997): 957.

109. Feshbach, M., "Dead Souls," 1999, op. cit.

110. Bohlen, C., "In the ruble crisis, even prisoners go hungry." *New York Times* (December 14, 1998): A3; and Stanley, A., "Russians lament the crime of punishment." *New York Times* (August 8, 1997): A1.

111. Remnick, D., "More bad news from the gulag." *The New Yorker* (February 12, 1999): 27–28.

112. These figures are derived from an unpublished Ministry of Interior memo, which I obtained and authenticated in June 1997.

113. Dugarova's numbers are as follows:

TB INCIDENCE RATES, BURYATIA

Year	Rate per 100,000, All Ages	Mortality	Rate per 100,000, Pediatric (under 14 years)
1991	39.2	5.6	15.3
1992	44.2	5.1	20.6
1993	50.3	7.5	27.8
1994	62.5	7.1	47.1
1995	123.8	9.6	41.2
1996	150.2	14.3	61.1

PROJECTED CASELOAD, TB, ULAN UDE
(Population=360,000)

Year	Active TB Cases, All Ages
1997	2,035
1998	2,543
1999	3,428
2000	4,285

114. An interesting exception to the Stiblo Model was South Africa, where DOTS failed, largely because of tensions between patients and nurses. See: Zwarenstein, M., Schoeman, J. H., Vundule, C., et al., "Randomised controlled trial of self-supervised and directly observed treatment of tuberculosis." *Lancet* (1998): 1340–43; and Garner, P., "What makes DOT work?" *Lancet* 352 (1998): 1326–27.

115. Figures from Sillaustu include:

RATE TB PER 100,000

Year	Finland	Estonia	Lithuania	Latvia
1990	15.5	26.7	39.5	32.5
1995	12.9	41.6	63.6	60.9
1996	11.0	50.7	63.6	60.9

116. The St. Petersburg TB scientists offered this data on the Leningrad Oblast's TB rates:

	1970	1975	1980	1985	1990	1995	1st 6 months, 1996
Overall incidence per 100,000	64.2	41.8	34.5	26.9	28.7	48.0	55.4
Overall percent annual mortality	3.7	5.0	5.5	7.4	7.4	14.9	11.3

CULTURE TUBERCULOSIS ASSAYS FOR DRUG RESISTANCE,
ST. PETERSBURG, 1996
(SAMPLE SIZE = 1,644)

Antibiotic(s)	% Resistant
Streptomycin, only	6.2
INH, only	6.2
Streptomycin + INH	14.7
Streptomycin + INH + ETU+Rif.	4.6
Rifampin, alone	0.4

CULTURE RESISTANCE ASSAYS, LENINGRAD OBLAST, 1996
(SAMPLE SIZE = 222)

Antibiotic(s)	% Resistant
Streptomycin, alone	21.2
INH, alone	10.8
Streptomycin + INH	22.6

117. On August 6, 1998, the Soros Foundation, PHRI, and Médecins Sans Frontières sent a joint letter to President Yeltsin urging that drastic measures be taken immediately to slow the spread of drug-resistant TB in Russian prisons. The letter told Yeltsin that his country's TB problem would never end as long as the jails served as breeding sites for superstrains of the bacteria.

118. In attendance were, among others, First Lady Hillary Rodham Clinton, U.S. Health and Human Services Secretary Donna Shalala, U.S. Agency for International Development head Brian Atwood, World Bank President James Wolfensohn, WHO Director-General GroHarlem Brundtland, and George Soros.

119. Farmer, P., in *Sentenced to Die? The Problem of TB in Prisons in East and Central Europe and Central Asia*, ed. by Stern, V. and Jones, R. London: Prison Reform International, 1999.

120. From the CD "Go Space," Leningrad Cowboys, Megamania, Denmark, 1996.

121. Headley, D., "HIV and AIDS in Russia." Charities Aid Foundation, Kent, U.K., 1996.

122. Pokrovsky, V., Eramova, I. J., Kuznetsova, I. I., et al., "Nosocomial transmission of human immunodeficiency virus in Elista, USSR." Provided by authors, 1998.

123. Romania's AIDS epidemic was sparked by a very similar incident, involving eventually more than 2,000 babies who were injected with HIV-contaminated, bloody needles. See Garrett, L., *The Coming Plague*, 1994, op. cit, pages 505, 612, 701, footnotes 105–7; Dressler, S., "Let the children die: AIDS in Romania." *AIDS Newsletter* (London) 11 (10) (1996): 1; and Apetrei, C., Buzdugan, I., Mitroi, I., et al., "Nosocomial HIV-transmission and primary prevention in Romania." *Lancet* 344 (1994): 1028–29.

124. Russia AIDS Centre. "HIV-infection surveillance in Russia in 1987–1996 (statistics)." Russia AIDS Centre, Moscow, 1997.

125. After 1991 most of the former Soviet states enacted tough AIDS laws that were sharply denounced by the international AIDS community. For a sense of what, in Western terms, is considered appropriate HIV-related legislation see: Gostin, L. O. and Lazzarini, Z., *Human Rights and Public Health in the AIDS Pandemic*. New York: Oxford University Press, 1997; and Mann, J., and Tarantola, D., *AIDS in the World II*. New York: Oxford University Press, 1996.

For samples of laws passed regionally after 1991 see: Rich, V. "Russia's anti-AIDS law." *Lancet* 344 (1994): 1289–90; Rich, V., "Russia's law on iatrogenic HIV infection." *Lancet* 344 (1994): 1562; Freeland, C. "Russia set to impose HIV tests on foreign visitors." *Financial Times* (London) (November 11, 1995): A1; Smolskaya, T. and Chaika, N., "HIV/AIDS surveillance in northwestern Russia, St. Petersburg." Pasteur Institute, 1996; and "The law on HIV/AIDS prevention of the Republic of Georgia," enacted March 21, 1995.

126. Ernberg, G. "HIV outbreak among injecting drug users in Sveltogorsk." UNAIDS letter to Pavel Kral, July 25, 1996; van der Laan, N., "HIV crisis in Belarus 'worse than Chernobyl.' " Electronic telegraph (www.telegraph.co.uk), December 2, 1996.

A similar chain of events transpired in Kaliningrad, where only one IVDU/HIV case was seen as of January 1996. By January 1998 there were 3,245 HIV cases in IVDUs.

See Pokrovsky, V., Savchenko, I. Y., Ladnaia N. N., et al., "A recent epidemic of HIV infection in Russia IVDUs." Twelfth International Conference on AIDS, Geneva, June 28–July 3, 1998.

127. Lilitsola, K., Tashkinova, I., Korovina, G., et al., "HIV-1 genetic subtype A/B recombinant strain causing an explosive IDU epidemic in Kaliningrad." Twelfth International Conference on AIDS, Geneva, June 28–July 3, 1998.

128. For more on the genetic diversity of HIV-1 strains in the ex-USSR see: Kozlov, A. P., Emeljanov, A. V., Verevochkin, S. V., et al., "Characteristics of early phase of HIV/AIDS epidemic." *Russian Journal of HIV/AIDS and Related Problems* 1 (1997): 225; Nabatov, A. A., Marsharsky, A. E., Emeljanov, A. V., et al., "HIV/AIDS epidemic among IVDUs in Ukraine: Different HIV-1 subtypes in different cities." *Russian Journal of HIV/AIDS and Related Problems* 1 (1997): 253; Pashkova, T. A., Shchelkanov, M. Y., Sakhuria, I. B., et al., "Phenotypic features and AZT-susceptibility of HIV-1 isolates from Russian patients." *Russian Journal of HIV/AIDS and Related Problems* 1 (1997): 254; Yaroslavtseva, N. G., Shchelkanov, M. Y., Eremin, V. P., et al., "Serological Homogeneity of HIV-1 from Svetlogorsk epidemic source (1996) in Byelarus." *Russian Journal of HIV/AIDS and Related Problems* 1 (1997): 257; Expert

Group of the Joint United Nations Programme on HIV/AIDS. "Implications of HIV variability for transmission: Scientific and policy issues." *AIDS* 11 (1997): 1–15; Loures, L. A. M. "HIV prevalence estimates at country level." UNAIDS memo to Vadim Pokrovsky, November 1, 1996; Bobkov, A., Cheingsong-Popov, R., Selimova, L., et al., "HIV-1 diversity in the former USSR." Tenth International Congress on Virology, August 11–16, 1996, Jerusalem.

129. Alter, M., "Hepatitis C in the United States." Presentation to Infectious Diseases Society of America conference, San Francisco, September 15, 1997. Alter noted that 25 percent of all liver transplants in America were performed because of hepatitis C infection; 70 percent of those infected with the virus develop chronic liver disease in the absence of a transplant. Ten percent develop hepatocellular carcinoma within thirteen to twenty-eight years postinfection. Up to 90 percent of all IV drug users in the United States were hepatitis C positive in 1997. Overall in the United States some four million people suffered chronic liver disease in the 1990s due to hepatitis C infection, or 1.8 percent of the population.

130. Russian Academy of Medical Sciences, State Report, 1996, op. cit.

131. Gogulenko didn't trust the Odessa blood bank supplies, either, because some transfusion recipients had developed hepatitis. So he, too, urged his physicians and nurses to give patients their blood, or to have patients bank supplies of their own blood before they underwent surgery. Officials in Kyiv admitted that none of the nation's blood supply was routinely tested for hepatitis C, and hepatitis B test kits were in short enough supply that some blood was certainly being given to patients without appropriate screening for that virus as well.

132. Zmushko, E. and Bolekhan, V. N., "HIV-infection in the Russian Federation military forces." Twelfth International Conference on AIDS, Geneva, June 28–July 3, 1998.

133. Wines, M., "Heroin Carries AIDS to a Region in Siberia," *The New York Times* (April 24, 2000): A1.

134. Garrett, L., 1994, op. cit., pages 493–98.

135. European agencies, both governmental and private, were very slow to recognize this trend and slower, still, in dealing with it. See: Open Society Institute. "Response to the illegal trafficking of women in Europe." *The Forced Migration Monitor* 27 (1999): 1; Bohlen, C., "Exotic imports have captured Italy's sex market." *New York Times* (July 9, 1997): A4; Specter, M., "Traffickers' new cargo: Naive Slavic women." *New York Times* (January 11, 1998): A1; "Giving the customer what he wants." *The Economist* (February 14, 1998): 21–23; Farah, D., "Russian mobs form Colombian alliances." *San Francisco Chronicle* (September 29, 1997): A1; Smacchia, C., Parolin, A., DiPerri, G., et al., "Syphilis in prostitutes from Eastern Europe." *Lancet* 351 (1998): 572; and "Europe's smuggled masses." *The Economist* (February 20, 1999): 45–46.

136. See the following table.

SAMPLE STD ESTIMATES, FORMER USSR AND EASTERN BLOC NATIONS

Country	Year	Population Group	Syphilis	Gonorrhea	Source
Georgia	1990	General	676	2,613	EURO/GPA
	1991	General	725	2,261	Mission to
	1992	General	730	1,809	Georgia
	1993	General	653	1,562	
	1994	General	883	2,100	

Country	Year	Population Group	Syphilis	Gonorrhea	Source
Estonia	1994	General		205 per 100,000	Ministry of Social Affairs, Estonia
Estonia	1990–1994	General	16-fold increase; 1994=852 per 100,000	Doubled; 1994=3,089 per 100,000	Deaconess Institute, Helsinki, Finland
Estonia	1994	Prostitutes	5.2% active infections	16.5% active infections	Deaconess Institute, Helsinki, Finland
Lithuania	1995	General	Incidence=100 per 100,000; 100-fold increase since 1988		UNAIDS, Geneva
Ukraine	1995	General	Incidence=5 per 100,000 in 1991; by 1995 it's 118 per 100,000. By 1996 it's 124: 100,000		UNAIDS, Geneva
Ukraine	1996	General	118:100,000 incidence		WHO European Regional Office
Kazakhstan	1996	General	123:100,000 incidence		WHO European Regional Office
Belarus	1996	General	147:100,000 incidence		WHO European Regional Office
Russia	1997	General	New case diagnosis declined by 6% in 1997. But total cases=356,000		First Russian Nurses' Congress, St. Petersburg, Nov. 1998
Russia	1996	Moscow	89,136 active cases: Rate is 60.24 per 100,000		Moscow City Department of Health
Russia	1995	General	256,296 active cases		Russian Ministry of Health
Russia	1996	General	376,084 active cases (47% increase over 1995)		Russian Ministry of Health
Russia	1991	General	Incidence is 7.2 per 100,000		Dr. Gennady Onyschenko
Russia	1996	General	Incidence is 254.2 per 100,000 (350% increase over period)		Dr. Gennady Onyschenko
Moldova	1997	Homeless children	One-third have syphilis		Moldova Ministry of Health
Ukraine	1991 1994 1995 1996		5:100,000 cases 65:100,000 cases 118:100,000 cases 124:100,000 cases		British Council Division, Calcutta

Country	Year	Population Group	Syphilis	Gonorrhea	Source
Ukraine	1990		5:100,000 (approx)		UNAIDS
	1991		10:100,000 (approx)		
	1992		20:100,000 (approx)		
	1993		40:100,000 (approx)		
	1994		70:100,000 (approx)		
	1995		120:100,000 (approx)		
Ukraine	1989	Women	7.6:100,000	63.5:100,000	UNICEF, WHO,
	1991		8.7:100,000	50.2:100,000	UNAIDS, UNDP
	1993		32.0:100,000	71.2:100,000	
	1995		112.6 100,000	59.4:100,000	
Ukraine	1989	Girls up to 16 years	13:100,000		UNICEF, WHO, UNAIDS, UNDP
	1991		23:100,000		
	1993		64:100,000		
	1995		229:100,000		
Ukraine	1991	Children ages 15–17	400 (approx)	2,700 (approx)	Ukraine Centre for AIDS Prevention
	1992		500 (approx)	3,200 (approx)	
	1993		1,000 (approx)	4,300 (approx)	
	1994		2,000 (approx)	3,500 (approx)	
	1995		3,400 (approx)	2,900 (approx)	
Ukraine	1991	Children up to 14 years	50 (approx)	525 (approx)	Ukraine Centre for AIDS Prevention
	1992		60 (approx)	625 (approx)	
	1993		100 (approx)	650 (approx)	
	1994		150 (approx)	850 (approx)	
	1995		350 (approx)	600 (approx)	
Ukraine	1989	Girls up to 14 years		551:100,000	UNICEF, WHO, UNAIDS, UNDP
	1991			506:100,000	
	1993			662:100,000	
	1995			588:100,000	
Ukraine	1989	Girls 15–16 years		—	UNICEF, WHO, UNAIDS, UNDP
	1991			1,568:100,000	
	1993			2,029:100,000	
	1995			1,531:100,000	
Ukraine	1994	General	118 per 100,000 incidence		AIDS Newsletter, London School of Hygiene and Tropical Medicine
Kazakhstan	1994	General	123:100,000 incidence		AIDS Newsletter, London School of Hygiene and Tropical Medicine
Belarus	1994	General	147:100,000		AIDS Newsletter, London School of Hygiene and Tropical Medicine

Country	Year	Population Group	Syphilis	Gonorrhea	Source
Moldova	1994	General	172:100,000		*AIDS Newsletter*, London School of Hygiene and Tropical Medicine
Russia	1994	General	173:100,000 (note: that is 175 times the rate that year in Scandinavia)		*AIDS Newsletter*, London School of Hygiene and Tropical Medicine
Russia	1997	Moscow	More than 20,000 cases (note: entire USA number that year was less than 17,000)		Moscow City Department of Health
Russia	1996	Moscow	Rate is 221.9 per 100,000		Moscow City Department of Health
Russia	1995	18–19-year-old females	Rate of active cases is 922 per 100,000		Moscow City Department of Health
Russia	1996	General	Rate of 519.7 per 100,000		Médecins du Monde, Moscow
Russia	1997	General	One in every 400 people had syphilis. Incidence rose 50-fold in 7 years.		WHO
Russia	1997	Children	40-fold increase in 7 years		WHO
Russia	1993–1994	Children under 14 years	173% increase		WHO
Russia	1987	General		75 cases per 100,000	University of London
Russia	1993	General		236 per 100,000	University of London
Russia	1987	Women		41,219 cases registered	University of London
Russia	1994	Women		113,684 cases registered	University of London
Russia	1995	General		164.9 per 100,000 registered	University of London
Russia	1996	General	387,704 cases (up from 6,234 cases in 1988)		Officially registered, Ministry of Health
Russia	1996	Females aged 18–19	Rate of 1,321 per 100,000		Officially registered, Ministry of Health

Country	Year	Population Group	Syphilis	Gonorrhea	Source
Russia	1996	Females aged 20–29	Rate of 919 per 100,000		Officially registered, Ministry of Health
Russia	1996	Males aged 18–19	Rate of 507 per 100,000		Officially registered, Ministry of Health
Russia	1996	Males aged 20–29	Rate of 916 per 100,000		Officially registered, Ministry of Health

137. Daigle, K., "Exposing the face of sex in Moscow." *The Moscow Times* (April 4, 1997): 20; and multiple street interviews with prostitutes.

138. Maksimovsky, E., *Moscow Prostitutes: An anti-brothel guidebook.* Moscow: Syravnika Press, 1996.

139. The line between organized crime and prostitution in the area profoundly limited public health access to these women. See, for example: Pyroyshkina, E., Presentation to the Twelfth International Conference on AIDS, Geneva, June 28–July 3, 1998; Stanley, A., "A tale of murder and sex slaves to stun Dostoyevsky." *New York Times* (August 28, 1997): A3; and Stanley, A., "With prostitution booming legalization tempts Russians." *New York Times* (March 3, 1998): A1.

140. Data from the Russian Ministry of Health, 1997.

141. Gerasimenko, op. cit; Renton, A., Ward, H., and Meheus, A., "Epidemiology, control and surveillance of syphilis and gonorrhea in the Russian Federation." Report to UNAIDS, March 12, 1996; and Tichonova, L., Borsenko, K., Ward, H., et al., "Epidemics of syphilis in the Russian Federation: Trends, origins and priorities for control." *Lancet* 350 (1997): 210–13.

142. All data derived from Russian Ministry of Health and Moscow Department of Health.

143. Russia Today Online. "Syphilis rise may worsen AIDS epidemic" (April 6, 1998).

144. Other figures for rising syphilis rates, obtained independent of local government agencies, appeared in Winceslaus, S. J., "Screening for Syphilis." *Lancet* 353 (1999): 1441; and Glass, N., "Syphilis cases are increasing in Czech Republic." *Lancet* 353 (1999): 992.

145. See World Health Organization. "Task force to curb sexually transmitted disease epidemic in Europe." Press Release EURO/03/98, Copenhagen, April 1998.

146. Sinyavsky, A., 1997, op. cit.

147. Gogulenko's data was as follows for his 1,120-bed hospital:

	1992	1993	1994	1995	1996
Bed Use Rate	354.7	338.6	338.7	342.6	359.5
Average Duration of Stay (days)	15.0	14.1	14.0	13.8	13.1
Mortality Rate (per 100 patients)	1.7	1.6	1.4	1.3	1.2
Number of Patients Successfully Treated and Sent Home	26,661	26,863	27,147	27,606	28,198

148. Associated Press. "Clinics vie for Russian health care" (February 17, 1995); Swarns, R. L. "Russia's cardiac patients, little care and grim prognosis." *New York Times* (September 24, 1996): A1; and Powell, B., "Heart to heart." *Newsweek* (September 16, 1996): 54–61.

149. Matlack, C., "Need surgery? Bring vodka and a bribe." *BusinessWeek* (March 7, 1997): 45; Spolar, C., "Polish health-care system is in critical condition." *Washington Post* (May 5, 1997): A1; Specter, M., "Citadel of Russia's wasteful health system." *New York Times* (February 4, 1998): A1; Kaplan, F., "Russian health crisis needs intensive care." *Boston Globe* (December 6, 1992): A1; Saffron, I., "New life the old way: Russia's birth houses reflect '50s." *Chicago Tribune* (May 19, 1996): 9; Simon, S., "Childbirth in Russia is miserable." *Los Angeles Times* (February 22, 1996): A1; and Bilmes, L. and Lindquist, J., "The bear has a sore head." *Financial Times* (London) (August 26, 1994): 1.

150. The class distinctions in quality of health care during Soviet times were *very* pronounced. And bribery—particularly of surgeons—was the norm. In many cases surgeons flat-out refused to operate in lieu of substantial cash payments. They may have been workers in the proletariat state, but they were also skilled professionals who thrived on an assumed pattern of corruption. See: Voslensky, M., *Nomenklatura: The Soviet Class, An Insider's Report*. Translated by Eric Nosbacher. New York: Doubleday & Co., 1984; and Smith, H., *The Russians*, 1973, op. cit.

151. Editorial. "Health in Russia is broke, but who is to fix it?" *Lancet* 353 (1999): 337; Burger, E. J., Field, M. G., and Twigg, J. L., "From assurance to insurance in Russian health care: The problematic transition." *American Journal of Public Health* 88 (1998): 755–58; and Sheiman, I., "Forming the system of health insurance in the Russian Federation." *Social Science and Medicine* 39 (1994): 1425–32.

152. Josephson, P. R., *New Atlantis Revisited: Akademgorodok, the Siberian City of Science*. Princeton, N.J.: Princeton University Press, 1997.

153. Saltykov, B. G., "Transformation of Soviet science (1992–96)." AAAS, Seattle, February 13–18, 1997.

154. Centre of Science Research and Statistics. "Social status of scientists in Russia." *Science* 275 (1997): 485.

155. Hamer, M., "East Germany's science breaks from the state." *New Scientist* (December 9, 1989): 15.

156. Hamer, M., "Breaking walls, building bridges." *New Scientist* (January 13, 1990): 33–34.

157. Whitehead, C., "The remaking of Czechoslovakian science." *New Scientist* (March 3, 1990): 26–29.

158. Stone, R., "Civil war leaves once-proud Georgian science in tatters." *Science* 272 (1996): 1581–82.

159. Koenig, R., "Spirited academy faces painful cuts, consolidation." *Science* 277 (1997): 175; and Koenig, R., "Eastern Europe's research gamble." *Science* 283 (1999): 22–26.

160. Stone, R., "Cash-starved researchers to undergo trial by peer review." *Science* 271 (1996): 1802–3.

161. Stone, R., "New minister sets lofty goals." *Science* 282 (1998): 1979–80.

162. Holden, C., "Russia's science spending diving toward new low." *Science* 283 (1999): 31.

163. Saltykov, B., op. cit.

164. Chuprikov, A. P., Linyov, A. N., and Martsenkovsky, I. A., *Lateral Therapy*. Kyiv: Zdorovie Publishers, 1994; and Merskey, H., "The Chuprikov file: Documents evaluating the

scientific work of Professor A. P. Chuprikov." Geneva Initiative on Psychiatry, Amsterdam, 1994.

165. The reader is referred for details to the Geneva Initiative's journal, *Mental Health Reforms*, published quarterly out of Amsterdam since 1996. Available from gip@euronet.nl.

166. Mehilane, L., "Mental health care reforms in the Baltic States." University of Tartu and Geneva Initiative, Amsterdam, 1996.

167. According to the World Bank the average monthly wage in Russia in 1996 was about $150, down by 10 percent from 1992 levels. Wages in Ukraine fell to an average of $80/month in 1997 with the total of backlogged unpaid salaries exceeding an entire year's worth for the nation. In Georgia wages dropped 17 percent between 1985 and 1995, hitting a mere $36 a month.

Even in Eastern European and Baltic countries where wages rose over the 1995–97 period, it had generally been at the expense of many jobs. By shrinking the sizes of their labor forces newly privatized industries became more competitive on the international market.

The average unemployment payment in Russia—when it was actually paid out—was only $35 a month, but Moscow calculated that subsistence required $57 a month. And unemployed workers who lost low-level jobs received only $12.50 each month.

168. But no one knows for sure because the government hasn't published such data since 1991.

169. "Psychology has practically disappeared in Russia since [World War II], and in the fall of 1948 physics was under fire. Statisticians dare not publish conclusions unpalatable to the Central Committee. It is possible that authoritarianism simply cannot allow the existence of the intellectual standards of free scientific inquiry." Zirkle, C., ed. *Death of Science in Russia*. Philadelphia: University of Pennsylvania Press, 1949.

170. Ostrander, S. and Schroeder, L., *Psychic Discoveries Behind the Iron Curtain*. New York: Bantam Books, 1970.

171. Polavets, V. and Bilynska, M., "Psychiatry problems related to religious boom in Ukraine in late '80s–early '90s." In documents on the Abolition and Prevention of Political Abuse of Psychiatry, Geneva Initiative, August-September 1995, Amsterdam.

172. Centers for Disease Control and Prevention. "Frequency of vaccine-related and therapeutic injections—Romania, 1998." *Morbidity and Mortality Weekly Report* 48 (1999): 271–74; Hutin, Y. F., Harpaz, R., Probeniuc, J., et al., "Transmission of hepatitis B virus in Moldova." Thirty-seventh meeting of the Interscience Conference on Antimicrobial Agents and Chemotherapy, Toronto, September 1997; Hutin, Y. F., Craciun, D., Ion-Nedelcu, N., et al., "Using surveillance data to monitor key aspects of the epidemiology of hepatitis B virus (HBV) infection in Romania." Thirty-sixth Annual Meeting of the Infectious Disease Society of America, Denver, November 1998; and Hutin, Y. J. F., "High frequency of therapeutic injections, Republic of Moldova." *Weekly Epidemiological Record* 11 (1999): 84–86.

173. Soyfer, V. N., "New light on the Lysenko era." *Nature* 339 (1989): 415–20; Medvedev, Z. A., *The Rise and Fall of T. D. Lysenko*. New York: Columbia University Press, 1969; Adams, M. B., "The Soviet experiment: Genetics, eugenics, and Lysenkoism, 1910–1990." *American Journal of Human Genetics* 49S (1991): 66; Shtilmark, F. R., and Sukhomirov, G. I., "On two trends ('schools') in the Soviet hunting science." *Biologicheskii* 96 (1991): 77–87; and several articles from the *Quarterly Review of Biology* 65 (1990) 413–78.

174. Malia, M., *The Soviet Tragedy: A History of Socialism in Russia, 1917–1991*. New York: The Free Press, 1994.

175. In essence, Lysenko and his supporters were Communist Lamarckians, though

they never gave themselves that appellation. Jean Baptiste Pierre Antoine Monet de Lamarck was a late-eighteenth-century French naturalist who believed organisms spontaneously acquired characteristics from their environment. For example, Lamarck argued, if an apple were placed in a sealed container for several days it would "become" a colony of worms. It would, he said, transmutate from one thing to another simply by being subjected to a new environment. Lamarck's ideas had long since been rejected by most of the world's scientific community, not just because they were at face value absurd, but due to the pioneering genetics efforts of Britain's Charles Darwin and Slovakia's Gregor Mendel.

Darwin demonstrated that species did evolve over time, but not as a result of spontaneous Lamarckian transmutations. Rather, he showed that mutant deviants always exist within any population and may come to dominate in the presence of powerful selection forces, such as predation or climate, that kill off the more common genetic forms of the species.

Mendel brought empiricism to genetics in the nineteenth century, showing in now famous studies of peas that traits were passed from parent to child in arithmetically predictable fashion, with some traits being dominant, others recessive. Mendel's experiments foreshadowed the later understanding that these traits were carried in DNA, organized in chromosomes, a set of which was passed by each parent into an egg, resulting in an offspring that possessed traits from each of its forebears.

176. In August 1948 Lysenko was given a privilege unusual for lab scientists—he addressed the Soviet Central Committee. His primary assertion was: "We, the representatives of the Soviet Michurinist concept, maintain that the inheritance of characteristics acquired by plants and animals in the process of their development is possible and necessary."

After Lysenko's speech the Central Committee did something unprecedented—it formally decreed what was "correct science," endorsing Lysenko's views.

177. Some experts maintain that every single Darwinist in the USSR died during the 1940s. See Malia, M., 1994, op. cit.

178. "Another refuge from Lysenko?" *Nature* 329 (1987): 797.

179. The point was stated succinctly by Zirkle in 1949: "When intellectual freedom does not exist, intellectual honesty becomes a liability, and the consequences for science are disastrous" (Zirkle, C., 1949, op. cit.).

And C. D. Darlington, two years earlier, summarized Lysenko's impact in stark terms: "In a word, after thirteen years of persecution, the great fellowship of Russian biological research, formed in the revolution, had been crushed and broken. . . . Never before has science been offered so many martyrs to its cause, men, too, honoured and beloved throughout the world" (Darlington, C. D., "Genetics in Russia after ten years of cold official warfare." *Nineteenth Century* 142 (1947): 157–68).

180. Some experts even argue that the growing "Chernobyl Syndrome" view in the region is a direct outgrowth of Lysenkoism. Malia labels it "metaphysical utopianism." See Malia, M., 1994, op. cit.

181. Stone, R., "Estonian researchers lead the way in science reform." *Science* 274 (1996): 29–30; and Martinson, H., *The Reform of R & D System in Estonia.* Estonian Science Foundation, Tallinn, 1995.

182. Holden, C., "Eastern Europe's social science renaissance." *Science* 283 (1999): 1620–22.

183. See, for example, Hammond, A., *Which World? Scenarios for the 21st Century.* Washington, D.C.: Island Press, 1998; and Yergin, D. and Gustafson, T., 1995, op. cit.

184. An April 1999 survey found Russian voters inclined, if permitted, to vote as follows:

10.1%	Party Our Home Is Russia (Chernomyrdin's party)
22.3%	Communist
6.9%	Yablokov (Yavlinsky)
11.2%	Zhirinovsky (Ultra-Nationalist)
4.3%	Lebed

See: *The Economist* (April 10, 1999): 48.

185. Feshbach, M., Georgetown University, 1997, op. cit.

186. See, for example: Human Resources Division, County Dept. III. "Staff appraisal report, Russian Federation, Community Social Infrastructure Project." The World Bank, Report No. 14977-RU, 1996, Washington, D.C.; World Bank. "Bank to lend over $880 million to Russia." *World Bank News* (June 12, 1997): 1–2; Office of International and Refugee Health, Gore-Chernomyrdin Commission. "Summary documentation from the fourth meeting of the GC Health Committee." Moscow, July 12, 1996; Rosenbaum, D. E., "Requests are to include more aid to Russia." *New York Times* (January 19, 1996): A15; and USAID Zdrav Reform Project. "NIS strategy development: Transforming traditions into pluralism and partnerships." U.S. Agency for International Development, 1996, Washington, D.C.

187. Burger, E. J., Field, M. G., and Twigg, J. L., 1998, op. cit.

188. One of Estonia's wunderkind health planners, young Maris Jesse, who ran the nation's insurance Sickness Fund, was more blunt: "We are always referring to the United States as a negative model. There is the attitude there that private is good and public isn't. We say, 'Well, that's not so good for public health!' "

CHAPTER FOUR

1. Callahan, D., *False Hopes: Why America's Quest for Perfect Health Is a Recipe for Failure.* New York: Simon and Schuster, 1998.

2. Caldwell, M., *The Last Crusade: The War on Consumption 1862–1954.* New York: Atheneum, 1988.

3. The burden of viral nosocomial infection was difficult to calculate. The CDC felt confident that blood screening and basic hospital hygiene had eliminated nosocomial spread of the AIDS virus, HIV, by 1985. But other blood-borne viruses, particularly hepatitis types B, C, and D, and herpes viruses, continued to spread in medical settings well into the 1990s. Vogt, M., Lang, T., Frösner, G., et al., "Prevalence and clinical outcome of hepatitis C infection in children who underwent cardiac surgery before the implementation of blood donor screening." *New England Journal of Medicine* 341 (1999): 866–870.

4. Blau, S. P. and Shimberg, E. F., *How to Get Out of the Hospital Alive.* New York: Macmillan, 1997.

5. Tenover, F. C. and Hughes, J. M., "The challenge of emerging infectious diseases." *Journal of the American Medical Association* 175 (1996): 300–304.

6. Jones, R. N. and Verhoef, J., Presentation to the 37th Interscience Conference on Antimicrobial Agents and Chemotherapy, Toronto, September 29, 1997.

7. The author interviewed Hamburg and other New York health experts on numerous occasions during the 1990s. Unless otherwise noted in this section, individuals' comments and observations were gleaned from those interviews.

8. Raad, I. and Darouchie, R. O., "Catheter-related septicemia: risk reduction," *Infection and Medicine* 13 (1996): 807–812; 815–816; 823. And Raad I., "Intravascular-catheter-related infections," *Lancet* 351 (1998): 893–898.

9. Austrian, R., "Confronting drug-resistant *Pneumococci.*" *Annals of Internal Medicine* 121 (1994): 807–809.

10. Gleason, P. P., Kapoor, W. M., Stone, R. A., et al., "Medical outcomes and anti-microbial costs with the use of the American Thoracic Society guidelines for outpatients with community-acquired pneumonia." *Journal of the American Medical Association* 278 (1997): 32–39.

11. Garrett, L., "Tough bugs thrive." *Newsday* (November 21, 1996): A20.

12. Patterson, J. E., "Making real sense of MRSA." *Lancet* 348 (1996): 836–837.

13. Boyce, J. M., Opal, S. M., Chow, J. W., et al., "Outbreak of multidrug-resistant *Enterococcus faecium* with transferable *vanB* class vancomycin resistance." *Journal of Clinical Microbiology* 32 (1994): 1148–1153; Fan, C., Moews, P. C., Walsh, C. T., et al., "Vancomycin resistance: Structure of D-alanine: D-alanine ligase at 2.3A resolution." *Science* 266 (1994): 439–443; Gilmore, M. S. and Hoch, J. A., "A vancomycin surprise." *Nature* 399 (1999): 524–527; and Novak, R., Henriques, B., Charpentier, E., "Penicillinase resistant *S. pneumoniae* with decreased vancomycin susceptibility." *Nature* 399 (1999): 590–593.

14. Farrag, N., Eltringham, I., and Liddy, H., "Vancomycin-dependent *Enterococcus faecalis.*" *Lancet* 348 (1996): 1581–1582.

15. Blau, S. P. and Shimberg, E. F., 1997, op. cit.; Bolognia, J. L. and Edelson, R. L., "Spread of antibiotic-resistant bacteria from acne patients to personal contacts—a problem beyond the skin?" *Lancet* 350 (1997): 972–973; Burnie, J. P. and Loudon, K. W., "Ciproloxacin-resistant *Staphylococcus epidermis* and hands." *Lancet* 349 (1997): 649; Caul, E. O., "Small round structured viruses: Airborne transmission and hospital control." *Lancet* 343 (1994): 1240–1241; Centers for Disease Control and Prevention, "Bronchoscopy-related infections and pseudoinfections—New York, 1996 and 1998." *Mortality and Morbidity Weekly Report* 48 (1999): 557–560; Centers for Disease Control and Prevention, "Multistate outbreak of hemolysis in hemodialysis patients—Nebraska and Maryland, 1998." *Mortality and Morbidity Weekly Report* 47 (1998): 483–484; Centers for Disease Control and Prevention, "Nosocomial group A streptococcal infections associated with asymptomatic health care workers—Maryland and California, 1997." *Mortality and Morbidity Weekly Report* 48 (1999): 163–166; Hilts, P., "Infection kills four infants, and hospital closes a unit." *New York Times* (September 16, 1997): A16; and Levitz, R. E., "Prosthetic-valve endocarditis caused by penicillin-resistant *Streptococcus otitis.*" *New England Journal of Medicine* 340 (1999): 1843–1844.

16. Columbia-Presbyterian, North Shore University Hospital in Manhasset, and Long Island Jewish Hospital.

See Lam, S., Singer, C., Tucci, V., et al., "The challenge of vancomycin-resistant enterococci: A clinical and epidemiologic study." *American Journal of Infection Control* 23 (1995): 170–180.

17. Rice, L., Presentation to the annual meeting of the Infectious Diseases Society of America, San Francisco, September 15, 1997.

18. Rahal, J., Presentation to the annual meeting of the Infectious Diseases Society of America, San Francisco, September 15, 1997.

19. The other preantibiotic era approach to killing bacteria involved the use of phages, or bacterial viruses. If properly grown and purified bacteriophages were harmless to human beings, but wiped out all members of a given species of bacteria. At the close of the nineteenth century Germany's Paul Erlich experimented with such phages, calling them "magic bullets" in the war against disease. A century later, fearing the approaching end of the antibiotic era, researchers in Tbilisi, Georgia, collaborated with Western drug companies in a race to again develop phages technology—before antibiotics were rendered truly useless. See Osborne, L., "A Stalinist antibiotic alternative," *New York Times Magazine;* 2000: February 6, 50–55.

20. Senate Committee on Investigations. *The Growing Menace of Bacterial Infections.* Albany: New York State Senate, 1999.

21. In addition to the Senate report, see Roberts, R., Tomasz, A., and Kreiswirth, B., *Antibiotic Resistance in New York City: A Growing Public Health Threat and a Proposal for Action.* New York: Bacterial Antibiotic Resistance Group, 1995.

22. For details spanning 1600 to 1776 in New York, Boston, Philadelphia, and other colonial cities, see Carlson, L. W., *A Fever in Salem.* Chicago: Ivan R. Dee Publisher, 1999; Duffy, J., *Epidemics in Colonial America.* Baton Rouge: University of Louisiana Press, 1953; Duffy, J., *A History of Public Health in New York City.* New York: Russell Sage Foundation, 1968; McKeown, T., *The Origins of Human Disease.* Cambridge, Mass.: Basil Blackwell, 1988; McKeown, T., *The Role of Medicine: Dream, Mirage, or Nemesis?* Princeton: Princeton University Press, 1979; McNeill, W. H., *Plagues and Peoples.* New York: Anchor Books, 1977; Porter, R., *The Greatest Benefit to Mankind.* New York: Harper Collins, 1997; Powell, J. M., *Bring Out Your Dead.* Philadelphia: University of Pennsylvania Press, 1949; and Watts, S., *Epidemics and History.* New Haven: Yale University Press, 1998.

23.

EPIDEMICS OF NEW YORK CITY: 1679–1873*
*(Not including Tuberculosis)

Year	Cause	# of Deaths	% of Population Killed
1679	Smallpox	Unknown	—
1689	Smallpox	Unknown	—
1702	Yellow Fever	570	12
1713	Measles	Unknown	—
1729	Measles	Unknown	—
1731	Smallpox	549	8
1732	Yellow Fever	Unknown	—
1743	Yellow Fever	217	1.5
1745	Smallpox	Unknown	—
1795	Yellow Fever	750	2
1798	Yellow Fever	>2,000	3.6
1805	Yellow Fever	262	0.3
1810	Cholera	146	0.15
1819	Yellow Fever	38	0.03
1822	Yellow Fever	388	0.28
1832	Cholera	3,513	1.5
1845	Smallpox	425	0.12
1847	Typhoid/Typhus	1,396	0.35
1848–49	Cholera	8,000	1.7
1851	Smallpox	586	0.11

Year	Cause	# of Deaths	% of Population Killed
1851	Scarlet Fever	627	0.12
1852	Smallpox	516	0.1
1853	Smallpox	681	0.1
1854	Smallpox	624	0.01
1854	Cholera	>450	0.08
1855	Yellow Fever	179	0.02
1871	Smallpox	805	0.08
1872	Smallpox	1,866	0.19
1873	Diphtheria	1,151	0.12
1874	Diphtheria	1,600	0.21
1874	Smallpox	484	0.047
1875	Smallpox	1,280	0.12
1875	Diphtheria	2,329	0.29

(Compiled from multiple sources, including Condran, G. "Changing patterns of epidemic disease in New York City." In D. Rosner, editor. *Hives of Sickness: Public Health and Epidemics in New York City*. New Brunswick, NJ: Rutgers University Press, 1995; Duffy, J. *A History of Public Health in New York City, 1625-1866*. New York: Russell Sage Foundation, 1968; Duffy, J. *Epidemics in Colonial America*. Baton Rouge: Louisiana State University, 1953; Emerson, H. and Hughes, H.E. *Populations, Births, Notifiable Diseases, and Deaths, Assembled for New York City, New York, 1866-1938, from Official Records*. New York: The DeLamar Institute of Public Health, Columbia University, 1941; and Rosenwaike, I. *Population History of New York City*. New York: Syracuse University Press, 1971.)

24. Duffy, J., *A History of Public Health in New York City*. New York: Russell Sage Foundation, 1968.

25. Burrows, E. G. and Wallace, M., 1999, op. cit.

26. Notably, "Account of the climate and diseases of New York." See Duffy, J., *The Sanitarians: A History of American Public Health*. Illini Books Edition. Chicago: University of Illinois Press, 1992; and Duffy, J., 1968, op. cit.

27. During the same period, New York City passed its own tough quarantine laws, opened New York Hospital, built a dispensary (located on the corner of Beekman and Nassau streets in Manhattan) for delivery of health care to the poor, and witnessed the opening of Bellevue Hospital, which would come under city control in 1805.

28. See Table: "New York City Average Annual Death Rates Per 100,000 People, 1804–1995" on pages 650–652.

29. Between 1840 and 1860, 4.5 million of Europe's poor landed in the U.S.'s eastern ports, swelling the already densely populated tenements and slums. More than 3.5 million of them never left New York. The following gives an overview of New York City's exponential rate of growth:

POPULATION OF NEW YORK CITY, 1650–1990

Year	Population	Year	Population	Year	Population	Year	Population
1650	1,000	1800	60,489	1860	813,669	1930	6,930,446
1698	4,937	1805	75,770	1865	871,583	1935	7,206,000
1703	4,375	1810	96,373	1870	942,292	1940	7,454,995
1712	5,840	1814	95,519	1875	1,041,886	1945	7,648,000
1723	7,248	1815	93,630	1880	1,206,299	1950	7,891,957
1731	8,622	1816	93,634	1885	1,377,085	1955	7,843,000
1737	10,664	1820	123,706	1890	1,515,302	1960	7,781,985
1746	11,717	1825	166,086	1895	1,787,412	1965	7,839,000
1749	13,294	1830	202,589	1900	3,437,202	1970	7,895,563
1756	13,046	1835	270,089	1905	4,121,678	1975	7,896,000
1770	21,000	1840	312,710	1910	4,766,883	1980	7,071,639
1771	21,863	1845	371,223	1915	5,224,591	1985	7,197,000
1786	23,610	1850	515,547	1920	5,620,048	1990	7,322,600
1790	33,131	1855	629,904	1925	6,323,190	1995	7,542,500

Note: Population figures before 1890 are for Old New York (Manhattan and the Bronx). Population figures after the 1898 unification are for Great New York City (the five boroughs: Manhattan, the Bronx, Brooklyn, Queens, and Staten Island). In 1993, 128,292 immigrants were legalized as residents of New York City under a single U.S. Department of Justice action.

Sources: Condran, G., "Changing patterns of epidemic diseases in New York City." In D. Rosner, editor, Hives of Sickness: Public Health and Epidemics in New York City. New Brunswick, N.J.: Rutgers University Press, 1995; Duffy, J., A History of Public Health in New York City, 1625–1866. New York: Russell Sage Foundation, 1968; Duffy, J., A History of Public Health in New York City, 1866–1966. New York: Russell Sage Foundation, 1974; Emerson, E., Supplement 1936–1953 to Population, Births, Notifiable Diseases, and Deaths, Assembled for New York City, New York. New York: DeLamar Institute of Public Health, Columbia University, 1941; Emerson, H. and Hughes, H. E., Populations, Births, Notifiable Diseases, and Deaths, Assembled for New York City, New York, 1866–1938, from Official Records. New York: DeLamar Institute of Public Health, Columbia University, 1941; Rosenwaike, I., Population History of New York City. New York: Syracuse University Press, 1971; Shupe, B., Stains, J., and Pandit, J., New York State Population, 1790–1980: A Compilation of Federal Census Data. New York: Neal-Schuman, 1987; and New York City and New York State Department of Health statistics.

30. In New York City, for example, typhoid fever claimed 1,396 lives in 1847; cholera killed another 5,071 (possibly 8,000) in the summer of '49; smallpox and typhoid fever both hit in 1851, killing 1,600 people; and cholera struck again the summer of '54, killing 2,501. These epidemics, coupled with alarmingly increasing maternal and child death rates, by 1855 drove the New York City mortality rate upwards to forty-eight deaths per year per one thousand people.

31. Puerperal fever is postpartum infection caused by any of a number of bacterial species. Typically, the women got infected as a result of the horrible standards of hygiene practiced by midwives and obstetricians.

32. Many observers argue persuasively that the need for large middle classes is fundamental to implementation of public health in any society that operates via an electoral or democratic process. The proper function of civil society requires that the populace feel genuinely invested in its future. Clearly, in the former Soviet Union nations, central Africa and India, middle classes are nearly nonexistent. All of these countries are marked by eco-

NEW YORK CITY AVERAGE ANNUAL DEATH RATES
PER 100,000 PEOPLE, 1804–1995

Year	Deaths	TB	Measles	Whooping Cough	Scarlet Fever	Diphtheria	Typhoid Fever	AIDS
1804–1809	2810	580	16	50.2	10	—	—	0
1810–1814	2290	620	13.5	64.3	—	—	—	0
1815–1819	2900	650	18.2	70.5	—	—	—	0
1820–1824	2710	540	63.6	46.9	—	—	—	0
1825–1829	2880	520	45.2	56.0	30	—	—	0
1830–1834	3560	620	44.4	59.4	130	—	—	0
1835–1839	2760	520	72.2	53.3	100	—	1.1	0
1840–1844	2620	450	33.6	35.5	100	—	6.1	0
1845–1849	3930	500	33.9	38.5	40	—	46.3	0
1850–1854	4070	490	53.7	38	100	—	22.1	0
1855–1859	3400	450	53.7	47.5	160	fn	25.2	0
1860–1865	2970	410	27.2	26.8	130	77.2	54	0
1870	2881	551	32.1	21.6	104.9	78.4	45.4	0
1875	2940	517.2	16	38.4	49.2	296	37	0
1880	2641	503.2	40	22.8	51	190	31.6	0
1885	2555	506.6	53.4	35.1	41.6	156	30.8	0
1890	2487	407.8	48.2	32.1	26.9	111	23.2	0
1895	2318	331.4	44.4	27.7	26.2	105	18	0
1900	2057	280	24	17	13	66	21	0
1905	1831	240	13	10	12	38	16	0

1910	1601	210	16	6	20	36	12	0
1915	1460	187	12	7	5	23	6	0
1920	1290	125.6	12.9	10.8	3.9	18.4	2.4	0
1925	1140	86.6	2	4.8	1.2	10.5	3.2	0
1930	1080	73.2	2.2	1.8	.8	2.8	.9	0
1935	1030	59.9	1.4	2	1.0	0.9	.5	0
1940	1020	48.6	<0.05	.7	.2	.1	.2	0
1945	1040	45.1	<0.05	.45	.07	.7	.1	0
1950	1000	29.4	2.2	<0.05	0	.1	<0.05	0
1955	1040	13.8	1.8	.3	0	0	0	0
1960	1110	10.4	.25	<0.05	<0.05	0	.1	0
1965	1110	7.6	<0.05	—	—	0	0	0
1970	1120	4.9	0.2*	—	—	0	0	0
1975	1020	4.7	0.2*	—	—	0	0	0
1980	1080	2.8	0.2*	—	—	0	0	<.01
1985	1040	1.0	1.0*	—	—	0	0	22.2
1990	1010	1.7	1.7*	—	—	0	0	60.3
1995	970	1.2	1.2*	—	—	0	0	91.5

fn = Diphtheria was first reported in 1857.

NOTE: Compilation of these 2 tables ("New York City Average Annual Death Rates" and "New York City Annual Death Rates") proved exceptionally difficult as historians are not in agreement on many data points. The known accuracy of population and mortality data varies from year to year. Different official reports give various data for the same years. Therefore, please note:

- Prior to the end of the Civil War data is presented as five-year averages;

- In 1898 New York City consolidated, incorporating all five boroughs. (See Table: "Population of New York City");

- Definitions and categorizations of diseases changed over time. Prior to the 19th century many illnesses had no given identity. TB/Tuberculosis/Consumption were the same. From 1870 forward this chart groups pulmonary and other presentations of the disease. Typhoid and paratyphoid were not specifically diagnosed, and were reported together for several decades. So were typhoid and typhus; so were diphtheria and croup.

- For 2 particular years, 1865 and 1890, population estimates are especially suspect: they are historically considered undercounted. (See: Rosenwaike, I., 1972, op. cit.)

- Childhood diseases, such as measles and diphtheria, were typically reported in age categories. In this chart, for the most part, we have grouped the reports across all ages.

Sources: Condran, G. "Changing patterns of epidemic disease in New York City." In D. Rosner, editor. *Hives of Sickness: Public Health and Epidemics in New York City.* New Brunswick, NJ: Rutgers University Press, 1995; Duffy, J. *A History of Public Health in New York City, 1625–1866.* New York: Russell Sage Foundation, 1968; Duffy, J. *A History of Public Health in New York City, 1866–1966.* New York: Russell Sage Foundation, 1974; Emerson, E. *Supplement 1936–1953 to Population, Births, Notifiable Diseases, and Deaths, Assembled for New York City, New York.* New York: DeLamar Institute of Public Health, Columbia University, 1941; Emerson, H. and Hughes, H.E. *Populations, Births, Notifiable Diseases, and Deaths, Assembled for New York City, New York, 1866–1938, from Official Records.* New York: The DeLamar Institute of Public Health, Columbia University, 1941; Jackson, K.T., editor. *The Encyclopedia of New York City.* New Haven: Yale University Press, 1995; New York City Department of Health, *Annual Reports*; New York Department of Health Website (http://www.health.state.ny.us/mysdoh); and Rosenwaike, I. *Population History of New York City.* New York: Syracuse University Press, 1971.

* Measles data for 1970, 1975, 1980, 1985, 1990, 1995 are for children under 5 years old only.

Note: see above note for Table, "New York City Average Annual Death Rates."

Sources: see above sources for Table, "New York City Average Annual Death Rates."

nomic and social stratifications similar to those seen in American cities in the mid-nineteenth century.

It might well be argued, then, that public health cannot exist in a democracy in the absence of a strong middle class. Of course, it could also be argued that democracy itself cannot exist in the absence of such a class force.

33. An excellent rendition of Chadwick's contributions can be found in the chapter entitled "Public Medicine" in Porter, R., *The Greatest Benefit to Mankind: A Medical History of Humanity*. New York: Norton, 1998.

34. Details can be found in Duffy, J., *The Sanitarians: A History of American Public Health*. Illini Books Edition. Chicago: University of Illinois Press, 1992.

35. "Nativists" were American-born whites who favored their rights in U.S. society over and above those of immigrants, African-Americans, and American Indians. As a rule, nativists were strongly anti-Semitic and racist in their beliefs, blaming "non-natives" for all social ills.

36. This was not so clearly the case in Europe at the time. In the mid-nineteenth century, Americans were far more moralistic and uncaring in their approaches to public health than were their European counterparts. For example, Porter tells us that Rudolf Virchow called upon German physicians to become "attorneys for the poor," and France's Jules Guérin announced the need for what he labeled "social medicine." In general, European public health leaders were far less judgmental of the sick and more politically engaged than were their American colleagues. See Porter, R., 1998, op. cit.

37. Public distrust of New York physicians grew to riot proportions in 1788. Rumors spread across working-class neighborhoods of ghoulish doctors who dug up the cadavers of their loved ones by moonlight and then cut up the bodies for medical experiments and anatomy studies. Fueled by a child's claim of having witnessed a New York Hospital doctor carving up the child's recently deceased mother, a mob of five-thousand people stormed Columbia College and New York Hospital, scattering terrified physicians and medical students before it. The doctors took refuge in the city jail, which the horde stormed with angry intent. Three rioters were killed when local militia fired their weapons in defense of the besieged physicians.

38. Starr, P., *The Social Transformation of American Medicine*. New York: Basic Books, 1982; Ludmerer, K. M., *Learning to Heal*. Baltimore: Johns Hopkins University Press, 1985; and Ludmerer, K. M., *Time to Heal*. New York: Oxford University Press, 1999.

39. In his previously cited books on medical education, Kenneth Ludmerer argues that as early as the 1830s French medical instructors had abandoned the rote memorization approach to training doctors in favor of direct contact with patients and problem solving. The handful of Americans who returned each year from such Parisian training knew how to examine a patient and even had a sense of diseases that focused on specific organs of the body. But well into the end of the nineteenth century, most American doctors, regardless of their "training," had no concept of the relationships between the organs of the body and disease, nor could they perform patient examinations and correctly reach even rudimentary diagnoses.

40. In the 1840s Ignaz Philipp Semmelweis, a Hungarian-born physician practicing in Vienna, conducted a brilliant experiment that would revolutionize medical hygiene. All over Europe and America at that time, mothers were developing puerperal fever after delivery. Painful infections in their vaginas and uteri would rapidly develop into sepsis and the new mothers would develop skyrocketing fevers, sink into delirium, and die.

Semmelweis noted in his Viennese hospital that some physicians and nurses had fewer puerperal fever patients than others. He experimented with a theory, dividing the obstetrics ward in half, maintaining standard practices on one side, and on the other side instructing all nurses, doctors, midwives, and visitors to scrub their hands and arms vigorously with soap and boiled water before touching the mothers or newborns. None of the mothers on the scrub side died of puerperal fever.

As word of the "Semmelweis technique" spread in Europe, physicians reasoned that such scrubbing might also reduce the incidence of postsurgical infections and bars of soap soon appeared in doctors' offices and hospital wards all over France, Austria, Germany, and England. But such was not the case in the United States.

41. Ludmerer, K. M., 1985, op. cit.

42. Quoted in Jordan, P. D., *The People's Health: A History of Public Health in Minnesota to 1948*. St. Paul: Minnesota Historical Society, 1953.

43. Jordan, P. D., *The People's Health: A History of Public Health in Minnesota to 1948*. St. Paul: Minnesota Historical Society, 1953.

44. Paul Starr offers this summary: "For if the sick are the source of infection, one way to prevent the spread of disease (a recognized function of public health) is to diagnose and cure the people who are ill (recognized functions of medicine). Extending the boundaries of public health to incorporate more of medicine seemed necessary and desirable to some public health officials, but as one might imagine, private practitioners regarded such extensions as a usurpation. Doctors fought against public treatment of the sick, requirements for reporting cases of tuberculosis and venereal disease, and attempts by public health authorities to establish health centers to coordinate preventive and curative medical services." See Starr, P., 1982, op. cit.

45. *Californios* were, originally, the California-born owners of large California ranches obtained by Mexican land grants. In the 1950s Walter O'Malley would cut a deal with the city of Los Angeles to move the Brooklyn Dodgers baseball team to California. The state would declare eminent domain, and at gunpoint National Guards rousted the descendants of the Californios out of Chavez Ravine so it could become the site of Dodger Stadium.

46. There is some dispute on that figure. Duffy says six hundred died. Condran argues the total was 1,137. See Duffy, J., 1968, op. cit.; and Condran, G. A., "Changing patterns of epidemic disease in New York City." In Rosner, D., editor, *Hives of Sickness: Public Health and Epidemics in New York City*. New Brunswick, N.J.: Rutgers University Press, 1995.

47. Starr, P., 1982, op. cit.

48. See Table: "New York City Mortality Rates Per 100,000," n. 68.

49. In 1878 yellow fever struck the towns and cities of the Mississippi Valley with ferocity. The death toll in hardest-hit Memphis exceeded 10 percent of the city's population, and New Orleans lost 5 percent of its population. Nearly every family in those cities buried at least one relative and grief left its sobering mark on the culture for years afterward.

The epidemic was handled the only way people knew how, by removing the sick from amid the well and, in severe outbreaks, completely depopulating entire cities, driving the terrified populace into the countryside. Such depopulation campaigns were, when necessary, executed at gunpoint by police, U.S. military units, and local militias in response to mayors and governors who earnestly believed that they were fulfilling their public health trust. Sadly, such actions often put people in even more direct contact with the mosquitoes that were the vectors of the disease.

Coming as this did just eight years after the end of the Civil War, the Mississippi Valley epidemic's toll in lives and dollars seems today almost unimaginable. As Khaled Bloom notes in his excellent book on the subject, most of the disaster took place in recently defeated southern states where, no doubt, the mosquitoes had gained breeding grounds as a result of war damage and the devastation of formerly Confederate infrastructures. When Hayes sent federal—a.k.a. Union—officials and troops to aid the beleaguered southern cities, it marked a bold gesture in the direction of reconciliation between the recently warring factions. See: Bloom, K. J., *The Mississippi Valley's Great Yellow Fever Epidemic of 1848*. Baton Rouge: Louisiana State University Press, 1993.

    50.

GERM DISCOVERIES
1873–1905

Disease	Named Organism or Germ	Year Discovered
Relapsing fever	Spirocheta recurrentis	1873
Anthrax	Bacillus anthracis	1876
Gonorrhea	Micrococcus gonorrhoeae	1879
Malaria	Plasmodium malariae	1880
Glanders	Bacillus mallei	1882
Asiatic cholera	Spirillum cholerae	1883
Diphtheria	Bacillus diphtheriae	1884
Cholera	Vibrio cholerae	1884
Pneumonia	Diplococcus pneumoniae	1884
Tuberculosis	Bacillus tuberculosis	1884
Typhoid fever	Bacillus typhosus	1884
Brucellosis	Bacillus melitensis	1887
Cerebrospinal meningitis	Micrococcus meningitidis	1887
Tetanus	Bacillus tetani	1889
Influenza (bacterial)	Bacillus influenzae	1892
Plague	Bacillus pestis	1894
Dysentery	Bacillus dysenteriae	1898
Syphilis	Treponoma pallidum	1905

Source: Ludmerer, K.M., *Learning to Heal*, op. cit., 1985; and multiple others.

    51. In his landmark paper, "Aetiology of Tuberculosis," Koch not only offered evidence that *Mycobacterium tuberculosis* was the cause of TB but also laid out the modes of transmission of the germ (which he mistakenly called a virus) and strategies for control of its spread.

    "As to the the method in which tuberculosis virus is transmitted from the diseased to the healthy no doubts can obtain. In consequence of shocks from coughing of the diseased person, little particles are rent from the cough sputum, sent into the air and so dispersed like dust. Now numerous experiments have taught that the inhalation of finely dispersed phthisic sputum not only makes those sorts of animals sensitive to tuberculosis, but also those capable of resistance to tuberculosis with absolute certainty. That man should be an exception to this is not to be supposed. It may, therefore, be taken for granted that when a healthy human being accidentally finds himself in the immediate neighborhood of the phthisically diseased, and inhales particles of sputum sent forth into the air, he can be infected by them." See Koch, R., "Aetiology of Tuberculosis." Translated by Rev. F. Sause. *American Veterinary Review* 13 (1889): 54–214.

52. For this section see Bates, B., *Bargaining for Life*. Philadelphia: University of Pennsylvania Press, 1992; Burrows, E. G. and Wallace, M., 1999, op. cit.; Bushel, A., *Chronology of New York City Department of Health 1655–1966*. New York City Department of Health, 1966; Caldwell, M., 1988, op. cit.; Debré, P., *Louis Pasteur*. Baltimore: Johns Hopkins University Press, 1998; Dubos, R. J., *The White Plague*. New Brunswick: Rutgers University Press, 1992; Duffy, J., *A History of Public Health in New York City: 1866–1966*. New York: Russell Sage, 1974; Duffy, J., 1992, op. cit.; Golden, J. and Rosenberg, C. E., *Pictures of Health*. Philadelphia: University of Pennsylvania Press, 1991; Golub, E. S., *The Limits of Medicine*. New York: Times Books, 1994; Jackson, K. T., 1995, op. cit.; Leavitt J. W.,*Typhoid Mary: Captive to the Public's Health*. Boston: Beacon Press, 1996; Leavitt J. W. and Numbers, R. L., 1985, op. cit.; Mullan, F., *Plagues and Politics*. New York: Basic Books, 1989; Rosner, D., editor, 1995, op. cit.; Ryan, F., *The Forgotten Plague*. New York: Little, Brown, 1993; Tomes, N., *The Gospel of Germs: Men, Women, and the Microbe in American Life*. Cambridge, Mass.: Harvard University Press, 1998; Trudeau, E. L., *An Autobiography*. New York: Lea and Febiger, 1915; Winslow, C. E. A., *The Life of Hermann M. Biggs*. New York: Lea and Febiger, 1929; and Whitson, S., *New York City 100 Years Ago*. Albuquerque: Sun Books, 1976.

53. Evans, R. J., *Death in Hamburg: Society and Politics in the Cholera Years 1830–1910*. Oxford: Clarendon Press, 1987.

54. "Lung Block" was bordered by Catherine, Cherry, Hamilton, and Market Streets.

55. In his book Riis defined a tenement: "Generally a brick building from four to six stories high on the street, frequently with a store on the first floor . . . four families occupy each floor, and a set of rooms consists of one or two dark closets, used as bedrooms, with a living room twelve feet by ten feet. The staircase is too often a dark well in the center of the house, and no direct through ventilation is possible, each family being separated from the other by partitions. Frequently the rear of the lot is occupied by another building of three stories high with two families on a floor."

Tenement estimates for 1890 found there were 37,000 such buildings in New York City, which at the time was Manhattan and the lower Bronx only. In these buildings dwelled 1.2 million people. As a result, New York City had the highest human population density found anywhere in North America, with 522 people per acre. Philadelphia in that year had a population density of 118 per acre, Chicago 83.5. See Crisci, M., *Public Health in New York City in the Late Nineteenth Century*. Bethesda: National Library of Medicine, History of Medicine Division, 1990.

56. See Sanger, M. and Russell, W., *Debate on Birth Control*. Girard, Kans.: Haldeman-Julius Company, 1921.

57. This period marked the beginning of toilet seat phobias, which, in the twentieth century, would extend to include polio and all sexually transmitted diseases, allowing syphilitics to tell their spouses they "got it from a public toilet." With the appearance of AIDS in the 1980s, toilet seat phobia would also embrace HIV.

This is hardly a solely American phenomenon. In the 1990s—one hundred years after the introduction of indoor plumbing—most families living in formerly Soviet countries would deliberately disconnect toilet seats, preferring to squat to avoid alleged contagion.

58. Bellew, "Hygeia." *Harper's Weekly*, vol. 25 (1881): 231.

59. The massive water and sewer projects undertaken in Chicago, for example, are

described in Cain, L. P., "Raising and watering a city: Ellis Sylvester Chesbrough and Chicago's first sanitation system." In Leavitt, J. W. and Numbers, R. L., 1985, op. cit.

60. New York City Department of Health, *Annual Report of the Department of Health of the City of New York*, 1905 (for 1870–1895), 1915 (for 1900–1915). Note that there is debate on these figures. See Free, E. and Hammonds, E. M., "Science, politics and the art of persuasion." In Rosner, D., editor, 1995, op. cit. By measurements focused on Manhattan's tenement areas, the change in diphtheria death rates was from an 1894 high of 785 deaths per 100,000 to just 300 deaths per 100,000 in 1900.

61. Delivered at the BMA's annual meeting in Montreal, Canada, Sept. 3, 1897.

62. Hiscock, I. V., "A survey of public health activities in Los Angeles County, California." *American Public Health Association*, 1928.

63. A Board of Health that would execute the duties of public health for the entire region was created for Los Angeles County in 1915, when the population was approaching 700,000 people. Though nowhere in the United States had a county-level health department until 1911, few had as crying a need for one as did Los Angeles.

64. For ten years Pomeroy's department tried to fulfill its mandate in the absence of any significant medical facility in Los Angeles County. The county's powerful real estate developers seemed devoid of concern about infrastructure matters such as water, hospitals, schools, and transportation. Los Angeles County would have nearly two million residents in 1925 when its first hospital opened.

But that was still in the future. Pomeroy's era muddled through with just four small scattered health clinics, a TB sanitarium, and a small network of roving public health nurses and food inspectors. Creation of a public health nursing profession was really a Los Angeles idea, born out of necessity. The county couldn't afford an equivalent squad of MDs, and any team of tax-supported doctors would have aroused the wrath of the AMA. For details, see "A new kind of nurse appears." In Rosen, G., *A History of Public Health*. Baltimore: Johns Hopkins University Press, 1993.

65. In 1900 some 40 percent of all deaths annually in New York City involved children under five years of age. A 1918 survey by Josephine Baker also found that 21 percent of all New York City schoolchildren were malnourished.

66. Mary Baker Eddy, founder of the Church of Christ, Scientist was born in New Hampshire in 1821. As a young woman she became a follower of Phineas Parkhurst Quimby, a mesmerist who used hypnotism, magnets, and communing with the spirits of the dead to heal. In 1866, Eddy created the belief system that would be known as Christian Science. Her ideas caught fire with the publication, in 1875, of her manifesto *Science and Health*.

By the late 1880s Eddy had followers all over the United States as well as in Canada and Europe. Her trained healers promised "all Manner of Diseases Cured—Without Medicine or Ceremony. 'Disease a Belief, Not a Reality.'—Remarkable Facts for Metaphysicians—The Science of Medicine Contradicted."

A key 1902 Los Angeles case involved Merrill Reed, a Christian Scientist who denied his ailing daughters diphtheria antitoxin. They died. Reed was charged with manslaughter. In a dubious landmark decision that would protect the church for four decades, the court ruled in favor of Reed. The reason: diphtheria antitoxin was, Reed's attorneys argued, an "experimental, unproven therapy."

The decision wounded the stature of both physicians and public health leaders in California. They had already suffered defeat in 1876 when the legislature voted to give homeopathic treatments equal status with allopathic.

The superior status of public health would not be established firmly in California until

1954, when Los Angeleno Christian Scientist Cora Sutherland, a schoolteacher, died of tuberculosis. She had consistently refused diagnosis and treatment. Her autopsy revealed lungs full of TB bacteria. Thereafter, all schoolteachers in Los Angeles were required to undergo TB testing.

Thirty years later, in 1988, the California Supreme Court finally overturned the 1902 Reed decision, finding against Christian Scientist parents who refused medical care for their children who died of meningitis. The Court ruled that parents did not have a legal right to martyr their own children.

Throughout the twentieth century, vaccination was a bone of contention between public health authorities and Christian Scientists. Between 1985 and 1994 four measles epidemics in the United States originated among groups of unvaccinated Christian Scientists.

For these and myriad other remarkable insights regarding the church, see Fraser, C., *God's Perfect Child: Living and Dying in the Christian Science Church*. New York: Metropolitan Books, 1999.

67. Writing for the majority, Justice Harlan said: "The liberty secured by the Constitution of the United States to every person within its jurisdiction does not impart an absolute right in each person to be, at all times and in all circumstances, wholly freed from restraint. . . . Real liberty for all could not exist under the operation of the principle which recognizes the right of each individual person to use his own, whether in respect of his person or his property, regardless of the injury that may be done to others."

The case involved an ordinance mandating vaccination of all residents of Cambridge, Massachusetts. Henning Jacobson refused and challenged the ordinance all the way to the Supreme Court. The Court ruled that Cambridge could, indeed, issue such an ordinance. On the other hand, the Court skirted the issue of enforcement. Refusers could be jailed, fined, detained, but not physically forced to accept a vaccine. The case was *Jacobson v. Massachusetts*, 197 US 11, 26 (1905). See also Leavitt, J. W., "Be safe. Be sure': Epidemic smallpox." In Rosner, D., editor, 1995, op. cit.

68. Winslow, C. E. A., 1929, op. cit.

69. Throughout 1902 two dozen white-uniformed Sanitary Police roamed the streets of New York City in search of health code violators, arresting 304 illegal dumpers, spitters, quarantine violators, and "overcrowders"—landlords who packed too many immigrants into one room—and squads of food inspectors destroyed 8,471,538 pounds of produce and meat.

70.

NEW YORK CITY MORTALITY RATES PER 100,000:
CHILDREN SELECTED CAUSES, 1900–1950

Year	Measles (under 5 years)	Whooping Cough (under 5 years)	Scarlet Fever (under 15 years)	Diphtheria (under 15 years)
1900	187.8	141.7	81.3	413.3
1905	116.2	91.2	39.6	129.1
1910	154.8	58.0	69.4	124.8
1915	116.7	73.5	19.5	85.7
1920	131.2	109.6	13.7	64.9
1925	23.6	55.6	4.5	39.8
1930	28.7	23.3	3.4	11.7
1935	22.8	32.1	4.5	4.0
1940*	6.5	12.0	1.7	1.9

Year	Measles (under 5 years)	Whooping Cough (under 5 years)	Scarlet Fever (under 15 years)	Diphtheria (under 15 years)
1945*	2.6	7.9	0.5	0.7
1950*	1.4	0.8	—	0.1

*1940, 1945, 1950 are average annual deaths per 100,000 children for the years 1936–1940, 1941–1945, and 1949–1951, respectively.

Sources: Emerson, H. and Hughes, H. E., *Population, Births, Notifiable Diseases, and Deaths, Assembled for New York City, New York, 1866–1938, from Official Records.* New York: DeLamar Institute of Public Health, Columbia University, January, 1941; New York City Department of Health, *Annual Reports* 1937 and 1959–60.

71. See Soper, G., "Curious career of Typhoid Mary." *Bulletin of the New York Academy of Medicine* 15 (1939). In 1910 a definitive demonstration of far longer carrier status was produced by English health officer Dr. Theodore Thomson. From 1896 to 1909 his Folkstone District suffered an epidemic that Thomson eventually traced to a milkman he designated "Mr. N." Though Mr. N. had never suffered typhoid fever, he carried the microbe and passed it to dozens of people with whom he had personal contact or who drank the milk he prepared. See Mortimer, P. P., "Mr. N. the milker, and Dr. Koch's concept of the healthy carrier." *Lancet* 353 (1999): 1354–56.

72. Mallon would, indeed, turn out to be a lifelong typhoid carrier, as are, as later studies would reveal, a minority of all people who recover from typhoid fever. Indeed, some people who have never contracted the disease, but were unknowingly infected, can also serve as lifelong carriers. Even a century later, many of *Salmonella typhi*'s impressive repertoire of tricks would remain mysterious. In this case, and many others, public health policy has by necessity been based on incomplete science. For an excellent view of mechanisms used by various *Salmonella* species see Strauss, E., "Anti-immune trick unveiled in *Salmonella.*" *Science* 285 (1999): 306–307.

73. By the time Mallon was rearrested, however, she had cooked at Sloane Hospital for five months and infected at least twenty-five people, two of whom died—bringing her total to fifty-one cases and three deaths. As before, when authorities confronted Mallon she fled, this time into nearby woods. Eventually captured after a police chase, Mallon was sent to Riverside Hospital on North Brother Island, where she died, embittered and alone, in 1938.

There was little public or media sympathy for "Typhoid Mary" Mallon. "Mary's status after her second arrest has been totally different from that which she possessed after her first," disease detective George Soper's account concluded. "This is true both as to the legal aspects and public sympathy. Whatever rights she once possessed as the innocent victim of an infected condition precisely like that of hundreds of others who were free, were now lost. She was now a woman who could not claim innocence. . . . She was a dangerous character and must be treated accordingly." Soper, G. A., 1919, op. cit.

The story of Mary Mallon's case is drawn from Baker, J., 1939, op. cit; Fee, E. and Hammonds, E. M., "Science, politics, and the art of persuasion." In Rosner, D., editor, 1995, op. cit.; Leavitt, J. W., 1996, op. cit.; Soper, G., 1939, op. cit.; and Sufrin, M., "The case of the disappearing cook." *American Heritage* (August 1970): 37–43.

74. Hookworm disease is caused by any of three parasites indigenous to North America, particularly in subtropic ecologies. Hookworm larvae can infect people by entering cuts on bare feet. Once inside the body, hookworms can cause anemia, weakness, and mental retardation.

In 1906, when the Rockefeller campaign began, experts already recognized that though treatment options were lousy, prevention was fairly simple. Shoes, socks, and long pants were sufficient barriers, in most cases. Hookworm was a disease of extreme poverty.

75. By 1916 there were fewer than five schools of public health in the United States, but there were more than 160 medical schools—demonstrating that curative medicine was already a more attractive pursuit than populationwide disease prevention.

76. Stevens, R., *In Sickness and in Wealth: American Hospitals in the Twentieth Century*. Baltimore: Johns Hopkins University Press, 1989.

77. Ludmerer, K. M., 1985, op. cit.

78. On the other hand, this professionalization hardened doctor's opposition to all forms of what they saw as meddling in how they practiced medicine. Lawrence D. Weiss neatly summarized this tension: "Physicians, pharmacists, and drug manufacturers viewed public health predominately through entrepreneurial eyes even during the early days of the development of public health institutions and activities. They supported public health as long as it funneled patients and customers into their offices, but the moment they saw public health as competition, they turned their backs."

See Weiss, L. D., *Private Medicine and Public Health: Profit, Politics, and Prejudice in the American Health Care Enterprise*. Boulder: Westview Press, 1997.

79. Ben-David, J., "Scientific productivity and academic organization in nineteenth century medicine." *American Sociological Review* 25 (1960): 830.

80. Golub, E. S., 1994, op. cit. Adult cases of polio were rare, presumably because over decades of life, older individuals were naturally immunized by sequential exposures. In 1916, of course, all but the wealthiest of adults would have been exposed during childhood, having consumed less than ideally filtered water. After the horrible summer of 1916, the Franklin Delano Roosevelt family left New York City each season for Campobello Island, hoping to avoid the polio scourge. It was there in August 1921 that the future president contracted an unusual case of adult-onset polio which paralyzed his legs for the rest of his life.

81. For this section on polio, see New York City Department of Health, *Annual Report of the Department of Health of the City of New York for the Calendar Year 1917*. New York, 1918; Duffy, J., 1968, op. cit.; Golub, E. S., 1994, op. cit.; Kraut, A. M., "Plagues and prejudice." In Rosner, D., editor, 1995, op. cit.; and Smith, J. S., *Patenting the Sun: Polio and the Salk Vaccine*. New York: William Morrow and Company, 1990.

82. Polio probably waned in 1917 because it had saturated the nonimmune population, causing disease in the most vulnerable and naturally vaccinating the rest. Over subsequent decades, scientists would offer many explanations for the cyclic nature of polio, generally failing to recognize the salient feature.

83. As quoted in Kyvig, D. E., *Repealing National Prohibition*. Chicago: Chicago University Press, 1979.

84. Gray, M., *Drug Crazy: How We Got into This Mess and How We Can Get Out*. New York: Random House, 1998; and Ramirez, J. S., "The tourist trade takes hold." In Beard, R. and Berkowitz, L. C., 1993, op. cit.

85. In New York City, for example, the going bribery rate was $400 a week to be divided among a list of officials for protection of a speakeasy and $40 a week to the local beat cop.

86. Duffy, J., 1974, op. cit.; and New York City Department of Health, *Annual Report of the Department of Health of the City of New York for the Calendar Year 1920*. New York, 1921.

87. In its 1920 annual report the department also noted that, "With the advent of

Prohibition, a number of cases of wood alcohol poisoning were discovered," offering a clear rationale for the involvement of medical, versus criminal, authority.

88. Because one of the larger early outbreaks surfaced in Spain, the 1918 epidemic was labeled "Spanish Influenza" by all but the Spanish. If a geographic moniker was necessary, "Kansas Flu" might have been more appropriate.

89. For this section, see Beveridge, W. I. B., "The chronicle of influenza epidemics." *History and Philosophy of Life Sciences* 13 (1991): 223–35; U.S. Bureau of the Census, *Historical Statistics of the United States, Colonial Times to 1970.* Bicentennial Edition. 93rd Cong., 1st sess., H. Doc. 93-78 (Part 1); Centers for Disease Control and Prevention, "Prevention and control of influenza." *Morbidity and Mortality Weekly Reports* 48 No. RR-4 (1999); Crosby, A. W., *Epidemic and Peace, 1918.* London: Greenwood Press, 1976; New York City Department of Health, *Annual Report of the Department of Health of the City of New York for the Calendar Year 1918* (see also the years 1919 and 1920). New York: 1919 (1920, 1921); Garrett, L., 1994, op. cit.; Hiscock, I. V., 1928, op. cit.; Hoehling, A. A., *The Great Epidemic.* Boston: Little, Brown, 1961; and Jordan, P. D., 1953, op. cit.

90. The overall impact on rates of death due to all causes was as follows, according to the U.S. Census Bureau:

AGE-ADJUSTED DEATH RATE (PER 1,000)

Year	Total	White Both Sexes	White Male	White Female	Nonwhite Both Sexes	Nonwhite Male	Nonwhite Female
1916	15.1	14.7	15.8	13.4	22.2	22.6	21.6
1917	15.3	14.7	16.0	13.4	23.4	24.1	22.7
1918	19.0	18.4	20.2	16.6	28.0	28.9	27.1
1919	14	13.4	14.1	12.8	20.5	20.3	20.8
1920	14.2	13.7	14.2	13.1	20.6	20.4	21.0
1921	12.7	12.2	12.7	11.6	18.2	18.0	18.6

91. Eyler, J. M., "The sick poor and the state." In Rosenberg, C. E. and Golden, J., editors. *Framing Disease: Studies in Cultural History.* New Brunswick, N.J.: Rutgers University Press, 1992.

92. The nation's gross national product was skyrocketing, from $16 billion dollars in 1860 to $65 billion in 1890. And by 1921 it would top $300 billion. During that period—a time of 19-fold growth in national wealth—average per-capita income rose only 5.8-fold. Why? Because it wasn't really America that got richer but an elite stratum at the top that amassed astonishing wealth.

93. Smith, D. B., *Health Care Divided: Race and Healing a Nation.* Ann Arbor: University of Michigan Press, 1999.

94. Dublin, L. I., "The health of the Negro." *Annals of the American Academy of Politics and Social Science* 140 (1928): 77–85.

95. White, R., *It's Your Misfortune and None of My Own: A New History of the American West.* Norman: University of Oklahoma Press, 1991.

96. Average life expectancy for a white boy born in the United States in 1925 was 57.6 years; for a white girl, 60.6 years. For "Negroes and others," as they were then classified by the U.S. Census Bureau, life expectancies that year were far lower: 44.9 years for boys and 46.7 years for girls. That figure was, of course, affected by their far greater infant mortality

rates: 110.8 per 1,000 for "Negroes and others" versus 68.3 per 1,000 for white babies. See U.S. Bureau of the Census, 1976, op. cit.

97. By 1920 public hospitals were the population's major medical providers nationwide, with charitable private hospitals playing a secondary role. In theory, all of these facilities were available equally to everyone. But that was not the case.

In his landmark 1910 report on medical education Abraham Flexner argued: "The medical care of the Negro race will never be wholly left to Negro physicians. Nevertheless, if the Negro can be brought to feel a sharp responsibility for the physical integrity of his people, the outlook for their mental and moral improvement will be distinctly brightened. The practice of the Negro doctor will be limited to his own race, which in turn will be cared for better by good Negro physicians than by poor white ones. But the physical well-being of the Negro is not only of moment to the Negro himself. Ten million of them live in close contact with sixty million whites. Not only does the Negro himself suffer from hookworm and tuberculosis; he communicates them to his white neighbors, precisely as the ignorant and unfortunate white contaminates him. Self-protection not less than humanity offer weighty counsel in this matter; self-interest seconds philanthropy." Smith, D. B., 1999, op. cit.

In advocating advanced university training for African-Americans, Flexner was a progressive individual for his time—in which only seven U.S. universities admitted African-Americans. But Flexner never questioned the rationales of the day for racial segregation of health care: in much of the United States in 1920 dark-skinned Americans were not only required to drink from water fountains that were separate from those used by light-skinned Americans, they were also forbidden access to the same clinics and hospitals, or wards within hospitals.

At the time, Jews and Catholics were also segregated out of the medical system, and few major universities would admit them to advanced degree programs. But long after those walls had fallen, African-Americans, Asian-Americans, American Indians, and Mexican-Americans would remain outside the system.

98. Starr, P., 1982, op. cit.

99. His 1920s books extolling the praises of science and public health were *Microbe Hunters, Hunger Fighters*, and *Men Against Death*.

100. De Kruif, P., *Why Keep Them Alive?* London: Jonathan Cape, 1936.

101. Hopkins, H. L., "Hunger is not debatable." *New York World Telegram* (July 30, 1935).

102. De Kruif, P., *The Fight for Life*. London: Jonathan Cape, 1938.

103. Ibid.

104. At the 1933 meeting of the Child Health Recovery Conference, de Kruif's jaw dropped when former New York City health commissioner Havens Emerson, then director of the Minneapolis School of Hygiene, said: "The professional do-gooders among the social workers have expressed concern over the future effects of the depression on public health, there is no support for the belief that the public health will be benefitted or damaged by the worldwide economic debacle."

105. Duffy, J., 1992, op. cit.

106. See "Changes in U.S. Life Expectancy" table on page 663.

107. Eyer, J. and Sterling, P., "Stress-related mortality and social organization." *The Review of Radical Political Economics*, Vol. 9 (1977).

108. Twenty-two federal hospitals closed (dropping from 310 in 1934 to 288 in 1931); 110 state hospitals were shut down (the total dropping from 632 in 1924 down to 522 in 1937); 153 local government hospitals were closed (from 924 such facilities in 1927 down to

CHANGES IN U.S. LIFE EXPECTANCY AT BIRTH
DURING THE GREAT DEPRESSION

Year	TOTAL			WHITE			"NEGRO AND OTHERS"		
	Both sexes	Male	Female	Both sexes	Male	Female	Both sexes	Male	Female
1927	60.4	59.0	62.1	62.0	60.5	63.9	48.2	47.6	48.9
1928	56.8*	55.6*	58.3*	58.4*	57.0*	60.0*	46.3*	45.6*	47.0*
1929	57.1	55.8	58.7	58.6	57.2	60.3	46.7	45.7	47.8
1930	59.7	58.1	61.6	61.4	59.7	63.5	48.1	47.3	49.2
1931	61.1	59.4	63.1	62.6	60.8	64.7	50.4	45.5*	51.5
1932	62.1	61.0	63.5	63.2	62.0	64.5	53.7	52.8	54.6
1933	63.3	61.7	65.1	64.3	62.7	66.3	54.7	53.5	56.0
1934	61.1*	59.3*	63.3*	62.4*	50.6*	64.6*	51.8*	50.2*	53.7*
1935	61.7	59.9	63.9	62.9	61.0	65.0	53.1	51.3	55.2
1936	58.5*	56.6*	60.6*	59.8*	58.0*	61.9*	49.0*	47.0*	51.4*
1937	60.0	58.0	62.4	61.4	59.3	63.8	50.3	48.3	52.5
1938	63.5	61.9	65.3	65.0	63.2	66.8	52.9	51.7	54.3
1939	63.7	62.1	65.4	64.9	63.3	66.6	54.5	53.2	56.0

* = decrease from the previous year
(Source: U.S. Census Bureau)

871 in 1937). Charitable private hospitals also suffered, dropping from 1,060 in 1926 to 969 in 1936 (91 closures). Stevens, R., 1989, op. cit.

109. For these and other Depression-era basic facts, see Badger, A. J., *The New Deal: The Depression Years, 1933–1940.* New York: Macmillan, 1989; Heckscher, A., *When La Guardia Was Mayor: New York's Legendary Years.* New York: W. W. Norton and Company, 1978; and McElvaine, R. S., *The Great Depression.* New York: Random House, 1984.

110. The first storm, in April 1935, blew about 40 million tons of topsoil off the farms of Oklahoma. Another duster, on May 11, carried off 300 million tons of soil and rendered 332 million acres of the Great Plains and Texas a giant bowl of useless dirt.

111. The Hoover administration supported the deportations and sent federal officials to the West to deport an additional 82,000 men of Mexican heritage between 1929 and 1933. The effort failed, of course, as would all such deportation campaigns: bad as the economy of the West was in the 1930s, Mexico's was worse. And during those years an estimated 500,000 Mexicans crossed the border to El Norte, settling in California, Arizona, New Mexico, Texas, and Colorado. In California, these immigrants crowded in among the estimated 300,000 dust bowl refugees who also became targets of discrimination and political strife. Kleppner, P., "Politics without parties: The western states, 1900–1984." In Nash, G. D. and Etuliaian, R., editors, *The Twentieth Century West.* Albuquerque: University of New Mexico Press, 1987.

112. Pomeroy, J. L., "County health administration in Los Angeles." *American Journal of Public Health* 11 (1921): 796–800; Rosen, G., "The impact of the hospital on the patient, the physician and the community." *Hospital Administration* 9 (1964): 15–33; and Rosen, G., "The first neighborhood health center movement." In Leavitt, J. W. and Numbers, R. L., 1985, op. cit.

113. Between 1930 and 1934 in the state of California 894 children died of whooping cough, for example. See Duffy, J., 1992, op. cit.

114. Dunshee, J. D. and Stevens, I. M., "Previous history of poliomyelitis in California." *American Journal of Public Health* 24 (1934): 1197–1200.

115. As far as is known by the author, no one saved a sample of the 1934 virus. Thus, the very unusual symptoms and low mortality rate seen during the Los Angeles epidemic remain mysterious.

116. See the following sources for further information on the 1934 outbreak: Aronowitz, R. A., "From myalgic encephalitis to yuppie flu." In Rosenberg, C. E. and Golden, J., editors, 1992, op. cit.; Bower, et al. "Clinical features of poliomyelitis in Los Angeles." *American Journal of Public Health* 24 (1934): 1210; Dunshee, J. D. and Stevens, I. M., 1934, op. cit.; and Stevens, I. M. "The 1934 epidemic of poliomyelitis in Southern California." *American Journal of Public Health* 24 (1934): 1213.

117. The "iron lung" had been invented in 1928 by Philip Drinker of Harvard University. Polio victims lay in a six-foot steel tube that breathed for them, pumping their paralyzed lungs and holding their bodies in an airtight seal. The devices hadn't made their way to Los Angeles by 1934 and were too expensive for most of America during the Great Depression. But by 1940 hospitals all over the country would have the Drinker respirators. The image of large open hospital wards filled with row-upon-row of the coffinlike devices would become a lasting legacy of American polio. See Henig, R. M., 1997, op. cit.; and Golden J. and Rosenberg, C. E., 1991, op. cit.

118. See Duffy's delineation, "The Great Depression and the war years," in Duffy, J., 1992, op. cit.

119. As quoted in McElvaine, R. S., 1984, op. cit.

120. San Francisco had a very sorry track record vis-à-vis the health of its Chinese

population. During the 1870s to 1890s, when nearly every other locality in the country saw its death and disease rates go down, San Francisco's rose, primarily due to a sequence of epidemics of smallpox and diphtheria. Part of the problem—perhaps the paramount mistake—was the policy of the city's department of health of blaming Chinese immigrants for every single epidemic.

Chinatown was like a walled-off city within a city, ignored by the department except as a target for vilification. The Chinese, understandably, resented the finger pointing and grew increasingly hostile toward the department. By 1900, department officials were complaining about hostile Chinese, while Chinatown's elders were instructing their community not to trust the government representatives. This, against the background of often brutal anti-Chinese sentiments that sparked lynchings and other violence against the Asian immigrants. It was a classic paradigm of social bigotry and mistrust serving to promote the spread of disease.

121. Mullan, F., 1989, op. cit.

122. The epidemic ultimately ended not through the intervention of Science, but of Nature. The great San Francisco earthquake and fire of 1906 leveled the rodents' hiding places and drove the surviving rats to starvation. But feral rodents would continue to harbor plague-infested fleas. Periodically throughout the twentieth century squirrels, in particular, would be sources of isolated bubonic plague human illnesses and deaths. Thus, it could be argued that Gage's determined opposition to anitplague action allowed *Yersinia pestis* to become newly endemic in California rodent populations.

123. Two agencies were created within USPHS: in future years they would transform into the National Institutes of Health and the Centers for Disease Control.

124. See, for example, Institute of Medicine, "The disarray of public health: A threat to the health of the public." *The Future of Public Health*. Washington, D.C.: National Academy Press, 1988.

125. Unfortunately, Congress set a time limit on the act, and all its funds dried up in 1929, just when the states suddenly desperately needed the federal handout. Despite the act's lofty purpose—improvement of the health and well-being of America's babies and small children—Sheppard-Towner ran into staunch opposition. The American Medical Association, true to its on-going practice of standing firmly against anything thought to take profits away from private physicians, decried the act as "socialistic." And three states—Massachusetts, Connecticut, and Illinois—declared the act unconstitutional, filing federal law suits to block its implementation on the grounds that no federal agency could tell a state how, or on what, it should spend its money. That those cases floundered in the courts, never reaching the U.S. Supreme Court, reflected the judiciary's belief that such protest was groundless. See Furman, B., *Profile of the United States Public Health Service, 1798–1948*. Washington, D.C.: Government Printing Office, 1973.

126. Mullan, F., 1989, op. cit. Congress continued debating and creating yet more agencies until 1930. Every time a powerful member of Congress got riled up about a health-related issue, bingo!, a new agency was born. In 1929, just weeks before the crash, for example, Congress created a Federal Bureau of Narcotics to deal with increasing drug addiction problems. It would eventually become the Drug Enforcement Administration and take a staunch criminalization approach to the issue of drug use.

127. Badger tells us that "between 1933 and 1937 the American economy grew at an annual rate of 10 percent, but output had fallen so low after 1929 that even this growth left 14 percent of the workforce unemployed. A recession in 1937 quickly shot the unemployment rate back up to 19 percent. Well into 1941 unemployment remained at over 10 percent." Badger, A. J., 1989, op. cit.

128. Among the many New Deal initiatives that affected health programs were Aid to Dependent Children (1933); the Civil Works Administration (1933); the federal Emergency Relief Administration (1933); the National Recovery Administration (1933); the Public Works Administration (1933); the Tennessee Valley Authority (1933); the Rural Electrification Administration (1935); the Works Progress Administration (1935); and the Social Security Act (1935). In the same period Congress passed a series of federal initiatives specific to health. They included the Venereal Diseases Act (1935); the National Cancer Act (1937); and the Venereal Diseases Control Act (1938).

129. One of the most colorful figures in the history of U.S. politics, La Guardia was an improbable hero. Just five feet one inch tall in his stocking feet, he had a high-pitched voice and was prone to often hilarious twists of speech—the author's favorite being: "I think the reporter should get his facts straight before he distorts them." But he would serve four terms as mayor of New York City, from 1934 to 1945, enjoying a popularity never rivaled by a major municipal politician before or since in the United States.

130. For details on the La Guardia administration, see Heckscher, A., 1978, op. cit.

131. For details, see Duffy, J., 1968, op. cit.

132. For example, health department food distribution system that was intended to prevent starvation in poor neighborhoods had been hijacked by gangsters and turned into a ghoulish profiteering operation. And along with credibility, department revenues were also way down. In 1927 its budget was $6,119,244. By 1933 it was just $4,600,000—a 25 percent drop. As politicians no longer felt public pressure in support of the department, it was easy to hack away at is paltry budget.

133. As quoted in Duffy, J., 1968, op. cit.

134. Ibid. Robert McElvaine argues that, in general, the New Deal was a boon for the health of African-Americans. He notes that during the 1930s their life expectancies improved and illiteracy rates among them fell from 16.4 percent to 11.5 percent. (McElvaine, R. S., 1984, op. cit.) The problem with that argument is that white life expectancies also improved between 1929 and 1940, and by the end of the Great Depression the gap between the races remained wide. In 1929 life expectancy at birth (genders combined) for whites was 58.6 years; for blacks it was 46.7 years. Thus, on average whites were living 11.9 years longer than African-Americans.

In 1940 white life expectancy was 64.2 years; for blacks it was 53.1 years. So whites were living 11.1 years longer than blacks. The gap had therefore been closed by barely 1 percent. (Based on data from the U.S. Census Bureau. I am forced to surmise black life expectancies, though the Bureau listed them in a category entitled "Negro and Other.")

135. While La Guardia's health commissioner, Dr. John Rice, was busy rebuilding the health department, Dr. Sigismund Goldwater was building up the city's hospital system, thanks again to New Deal money. In two years he constructed three new hospitals and upgraded facilities in several older ones.

136. New York City Department of Health, *Annual Report of the Board of Health of the City of New York.* New York, 1938.

137. Badger A. J., 1989, op. cit.

138. As quoted in McElvaine, R. S., 1984, op. cit.

139. Badger, A. J., 1989, op. cit.; de Kruif, P., 1938, op. cit.; McElvaine, R. S., 1984, op. cit.; and Starr, P., 1982, op. cit.

140. De Kruif, P., 1938, op. cit.

141. Dubos, R., *Mirage of Health.* Garden City, New York: Doubleday Anchor, 1961.

142. U.S. Bureau of the Census, 1976, op. cit.

143. Some public health leaders believed that they had pushed TB rates down as low

as possible. They argued that tuberculosis would always be in the environment and could not be further limited through then-standard control measures. Some openly doubted that patient identification and isolation procedures were even responsible for the TB decline witnessed since 1900. See, for example, Frost, W. H., "How much control of tuberculosis?" *American Journal of Public Health* 27 (1937): 759–766.

144. U.S. Bureau of the Census, *County Data Book*. Washington, D.C.: Government Printing Office, 1947.

145. The major company responsible for infrastructure contracts was the Henry J. Kaiser Corporation and its subsidiary, Permanente Metals. Over the war years Kaiser won about a quarter billion dollars' worth of contracts. And the same company would later build California's health care HMO infrastructure, the massive Kaiser-Permanente system.

146. The Bracero farmworker program imported a quarter million temporary farmworkers from Mexico. Another two hundred thousand Mexicans entered California illegally during that time, most also ending up working the agricultural fields.

African-Americans also benefited from Southern California's war wealth—they found employment in the defense industry. Some 340,000 blacks moved to Los Angeles between 1940 and 1945, and most of them settled in a neighborhood of central Los Angeles called Watts. These migration estimates are garnered from the previously cited 1976 Bureau of the Census publication and from White, R., 1991, op. cit.

As racial tensions rose in Los Angeles during the war, Japanese- and Mexican-Americans were the primary targets: in 1943 white soldiers on duty in Southern California roamed Chavez Ravine beating up the neighborhood's zoot suit–wearing young Hispanics. Japanese-Americans, falsely accused of planning espionage or posing a threat to national security, were rounded up en masse just two months after Pearl Harbor and sent to remote detention camps.

147. Ainsworth, A., 1946. As quoted in Gottlieb, R. and Wolt, I., 1977, op. cit.

148. At the beginning of the century, Los Angelenos had been well served by the Big Red rail system. But during the Great Depression ownership of the Big Red system changed, its routes were gradually reduced, and by 1940 it was merely a memory. The saga of this demise is a sorry and a complicated one. In 1947 the U.S. Department of Justice brought charges against General Motors alleging that the company conspired with a variety of Los Angeles real estate and rail interests to destroy Big Red, committing the region to exclusive automobile use. GM executives were found guilty, but suffered no significant penalties.

149. When I grew up in Los Angeles County two decades later, these terribly boring recesses were routine. Promising young athletes were preferentially assigned to early morning physical education classes so that they would exercise during times of lower smog levels.

150. Rosen, G., 1993, op. cit.

151. Ultimately air pollution levels in Southern California would come down as a result of several factors, all of which were largely outside the influence of public health authorities. Steel production moved overseas, the petroleum industry, under federal pressure, lowered the lead and sulfur contents of gasoline, automobiles became more fuel efficient. Under the 1970 Clean Air Act, Congress granted the EPA strong regulatory powers with which to watchdog and pressure the auto and petrochemical industries. And in the 1990s Los Angeles County set in motion laws requiring twenty-first-century phase-out of all fossil fuel–powered automobiles.

152. Jordan, P. D., 1953, op. cit.

153. Ibid.

154. The term *venereal* disappeared from public health terminology in the 1970s and was replaced by the phrase *sexually transmitted disease*, or STD. The word *venereal* was

derived from the Latin word *venereus*, or "of Venus," and referred specifically to heterosexual intercourse. By the 1970s the highest incidence rates of nearly every sexually transmitted infection in the United States were seen not among heterosexuals, however, but among gay men. Thus, public health leaders stopped using the limiting expressions VD and venereal, replacing them with the broader term.

155. U.S. Bureau of the Census, 1976, op. cit.

156. Sexual diseases were, according to Harvard medical historian Allan Brandt, defined as "a uniquely sinful disease . . . of moral decay. Behavior—bad behavior at that—is seen as the cause of venereal disease. These assumptions may be powerful psychologically, and in some cases they may influence behavior, but so long as they are dominant—so long as disease is equated with sin—there can be no magic bullet." Brandt, A. M., *No Magic Bullet: A Social History of Venereal Disease in the United States Since 1890*. New York: Oxford University Press, 1985.

157. This sorry state of affairs persisted throughout the twentieth century, and limited STD control programs for decades. By the 1990s the moralistic American society would, for example, have a gonorrhea rate of 150 cases per 100,000. In contrast, the sexually far freer and less moralistic Swedish society would at the same time have a rate of only 3 per 100,000— fifty times lower. See Institutes of Medicine, *The Hidden Epidemic: Confronting Sexually Transmitted Diseases*. Washington, D.C.: National Academy Press, 1996.

158. Brandt, A. M., 1985, op. cit.

159. For further information on the Tuskegee syphilis experiment and its ramifications, see Annas, G. J. and Grodin, M. A., "Apology is not enough." *Boston Globe* (May 18, 1997): Focus C-1; Bowman, J. E., Corbie-Smith, G., Lurie, P., Wolfe, S. M., Caplan, A. L., Annas G. J., Fairchild, A. L., and Bayer, R., Letters in response to "Tuskegee as metaphor." *Science* 285 (1999): 47–50; Brandt, A. M., "Racism and research: The case of the Tuskegee syphilis study." In Leavitt, J. W. and Numbers, R. L., 1985, op. cit.; Clinton, W. J., "Apology." Delivered May 16, 1997, at Tuskegee University, Alabama; U.S. Department of Health Education and Welfare, *Final Report of the Tuskegee Syphilis Study Ad Hoc Advisory Panel*. Washington, D.C.: Government Printing Office, 1973; Fairchild, A. L. and Bayer, R., "Uses and abuses of Tuskegee." *Science* 284 (1999): 919-921; Glenn, J. "Remarks on S. 193." *U.S. Congressional Record*, January 22, 1997; Heller, J., "Tuskegee syphilis experiment." Associated Press, July 24, 1972; Jones, J. H., *Bad Blood: The Tuskegee Syphilis Experiment*. New York: Free Press, 1981; Kampmeir, R. H., "Final report on the Tuskegee syphilis study." *Southern Medical Journal* 67 (1974): 1349–1353; Kampmeier, R. H., "The Tuskegee study of untreated syphilis." *Southern Medical Journal* 65 (1972): 1247–1251; Smith, D. B., 1999, op. cit.; and Stolberg, S. G., " 'Unchecked' experiments on people raise concern." *New York Times* (May 14, 1997): A1.

160. On May 16, 1997, President William Jefferson Clinton would apologize to the nation for the USPHS syphilis experiment. In his apology, presented at Tuskegee University, President Clinton said: "The eight men who are survivors of the study are a living link to a time not so very long ago that many Americans would prefer not to remember but we dare not forget. It was a time when our nation failed to live up to its ideals, when our nation broke the trust with our people that is the very foundation of our democracy. . . . An apology is the first step. . . . We need to do more to ensure that medical research practices are sound and ethical, and that researchers work more closely with communities."

161. Garrett, L., 1994, op. cit.

162. U.S. Bureau of the Census, 1976, op. cit.

163. Garrett, L., 1994, op. cit.

164. U.S. Bureau of the Census, 1976, op. cit.

165. Ryan, F., 1993, op. cit.

166. Another World War II U.S. military innovation was the use of chloroquine for treatment of malaria, coupled with DDT and 2,4-D pesticides for eradication of disease-carrying mosquitoes and lice. Both technologies initially proved as miraculously successful as had penicillin and were immediately put to vigorous civilian use. In the malarial southern states the double wallop of pesticides and chloroquine was phenomenally successful. By 1952 the USPHS would declare the disease eradicated from North America. For a detailed history of U.S. malaria control efforts, see Garrett, L., 1994, op. cit.; Institute of Medicine. *Malaria: Obstacles and Opportunities.* Washington, D.C.: National Academy Press, 1991; and Wernsdorfer, W. H. and McGregor, I., *Malaria: Principles and Practice of Malariology.* Edinburgh: Churchill Livinstone, 1988.

167. Stevens, R., 1989, op. cit.

168. In 1946 American women gave birth to 3.4 million babies; 1947, '48, '49, '50, and '51 each welcomed another 3.8 million babies; in 1952 some 3.9 million Americans were born; and every year from 1954–64 another 4 million American babies arrived.

169. Stevens, R., 1989, op. cit.

170. Weiss, L. D., 1997, op. cit.

171. Stevens, R., 1989, op. cit.

172. The union militancy of the 1930s was consolidated during the postwar 1940s into a handful of extremely powerful unions that absorbed or virtually eliminated smaller labor organizations. The AFL-CIO, Teamsters, ILO, and other enormous unions' chief demands were not worker control but higher wages, longer paid vacations, job safety, forty-hour work weeks, and benefits packages that included pensions and medical insurance. By 1950, 15 million American workers were union members; by 1960 the number topped 17 million. See Lichtenstein, N., "Labor in the Truman Era: Origins of the 'private welfare state.' " In Lacey, M., editor. *The Truman Presidency.* Woodrow Wilson International Center for Scholars. New York: Cambridge University Press, 1989.

173. This number comes from the previously cited U.S. Census tracts, published in 1976. The data reveal that total health spending in the United States, both public and private, rose by only $300 between 1928 and 1940, and by about $1.5 million between 1940 and 1945. In 1948 total health spending hit $10.6 billion, of which a third was hospital care. (In 1929 hospital care had constituted only one sixth of the $3.6 billion the nation spent on health.)

By 1955 Americans were spending $17.7 billion on health, a third of which, $5.9 billion, was for hospital costs. In 1960 they again spent about a third of their health dollars on hospitals, or almost $9.1 billion. In 1970 health spending would top $71.5 billion and nearly 40 percent of that would be spent in hospitals. (These hospitalization figures do not include nursing homes, long-term care, or physician's services and pharmaceuticals.)

174. See U.S. Congressional Budget Office, *Containing Medical Care Costs Through Market Forces.* Washington, D.C.: Government Printing Office, 1982.

175. In 1940 nearly all of the $2.9 billion in personal health expenditures in the United States was paid out of pocket by individual patients or their families. In 1948 about 10 percent of the $6.8 billion in personal health payments was covered by private insurance. By 1950 insurance would be picking up 14 percent of the tab; in 1960 it would cover 38 percent. And by 1970 fully two-thirds of all personal health dollars would be covered by private insurance.

176. Stevens, R., 1989, op. cit.

177. Jones, L., *Great Expectations: America and the Baby Boom Generation.* New York: Coward, McCann & Geoghegan, 1980.

178. Under the Jones Act of 1917 Puerto Ricans had the right to U.S. citizenship and could freely reside in America. Tuberculosis case rates rose in the city during the 1940s, partly because of this influx of immigrants. Thanks to the department's dissemination of free

antibiotics to indigent TB sufferers, however, death rates in New York fell from 44.8 per 10,000 in 1941 to 35.7 in 1948. With Manhattan case rates topping 200 per 100,000 in 1948, however, the decline in deaths was not, alone, sufficient cause for celebration. The highest case rates—approaching 400 per 100,000—were among immigrants from Puerto Rico and other Caribbean countries. The lowest 1948 ratios—176 per 10,000—were among native-born African-Americans.

179. New York Department of Health, 1949, op. cit.

180. Leavitt, J. W., "Be safe. Be sure. New York City's experience with epidemic smallpox." In Rosner, D., 1995, op. cit; and Duffy, J., 1968, op. cit.

181. New York Department of Health, 1949, op. cit.

182. See U.S. Census Bureau, 1976, op. cit; and Smith, J. S., 1990, op. cit.

183. See Robin Marantz Henig's account of the Nobel-winning and subsequent research by Weller, Enders, and Robbins in her previously cited 1997 book.

184. Established in 1941, the Public Health Research Institute, or PHRI, was jointly funded by a variety of charities and the New York City Department of Health. Its original director, Dr. Thomas Rivers, was one of the most renowned virologists of the day. Originally the city contributed $100,000 a year to PHRI, a not inconsiderable sum in 1941. Mayor La Guardia doubled that sum, and by 1945 PHRI was the most important center of its kind in the United States, possibly worldwide.

185. The children who were Polio Pioneers were accorded hero status and received considerable media coverage. Many of them still today proudly display their Polio Pioneer buttons.

186. For details about the travails of the polio clinical trials, see Smith, J. S., 1990, op. cit.

187. Ibid. In 1954 the U.S. national polio rate was 23.9 cases per 100,000 people. The incidence fell 27 percent in 1955 and by 1957 was down to just 3.2 cases per 100,000 people.

188. In a comprehensive analysis by the Institute of Medicine it was found that the risk of contracting paralytic polio from Sabin's oral vaccine was 1:520,000 for the first dose, and 1:12,300,000 for each subsequent booster. See Institute of Medicine, Stratton, K. R., Howe, C. J., and Johnston, R. B., editors. *Adverse Events Associated with Childhood Vaccines: Evidence Bearing on Causality*. Washington, D.C.: National Academy Press, 1993.

189. Nickum, C., "Malaria transmitted by hypodermic syringe." *Journal of the American Medical Association* 100 (1933): 1401–1402.

190. Halpern, M., "Malaria among drug addicts in New York City; epidemic of aestivo-autumnal and quartan malaria by use of contaminated hypodermic syringes." *Public Health Reports* 49 (1934): 421–423.

191. Capps, R. B., Sborov, V., and Scheifly, C. H., "Syringe-transmitted epidemic of infectious hepatitis, with observations regarding incidence and nature of infectious donors." *Journal of the American Medical Association* 136 (1948): 819–824; Darmady, E. M. and Hardwick, C., "Syringe-transmitted hepatitis." *Lancet* 2 (1945): 106; Findlay, G. M., "Infective hepatitis in West Africa; syringe-transmitted hepatitis." *Monthly Bulletin Min. Health and Public Health Lab Service* 7 (1948): 32–39; Hughes, R. R., "Post-penicillin jaundice." *British Medical Journal* 2 (1946): 685–688; Laird, S. M., "Prevention of syringe-transmitted hepatitis." *British Journal of Venereal Diseases* 22 (1946): 29–40; Laird, S. M., "Syringe-transmitted hepatitis." *Glasgow Medical Journal* 28 (1947): 199–219; Marcussen, P. V., "Syringe-transmitted hepatitis in venereologic clinic." *Nordic Medicine* 40 (1948): 1760–1763; Martini, G. A., "The homologous serum-hepatitis." *Deutsche Med. Wehnschr.* 74 (1949): 568–572; Memo of medical officers, Ministry of Health, "Role of syringes in the transmission of jaundice." *Lancet* 2 (1945):

116–119; Morton, R. S., "Syringe-transmitted jaundice." *British Journal of Medicine* 2 (1948): 938–939; Paul, J. R. and Havens, W. P., "Recent advances in study of infectious hepatitis and serum." *Tr. A. Amer. Physicians* 59 (1946): 133–141; Sherwood, P. M., "Outbreak of syringe-transmitted hepatitis with jaundice in hospitalized diabetic patients." *Annals of Internal Medicine* 33 (1950): 380–396; and Willcox, R. R., "Effects of syringe transmitted jaundice on outcome of treatment of yearly syphilis." *British Journal of Venereal Diseases* 23 (1947): 121–123.

192. Garrod, L. P., "Nature of meningitis following spinal anesthesia and its prevention." *British Medical Bulletin* 4 (1946): 106–108; Harris, R. C., Buxbaum, L., and Appelbaum, E., "Secondary *Bacillus pscocyaneus* infection in meningitis following intra-thecal penicillin therapy." *Journal of Laboratory and Clinical Medicine* 3 (1946): 1113–1120; Harturg, K., "Meningitis reactions caused by syringe transmitted tuberculin during therapy of tuberculosis meningitis." *Deutsche Med. Wchnschr.* 80 (1955): 195–196; and Pestel, M., "Tuberculosis transmitted by syringe." *Presse Méd.* 61 (1953): 551.

193. Baer, M. H., Fancher, J., et al., "Are organisms introduced into vials containing medication when air is injected?" *Nursing Research* 2 (1953): 23–32; Christol, D., "Transmission of infections by contaminated syringes." *Presse Méd.* 57 (1949): 1109–1112; and Taylor, E. M. and Maloney, P. J., "Sterilization of plastic syringes by formalin vapor." *Canadian Medical Association Journal* 61 (1949): 621–622.

194. McCloskey, B. P., "Report of an investigation into an outbreak of poliomyelitis in a small town remote from Melbourne." *Medical Journal of Australia* 1 (1951): 612–613.

195. Hertzberger, E., "Mass vaccination and mobile syringe service in relation to problem of serum hepatitis." *Nederl. Tidijschr. Genseek.* 97 (1953): 1906–1909; and Gross, W. O., "Pure vaccine dose in spite of using one common syringe; new construction for prevention of inoculation hepatitis and poliomyelitis." *Deutsche Med. Wchnschr.* 79 (1954): 829–831.

196. Guyer, B., Bisong, A., et al., "Injections and paralytic poliomyelitis in tropical Africa." *Bulletin of the World Health Organization* 58 (1980): 285–291; Wyatt, H., "Provocation poliomyelitis; neglected clinical observations from 1914 to 1950." *Bulletin Hist. Med.* 55 (1981): 543–557; and Wyatt, H. V., "The popularity of injecting in the Third World: Origins and consequences for poliomyelitis." *Social Science and Medicine* 19 (1984): 911–915.

197. Garrett, L., 1994, op. cit.

198. Jezek, Z., Arita, I., et al., "Four generations of probable person-to-person transmission of human monkeypox." *Journal of Epidemiology* 123 (1986): 1004–1012.

199. Hooper, E., *The River*. New York: Random House, 1999; Mann, J. M., Francis, H., et al., "HIV seroprevalence in pediatric patients 2–14 years of age." *Pediatrics* 78 (1986): 673–677; and Mann, J. M., Francis, H., et al., "HIV seroprevalence among hospital workers in Kinshasa, Zaire." *Journal of the American Medical Association* 256 (1986): 3099–3102.

200. Institute of Medicine, *The Children's Vaccine Initiative: Achieving the Vision.* Washington, D.C.: National Academy Press, 1993; and Institute of Medicine, *Adverse Events Associated with Childhood Vaccines*, 1993, op. cit.

201. World Bank. *World Development Report 1993: Investing in Health.* New York: Oxford University Press, 1993.

202. In 1947 Truman pushed through passage of the National Security Act to create two key agencies: the National Security Council (NSC) and the Central Intelligence Agency (CIA).

203. The United States successfully detonated its first hydrogen bomb on the Pacific atoll of Bikini in 1952; the Soviets followed suit in Siberia nine months later.

204. Halberstam, D., *The Fifties*. New York: Villard Books, 1993.

205. The best source of information regarding Chargoff's numbers, DNA, and the basis of modern biology is Watson, J. D., Hopkins, N. H., Roberts, J. W., et al., *Molecular Biology of the Gene*. Fourth edition. Menlo Park: Benjamin/Cummings, 1987.

206. Upton, A. C., "Radiation Carcinogenesis." In Holland, J. F. and Frei, E., *Cancer Medicine*. Second edition. Philadelphia: Lea and Freberger, 1982.

207. The author interviewed Linus and Ava Helen Pauling on three occasions during the late 1970s and 1980s and attended several speeches he gave three decades after these events, reflecting on the nuclear fallout struggle. The author also interviewed Edward Teller three times between 1981 and 1988, while a reporter for National Public Radio. See also Pauling, L., *No More War!* New York: Dodd, Mead, 1958; Pauling, L., *Linus Pauling on Science and Peace*. New York: Fund for the Republic, 1964; and Goertzel, T. and Goertzel, B., *Linus Pauling: A Life in Science and Politics*. New York: Basic Books, 1995.

208. Teller often said this in interviews at the time. See Rhodes, R., *The Making of the Atomic Bomb*. New York: Simon and Schuster, 1986.

209. The soldiers and civilians around Totskoye were killed either by the blast or, more slowly, by radiation sickness and cancer. Swiftly covered up by the KGB, none of this was revealed until after the fall of the Soviet Union.

210. In Rhodes, R., 1986, op. cit. Between 1946 and 1962 the United States conducted surface tests of 299 nuclear weapons. More than 200,000 civilians and U.S. military personnel were exposed directly to radiation in those tests. A roughly equal number of surface tests were conducted during those years by the Soviet Union, and fewer by France, England, and China. None of those governments allowed independent medical assessments of the hundreds of thousands of people who were exposed to radiation from the bombs. And details of studies done by the Atomic Energy Commission in the United States and by its counterparts in the other nuclear nations were classified, cloaked in national security secrecy.

211. In 1962 the *New England Journal of Medicine* published a landmark piece that had a profound impact on physicians and nurses in the United States. The journal used a Joint Congressional Committee on Atomic Energy study on the effects of nuclear war as the basis for a blow-by-blow hypothetical account of a nuclear attack upon Boston. Few physicians who read the article could imagine how medical services in any city could handle such a catastrophe. See Hiatt, H. H., "The clinical picture." In Adams, R. and Cullen, S., editors. *The Final Epidemic*. Chicago: Education Foundation for Nuclear Science, 1981.

212. Patterson, J. T., *Great Expectations: The United States, 1945–1974*. New York: Oxford University Press, 1996.

213. See U.S. Arms Control and Disarmament Agency. *Effects of Nuclear War*. Washington, D.C.: Government Printing Office, 1979; Goen, R. L., Brown, S. L., Clark, E. D., et al., Stanford Research Institute. *Analysis of National Entity Survival*. Sponsored by the Office of Civil Defense (SRI 7979-007), November, 1967; Mitchell, H. H., The Rand Corporation. *Guidelines for the Control of Communicable Disease in the Postattack Environment*. Sponsored by the Atomic Energy Commission (RM-5090-TAB), August, 1966; Mitchell, H. H., The Rand Corporation. *Plague in the United States: An Assessment of Its Significance as a Problem Following a Thermonuclear War*. Sponsored by the Atomic Energy Commission (RM-4868-TAB), June, 1966; Mitchell, H. H., The Rand Corporation. *The Problem of Tuberculosis in the Postattack Environment*. Sponsored by the U.S. Air Force (RM-5362-PRB), June 1967; Pogrund R. S., The Rand Corporation. *Nutrition in the Postattack Environment*. Sponsored by the Atomic Energy Commission (RM-5052-TAB), December, 1966; Johnson, T. and Johnston, D. R., Research Triangle Institute. *Vector-borne Disease and Control*. Sponsored by the Office of Civil Defense (R-OU-303), June 1968; and Voors, A. W., Research Triangle Institute. *Epi-*

demiological Considerations for the Prevention of Post Nuclear Attack Epidemics. Sponsored by the Office of Civil Defense (RM-OU-332-4), October, 1967.

For a nongovernmental perspective, see Adams, R. and Cullen, S., editors, 1981, op. cit.

214. Garrett, L., "Facilities in city did tests in 1950s." *Newsday* (December 19, 1993): Al.

215. National Research Council, *A Review of the Department of Energy Classification Policy and Practice.* Washington, D.C.: National Academy of Sciences, 1995; and National Academy of Sciences, *Finding the Balance: National Security and Scientific Openness.* Washington, D.C.: National Academy of Sciences, 1999.

216. It must be noted that organizations of American and Soviet physicians formed in the 1970s and eighties to express mutual concern about the public health horrors of nuclear war. Chief among them was the International Physicians for the Prevention of Nuclear War, which won the Nobel Peace Prize in 1985. Sharing in that honor were in the Soviet Union Dr. George Kistiakowsky and Evgeni Chazov and in the United States Dr. Bernard Lown and others.

217. In 1982, based on the meager and flawed information at its disposal, the World Health Organization estimated that a thermonuclear exchange between the United States and USSR would directly and indirectly—via radiation, epidemics, and starvation—kill two billion people. That estimate was adjusted upward in the later 1980s when a group of astronomers, physicists, atmospheric researchers, and vulcanologists set forth the nuclear winter hypothesis. In their scenario, blasts involving bombs in excess of 100 kilotons would trigger an Ice Age few species would survive.

218. In 1961 Mahoney's successor, Dr. Leona Baumgartner, stated her position on the nuclear fallout question and how it affected New Yorkers: "Widespread realization of the potential hazards of ionizing radiation grew out of atomic bomb development. While some persons and groups tried to arouse public interest and concern in problems of fallout, there were those persons and groups who tried to minimize such dangers. Their attitude was represented by those who feel it is now quite clear that the problem of fallout radiation in its various forms is one with which we must learn to live; we have no choice.

"Public discussion of fallout radiation did have the effect of calling some people's attention to the fact that there are other forms of radiation which constitute a public health problem. . . . These people felt that when the total amount of radiation to which people are exposed increases, it is both common sense and sound public health practice to take measures to reduce the amount of radiation which can be controlled."

See the commissioner's remarks in New York City Department of Health, *Report of the Department of Health, the City of New York for the Years 1959–60.* New York, 1961.

219. American Public Health Association, *Study of the Department of Health, City of New York, for the Mayor's Committee on Management Survey.* Washington, D.C., 1952.

220. Hardly anyone had a television set in 1949 in the United States. But by 1952 some 15.2 million Americans had a TV and by 1955 the number had grown to some 32 million. This had a profound impact upon news, opinion, and information. See, for example, Curtin M., *Redeeming the Wasteland.* New Brunswick: Rutgers University Press, 1995.

221. By the 1990s the average American was watching four hours of television a day and rated TV as the number one vehicle responsible for shopping and voting decisions. See Kuttner, R., *Everything for Sale.* New York: Alfred A. Knopf, 1998. A Twentieth Century Fund book.

222. Duffy, J., 1968, op. cit.

223. New York City Department of Health. *Report of the Department of Health, the City of New York for the Years 1955–56.* New York, 1957.

224. Ibid.

225. Institute of Medicine, *Treating Drug Problems.* Washington, D.C.: National Academy of Sciences, 1990.

226. Baumgartner, L., in New York City Department of Health, 1961, op. cit.

227. Duke, S. B. and Gross, A. C., *America's Longest War: Rethinking Our Tragic Crusade Against Drugs.* New York: G. P. Putnam's Sons, 1993.

228. Gray, M., 1988, op. cit.

229. Patterson, J. T., 1996, op. cit.

230. GNP numbers were as follows:

(in billions of 1958-adjusted dollars)

1950	$355.3
1957	$452.5
1960	$487.7
1966	$658.1
1970	$722.5

Per capita GNP also rose radically:

(in 1958-adjusted dollar values)

1940	$1,720
1950	$2,342
1960	$2,699
1970	$3,555

Source: Patterson, J. T. ibid.

231. In the early 1950s the National Association for the Advancement of Colored People (NAACP) went to the courts, suing for equal rights to education, jobs, and housing. In the most dramatic case, *Brown v. Board of Education*, the Supreme Court ruled to desegregate the nation's public schools. In its opinion the court opined that segregation "generates a feeling of inferiority as to the status in the community that may affect their hearts and minds in a way unlikely ever to be undone." A succession of landmark legal decisions followed, knocking down most of the old "Jim Crow" laws that had segregated everything from water fountains to cemeteries in the United States since the Civil War. A century of legal segregation was being overturned.

232. See Williams, J., *Eyes on the Prize: America's Civil Rights Years, 1954–1965.* New York: Viking, 1987.

233. Cited in Dickstein, M., *Gates of Eden.* Cambridge, Mass.: Harvard University Press, 1997.

234. Smith, D. B., 1999, op. cit.

235. Ibid.

236. For a very good, detailed history of the legal claims and racialist policies of hospitals and medical societies during this period, see Smith, D. B., 1999, op. cit.

237. Ibid. Black physicians realized, however, that, limited as it was, HEW represented their only court of appeal. The AMA consistently defended the white privileges of its southern

members, and only begrudgingly admitted African-Americans into its fraternity. Nor did it revoke the charters of state chapters that refused admission to black doctors. That action would not be taken until 1966. And the AMA would not recognize the courage of black physicians who fought to desegregate the health system—and the American Medical Association—until 1989, more than 120 years after Abraham Lincoln signed the Emancipation Proclamation.

238. Johnson, L. B., "Address Before a Joint Session of Congress." November 27, 1963.

239. *Simkins v. Moses H. Cone Memorial Hospital.* 323 F 2d. 959, 970 n. 23 (1963).

240. Ibid.

241. Walen, C. and Walen, B., *The Longest Debate: A Legislative History of the 1964 Civil Rights Act.* Washington, D.C.: Seven Locks Press, 1985.

242. U.S. involvement in Vietnam dated to the Truman administration, which, beginning in 1947, provided funds and military advisors to aid French anti-Communist activities in colonial Vietnam. By 1961, with U.S. advisors having played discreet roles in the Vietnam conflict for seven years, Kennedy ordered a clandestine escalation. In 1963 South Vietnamese president Ngo Dinh Diem was assassinated, prompting Kennedy to order some eight thousand troops into Vietnam. Still labeled "advisors," these special forces were not, technically, at war.

During Johnson's administration, the war escalated steadily, especially following a bomb blast at a U.S. base in Vietnam in early 1965. By December '65 there were 184,000 U.S troops in Vietnam. The sum reached 450,000 by the end of 1966 and half a million in 1967. By early 1968 an estimated 130,000 U.S. military personnel were dead, wounded, or missing in action.

By November 1967, LBJ's approval rating was below 26 percent in national polls and few Americans believed that the administration or the Pentagon had a winnable strategy in place. On March 3, 1968, a thoroughly exhausted and defeated Lyndon Baines Johnson announced that he would step down at the end of his term, not seeking reelection. The war would continue under the Nixon administration, ending on May 1, 1975, as defeated South Vietnamese leaders and U.S. personnel scrambled onto the roof of the U.S. Embassy in Saigon to board the helicopters that offered their only means to escape advancing NLF troops.

243. Goodwin, D. K., *Lyndon Johnson and the American Dream.* New York: Harper and Row, 1976.

244. Numbers, R. L., "The third party: Health insurance in America." In Leavitt, J. W. and Numbers, R. L., 1985, op. cit.

245. A term invented by the American Medical Association but widely popularized by the Church of Christ, Scientist, during the early twentieth century. In California, physicians' opposition to competition and middle-class abhorrence of "commie medicine" may have reached its zenith in the 1930s when the Great Depression hit, and middle-class residents of Kern County flooded the public hospital and attendance at private facilities plummeted. The doctors cried unfair competition, and local anti–"socialized medicine" forces declared that Kern County had de facto created a universal health care system. California's supreme court ruled in 1934 that county hospitals statewide could *only* render care to impoverished patients. In other words, the court said public hospitals weren't for the middle class. That ruling went unchallenged for nearly four decades, radically skewing health care in California for the rest of the century. See "The political creation of the voluntary ideal." In Stevens R., 1989, op. cit.

246. In 1904 Biggs wrote: "It is estimated that the value of every life on the average in this country is not less than $2,000; the cost of each life to the community at twenty years of

age is at least that amount. The six thousand deaths from tuberculosis saved during the last year as compared with the number which would have occurred had the death rate been the same as it was in 1886, means the saving in the city of lives worth twelve million dollars. If we add to this sum the cost of sickness and the loss of the services and wages of these persons during the long illness, averaging at least six months, we have an additional cost of at least $300, making $1,800,000 more, or a total saving to the city during 1902, as compared to 1886 . . . of nearly $14,000,000. The total appropriation made by the Board of Estimate for the maintenance of the Department of Health for the year 1902 was $984,391.48. There can be no question, I believe, as to the fact that no expenditure made by a nation, city or community brings such large returns to the community in health, happiness and prosperity as that made for the conduct of its sanitary affairs. These expenditures bring returns not of three or five or even ten percent, but of one hundred, five hundred, and one thousand percent."

It was a classic cost/benefit rationale for public health, written eight decades before such monetary arguments would become essential components of all government health programs. New York City Department of Health, 1904, op. cit.

247. McKeown, T., 1979, op. cit.

248. All these life expectancy data come from U.S. Bureau of the Census, 1976, op. cit.

249. By 1970 average life expectancies at birth would be 59.9 years for men and 63.9 for women. Remaining years for sixty-year-old Americans would average 31.9 for men and 38.3 for women. In 1995 average life expectancies at birth were 72.5 years for men and 78.9 years for women. Men would have gained 11.7 years since 1970; women, 13.7 years.

250. Evans, R. G. and Stoddart, G. L., "Producing health, consuming health care." In Evans, R. G., Barer, M. L., and Marmor, T. R., *Why Are Some People Healthy and Others Not?* New York: Aldine de Gruyter, 1994.

251. Dr. Leona Baumgartner, New York City Commissioner of Health, 1961, in Baumgartner, L., 1961, op. cit.

252. That question remains highly debatable today. As the world faces a resurgent tuberculosis epidemic—particularly in Russia—it is critical to understand to what degree antibiotics versus environmental factors (housing, nutrition, etc.) can play a role in control of TB. Many explanations have been forwarded, including sanitariums, nutrition, and housing, but there remains today no consensus as to what factor(s) pushed TB incidence down during the first half of the twentieth century.

See McKeown T., 1979, op. cit.; and Evans, R. G. and Stoddart, G. L., 1994, op. cit.

253. See Garrett, L., 1994, op. cit.; and Webster, R. G., "Influenza." In Morse, S. S., *Emerging Viruses.* New York: Oxford University Press, 1993.

254. Dubos, R., 1961, op. cit.

255. One way to picture the dilemma is to ask, "Did the massive medicalization of society after 1965 push the population's health significantly beyond the trajectory it had already been on since 1900?"

256. Some such linkages would, indeed, emerge, because their overlapping interests so clearly put Medicaid, Medicare, AFDC, and other poverty programs in logical conjunction at the local level. But they would be a matter of happenstance, not of high-level planning.

257. Gornick, M., "Ten Years of Medicare: Impact on the Covered Population." *Social Security Bulletin* 39 (July 1976): 19.

258. Starr, P., 1982, op. cit.

259. Matusow, A., *The Unraveling of America: A History of Liberalism in the 1960s.* New York: Harper and Row, 1964.

260. Stevens, R., 1989, op. cit.

261. Between 1964 and 1981 the average costs of treating some procedures rose as follows:

Procedure/Illness	Percent of Cost Increase
Breast cancer	324
Childbirth	313
MI (heart attack)	420
Appendicitis	350

See Scitovsky, A. A. and McCall, N., "Changes in the Cost of Treatment of Selected Illnesses, 1951–1964–1971." *Health Policy Program, Palo Alto Medical Research Program*, 10 (August 1975): 17.

262. Smith, D. B., 1999, op. cit.

263. U.S. Census of Housing, 1966; *Los Angeles Times*. Marketing Research Department. *Market Data: Los Angeles Marketing Area, 1969*; U.S. Bureau of the Census. "Characteristics of the South and of East Los Angeles Areas, November 1965." *Current Population Reports*. Series P-23. No. 18. Washington, D.C., 1966.

264. Since World War II the densities of both neighborhoods had steadily increased as blacks migrated from the Deep South to Los Angeles and Hispanics flowed in from Mexico. The most densely populated neighborhood, Watts, had 14,000 residents per square mile, compared to the county average of 1,744.

265. These and subsequent Los Angeles health statistics come from Merrill, M. H., *Future Directions for Health Services: County of Los Angeles/1970*. Los Angeles: Los Angeles County Board of Supervisors, 1970.

266. Ibid.

267. White, R., 1991, op. cit.

268. The driver was twenty-one-year-old Marquette Frye. He was pulled over by LAPD officers in front of his home and Frye's family got into a shouting match with the officers. The officers placed the entire family under arrest, which sparked the riotous response of their neighbors.

269. Ibid. An estimated 30,000 citizens had participated in the riots, and another 60,000 had stood watch, often egging the rioters on with cries of "Burn, baby, burn!" Patterson, J. T., 1996, op. cit. No one, from the reporters on the scene for the *Los Angeles Times* to President Johnson, could view that outpouring of rage without realizing that something in America was terribly, terribly wrong. Governor's Commission on the Los Angeles Riots, *Violence in the City—An End or a Beginning?* Sacramento, 1965. At all tiers of government, the Watts riots forced a period of soul-searching and reappraisal. For white California voters, the riots, coupled with widespread unrest on the state's university campuses, seemed to cry out for a tough response. In 1966 the electorate rejected liberal incumbent Governor Pat Brown in favor of ultra-conservative ex–movie star Ronald Reagan.

270. For more details on Los Angeles County government, see Abernathy, B. and White, A., "The Invisible Growth Machine." *Los Angeles Times* West (May 28, 1972): 7–15.

271. According to Abernathy and White, the supervisors oversaw a 1972 budget of $2.7 billion. At their disposal were 72,000 county employees, 768 buildings (with 300 more in the planning stages), 11 miles of beachfront property, and the largest county jail in the world (housing 200,000 inmates annually) staffed by the world's biggest county police force (4, 553 officers).

272. Between 1913 and 1972 only twenty men (and no women) served as Los Angeles County supervisors.

273. Merrill, M. H., 1972, op. cit.

274. Ibid.

275. Though first seen acutely in Los Angeles, the ER crisis became a national phe-nomenon that by the end of the 1980s constituted a life-threatening fiscal drain on many urban public hospitals. By 1995 there would be 5,700 ER units in the United States, treating 90 million people a year. By far the majority of them were publicly funded facilities. See Weiss, L. D., 1997, op. cit.

276. In 1968 the county spent $215 million on hospital care and upkeep, $23 million on public health programs, and $16 million on mental health programs.

277. Even before the closure of state institutions, the ranks of L.A.'s needy mentally ill had been growing. They represented 79,133 patient visits to county facilities in 1963 and 566,013 in 1968.

278. Merrill, M. H., 1972, op. cit.

279. Brandt, A. M., 1987, op. cit.

280. In 1948 psychologist Alfred Kinsey released his first of several controversial re-ports on sexual behavior in the United States. Kinsey found that nearly half of all college-aged men he interviewed that year had had premarital sex. In 1953 Kinsey released a similar report on college women, 20 percent of whom had had premarital sexual intercourse. By 1968 those numbers were up to 55 percent for men and 44 percent for women.

Kinsey, A., *Sexual Behavior in the Human Female* and *Sexual Behavior in the Human Male*. Philadelphia: W. B. Saunders, 1948. The Kinsey reports were later followed by the far more controversial studies by William Masters and Virginia Johnson, *Sexual Response* in 1966 and *Human Sexual Inadequacy* in 1970.

281. For examples, see Friedan, B., *The Feminine Mystique*. New York: Norton, 1963; Gitlin, T., *The Sixties: Years of Hope, Days of Rage*. New York: Bantam Books, 1987; Millet, K., *Sexual Politics*. New York: Simon & Schuster, 1990; Greer, G., *The Female Eunuch*. New York: McGraw-Hill, 1971.

282. Garrett, L., 1994, op. cit.

283. Minnesota Department of Health, *Healthy People: The Minnesota Experience*. Minneapolis: Minnesota Center for Health Statistics, 1982.

284. I have written extensively elsewhere about the STD trends that preceded emer-gence of AIDS. I refer readers to Garrett, L., 1994, op. cit.; and Brandt, A. M., 1987, op. cit.

285. Carson, R., *Silent Spring*. Boston: Houghton Mifflin, 1962.

286. The Environmental Protection Agency (EPA, created in 1970), the Food and Drug Administration (FDA), the Occupational Safety and Health Administration (OSHA), the Na-tional Institute of Occupational Safety and Health (NIOSH), the Centers for Disease Control and Prevention (CDC), and the National Cancer Institute (NCI).

287. U.S. Bureau of the Census, 1976, op. cit.

288. Mullan, F., 1989, op. cit.

289. U.S. Surgeon General's Advisory Committee on Smoking and Health, *Smoking and Health: Report of the Advisory Committee to the Surgeon General of the Public Health Service*. PHS No. 1103. Washington, D.C.: Government Printing Office, 1964.

290. Hilts, P., *Smokescreen: The Truth Behind the Tobacco Industry Cover-Up*. Reading, Mass: Addison-Wesley, 1996; Kluger, R., *Ashes to Ashes: America's Hundred-Year Cigarette War, the Public Health and the Unabashed Triumph of Philip Morris*. New York: Alfred A. Knopf, 1996; and Orey, M., *Assuming the Risk: The Mavericks, the Lawyers and the Whistle-Blowers Who Beat Big Tobacco*. Boston: Little, Brown, 1999.

By the mid-sixties more than half of all men and a third of all women in the United States were cigarette smokers.

291. For example, Larry Agran's 1977 bestseller *The Cancer Connection* (New York: Houghton Mifflin) makes *no* references to tobacco or smoking, attributing 90 percent of all U.S. cancer incidence to environmental and occupational pollutants.

The cigarette versus pollution dilemma was better stated in 1973 by chemist Jeanne Stellman and physician Susan Daum. See Stellman, J. M. and Daum, S. M., *Work Is Dangerous to Your Health*. New York: Vintage, 1973.

292. Koop, C. E., *Koop: The Memoirs of America's Family Doctor*. New York: Random House, 1991.

293. In the 1980s California and Massachusetts pioneered the most successful anti-smoking campaigns, deploying Madison Avenue techniques. Both states levied heavy taxes on tobacco sales and used the revenue to purchase prime television time and billboard space for highly sophisticated, often ironic, ads. The ad campaigns proved effective in reducing smoking levels in the two states below those in the rest of the United States, and in reducing the numbers of new smokers emerging annually among teenagers. See Centers for Disease Control and Prevention, "Cigarette smoking before and after an excise tax increase and antismoking campaign." *Morbidity and Mortality Weekly Report* 45 (1996): 966–970.

294. For a very accessible delineation of the biology of tobacco addiction, see Goldstein, A., *Addiction: From Biology to Drug Policy*. New York: W. H. Freeman, 1994.

295. Koop, C. E., 1991, op. cit.

296. Centers for Disease Control and Prevention, "Cigarette smoking—attributable mortality and years of potential life lost—United States, 1990." *Morbidity and Mortality Weekly Report* 42 (1993): 645–649. The CDC also estimated that if 1990 smoking levels continued, the generation born between 1978 and 1995 would eventually suffer 5 million deaths due to smoking, costing $50 billion a year in medical treatment and $1.4 billion annually in lost productivity and other indirect costs.

297. U.S. Department of Health and Human Services, *Healthy People 2010 Objectives: Draft for Public Comment*. Washington, D.C.: Office of Public Health and Science, 1998.

298. Office of Smoking and Health, *Reducing the Health Consequences of Smoking: 25 Years of Progress. A Report to the Surgeon General*. DHHS Pub. No. 89-8411. Washington, D.C.: U.S. Department of Health and Human Services, 1989.

299. U.S. Public Health Service, *Healthy People 2000*. Washington, D.C.: U.S. Department of Health and Human Services, 1990.

300. Heuper, W. C., *Occupational and Environmental Cancers of the Urinary System*. New Haven: Yale University Press, 1969. The du Pont company acknowledged in 1976 that 339—17 percent—of the 2,000 dye workers who had used these two chemicals between 1919 and 1955 developed bladder cancer. By any measure, that was a phenomenal and tragic cancer rate.

301. Without cheap and reliable ways to measure levels of not only pollutants but also their often more lethal chemical breakdown products, the state and federal regulatory agencies were chewing at the problem with toothless gums. According to the U.S. Toxic Chemical Release Inventory, some eighteen years after creation of the EPA, 2.6 billion pounds of toxic chemicals would still be released in the environment annually, including 0.24 billion pounds of compounds that were classified as human carcinogens. National air pollution standards would go unmet at 101 sites (including Los Angeles County and metropolitan New York), routinely exceeding permissible levels of carbon monoxides and ozone. And the American Lung Association would conclude that in the United States air pollution was annually responsible for up to 120,000 premature deaths and medical costs of $50 billion a year. Air pollution would be named the chief cause of a U.S. asthma epidemic throughout the later twentieth century, with asthma hospitalization rates among children rising from about 180

per 100,000 youngsters in 1970 to 284 per 100,000 in 1987. American Lung Association, *Health Care Costs of Air Pollution*, third edition. New York: American Lung Association, 1990; National Heart, Lung and Blood Institute, *Infomemo* (December 1989; U.S. Department of Health and Human Services, *Healthy People 2000*, 1990, op. cit.

302. For examples of various positions, see Agran L., 1977, op. cit.; Arrow, K. J., Cropper, M. L., Eado, G. C., et al., "Is there a role for benefit-cost analysis in environmental, health and safety regulation?" *Science* 272 (1996): 221–222; Burke, T. A., Shalauta, N. M., and Tran, N. L., "Strengthening the role of public health in environmental policy." *Policy Studies Journal* 23 (1995): 76–85; Centers for Disease Control and Prevention, "Public health focus: Effectiveness of disease and injury prevention." *Morbidity and Mortality Weekly Report* 46 (1997): 73–76; Committee on the Institutional Means for Assessment of Risks to Public Health. Commission on Life Sciences. National Research Council. *Risk Assessment in the Federal Government: Managing the Process*. Washington, D.C.: National Academy Press, 1983; Lare, L. B., "Fixing the system." In Burke, T. A., Tran, N. L., et al, editors, *Regulating Risk: The Science and Politics of Risk*. Washington, D.C.: International Life Sciences Institute Press, 1993; Mott, L. and Snyder, K., *Pesticide Alert: A Guide to Pesticides in Fruits and Vegetables*. San Francisco: Sierra Club Books, 1987; *National Resources Defense Council v. Environmental Protection Agency* 824F .2d 1211 (D.C. Cir., 1987); Oakley, G. P. and Heath, C. W., "Cancer, environmental health, and birth defects—examples of new directions in public health practice." *American Journal of Epidemiology* 144 (1996): S58–S64; Pershagen, G., "Environmental epidemiology in public health." *Lancet* 352 (1998): 417; Rabe, B. G., *Fragmentation and Integration in State Environmental Management*. Washington, D.C.: The Conservative Foundation, 1986; Silbergeld, E. K., "A proposal for overcoming paralysis in improving risk regulation." In Burke, T. A., et al., editors, 1993, op. cit.; Stellman, J. M. and Daum, S. M., 1973, op. cit.; Thacker, S. B., Stroup, D. F., and Parrish, G., et al., "Surveillance in environmental public health: Issues, systems, and sources." *American Journal of Public Health* 86 (1996): 633–638; Van Den Bosch, R., *The Pesticide Conspiracy*. New York: Doubleday, 1978; Weir, D. and Schapiro, M., *Circle of Poison*. San Francisco: Institute for Food and Development Policy, 1981.

303. U.S. Department of Health and Human Services, *Healthy People 2000*, 1990, op. cit.

304. The landmark history of the Pill by Barbara Seaman was recently re-released in a twenty-fifth anniversary edition: Seaman, B., *The Doctors' Case Against the Pill*. Twenty-fifth Anniversary edition. New York: Hunter House, 1995.

305. By 1964 there were reports of thirty-seven deaths on file at the FDA. By 1968 the FDA had been receiving twenty to forty death reports per year. In 1968 the FDA ordered Searle and other birth control manufacturers to put warnings inside packages of the Pill: "Be alert to earliest manifestations of thrombotic disorders," the warning began, detailing the apparent risks.

306. Murad, F. and Kuret, J. A., "Estrogens and progestins." In Gilman, A. G., Rall, T. W., Nies, A. S., et al., *The Pharmacological Basis of Therapeutics*. Eighth edition. New York: Pergamon Press, 1990.

307. For details on the DES saga, see Dutton, D. B., 1988, op. cit.; Institute of Medicine, *Drug Efficacy Study*. Washington, D.C.: National Academy Press, 1967; Henig, R. M., 1997, op. cit.; Meyers, R., *DES: The Bitter Pill*. New York: Putnam, 1983; and Subcommittee of the Committee on Government Operations. House of Representatives. 92nd Cong., 1st Sess. November 11, 1971.

308. Herbst, A. L., Ulfelder, H., and Poskanzer, D. C., "Adenocarcinoma of the vagina." *New England Journal of Medicine* 284 (1971): 878–881.

309. By 1998 the company would only recommend use of DES for two purposes: treatments of breast and prostate carcinomas. And it would specifically warn, in bold type: "DIETHYLSTILBESTEROL SHOULD NOT BE USED FOR ANY PURPOSE DURING PREGNANCY. ITS USE MAY CAUSE SEVERE HARM TO THE FETUS." *Physicians Desk Reference.* Forty-third edition. Oradell, N.J.: Medical Economics Company, 1989.

310. Dutton, D. B., *Worse Than the Disease: Pitfalls of Medical Progress.* New York: Cambridge University Press, 1988. Dutton notes: "The DES story raises a number of larger issues about medicine's role in society and the limits of regulatory safeguards. It reveals a pattern of deeply ingrained optimism about the benefits of medical science in solving perceived social needs, a cultural outlook shared by groups as diverse as doctors, farmers, scientists, and college coeds. So great was the optimism enveloping DES that it allowed an almost willful disregard of the abundant evidence of risk."

The FDA also appeared to come up short in its regulation of artificial sweeteners. In 1969, based only on laboratory animal studies, it found cyclamates to be carcinogenic and banned their sale in the United States. But in 1977, when faced with even stronger evidence of laboratory-tested carcinogenicity for the next big sweetener, saccharin, the FDA responded to public support of the noncaloric sweetener and allowed it to remain on the market. Henig, R. M., 1997, op. cit.

311. Patterson, J. T., 1996, op. cit.

312. "Nixon proposals vs. 'Health Security': The issues shape up." *Hospital Practice* (April 1971): 22–38.

313. Fein, R., "What direction for national health insurance?" *Hospital Practice* (August 1970): 67–72.

314. "Nixon proposals vs. 'Health Security': The issues shape up," 1971, op. cit.

315. Starr, P., 1982, op. cit.

316. For a thumbnail history of HMOs, see Mayer, T. R. and Mayer, G. G., "HMOs: Origins and development." *New England Journal of Medicine* 312 (1985): 590–594.

317. Senators Abe Ribicoff, a Connecticut Democrat, and Russell Long, a conservative Louisiana Democrat, offered the Catastrophic Health Insurance and Medical Assistance Reform Act of 1973. It was backed by Nixon's presidential opponent, Senator George McGovern, a South Dakota Democrat.

318. The Medicredit plan, which offered vouchers for health care so that consumers could shop around to private doctors.

319. The AHA wanted the Hill-Burton Act extended and provisions lifted that LBJ had amended to the act. Those provisions required recipient medical facilities to offer free care to indigent patients, comprising a minimum of 5 percent of their clientele.

320. The Democrat's McGovern campaign had several offices inside the Watergate Hotel in Washington, D.C. A team calling themselves "the Plumbers" broke into those offices with the intent to steal campaign information and place electronic eavesdropping devices. They were arrested for simple thievery, but a trail of disclosures over subsequent months, largely in the pages of the *Washington Post*, revealed that the Plumbers were in the employ of the Campaign to Reelect the President, and orders for their activities, as well as other subterfuges against the Democrats, had come directly from the White House. In 1973 these revelations unfolded almost daily, all but paralyzing the administration as it scrambled to destroy evidence, cover its tracks, and concoct false defenses to deliver to Congress. By 1974 many members of Nixon's own party leadership were calling for his resignation or impeachment, and members of his administration faced indictment. It was under this cloud that Nixon resigned in August, 1974.

321. Mayer, T. R. and Mayer, G. G., 1985, op. cit.

322. For a sense of the changes then under way see "Administration seeks to shift Medicare cuts to elderly." *Hospital Practice* (March 1973): 182–187; "Auditing ambulatory care." *Hospital Practice* (June 1974): 155–160; Gold, M. R. and Rosenberg, R. G., "Use of emergency room services by the population of a neighborhood health center." *Health Services Reports* 89 (1974): 65–70; "Kennedy-Mills: A new pairing on the health insurance front." *Hospital Practice* (June 1974): 176–184; "The kidney care issue: A test for national health insurance?" *Hospital Practice* (April 1973): 49–59; "The Nixon budget crisis—one medical school's 'share.'" Editorial. *Hospital Practice* (August 1973): 4–5; "Two senators offer 'middle way' national health insurance package." *Hospital Practice* (January 1974): 209–210; Weil, M. H. and Carlson, R. W., "Priorities governing the care of the critically ill." *Hospital Practice* (September 1976): 67–76; and "Will health care price freeze, warm, or chill the voters?" *Hospital Practice* (September 1972): 167–171.

323. Rogers, D. E. and Blendon, R. J., "The changing American health scene: Sometimes things get better." *Journal of the American Medical Association* 237 (1977): 1710 –1714.

324. As quoted in Baum, D., *Smoke and Mirrors: The War on Drugs and the Politics of Failure.* Boston: Little, Brown, 1996.

325. Ibid.

326. Ibid.

327. National Commission on Marijuana and Drug Abuse, *Evaluating the Social Impact of Drug Dependence.* Washington, D.C., 1972.

328. In 1989 James Ostrowski of the Cato Institute estimated the following had been true every year since 1969:

Drug	Number of Users	Deaths Annually	Death Rate Per 100,000
Tobacco	60 million	390,000	650
Alcohol	100 million	150,000	150
Heroin	500 thousand	400	80
Cocaine	5 million	200	4

See Duke, S. B. and Gross, A. C., 1993, op. cit.

A differing estimate of drug use rates put the number of heroin users in 1955 at about fifty-five thousand and the total in 1987 at 1.5 million. Those figures would indicate that Nixon's War on Drugs policy had utterly failed. See Institute of Medicine, *Treating Drug Problems.* Vol. I. Washington, D.C.: National Academy Press, 1990.

329. Payne, L., Royce, K., Greene, B., et al., *The Heroin Trail.* New York: Holt, Rinehart and Winston, 1974.

330. Duke, S. B. and Gross, A. C., 1994, op. cit.

331. There was little data to support this idea. Heroin users were not, in reality, significantly more crime-prone than the rest of society and often less prone to commit felony crimes than was the adult norm in the community in which they resided. See Institute of Medicine, 1990, op. cit.

332. Eventually the Special Action Office was dovetailed into the National Institute on Drug Abuse (NIDA), created in 1973.

333. Massing, M., *The Fix: Under the Nixon Administration America Had an Effective Drug Policy. WE SHOULD RESTORE IT. (Nixon Was Right).* New York: Simon and Schuster, 1998.

334. Because the author and others have detailed these emerging diseases issues elsewhere, the presentation here is deliberately superficial. For more information on infectious

diseases issues during the 1960–1990 time frame, see Biddle, W., *A Field Guide to Germs*. New York: Henry Holt, 1995; Centers for Disease Control and Prevention. *CDC and the Smallpox Crusade*. Washington, D.C.: U.S. Department of Health and Human Services, 1987; Fenner, F., Hendersen, D. A., Arita, I., et al. *Smallpox and Its Eradication*. Geneva, World Health Organization, 1988; Foege, W. H., "Alexander D. Langmuir—his impact on public health." *American Journal of Epidemiology* 144 (1996): S11–S15; Garrett, L., 1994, op. cit.; Henig, R. M., *A Dancing Matrix*. New York: Alfred Knopf, 1993; Institute of Medicine, *Emerging Infection: Microbial Threats to Health in the United States*. Washington, D.C.: National Academy Press, 1992; Karlen, A., *Man and Microbes*. New York: Putnam, 1995; McCormick, J. B. and Fisher-Hoch, S, *Level 4:Virus Hunters of the CDC*. Atlanta: Turner, 1996; Morse, S. S., editor, 1993, op. cit.; Preston, R., *The Hot Zone*. New York: Random House, 1994; Regis, E., *Virus Ground Zero*. New York: Pocket Books, 1996; and Wilson, M. E., Levins, R., Spielman, A., "Disease in Evolution." *Annals of the New York Academy of Sciences* 740 (1994).

335. This is, of course, described in greater detail in Chapter 2 of this book and in the chapter entitled "Yambuku" in Garrett, L., 1994, op. cit.

336. For more about smallpox eradication, see Chapter 5 of this book and the smallpox selections cited above.

337. Neustadt, R. E. and Fineberg, H. V., *The Swine Flu Affair: Decision-Making on a Slippery Slope*. Washington, D.C.: U.S. Department of Health, Education and Welfare, 1978.

338. The CDC had no way of knowing whether the 1976 virus was, indeed, anything like the 1918 one because there was no sample of the old killer to which they could compare the new influenza. But because both flus induced antibody reactions against pig antigens in infected people, there was a worrisome swine link between the two. Flu strains that had arisen from pigs were thought by experts to be the most dangerous to people.

339. Guillan-Barré syndrome was a poorly understood nerve disorder that led to inflammation of major nerves, paralysis, pain, and other neurological symptoms. Nobody knew the cause of Guillan-Barré syndrome, but a certain number of people came down with it all the time. By examining thousands of medical records, Osterholm determined that there had been a slight increase in the number of Guillan-Barré cases among vaccine recipients in Minnesota compared to those who declined to get the flu immunization. The difference was 9.7 additional syndrome cases per one million vaccinated Minnesotans.

Safranek, T. J., Lawrence, D. N., Kurland, L. T., et al., "Reassessment of the association between Guillan-Barré Syndrome and receipt of Swine Influenza vaccine in 1976–1977: Results of a two-state study." *American Journal of Epidemiology* 133 (1991): 940–951.

340. See Bloom, B. R., "The United States needs a national vaccine authority." *Science* 265 (1994): 1377–1380; Citizens Against Government Waste, *An Ounce of Prevention: Why Congress Should Repeal the Vaccines for Children Program*. Washington, D.C.: Citizens Against Government Waste, 1994; Cohen, J., "Bumps on the vaccine road." *Science* 265 (1994): 1371–1375; Douglas, G. R., "The Children's Vaccine Initiative: Will it work?" *Journal of Infectious Diseases* 168 (1993): 269–274; Gibbons, A., "Children's Vaccine Initiative stumbles." *Science* 265 (1994): 1376–1377; Institute of Medicine, *The Children's Vaccine Initiative: Achieving the Vision*. Washington, D.C.: National Academy Press, 1993; Katz, S. and Gellin, B. G., "Measles vaccine: Do we need new vaccines or new programs?" *Science* 265 (1994): 1391–1392; Nowak, R., "U.S. national program is going nowhere fast." *Science* 265 (1994): 1374–1376; Pear, R., "Serious troubles are found in federal vaccine program." *New York Times* (July 17, 1994): A16; Sternberg, S. "Bottleneck keeps existing vaccine off market." *Science* 266 (1994): 22–23; U.S. Department of Health and Human Services, *Disease Prevention through Vaccine Development and Immunization: The U.S. National Vaccination Plan—1974*. Washington, D.C.: National Vaccine Program Office, 1994; U.S. General Accounting Office. *Vac-*

cines for Children. GAO/PEMD-95-22. Washington, D.C.: Government Printing Office, 1995; "Vaccines: Big shots." *The Economist* (May 9, 1998): 63; Vagelos, P. R., "A shot in the (wrong) arm." *New York Times,* (April 20, 1993): editorial; and World Health Organization, *State of the World's Vaccines and Immunization.* Geneva: World Health Organization, 1996.

341. Hilleman, M., Presentation to the Institute of Medicine, October 6, 1995.

342. In 1987 the National Academy of Sciences convened a high-powered meeting to discuss strategies for developing a vaccine against HIV. The shadow of the swine flu fiasco eleven years previously hung over the meeting as scientists argued how to perform the seemingly impossible task of generating a safe, 100 percent effective vaccine against a retrovirus.

Scientists interjected comments regarding the far greater genetics and molecular biology capabilities of 1987, versus those that were at Salk's disposal for polio in 1950.

"I'm sure you could genetically engineer anything," Maurice Hilleman of Merck pharmaceutical company said. "But who would take liability? Who could guarantee a [virus] vaccine wouldn't recombine in a patient? It comes down to law. The science is good, but the possibility of providing safety insurmountable."

343. Influenza is an avian virus normally found in migratory aquatic birds. In its avian-adapted form, the virus is rarely infectious to human beings and can never, so far as is known, spread from person to person. Human epidemics involve an intermediary species, typically pigs, in which the avian influenza reproduces and mutates into a form adapted to mammals.

China offers ideal circumstances for such viral events because most rural and even urban households raise ducks and pigs, usually housed beside one another in crowded pens. See Webster, R. G., "Influenza." In Morse, S., 1993, op. cit.

344. Cox, N., Comments to the World Health Organization/National Institutes of Allergy and Infectious Diseases (WHO/NIAID) meeting, "Pandemic Influenza: Confronting a Re-emergent Threat," Bethesda, Maryland, December 11–13, 1995.

345. Prior to 1991 the U.S. military had a vast flu surveillance network of its own that took advantage of troop placement in far flung places to sample emerging flu strains. This served as a strong complement to the civilian WHO system. But following the collapse of the Soviet Union, Congress ordered several rounds of budget reductions for the Department of Defense. One of the casualties of this was the military influenza network which, by 1999, had been gradually phased out to a point where it was meager-to-nonexistent, according to the U.S. Army.

346. Meltzer, M. and Cox, N., Data presented at the First International Conference on Emerging Diseases, Atlanta, Georgia, March 8, 1998. Kolata, G. *Flu.* New York: Farrar, Straus Giroux, 1999.

347. Patriarca, P., Comments to the WHO/NIAID meeting, 1995, op. cit.

348. Dowdle, W., Comments to the WHO/NIAID meeting, 1995, op. cit.

349. This is described in greater detail in Garrett, L., 1994, op. cit.

350. Centers for Disease Control and Prevention. *Summary of Notifiable Diseases, United States, 1997.* Atlanta: U.S. Department of Health and Human Services, CDC, 1997.

351. Carter, J., *Keeping Faith: Memories of a President.* New York: Bantam, 1982.

352. The details were as follows: at four o'clock in the morning a water pump for the reactor cooling system shut down. The reactor continued to run at full power. This allowed superhot water to build up in the system, creating explosive pressure. An automatic pressure release gauge vented the radioactive steam and shut down the reactor. The pressure gauge failed to close, as it was supposed to in such incidents. Radioactive steam and water continued gushing out of the system. Back-up cooling switches failed to automatically switch on to counter the steam pressure, but control panel readings mistakenly indicated that cooling was under way. With the core still superhot, another emergency system poured coolant into

the core, but power plant engineers misunderstood what was going on and shut off that back-up cooler pump. Steam spewed out and a primary fuel rod cracked. Meltdown started, and radioactive gases were emitted into the air outside the power plant.

To understand how such power plants work, see Nero, A. V., *A Guidebook to Nuclear Reactors*. Berkeley: University of California Press, 1979.

353. Further fueling suspicions were Jimmy Carter's background and the energy crisis. Carter had served as an engineer on a nuclear submarine while in the U.S. Navy and was supportive of the nuclear power industry. And the ongoing energy crisis had prompted special considerations from Congress for the nuclear industry.

354. Booth, W., "Postmortem on Three Mile Island." *Science* 238 (December 4, 1987); Del Tredici, R., *The People of Three Mile Island*. San Francisco: Sierra Club Books, 1980; Gray, M., "What really happened at Three Mile Island." *Rolling Stone* (May 17, 1979); May, J. *Nuclear Age*. New York: Pantheon Books, 1989; Stephens, M., *Three Mile Island*. New York: Junction Books, 1980; and Torrey, L., "The week they almost lost Pennsylvania." *New Scientist* (April 4, 1979).

355. Days after the Shah of Iran, a long-standing U.S. ally, arrived in the United States for medical treatment, his rule was overthrown in Iran and student militants seized the U.S. Embassy, taking the entire staff hostage. The new Iranian government of Ayatollah Khomeini gave the students its full support and the hostages remained in captivity inside the embassy throughout the rest of 1979 and all of 1980, On September 22, 1980, the Iraqi government of Saddam Hussein invaded Iran, sparking the bloodiest Middle East conflict of the twentieth century. Possibly because it had its hands full with that war, Iran agreed to release the U.S. hostages. It did so on the day of Ronald Reagan's inauguration, snatching, in a final gesture of humiliation, the credit from Carter.

As a result of the Iran and Iraq tensions, the crisis of oil pricing and availability worsened during the Carter years. And that fed inflation.

356. Carter, J., 1982, op. cit.

357. Ibid.

358. Starr, P., 1982, op. cit.

359. "It's time to operate." *Fortune* 81 (1970): 79.

360. Folland, S., Goodman, A. C., and Stano, M., *The Economics of Health and Health Care*. New York: Macmillan, 1993.

361. Feldman, R., "Competition among physicians, revisited." *Journal of Health, Politics, Policy and Law* 13 (1988): 239–261; McMenamin, P., "A crime storm from Medicare Part B." *Health Affairs* (Winter 1988): 94–101; and Rice, T. H., "The impact of changing Medicare reimbursement rates on physician-induced demand." *Medical Care* 21 (1983): 803–815.

362. Cooper, B. and Rice, D., *The Economic Cost of Illness Revisited*. Washington, D.C.: National Center for Health Statistics, U.S. Public Health Service, HEW, 1976.

363. *Source*: Health Care Financing Administration.

364. Ibid.

365. Dorothy Rice kindly provided me with her data on June 10, 1983, during an interview. Her numbers were as follows:

Covered Percentages	1950	1960	1970	1980
From philanthropy and industry	2.9	2.3	1.6	1.4
From government	22.4	21.8	34.4	40.4
From private health insurance	9.1	21.1	24.1	26.2
Direct out-of-pocket payment	65.5	54.9	40.0	32.0

366. As early as 1970 some hospitals were getting away with billing Medicare and private insurance companies $500 a day for hospital rooms. While these were intensive care rooms, in 1970 that sum could have rented out an entire floor of the poshest hotel in Manhattan, complete with servants, room service, and a panoramic view of Central Park. See "Intensive care units and the $500-a-day hospital." *Hospital Practice* (August 1971): 22–31.

367. Krant, M. J., "The organized care of the dying patient." *Hospital Practice* (January 1972): 101–108. By 1965 nearly half of all deaths were occurring in hospitals, compared to a third in 1937. Scitovsky, A. A., " 'The high cost of dying': What do the data show?" *Milbank Quarterly* 62 (1984): 591–608. Within just two years of its enactment, the 5 percent of Medicare recipients who died were absorbing 22 percent of all the program's expenditures. Piro, P. A. and Lutins, T., "Utilization and reimbursement under Medicare for persons who died in 1967 and 1968." *Health Insurance Statistics*. Pub. No. SSA-74-11702. Washington, D.C.: U.S. Department of Health, Education and Welfare, October 17, 1969. A 1978 study got similar results: 5.9 percent of the Medicare population, mostly terminally ill patients, that year absorbed 27.9 percent of the agency's health expenditures. Lubitz, J. and Prihoda, R., "The use and costs of Medicare services in the last two years of life." *Health Care Financing Review* 5 (1984): 117–131.

368. "Can 'health maintenance' plan brake runaway Medi-costs?" *Hospital Practice* (May 1970): 19–28.

369. Carter, J., 1982, op. cit.

370. According to economist William Hsiao of the Harvard School of Public Health, total spending to sway public opinion and Congress on health policy ran at about $16 million a year. The money came from large employers who had huge numbers of employees on health insurance (e.g., IBM, GM, GE, etc.), organizations of small businesses, organized labor, the insurance industry, the AMA, the American Hospital Association, and the pharmaceutical industry.

371. These were published by HEW as *Objectives for the Nation* (1979), *The Surgeon General's Report on Health Promotion and Disease Prevention* (1979), and *Objectives for the Nation* (1980).

372. The Valentine Brothers, "Money's Too Tight (to mention)," 1973. Adapted by Simply Red, 1988. BMI.

373. McBeath, W. H., Opening remarks, annual meeting of the American Public Health Association. New York, October 1, 1990.

374. Reagan, R., *Speaking My Mind*. New York: Simon and Schuster, 1989.

375. Center for Health Statistics, *Health Data Summaries for California Counties 1980*. Sacramento: Department of Health Services, State of California, 1981; Centers for Disease Control and Prevention, "Motor-vehicle safety: A 20th century public health achievement." *Morbidity and Mortality Weekly Report* 48 (1999): 369–374.

376. In 1980 there were a total of 119,681 births and 68,018 reported abortions, meaning that 36 percent of all pregnancies were being terminated. A racial breakdown of abortions cannot be found, but generally, in California, abortion rates were highest among white women.

377. Janis, J. M. and Walker, A., "An approach to monitoring the health status of Los Angeles County residents." Los Angeles: UCLA School of Public Health, April 1983; Center for Human Statistics, *Health Data Summaries for California Counties*. Sacramento: California State Department of Health. For the years 1960, 1970, 1980, 1982, 1983.

378. See "Los Angeles County Childbirth Trends 1978–88" table on page 687.

379. Another way to look at the racial disparity was to compare rates of improvement

LOS ANGELES COUNTY CHILDBIRTH TRENDS
1978–88

Year	Births under 2500 grams (%)	Mothers unwed (%)	No or inadequate prenatal care (%)	Mothers under 20 yrs of age (%)	Mothers with <12 years education (%)	Infant mortality, all races (deaths per 1,000)	Infant mortality, black (deaths per 1,000)
1978	6.8	24.1	8.6	15.6	—	12.6	22.6
1980	6.1	25.0	4.8	14.3	40.1	11.9	21.49
1982	6.2	27.5	5.2	13.1	40.1	11.7	20.9
1984	6.4	30.1	5.6	11.8	40.1	10.5	18.6
1986	6.4	33.6	6.3	11.7	40.1	10.8	20.6
1988	6.3	35.0	5.8	11.5	—	10.0	19.8

(Source: Los Angeles County Department of Health)

in infant mortality. Between 1970 and 1980 infant mortality declined in L.A. County as follows:

	Percent of Disease
Whites	36.5
Nonwhites (Hispanics)	35.8
Blacks	21.6
Asians and "Others"	44.1
TOTAL DECLINE	34.6
Difference between Blacks and Total	−13.0
Difference between Blacks and Whites	−14.9
Difference between Blacks and Nonwhites (Hispanics)	−13.6
Difference between Blacks and Asians (and "Others")	−22.5

Sources: Ibid.

380. In 1980 5.2 percent of white babies were born weighing less than 2,500 grams (or 5.5 pounds). Twelve percent of African-American babies were born weighing less than that amount.

381. U.S. Bureau of the Census, *World Population Profile: 1994*. Washington, D.C.: U.S. Department of Commerce, 1994.

382. Los Angeles would continue to have trouble getting its children fully vaccinated. In 1982 about 21 percent of kindergartners weren't fully immunized. By 1985 that number had come down to 15.1 percent, thanks in large part to a big vaccination campaign in Spanish. In 1987 just over 11 percent of the kindergartners were inadequately vaccinated.

And then the figure stagnated, holding at 11–12 percent for several years.

383. World Health Organization. *World Health Report, 1984*. Geneva, WHO, 1984.

384. Gonorrhea rates in Los Angeles had consistently exceeded both statewide and U.S. rates for twenty years. By 1980 L.A. County had a rate of 683.7 per 100,000. California's was 574.1. For the United States it was 443.3. Syphilis rates had shown a more variable trend, but an overall increase in Los Angeles for twenty years, and, again, L.A. rates had always exceeded both California and national averages.

See Janis, J. M. and Walker, A., 1983, op. cit; U.S. Center for Human Statistics, 1960, 1970, 1980, 1982, 1983, op. cit.

385. In 1979 the county collected $1.1 billion in Medicare monies (averaging $1,552 per Medicare client that year), and handled 942,486 Medi-Cal cases per month, billing the state about $1.2 billion. By 1981 the county's Medicare income jumped to $1.6 billion, averaging $2,175 per recipient. And the county took in $1.5 billion in Medi-Cal reimbursements, averaging $3,012 per Medi-Cal client. Janis, J. M. and Walker, A., 1983, op. cit; U.S. Center for Human Statistics, 1980, 1982, op. cit.

386. During the Reagan presidency, his home state would prosper as the number one recipient of military contracts, averaging $100 billion each year. By 1983 California's defense contract payroll would top $8 billion, most of it paid out to workers in Los Angeles County. U.S. Bureau of the Census, *Statistical Abstract of the United States*. Washington, D.C.: U.S. Department of Commerce, 1984.

387. Savage, J. D., *Balanced Budgets and American Politics*. Ithaca: Cornell University Press, 1988.

388. Reagan, R., 1989, op. cit.

389. Ginzberg, E., *Tomorrow's Hospital: A Look to the Twenty-first Century*. New Haven: Yale University Press, 1996.

390. Savage, J. D., 1988, op. cit.

391. The corps offered two enticing options to medical students. Those who contracted to work in the corps after completion of their studies got federally subsidized medical education. And service in the corps was grounds for draft deferral from the armed forces.

392. Ambler, M., "Taking care of our own: Training Indians to heal Indians." *Tribal College* 5 (1994): 10–16.

393. Associated Press, "U.S. refines rules for Indian Service." October 4, 1987.

394. United Press International, "Report tells of poor doctoring for the Indians." October 7, 1987.

395. In part this represented a shift, as more people went to tribal-run clinics rather than the IHS hospitals. See Indian Health Services, *Chart Series Book.* Washington, D.C.: U.S. Department of Health and Human Services, April 1987.

396. Interviews with IHS and Navajo health experts were conducted by the author in New Mexico, Arizona, Los Angeles, and Washington, D.C., from September through November of 1987.

397. Cannon, L., *President Reagan: The Role of a Lifetime.* New York: Simon and Schuster, 1991.

398. Interestingly, Reagan was operating contrary to what polls revealed to be clear public opinion in these matters. For example, a poll sponsored by the AMA asked: "If there were less government regulation of health care, in your opinion what would probably happen to the quality of health care?" And the results were, over two years:

Percent of Respondents Who Thought It Would:	1979	1981
Improve a great deal	5	3
Improve somewhat	13	19
No change	25	20
Decline a great deal	11	10
Decline somewhat	29	33
DK (don't know)	17	15

Even more revealing were American's views on national health insurance. A *New York Times*/CBS poll conducted over five years asked: "Do you favor or oppose . . . national health insurance, financed by tax money, and paying for most forms of health care?" And the responses were:

	August 1976	July 1977	February 1980	March 1980	April 1981
Percent in favor	49	60	50	46	52
Percent opposed	39	33	41	43	37
Percent no opinion	9	7	9	11	11

See Shapiro, R. Y. and Young, J. T., "The polls: Medical care in the United States." *Public Opinion Quarterly* 50 (1986):418–428.

399. Nathan, R. P. and Omenn, G. S., "What's behind those block grants in health?" *New England Journal of Medicine* 306 (1982): 1057–1060; and Brooks, E. F., DeFriese, G. H., Miller, C. A., et al., "A survey of local public health departments and their directors." *American Journal of Public Health* 67 (1977): 931–939.

400. Miller, C. A., Brooks, E. F., DeFriese, G. H., et al, 1977, op. cit.

401. Association of State and Territorial Health Officials, *Inventory of Programs and*

Expenditures. Washington, D.C.: National Public Health Reporting System, HEW, for the years 1974, 1776, 1978, 1980, 1981, and 1982.

402. Beyle, T. L. and Dusenbury, P. J., "Health and Human Services block grants: The state and local dimension." *State Government SSI* (1982): 2–13.

403. DeFriese, G. H., Hetherington, J. S., Brooks, E. F., et al., "The program implications of administrative relationships between local health departments and state and local government." *American Journal of Public Health* 71 (1981): 1109–1115; Gilbert, B., Moos, M. K., and Miller, C. A., "State-level decision making for public health: The status of boards of health." *Journal of Public Health Policy* 3 (1982) 51–61; Institute of Medicine, *The Future of Public Health*. Washington, D.C.: National Academy Press, 1988; Lockwood, S. A. and Malvitz, D. M., "Trends in state agency oral health and public health expenditures, 1984 through 1989." *American Journal of Public Health* 85 (1995): 1266–1268; Miller, C. A., Moore, K. S., and Richards, T. B., "The impact of critical events of the 1980s on core functions for a selected group of local health departments." *Public Health Reports* 108 (1993): 695–700; and Miller, C. A., Gilbert, B., Warren, D. G., et al., "Statutory authorizations for the work of local public health departments." *American Journal of Public Health* 67 (1977): 940–945.

404. Iglehart, J. K., "Medical care of the poor—a growing health problem." *New England Journal of Medicine* 313 (1985): 59–64.

405. Joe. T. C. W., "Arbitrary access to care: the case for reforming Medicaid eligibility." *Health Affairs* 4 (1985): 59–74.

406. Ginzberg, E., 1996, op. cit.

407. Stevens, R., op. cit, 1999.

408. Ibid.

409. Muñoz, E., Laughlin, A., Regan, D. M., et al., "The financial effects of emergency department-generated admissions under prospective payment systems." *Journal of the American Medical Association* 254 (1985): 1763–1771; Norton, E. C. and Staiger D. O., "How hospital ownership affects access to care for the uninsured." *RAND Journal of Economics* 25 (1994): 171–185; and Stern, R. S. and Epstein, A. M., "Institutional responses to prospective payment based on Diagnosis-Related Groups." *New England Journal of Medicine* 312 (1985): 621–627.

410. Wennenberg, J. E., McPherson, K., and Caper, P., "Will payment based on Diagnosis-Related Groups control hospital costs?" *New England Journal of Medicine* 311 (1984): 295–300.

411. Dentzer, S., Hager, M., Zuckerman, S., et al., "Hospitals take the cure." *Newsweek* (July 2, 1984): 56–65.

412. Feder, J., Hadley, J., and Zuckerman, S., "How did Medicare's Prospective Payment System affect hospitals?" *New England Journal of Medicine* 317 (1987): 867–873; Prospective Payment Assessment Commission, *Medicare and the American Health Care System*. Report to Congress, Washington, D.C., June 1992. Stephen Shortell and Edward Hughes focused on sixteen common procedures performed on Medicare patients (e.g., mastectomies, emergency cardiac resuscitation, coronary bypass surgery, and hip replacements) and looked at death rates in patients who underwent the procedures at various facilities nationwide. The average death rate, all procedures combined, was 11 percent; but in some facilities only 6.5 percent died, while in others as many as 15.5 percent succumbed. The death rates were found to follow a geographic pattern, with the highest rates occurring in the least regulated, most highly competitive markets. At least one study found that in parts of the country where such profitable hospital practices had blossomed in a market that was highly competitive and not closely regulated by local or state government, more patients died. Shortell, S. and

Hughes, E. F. X., "The effects of regulation, competition, and ownership on mortality rates among hospital inpatients." *New England Journal of Medicine* 318 (1988): 1100–1107.

413. Wikler, D., "Who should be blamed for being sick?" *Health Education Quarterly* 14 (1987): 11–25.

414. Davis, K. and Rowland, D., "Uninsured and underserved: inequalities in health care in the United States." *Milbank Quarterly* 61 (1983): 149–176.

415. Farley, P. J., "Who are the underinsured?" *Milbank Quarterly* 63 (1985): 476–503.

416. The Congressional Budget office projected three scenarios for 2000 and 2002, based on different economic assumptions:

Year 2000:

Best case scenario	42.6 million uninsured
Middle scenario	46.1 million uninsured
Worst case scenario	58.8 million uninsured

Year 2002:

Best case scenario	43.8 million uninsured
Middle scenario	48.7 million uninsured
Worst case scenario	66.8 million uninsured

See Schroeder, S., "The medically uninsured—will they always be with us?" *New England Journal of Medicine* 334 (1996): 1130–1133.

The U.S. Census Bureau also predicted increases in uninsured Americans. U.S. Bureau of the Census, *Sourcebook of Health.* Washington, D.C.: Department of Commerce, 1994.

417. U.S. Public Health Service, *U.S. Immunization Survey.* Washington, D.C.: Centers for Disease Control, GPO, 1978.

418. Interview with the author, 1984.

419. Lurie, N., Ward, N. B., Shapiro, M. F., et al., "Termination from Medi-Cal—does it affect health?" *New England Journal of Medicine* 311 (1984): 480–484.

420. Interview with the author, International Cancer Congress, Seattle, September 1981.

421. Burkitt, D. P., "Etiology and prevention of colorectal cancer." *Hospital Practice* (February 1984): 67–77.

422. Interview with the author, International Cancer Congress, Seattle, September 1981.

423. Bjelke, E., "Dietary vitamin A and human lung cancer." *International Journal of Cancer* 15 (1975): 561; Greenwald, P., "Manipulation of nutrients to prevent cancer." *Hospital Practice* (May 1984): 119–134; Mettlin, C., Graham, S., and Swanson, M., "Vitamin A and lung cancer." *Journal of the National Cancer Institute* 62 (1979): 1435; Peto, R., "Can dietary beta-carotene materially reduce human cancer rates?" *Nature* 290 (1981): 201; Wald, N., "Low serum-vitamin-A and subsequent risk of cancer: Preliminary results of a prospective study." *Lancet* 2 (1980): 813; and Willett, W. C., "Relation of serum vitamins A and E and carotenoids to the risk of cancer." *New England Journal of Medicine* 310 (1984): 430–435.

424. For examples of the thinking about viruses, oncogenes, and carcinogenesis during the early 1980s, see Baltimore, D., "Retroviruses and cancer." *Hospital Practice* (January 1978): 49–57; Bishop, J. M., "Enemies within: The genesis of retrovirus oncogenes." *Cell* 23

(1981): 5–6; Bishop, J. M., "The molecular biology of RNA tumor viruses: A physician's guide." *New England Journal of Medicine* 303 (1980): 675–682; Bishop, J. M., "The molecular genetics of cancer." *Science* 235 (1987): 305–311; Bishop, J. M., "Oncogenes." *Scientific American* 246 (1982): 80–92; Dulbecco, R., "From the molecular biology of oncogenic DNA viruses to cancer." *Science* 192 (1976): 437; Kasid, A., Lippman, M. E., Papageorge, A. G., et al., "Transfection of v-ras^H DNA into MCF-7 human breast cancer cells bypasses dependence on estrogen for tumorigenicity." *Science* 228 (1985): 725–728; Nahmias, A. J. and Hall, C. B., "Diagnosis of viral diseases—today and tomorrow." *Hospital Practice* (April 1981): 49–61; Varmus, H. E., "Form and function of retroviral previruses." *Science* 216 (1982): 812–820; and Yunis, J. Y., Frizzera, G., Oken, M. M., et al., "Multiple recurrent genomic defects in follicular lymphoma: A possible model for cancer." *New England Journal of Medicine* 316 (1987): 79–84.

425. National Research Council, *Diet and Nutrition.* Washington, D.C.: National Academy Press, 1982.

426. Wynder, E. L., Hall, N. E. L., and Polansky, M., "Epidemiology of coffee and pancreatic cancer." *Cancer Research* 43 (1983): 3900–3906; "Decaffinating and cancer." *San Francisco Chronicle* (June 18, 1982): A6.

427. Stolberg, S. G., "Fiber does not help prevent colon cancer, study finds." *New York Times* (January 21, 1999): A14.

428. Holmes, M. D., "No apparent relationships between total fat intake or consumption of certain types of fat and breast cancer risk." *Journal of the American Medical Association* 281 (1999): 914–920.

429. Rehak, M., "To drink or not to drink." *New York Times Sunday Magazine* (March 14, 1999): 20.

430. Marmot, M. G., "From alcohol and breast cancer to beef and BSE—improving our communication of risk." Editorial. *American Journal of Public Health* 86 (1996): 921–923.

431. Marmot, M. G. and Mustard, J. F., "Coronary heart disease from a population perspective." In Evans, R. G., et al., 1994, op. cit.

432. American Heart Association, *Heart and Stroke Statistical Update.* Dallas: American Heart Association, 1999. The same pattern was *not* followed in the Soviet Union and Warsaw Pact countries. There, the post–World War II upsurge in cardiac disease was more subtle, partly because the rates were already high in the 1930s. These countries saw their rates continue to climb in the 1980s, largely because tobacco use soared and dietary fat was unchanged. And then male cardiac death rates skyrocketed after the 1991 collapse of the Soviet Union. See Chapter 3 of this book.

433. Kochanek, K. D., Maurer, J. D., Rosenberg, H. M., "Why did black life expectancy decline from 1984 through 1989 in the United States?" *American Journal of Public Health* 84 (1994): 938–944.

For example 43.9 percent of white male adults suffered hypertension during the period 1976–1980 compared to 48.7 percent of black males. And by 1994 white male hypertension prevalence had dropped to 24.4 percent versus 35 percent in black men. The female differential was sharper. White females had a prevalence of 32.1 percent in the period 1976–1980 and 19.3 percent by 1994. Black females went from a 47.6 percent prevalence to 34.2 percent.

But when Hispanics and Asians are thrown into the data base, it's clear that the dichotomy is broader than just black/white. Asians consistently have had very low hypertension rates. And among Hispanics during the period 1970–1994, the prevalences held at 22 to 25 percent in both men and women, with no significant changes over time. (*Source:* American Heart Association, 1999, op. cit.)

Some have blamed the problem on poverty, but that differential seems to disappear when black and Hispanic prevalences are matched by socioeconomic status: blacks of all classes have higher hypertension rates. Access to health care is clearly poorer for blacks versus whites, but not necessarily for blacks versus Hispanics. There is evidence that blacks are less likely to be treated with aggressive therapy, such as cardiac bypass surgery or transplants, which could affect their death rates. But that could not explain higher hypertension rates. Genetic explanations were also sought, without satisfaction.

From a public health point of view, the lack of clear understanding of the roots of the disparity made prevention efforts dubious: if one doesn't know *why* black Americans have more heart disease, how can one, with certitude, determine whether it is best to expend scarce resources and public health credibility targeting diet, stress, obesity, exercise, or other factors for behavioral changes in the African-American community?

See Bhopal, R. and Donaldson, L., "White, European, Western, Caucasian or what? Inappropriate labeling in research on race, ethnicity, and health." *American Journal of Public Health* 88 (1998): 1303–1307; Blendon, R. J., Aiken, L. H., Freeman, H. E., et al., "Access to medical care for black and white Americans." *Journal of the American Medical Association* 261 (1989): 278–281; Centers for Disease Control and Prevention, "Health beliefs and compliance with prescribed medication for hypertension among black women—New Orleans, 1985–86." *Morbidity and Mortality Weekly Report* 39 (1990): 701–704; Centers for Disease Control and Prevention, "Report of the Secretary's Task Force on black and minority health." *Morbidity and Mortality Weekly Report* 39 (1990): 701–704; Centers for Disease Control and Prevention, "Report of the Secretary's Task Force on black and minority health." *Morbidity and Mortality Weekly Report* 3 5 (1986): 109–113; Collins, K. S., Hall, A., and Neuhaus, C., *U.S. Minority Health: A Chartbook.* New York: The Commonwealth Fund, 1999; Fessendon, F., "A difference of life and death." *Newsday* (November 29, 1998): Al; Fresco, R., "Long frustrating delay for a kidney." *Newsday* (December 1, 1998): A7; Fullilove, M. T., "Comment: Abandoning 'race' as a variable in public health research—an idea whose time has come." *American Journal of Public Health* 88 (1998): 1297–1298; Geronimus. A. T., Bound, J., Waidmann, T. A., et al., "Excess mortality among blacks and whites in the United States." *New England Journal of Medicine* 335 (1996): 1552–1558; Gordon, H. S., Harper, D. L., and Rosenthal, G. E., "Racial variation in predicted and observed in-hospital death." *Journal of the American Medical Association* 276 (1996): 1639–1644; Gorey, K. M. and Trevisan, M., "Secular trends in the United States black/white hypertension prevalence ratio: Potential impact of diminishing response rates." *American Journal of Epidemiology* 147 (1998): 95–102; McCord, C. and Freeman, H. P., "Excess mortality in Harlem." *New England Journal of Medicine* 322 (1990): 173–177; Schulman, K. A., Berlin, J. A., Harless, W., et al., "The effect of race and sex in physicians' recommendations for cardiac catheterization." *New England Journal of Medicine* 340 (1999): 618–626; Stevens, C., "System, Race, and Suspicion Promote Medical Disparities." *Detroit News and Free Press* (December 10, 1995): Metro P1; and Wallace, R. and Wallace, D., "Origins of public health collapse in New York City: The dynamics of planned shrinkage, continuous urban decay, and social disintegration." *Bulletin of the New York Academy of Medicine* 66 (1990): 391–434.

434. Low-density lipoprotein cholesterol, or LDL, was shown during the late 1970s and early eighties to be able to attach to the linings of blood vessels and arteries, forming plaques. These plaques, unless "scrubbed" away by HDLs (the "good" cholesterol), grew and compounded with time as more LDL-cholesterol entered the blood stream, its production by the liver fueled by ingestion of saturated fats. Eventually, the vessels would thicken, offering less space for blood flow. An individual then had atherosclerosis, or "hardening of the arteries," and was at very high risk of suffering a heart attack or stroke.

435. Brody, J. E., *Jane Brody's Good Food Book.* New York: W. W. Norton, 1985; Brody, J. E., *Jane Brody's Nutrition Book.* New York: W. W. Norton, 1981; Butrum, R. R., Clifford, C. K.,

and Lanza, E., "NCI Dietary Guidelines: Rationale." *American Journal of Clinical Nutrition* 48, Supplement (1988): 888–895; U.S. Departments of Agriculture and Health and Human Services, *Dietary Guidelines for Americans.* Washington, D.C.: U.S. Departments of Agriculture and Health and Human Services, 1985; U.S. Food and Drug Administration, Division of Consumer Studies, *Health and Dietary Survey* (1988), unpublished; Life Sciences Research Office, Federation of American Societies for Experimental Biology, *Physiologic Effects and Health Consequences of Dietary Fiber.* Bethesda: Federation of American Societies for Experimental Biology, 1987; National Heart, Lung and Blood Institute, *The Report of the Expert Panel on Population Strategies for Blood Cholesterol Reduction.* Washington, D.C.: U.S. Department of Health and Human Services, 1990; National Research Council, *Diet and Health: Implications for Reducing Chronic Disease Risk.* Washington, D.C.: National Academy Press, 1989; U.S. Public Health Service, *The Surgeon General's Report on Nutrition and Health.* Pub. No. 88–50210. Washington, D.C.: U.S. Department of Health and Human Services, 1988; and Sussman, V., *The Vegetarian Alternative.* Emmaus, Penn.: Rodale Press, 1978.

436. The breakdown in 1980 was as follows:

Population Groups (all over 20 years of age)	Percent Overweight
Low-income women	37
African-American women	44
Mexican-American women	39
Puerto Rican women	37
American Indians, male and female	Up to 75
Men, all races	24

Source: Centers for Disease Control, *National Health and Nutrition Examination Survey.* Washington, D.C.: U.S. Department of Health and Human Services, yearly 1970–1980.

During the 1980s and nineties economic and cultural changes in the United States would leave families with less time to cook, so they would eat more often at restaurants or fast-food chains where foods typically contained more fat. Average out-of-home meals presented 38 percent of their calories in the form of fat; 13 from saturated fats.

437. For example, a person's total cholesterol count might be 220, which wasn't great. But if 35 percent or more of that count was made up of HDL (high density lipoprotein) rather than the worrisome LDL, a physician would be ill-advised to intervene. And there were a host of other dietary chemicals—triglycerides, niacin, caffeine, alcohol, apo-B, estrogens, calcium—that also played roles in determining an individual's risk for heart disease. There were even families that seemed generally resistant both to weight gain and build-up of cholesterol, regardless of what foods they ate.

438. Callahan, D., *False Hopes: America's Quest for Perfect Health Is a Recipe for Failure.* New York: Simon & Schuster, 1998.

439. The economic value of health improvements due to prevention was expressed by Harvard University's David Cutter and Elizabeth Richardson as follows: "We define 'health capital' as the discounted value of the current and future utility associated with individual health. We measure health capital empirically using data on mortality and morbidity from chronic disease. Our estimates suggest that health capital at birth increased by about $100,000 between 1970 and 1990, and health capital at age 65 increased by about $160,000. The greater increase for the old is because most of the improvements in health are a result of decreased mortality from cardiovascular disease. . . ."

See Cutter, D. M. and Richardson, E., *Measuring the Health of the United States Pop-*

ulation. Washington, D.C.: Brookings Institute, Brookings Papers on Economic Activity, Microeconomic Edition, 1997.

440. Kindig D. A., *Purchasing Population Health: Paying for Results*. Ann Arbor: University of Michigan Press, 1997.

441. GISSI-Prevenzione Investigators, "Dietary supplementation with n-3 polyunsaturated fatty acids and vitamin E after myocardial infarction: Results of the GISSI-Preventione trial." *Lancet* 354 (1999): 447–455.

Nor, as it turned out, did omega-3 fat from fish lower breast cancer risk, as previously thought. See Holmes, M. D., "Lower fat consumption not associated with decreased breast cancer risk." *Journal of the American Medical Association* 281 (1999): 914–920.

442. Some fish looked helpful for the heart, e.g. salmon. Other types seemed to offer little benefit, e.g. tuna. The key would, at least according to 1990s research, be omega-3 fatty acids. The list goes on. See *Time* magazine's handy summary: Lemonick, M. D., "Eat your heart out." *Time* magazine (July 19, 1999): 40–52.

443. The author will here present only a superficial view of TSS, as a lengthy analysis of the disease's emergence appears in the chapter entitled "Feminine Hygiene" in Garrett, L., 1994, op. cit.

444. See Centers for Disease Control, "Update: Toxic-Shock Syndrome in the United States." *Journal of the American Medical Association* 20 (1983): 1017; Institute of Medicine, *Toxic Shock Syndrome: Assessment of Current Information and Future Research Needs*. Washington, D.C.: National Academy Press, 1982; Schlievert, P. M., Shands, K. M., Dan, B. B., et al., "Identification and characterization of an exotoxin from *Staphylococcus aureus* associated with Toxic-Shock Syndrome." *Journal of Infectious Diseases* 143 (1981): 509–516; and Schlievert, P. M., Bettin, K. M., and Watson, D. W., "Purification and characterization of Group A streptococcal pyrogenic exotoxin Type C." *Infection and Immunology* 16 (1977): 673–679.

445. In 1982 a man or woman aged thirty-five years could expect to live the following numbers of additional years of life, on average:

	ADDITIONAL LIFE EXPECTANCIES	
	Male, age 35 years	Female, age 35 years
Minnesota	41.4	47.2
U.S.A.	37.7	44.4
Denmark	38.8	44.1
Finland	35.2	42.8
Norway	39.5	45.1
Sweden	39.6	45.3
Poland	35.4	42.4
German Democratic Republic*	36.8	41.3
Federal Republic of Germany**	37.2	43.0
Canada	38.5	45.1
Japan	40.3	45.0

*What was called East Germany until 1989.
**Called West Germany until 1989.
Source: Minnesota Department of Health

446. Minnesota Planning, *Line Item*. St. Paul: Minnesota Planning, December 1994.

447. In 1968 the Minnesota Department of Health's budget was $4,110,256, of which $1,794,124 came from local and state sources and $2,316,132 was federally derived.

448. State and local contributions to the Minnesota Department of Health budget in 1985 totaled $30,750,200. The federal tally was $38,206,500.

449. In 1998 Minnesota Department of Health revenues would break down as $120,321,297 from state and local sources; $107,280,502 federal. Yet the health department did suffer during the Reagan years, as even generous Minnesotans struggled to compensate for changes being made in Washington. Between 1980 and 1983 the department lost 17 percent of its full-time employees, and staffing did not regain 1980 levels until 1987.

450. White, K. E, Hedberg, C. W., Edmonson, L. M, et al., "An outbreak of Giardiasis in a nursing home with evidence for multiple modes of transmission." *Journal of Infectious Diseases* 160 (1989): 298–304.

451. MacDonald, K. L., White, K. A., Heiser, J., et al., "Evaluation of a sick child day care program: lack of detected increased risk of subsequent infections." *Pediatric Infectious Disease Journal* 9 (1990): 15–20.

452. *E. coli* became popularly known as the "Jack-in-the-Box bug" after it turned up in hamburgers sold by that fast-food chain in Washington State in 1993. But outbreaks had occurred all over the United States, and Jack-in-the-Box had no particular association with the epidemics. In the outbreaks in Washington, Idaho, Nevada, and California, where more than seven hundred children contracted the disease, 178 were hospitalized and four died. Washington state health authorities determined that the cases in all four states were linked to the same hamburger supplier. And, terrifyingly, found that as few as fourteen *E. coli* 0157: H7 bacteria in an undercooked hamburger patty were sufficient to cause hemolytic uremic syndrome. See Swerdlow, D., 1994, op. cit.; and "The emergence of *Escherichia coli* 0157:H7 infection in the United States." Editorial. *Journal of the American Medical Association* 269 (1993): 2264–2266.

453. Swerdlow, D., Comments to the USDA, *E coli* 0157 Conference. Washington, D.C., July 11–13, 1994.

454. Belongia, E. A, MacDonald, K. L., White, K. E., et al., "Outbreak of *Escherichia coli* 0157:H7 colitis associated with precooked hamburgers." Twenty-ninth Interscience Conference on Antimicrobial Agents and Chemotherapy, Houston, Texas, September 17–20, 1989; Belongia, E. A., MacDonald, K. L., Blaser, M. T., et al., "Outbreak of *Escherichia coli* 0157:H7 in a day care center: Patterns of transmission and control methods." Twenty-ninth Interscience Conference on Antimicrobial Agents and Chemotherapy, Houston, Texas, September 17–20, 1989; Griffin, P. M. and Tauxe, R. V., "The epidemiology of infections caused by *Escherichia coli* 0157:H7, other enterohemorrhagic *E. coli*, and the associated hemolytic uremic syndrome." *Epidemiologic Reviews* 13 (1991): 60–98; MacDonald, K. L., O'Leary, M. J., Cohen, M. L., et al., "*Escherichia coli* 0157:H7, an emerging gastrointestinal pathogen: Results of a one-year, prospective, population-based study." *Journal of the American Medical Association* 259 (1988): 3567–3570; Martin, D. L., MacDonald, K. L., White, K. E., et al., "The epidemiology and clinical aspects of the Hemolytic Uremic Syndrome in Minnesota." *New England Journal of Medicine* 323 (1990): 1161–1167; and Riley, L. W., Remis, R. S., Helgerson, S. D., et al., "Hemorrhagic colitis associated with a rare *Escherichia coli* serotype." *New England Journal of Medicine* 308 (1983): 681–685.

455. In 1996 Japan would suffer a huge epidemic involving ten thousand cases that would prompt closure of schools all over the nation. After years of investigation, U.S. and Japanese researchers would determine that the outbreak originated in Idaho at a daikon seed farm. Cow manure from *E. coli*–infected animals was used to fertilize the radishes, the seeds of which were sold to Japanese daikon growers. And the seeds contained dormant *E. coli*, which readily colonized sprouts that grew from the seeds. Since daikon is consumed un-

cooked, the *E. coli* in those sprouts was even more dangerous than that found in partially cooked burgers.

See Brever, T., Shapiro, R., Hall, W., et al., "*Escherichia coli* 0157:H7 first linked to consumption of alfalfa sprouts." First International Conference on Emerging Infectious diseases, Atlanta, March 8–11, 1998; Efron, S. "Food poisoning outbreak causes alarm." *Los Angeles Times* (July 23, 1996): A1; Garrett, L., "Mutant superbug strikes in Japan." *Newsday* (July 24, 1996): A4; Garrett, L., "Superbug raging in Japan; experts baffled." *Newsday* (July 26, 1996): A20; Garrett, L., "U.S. to aid Japan on *E. coli.*" *Newsday* (July 27, 1996): A7; Garrett, L., "Unsolved mystery plagues Japan." *Newsday* (July 26, 1996): A20; Gutierrez, E. and Netley, G., "Japanese *Escherichia coli* outbreak is still puzzling health officials." *Lancet* 348 (1996): 540; Itoh, Y., Sugita-Konishi, Y., Hara-Kudo, Y., et al., "Experimental contamination of radish sprouts with enterohemorrhagic *Escherichia coli* 0157." First International Conference on Emerging Infectious Diseases, Atlanta, March 8–11, 1998; Kageyama, Y., "Search for Japanese food poisoning cause hits stalemate." *Associated Press.* (August 7, 1996); Veno, T., "Japan admits failure in food poisoning investigation." *Reuter* (August 7, 1996); Watanabe, H., Wada, A., Inagaki, Y., et al., "Outbreaks of enterohemorrhagic *Escherichia coli* 0157:H7 infection by two different genotype strains in Japan, 1996." *Lancet* 348 (1996): 831–832; and Yamaguchi, N., "Two die in Japan food poisoning." *Reuter* (July 23, 1996).

456. Cannon, L. 1991, op. cit.

457. Address to the annual National Gay and Lesbian Health Conference. Washington, D.C., July 25, 1988, and interview comments afterward.

458. It is beyond the scope of this book to detail the long list of frustrations, monetary problems, political intrigues, and intellectual obstacles responsible for the utter failure in the pursuit of an HIV vaccine. Despite many highly optimistic statements over the years, made by authorities to the general public and to Wall Street, nobody by the end of the century had a product in hand that held the promise of doing for HIV what Salk's vaccine had done for polio. To understand some of the reasons why, see Cohen, J., "Glimmers of hope from the bottom of the well." *Science* 285 (1999): 656–657; Cohen, J., *Shots in the Dark: The Wayward Search for an AIDS Vaccine*, to be published in 2000, manuscript shared by author; Institute of Medicine, *The Potential Value of Research Consortia in the Development of Drugs and Vaccines Against HIV Infection and AIDS*. Washington, D.C.: National Academy Press, 1988; and various authors, "AIDS: The Unanswered Questions." *Science* 260 (1993): 1219–1293.

459. Institute of Medicine, *Confronting AIDS*. Washington, D.C.: National Academy Press, 1988; Mann, J. M., Tarantola, D. J., and Netter, T. W., editors, *AIDS in the World.* Cambridge, Mass.: Harvard University Press, 1992; National Research Council, *AIDS: The Second Decade*. Washington, D.C.: National Academy Press, 1990; National Research Council, *AIDS: Sexual Behavior and Intravenous Drug Use*. Washington, D.C.: National Academy Press, 1989; Nichols, E. K., *Mobilizing Against AIDS*. Washington, D.C.: National Academy Press, 1986; Sepulveda, J., Fineberg, H., and Mann, J. M., editors, *AIDS: Prevention Through Education*. Boston: published privately by computer, 1986.

460. Institute of Medicine, *Contronting AIDS*, 1988, op. cit.

461. The blood bank and blood products industry, in particular, stalled attempts to clean up the blood supply, allowing thousands of Americans to become infected as a result of transfusions or use of blood factors. Once they realized they would have to give in or face enormous lawsuits, the industry took two postures. First, it discreetly exported unscreened blood products, spawning HIV epidemics in Japan and other countries. And second, it agreed to "voluntary" screening efforts but opposed all forms of legally mandated screening. The Reagan FDA allowed this, and mandatory screening was not instituted until more than a

decade after the epidemic was first recognized. See Garrett, L., 1994, op. cit.; and Starr, D., *Blood: An Epic History of Medicine and Commerce.* New York: Alfred A. Knopf, 1998.

462. See National Center for Health Statistics, "AIDS knowledge and attitudes for May and June 1988." *Advancedata* 160 (1988): 1–5; and Garrett, L., in Sepulveda, J., et al., editors, 1989, op. cit.

463. For example, many activists argued that AIDS conferences should not be held in countries that had immigration policies that discriminated against people who were HIV positive. This apparently laudable position was supported by prominent public health leaders, until it became clear that this excluded the United States, nearly all Asian and African countries, and much of Europe. This forced conference organizers to convene meetings in nations that were extremely expensive places to visit—Sweden, Switzerland, Japan. For people from developing countries this amounted to a fiscal exclusionary policy put in place merely to appease a small number of activists from the United States, Canada, and Western Europe. Though nations did not change their policies, eventually AIDS meetings were held all over the world, regardless of immigration policies.

464. Comments made at the American Blood Bank Meeting, Washington, D.C., November 1985.

465. Based on the data that they were able to obtain, the CDC thought that the average HIV-infected individual had a 45 percent chance of dying, and that death ensued two years after infection. Based on the reported AIDS cases, Curran's group also felt that gay men were the only large risk group, with injecting drug users and their sex partners representing less than 10 percent of HIV cases. They estimated the national AIDS case rate to be 0.1 per 100,000 Americans; but 1,000 per 100,000 San Francisco gay men.

466. Curran, J., "Summary of meeting on AIDS and the bathhouses, with medical experts and representatives of the S. F. medical community." San Francisco, September 25, 1984, unpublished.

467. Moss addressed the superior court subsequent to legal challenges of actions the city had taken to try to curb spread of HIV by closing gay bathhouses. Moss, A. R., statement before San Francisco Superior Court Judge Roy Wonder, October 15, 1984.

468. On January 6, 1988, Governor Cuomo ordered all prenatal treatment sites statewide to encourage pregnant women to get HIV tests. This followed recognition that mandated anonymous screening of newborns statewide showed that in 1987 fully 1 percent were born HIV positive.

469. Carroll, M., "To combat AIDS, New York may order bathhouses shut." *New York Times* (October 25, 1985): B1.

470. Between 1983 and 1988, New York City's excess mortality rate increased by 5 percent due to AIDS. In 1988 in the city 3,739 people died of the disease. It was just the beginning. As of November 1989, some 22,200 AIDS cases had been reported in New York City since the epidemic's beginning, and AIDS was the leading cause of death for men aged thirty to forty-nine years and women aged twenty to thirty-nine years.

See Smith, P. F., Mikl, J., Hyde, S., et al., "The AIDS epidemic in New York State." *American Journal of Public Health* 815 (1991): 54–60.

471. Kramer, L., *Report from the Holocaust.* New York: St. Martins, 1994,; Nussbaum, B., *Good Intentions.* New York: Atlantic Monthly Press, 1990; and Shilts, R., *And the Band Played On.* New York: St. Martins, 1986.

472. New York State Department of Health. *AIDS in New York State.* Albany: New York State Department of Health, 1989.

473. Centers for Disease Control and Prevention, "Update: Reducing HIV transmission in intravenous-drug users not in drug treatment—United States." *Morbidity and Mor-*

tality Weekly Report 39 (1990): 529–538; U.S. General Accounting Office, *Needle Exchange Programs: Research Suggests Promise as an AIDS Prevention Strategy.* GAO/HRD-93-60. Washington, D.C.: House of Representatives, 1993; Kaiser Family Foundation, *Needle and Syringe Availability and Exchange for HIV Prevention.* Menlo Park: Kaiser Family Foundation, 1992; Vlahov, D., Muñoz, A., Anthony, J. C., et al., "Association of drug injection patterns with antibody to Human Immunodeficiency Virus Type 1 among intravenous drug users in Baltimore, Maryland." *American Journal of Epidemiology* 132 (1990): 847–856; and Wilson, B. L., "Dirty needles and the AIDS dilemma." *Governing* (April 1992): 22–23.

474. "Let's move quickly in battling AIDS." Editorial. *USA Today* (March 3, 1988): 10A.

475. Hahn, R. A., Onorato, I. M., Jones, S., et al, "Prevalence of HIV infection among intravenous drug users in the United States." *Journal of the American Medical Association* 261 (1989): 2677–2684; and Wysowski, D. K., Schober, S. E., Wise, R. P., et al., "Mortality attributed to misuse of psychoactive drugs, 1979–1988." *Public Health Reports* 108 (1993): 565–570.

476. In 1988 in New York City, for example, 38.5 percent of injecting drug users who entered a treatment center were HIV positive, 44 percent of those who acknowledged sharing needles were infected. Overall, by then New York City had an estimated HIV population of 235,000 people, at least a third of whom had acquired their infections through needle sharing. New York State Department of Health, 1989, op. cit.

477. Reagan, R., "Remarks on signing Executive Order 12368, concerning drug abuse policy functions." White House, June 24, 1982.

478. Gray, M., 1998, op. cit.

479. In lieu of due process and criminal proceedings, federal and local agencies could try to force suppliers out of business by seizing individuals' lands and personal vehicles or assets. Agencies could sell these items to fund further police operations—all without a trial or actual proof that the individuals were illegal drug manufacturers or suppliers.

480. Wysowski, D. K., et al, 1993, op. cit.

481. Baum, D., 1996, op. cit.

482. Davidson, J., "Cries for help." *Wall Street Journal* (September 4, 1990): A1.

483. Institute of Medicine, ibid.

484. New York Academy of Sciences, *Statement on AIDS Initiatives in Drug Treatment, Services in New York City.* New York City: Academy of Sciences, May 30, 1991.

485. Duke, S. B. and Gross, A. C., *America's Largest War: Rethinking Our Tragic Crusade Against Drugs.* New York: Putnam Books, 1994.

486. Levine, D. B. and Sobel, J. D., *Infections in Intravenous Drug Abusers.* New York: Oxford University Press, 1991; and Institute of Medicine, *Treating Drug Problems.* Vol. I. Washington, D.C.: National Academy Press, 1990.

487. Though the later, more expensive marijuana was likely to have been bred for higher levels of tetrahydrocannabinol, or THC, which meant that most smokers could get high on a lot less of the substance.

488. Prices for *all* forms of cocaine fell sharply, due in large part to great acceleration in supply provision from Latin America. In 1979 a pure gram of cocaine cost $780; by 1987 it could be had for just $142. See Trebach, A. S. and Zeese, K. B., editors, *The Great Issues of Drug Policy.* Washington, D.C.: Drug Policy Foundation, 1990.

489. Duster, T., "Pattern, purpose, and race in the drug war." In Reinarman, C. and Levine, H. G., editors, *Crack in America.* Berkeley: University of California Press, 1997; Baum, D., 1996, op. cit.; Gray, M., 1998, op. cit.; and Massing, M., 1998, op. cit.

490. Kozel, N. J. and Adams, E. H., "Epidemiology of drug abuse: An overview." *Science* 234 (1986): 970–974.

491. Institute of Medicine, *Homelessness, Health, and Human Needs.* Washington, D.C.: National Academy Press, 1988.

492. Wallace, D. and Wallace, R., *A Plague on Your House: How New York Was Burned Down and National Public Health Crumbled.* New York: Verso, 1998.

493. Bourgois, P., "In Search of Horatio Alger." In Reinarman, C. and Levine, H. G., 1997, op. cit.; Myers, S. L., "Crime, entrepreneurship, and labor force withdrawal." *Contemporary Policy Issues* X (1992): 84–97; and Prothrow-Stith, D., *Deadly Consequences.* New York: HarperCollins, 1991.

494. *National Household Survey on Drug Abuse, 1985.* Washington, D.C.: National Institute on Drug Abuse, 1986.

495. Kleiman, M. A. R., 1992, op. cit.; and Reinarman, C. and Levine, H. G., "The crack attack." In Reinarman, C. and Levine, H. G., 1997, op. cit.

496. Reinarman, C. and Levine, H. G., 1997, op. cit.

497. Minnesota § 152.025 statute.

498. The case was *State of Minnesota v. Gerard Jerome Russell, Deshone Armstead, Michael Odell Johnson, Steve Antonio Morrison and James NMN Alderson.* Supreme Court of Minnesota, December 13, 1991, Nos. C#-91-22, C7-91-203. See details of this and other legal cases related to crack in Glasser, I. and Segal, L., "Civil rights and liberties." In Reinarman, C. and Levine, H. G., 1997, op. cit.

499. See "Arrests, Minnesota, All Ages by Race, 1985–1995" table on page 701.

500. Duffy, M. and Goodgame, D., *Marching in Place: The Status Quo Presidency of George Bush.* New York: Simon & Schuster, 1992.

501. The *Washington Post* published details on the arrest that led to that Baggie being in President Bush's hands. Teenager Keith Jackson was lured from the other side of the District of Columbia to Lafayette Park by DEA agents who bought the crack and arrested Jackson specifically so that Bush would be able to say that the park across from the White House was a haven for drug dealers. It was not. See Isikoff, M., "Drug buy set up for Bush speech: DEA lured seller to Lafayette Park." *Washington Post* (September 22, 1989): A1.

502. National Criminal Justice Commission. Donziger, S. R., editor, *The Real War on Crime.* New York: Harper Perennial, 1996.

503. The National Criminal Justice Commission (ibid.) noted the following startling points:

- In 1993, on an average day, one out of every three black males aged 20–29 was in prison, jail, or on parole.
- One-third of African-American men aged 20–29 years in Los Angeles were behind bars in 1991.
- On any given day in 1991, 56 percent of 18- to 35-year-old black men in Baltimore and 42 percent of their counterparts in Washington, D.C., were under criminal justice supervision.
- One out of every three black men aged 18–21 in the nation's capitol was arrested and indicted in 1991.
- On any given day in 1989, one out of every four African-American men aged 20–29 in the United States was either in prison, jail, or on parole.
- In 1991 the Denver Police Department compiled a list of "suspected gang members." It contained the names of two of every three males in the community who were African-American and between the ages of 12 and 24 years. There were 5,500 names on the list, though local gang membership was said to number no more than 250.

ARRESTS, MINNESOTA, ALL AGES
BY RACE, 1985–1995

ALLEGED CRIME	1985			1990			1995		
	WHITE	AFRICAN AMERICAN	TOTAL	WHITE	AFRICAN AMERICAN	TOTAL	WHITE	AFRICAN AMERICAN	TOTAL
Homicide	41	26	76	43	60	139	73	106	216
Rape	282	122	435	313	179	546	724	249	1,047
Robbery	342	360	784	320	596	1,048	459	954	1,514
Aggravated assault	1,623	727	2,641	2,335	1,054	3,819	2,431	1,392	4,326
Burglary	3,922	500	4,718	3,442	558	4,366	3,399	588	4,295
Larceny	18,417	2,959	22,831	19,775	3,797	25,193	19,384	5,084	26,451
Weapons	1,130	223	1,411	1,052	377	1,526	1,868	1,053	3,122
Prostitution	518	343	918	699	723	1,513	463	402	946
Narcotics	4,765	459	5,372	5,266	1,825	7,307	10,855	3,665	15,058
Family/Children	267	22	312	363	58	445	619	137	808
GRAND TOTAL	121,553	14,985	144,235	148,928	22,940	181,887	179,582	36,796	231,049
Arrests, White (%)	84			81.9			77.7		
Arrests, African American (%)		10.4			12.6			15.9	
Population that is African American (%)		1.8			2.4			2.8	

Source: Minnesota Planning, Criminal Justice Statistical Analysis Center

504. Though thoroughly discounted in scientific data, there continued to be assertions regarding the "innate character" of the arrestees. Nearly all of the increase in arrests was, however, for nonviolent crimes, such as possession of drugs or of drug paraphernalia, sale of drugs to undercover agents, small-time unarmed robberies aimed at obtaining cash for drugs. During this time, for example, New York City experienced a rash of auto break-ins in which a car window was smashed and the stereo system torn from the dashboard and sold or exchanged for a pipe of cocaine.

505. Trebach, A. S. and Zeese, K. B., editors. *The Great Issues of Drug Policy*. Washington, D.C.: Drug Policy Foundation, 1990.

506. Baum, D., 1996, op. cit.

507. Tonry, M., *Malignant Neglect*. New York: Oxford University Press, 1995; and Glasser I. and Siegal, L., 1997, op. cit.

508. Free, M. D., *African Americans and the Criminal Justice System*. New York: Garland, 1996.

509. These comments were made in all seriousness by LAPD chief Daryl Gates and Drug Czar Bennett in 1989. See Baum, D., 1996, op. cit.

510. In this section, these and other quotations from scientists came from interviews conducted by the author in 1989.

511. Further examples of the state of scientific understanding in the early 1990s of cocaine/crack effects on the human body include: "Cocaine treatment is said to cause paranoia." *Associated Press* (October 27, 1982); Becker, G. S. and Murphy, K. M., "A theory of rational addiction." *Journal of Political Economy* 96 (1988): 675–700; Cregler, L. L. and Mark, H., "Medical complications of cocaine abuse." *New England Journal of Medicine* 315 (1986): 1495–1500; Fisher, M., "A neural short circuit." *Washington Post* (July 31, 1988): A1; Gawin, F. H. and Ellinwood, E. H., "Cocaine and other stimulants."*New England Journal of Medicine* 218 (1988): 1173–1182; Isner J. M., Estes, M. N. A., Thompson, P. D., et al, "Acute cardiac events temporally related to cocaine abuse." *New England Journal of Medicine* 315 (1986): 1438–1443; Jonsson, S., O'Mera, M., and Young, J. B., "Acute cocaine poisoning." *American Journal of Medicine* 75 (1983): 1081–1084; Levine, S. R., Brust, J. C. M., Futrell, N., et al., "Cerebrovascular complications of the use of the 'crack' form of alkaloidal cocaine." *New England Journal of Medicine* 323 (1990): 699–704; Marzuk, P. M., Tardiff, K., Leon, A. C., et al., "Prevalence of recent cocaine use among motor vehicle fatalities in New York City." *Journal of the American Medical Association* 263 (1990): 250–256; Mello, N. K., Mendelson, J. H., Bree, M. P., et al., "Buprenorphine suppresses cocaine self-administration by Rhesus monkeys." *Science* 245 (1989): 859–862; Minor, R. L., Scott, B. D., Brown, B. D., et al., "Cocaine-induced myocardial infarction in patients with normal coronary arteries." *Annals of Internal Medicine* 115 (1991): 797–806; Nademanee, K., Gorelick, D. A., Josephson, M. A., et al., "Myocardial ischemia during cocaine withdrawal." *Annals of Internal Medicine* 111 (1989): 876–880; and Pollock, D. A., Holmgreen, P., Lui K. J., et al., "Discrepancies in the reported frequency of cocaine related deaths, United States, 1983 through 1988." *Journal of the American Medical Association* 266 (1991): 2233–2271.

512. Chasnoff, I. J., "Drug use in pregnancy." *New York State Journal of Medicine* (May 1989): 255; Handler, A., Kistin, N., Davis, F., et al., "Cocaine use during pregnancy: Perinatal outcomes." *American Journal of Epidemiology* 133 (1991): 818–824; Kaye, K., Elkind, L., Goldberg, D., et al., "Birth outcomes for infants of drug abusing mothers." *New York State Journal of Medicine* (May 1989): 256–261; Morgan, J. P. and Zimmer, L., "The social pharmacology of smokeable cocaine." In Reinarman, C. and Levine H. G., 1997, op. cit.; Siegal, L. "The pregnancy police fight the War on Drugs." In Reinarman, C. and Levine H. G., 1997, op. cit.; Toufexis, A., "Innocent victims." *Time* magazine (May 13, 1991): 56–63; and Woods, J. R.,

Plessinger, M. A., Clark, K. E., "Effect of cocaine on uterine blood flow and fetal oxygenation." *Journal of the American Medical Association* 257 (1987): 957–961.

513. Donziger, S. R., 1996, op. cit.; Nadelman, E. A., "Drug prohibition in the United States: Costs, consequences, and alternatives." *Science* 245 (1989): 939–946; and Trebach, A. S. and Zeese, K. B., 1990, op. cit.

514. Joseph, S. C., "A methadone clone for cocaine." *New York Times* (January 11, 1989): Op-Ed. A:17.

Because of the pain of the "crash" coming off a cocaine high, nearly all crack users were also using drugs that eased them through the emotional troughs between cocaine highs: alcohol, Valium, quaaludes, marijuana, and heroin. As a result, said Harvard's Scott Lucas, cocaine treatment "is a mess" and actually involved care of several simultaneous addictions, each of which altered the chemistry of the brain.

All psychoactive drugs exert their effects by latching on to various receptors in the brain that normally regulate such things as sleep, dreams, and visual stimulation. Many scientists believed cocaine attacked the dopamine receptor, but there was evidence that other receptors, particularly serotonin, might be targets.

Although the target remained a mystery, scientists were trying a variety of dopamine or serotonin-related drugs in cocaine treatment. Some, such as carbamazepine, were normally used for epilepsy. Bromocriptine, which was meant for treatment of Parkinson's disease, was touted by researchers at the Scripps Clinic in California and the University of Maryland.

Jeffrey Rosecan found that the antidepressant imipramine helped reduce cocaine cravings in some people, and saw promise with its chemical cousin, desipramine.

In 1989 Frank Gawin of Yale University published striking success with the use of flupenthixol decanoate. Gawin treated ten crack users in the Bahamas and said he was able to reduce cravings in all but one. After five months, four of the individuals remained off cocaine. (Gawin, F. H., Allen, D., Humblestone, B., "Outpatient treatment of 'crack' cocaine smoking with flupenthixol decanoate." *Archives of General Psychiatry* 46 [1989]: 322–325.) The study, however, was quite small, and the apparent success of the treated individuals was not compared to an untreated control population.

515. Goldstein, P. J., Brownstein, H. H., Ryan, P. J., et al., "Crack and homicide in New York City." In Reinarman, C. and Levine, H. G., 1997, op. cit.

516. Glasser, I. and Siegel, L., 1997, op. cit.

517. Police Commissioner Lee Brown ordered creation of a Drugbusters program under which cops and community representatives had meetings and coordinated their activities. The TNT was required to tell Drugbusters in advance of planned raids: some community members simply tipped off the targeted dealers. It would be revealed in 1993 that police in several precincts had become thoroughly corrupt over the years. Internal reviews would lead to dozens of arrests and many more firings of NYPD officers, especially those who worked Harlem and eastern Brooklyn precincts.

Dinkins also increased by ten thousand the number of treatment slots available in the city for cocaine users, but this fell far short of the estimated one hundred thousand New York needed. And success rates were very low because most "treatments" lasted only seven days and did not offer housing away from the drug-use environment. Rainone, G., Frank, B., Kott, A., et al., *Crack Users in Treatment.* Albany: New York State Division of Substance Abuser Services, 1987; and Massing, M., 1998, op. cit.

518. Scott, J., "L. A.'s battle against AIDS." *Los Angeles Times* (February 26, 1988): Part II, 1.

519. Not surprisingly, many in the black community began to refer to genocide: Is

this an insidious plan designed to cause a rise in mortality rates of marginalized groups? Is this a plan to erode the traditional values and culture that support the development of a strong black community? Is the expected result of present drug policies the withdrawal from productive spheres of economic life, self-defeating and destructive behaviors by these marginalized groups? How is it that young males in the marginalized population are killing one another at such alarming rates that the ability of the population to reproduce itself is effectively eliminated?

"What internationally recognized term would best describe this process?" the Drug Policy Foundation asked. Perhaps, it answered, "genocide."

See Trebach, A. S. and Zeese K. B., editors, 1990, op. cit.

520. Booth, R. E., Walters, J. K., Chitwood, D. D., et al., "HIV risk-related sex behaviors among injection drug users, crack smokers, and injection drug users who smoke crack." *American Journal of Public Health* 83 (1993): 1144–1148; Diaz, T. and Chu, S. Y., "Crack cocaine use and sexual behavior among people with AIDS." *Journal of the American Medical Association* 269 (1993): 2845–2846; Fullilove, R. E., Fullilove, M. T., Bowser, B. P., et al., "Risk of sexually transmitted disease among black adolescent crack users in Oakland and San Francisco, Calif." *Journal of the American Medical Association* 263 (1990): 851–855; Knox, R. A., "AIDS experts track the cocaine connection." *The Boston Globe* (June 14 1988): A5; and Lazare, D., "Crack and AIDS: The next wave?" *Village Voice* (New York) (May 8, 1990): 29.

521. Chaisson, R. E., Bacchetti, P., Osmond, D., et al., "Cocaine use and HIV infection in intravenous drug users in San Francisco." *Journal of the American Medical Association* 261 (1989): 561–565; Garrett, L., "New AIDS cocaine connection." *Newsday* (January 27, 1989): A3; and Lambert, B., "AIDS peril grows for cocaine users." *New York Times* (November 28, 1988): A15.

522. Centers for Disease Control and Prevention. *On the Front Lines: Fighting HIV/AIDS in African-American Communities.* U.S. Department of Health and Human Services, August, 1999.

523. Hertzman, C., Frank, J., and Evans, R. G., "Heterogeneities in health status." In Evans, R. G., et al, 1994, op. cit.

524. Callahan, D., 1998, op. cit.

525. A quarter of the cases and deaths were babies too young to immunize; so if their neighbors or siblings had measles, these infants were helpless when exposed to the virus. See Benenson, A. S., editor, *Control of Communicable Diseases Manual*, sixteenth edition. Washington, D.C.: American Public Health Association, 1995; and LeBaron, C. W., Birkhead, G. S., Parsons, P., et al., "Measles vaccination levels of children enrolled in WIC during the 1991 measles epidemic in New York City." *American Journal of Public Health* 86 (1996): 1551–1556.

526. LeBaron, C. W., et al., 1996, op. cit.

527. Centers for Disease Control and Prevention, "Physician vaccination referral practices and vaccines for children—New York, 1994." *Morbidity and Mortality Weekly Report* 44 (1995): 3–6; Dietz, V., Zell, E., Eddins, D., et al, "Vaccination coverage in the USA." *Lancet* 344 (1994): 1439–1440; Institute of Medicine, *Adverse Events Associated with Childhood Vaccines.* Washington, D.C.: National Academy Press, 1993; Manning, A. "Kids in USA get 21 shots before start of 1st grade." *USA Today* (August 3, 1999): A1; Preston, N. W., "Pertussis vaccination: Neither panic nor complacency." *Lancet* 344 (1994): 491–492; and "3 million in U.S. are at risk of measles from skipping vaccine, health officials say." *Associated Press* (August 13, 1995).

528. Centers for Disease Control and Prevention, "National, state, and urban area

vaccination coverage levels among children aged 19–35 months—United States, January-December 1995." *Morbidity and Mortality Weekly Report* 46 (1997): 176–182.

529. Centers for Disease Control and Prevention, "Summary of notifiable diseases, United States 1997." *Morbidity and Mortality Weekly Report* 46 (1997): full issue #54.

530. Centers for Disease Control and Prevention, "Epidemiology of measles—United States, 1998." *Morbidity and Mortality Weekly Report* 48 (1999): 749–753.

531. In most of the cases, the ailing individual had received no vaccine, or just one of the three required for full protection. Or the victim was a baby in a household that had a carrier or a case involving an older child. Worsening matters was indication that one type of pertussis vaccination offered less-than-ideal protection.

See Centers For Disease Control and Prevention, "Resurgence of pertussis—United States, 1993." *Morbidity and Mortality Weekly Report* 42 (1993) 952–965; and Christie, C. D. C., Marx, M. L., Marchant, C. D., et al., "The 1993 epidemic of pertussis in Cincinnati." *New England Journal of Medicine* 331 (1994): 16–21.

532. In 1992 HHS Secretary Donna Shalala practically begged physicians to take child immunization seriously. She said that "now is the time for individual health care providers to demonstrate their level of commitment" to child health. And she acknowledged that only 44 percent of American children were fully vaccinated. See Shalala, D. E., "Giving pediatric immunizations the priority they deserve." *Journal of the American Medical Association* 269 (1993): 1844–1845.

Yet physicians, made anxious by a lengthening list of recommended vaccines, demurred. As did millions of parents. When state health departments tried to remedy the situation by keeping track of which children were vaccinated and mailing reminders to forgetful parents, they ran straight into the Christian Coalition. Such record keeping, the Christian Coalition argued, was an example of Big Brother government intruding into private lives. See "Effort to increase child immunization is under attack in Idaho." *New York Times* (March 7, 1999): A25.

See "Big shots." *The Economist* (May 9, 1998): 63; Gilbert, S, "New study supports effectiveness of little used chickenpox vaccine." *New York Times* (November 4, 1997): B8; Keusch, G. T. and Cash, R. A., "A vaccine against rotavirus—when is too much too much?" *New England Journal of Medicine* 337 (1997): 1228–1229; Pollak M., "Doctors Fighting Backlash Over Vaccines." *New York Times* (April 27, 1999): F7; and "Rash worries." *The Economist* (April 11, 1998): 63–64.

533. For further discussion of the Persian Gulf conflict, Operation Desert Storm, and biological warfare, see Chapter 5 of this book.

534. Duffy, M. and Goodgame, D., 1992, op. cit.

535. Ibid.

536. Salive, M. E., Vlahov, D., and Brewer, T. F., "Coinfection with tuberculosis and HIV-1 in male prison inmates." *Public Health Reports* 105 (1990): 307–310.

537. For details on the TB resurgence of 1989–1992, see Garrett, L., 1994, op. cit., the chapter entitled "Thirdworldization." The details will not be repeated here.

538. In congressional hearings on April 2, 1992, New York Congressman Ted Weiss asked CDC director Dr. William Roper to detail the recent TB budgets. Roper's rundown was as follows:

Year	CDC Request (in $ millions)	Actual Appropriation Received (in $ millions)
1998	$ 5	$ 4
1989	$25	$ 7

Year	CDC Request (in $ millions)	Actual Appropriation Received (in $ millions)
1990	$29	$ 7
1991	$34	$ 8
1992	$35	$12

In 1992, NIAID director Anthony Fauci told Weiss at the hearing, the entire NIH tuberculosis research budget was $5.1 million, but as the drug-resistant TB epidemic unfolded, he requested an addition $4.1 million for that year. And for 1993 Fauci sought $33 million.

539. All of the details in this section that are not covered in *The Coming Plague* or in the bibliographic citations of that book are based on reporting and interviews by the author, unless otherwise noted. In addition, see Annas, G. J., "The impact of health policies on human rights: AIDS and TB control." In Mann, J. M., et al., 1999, op. cit.; Centers for Disease Control and Prevention, "Tuberculosis elimination revisited: Obstacles, opportunities, and a renewed commitment." *Morbidity and Mortality Weekly Report* 48: (1999): RR-9 (special issue); Centers for Disease Control and Prevention, "Tuberculosis outbreaks in prison housing units for HIV-infected inmates in California, 1995–1996." *Morbidity and Mortality Weekly Report* 48 (1999): 79–82; Farmer, P., *Infections and Inequalities: The Modern Plagues.* Berkeley: University of California Press, 1999; Gasner, M. R., Maw, K. L., Feldman, G. E., et al., "The use of legal action in New York City to ensure treatment of tuberculosis." *New England Journal of Medicine* 340 (1999): 359–366; Layton, M., Henning, K. J., Alexander, T. A., et al., "Universal radiographic screening for tuberculosis among inmates upon admission to jail." *American Journal of Public Health* 87 (1997): 1335–1337; Lerner, B. H. and Rothman, D. J., "Legal action to ensure treatment of tuberculosis." *New England Journal of Medicine* 341 (1999): 130–131; Moore, M., Onorato, I. M., McCray, E., et al., "Trends in drug-resistant tuberculosis in the United States, 1993–1996." *Journal of the American Medical Association* 278 (1997): 833–837; Reichman, L. B., "Defending the public's health against tuberculosis." *Journal of the American Medical Association* 278 (1997): 865–867; and Wallace, D. and Wallace, R., 1998, op. cit.

540. See Belkin, L. "A brutal cure." *New York Times Sunday Magazine* (May 30, 1999): 34–39; and Sachs, S., "90 asylum seekers at center are infected by man with TB." *New York Times* (July 31, 1995): B5.

541. Dye, C., Garnett, G. P., Sleeman, K., et al., "Prospects for worldwide tuberculosis control under the WHO DOTs strategy." *Lancet* 352 (1998): 1886–1891. In 1998 WHO officially was notified of 3.81 million cases of active TB worldwide, with 85 percent of the nations filing reports. This was certainly a gross underestimate, as few nations had accurate TB surveillance and reporting systems in place in 1998 and most nations had political and economic reasons for downplaying the sizes of their epidemics. Dye's group estimated that for that year the true global TB burden was 7.96 million new cases plus 16.2 million chronic tuberculosis sufferers, with 1.87 million dying. The global case fatality rate, they estimated, was 23 percent per year of all active TB cases, with highest death rates occurring in nations with large HIV epidemics.

542. Just five years later, Hamburg's limited powers and the overall restraints placed on public health authorities would face an interesting new legal and ethical quandary: genetics and crime. America would be fixated on so-called rampage killings in which individuals went on terrifying murder sprees, typically targeting schoolmates or coworkers. Studies of such killings would reveal that nearly all were committed by people who had long histories of mental illness. Perhaps a third were diagnosed schizophrenics who had stopped taking their medication.

Blurring the lines between public health and law enforcement, researchers were fast identifying the genes responsible for such mental illness. And looming on the millennial horizon was talk of compelling medication of all genetically identified schizophrenics and psychotics as a matter of "public health," e.g., to protect the population at large against rampage killers.

See Goodstein, L. and Glaberson, W., "The well-marked road to homicidal rage." *New York Times* (April 10, 2000):A1.

543. Contributing to the decline of TB in New York City and nationwide was Highly Active Anti-Retroviral Therapy, or HAART, for HIV treatment. Introduced in 1996, HAART greatly enhanced the health of most HIV patients who took the medicine, rendering them *far* less vulnerable to tuberculosis.

544. In laboratory studies done at Colorado State University, scientists infected mice with the Tennessee microbe, comparing their reactions to mice infected with the "W" strain from New York. The"W"-infected group of mice grew 10^3 bacilli in their lungs in ten days. In the same time, the Tennessee–TB infected mice grew one thousand times more microbes.

The CDC's Sandra Valway noted that similarly astonishing rates of growth were seen when the new TB bacteria were cultured in lab dishes on human cells, and she remarked that "lab workers say they have never seen anything like this."

545. Much harder to treat were a flurry of group "W" strain outbreaks that occurred inside hospitals all over the United States, spread via contaminated bronchoscopes that had been used over and over again to examine patients' lungs. Agerton, T., Valway, S., Gore, B., et al., "Transmission of highly drug-resistant strain (strain W1) of *Mycobacterium tuberculosis." Journal of the American Medical Association* 278 (1997): 1073–1077; and Michele, T. M., Cronin, W. A., Craham, N. M., et al., "Transmission of *Mycobacterium tuberculosis* by a fiberoptic bronchoscope." *Journal of the American Medical Association* 278 (1997): 1093–1095.

546. For summaries, see Morse, S., 1993, op. cit.

547. For more details see: Henig, R. M., 1993, op. cit.; and Garrett, L., 1994, op. cit.

548. Institute of Medicine, 1988, op. cit.

549. The report concluded that "the dilemma faced by public health is how to take on the new challenges while continuing its work to contain long-existing problems. Public health leaders have not succeeded in making clear that both aspects of public health must be tackled vigorously. All too often, political leaders push short-term 'solutions' to various health crises without reference to the knowledge base that exists for sound programs. The general public is confused. The result is a hodgepodge of fractionated interests and programs, organizational turmoil among new agencies, and well-intentioned but unbalanced appropriations—without coherent direction by well-qualified professionals."

550. Weiss, L. D., *Private Medicine and Public Health.* Boulder: Westview Press, 1997.

551. Ibid.

552. Robert Wood Johnson Foundation, *Access to Health Care in the United States: Results of a 1986 Survey.* Special Report No. 2. New York: Robert Wood Johnson Foundation, 1987; and Robert Wood Johnson Foundation, *Announcing the Health Care for the Uninsured Program.* New York: Robert Wood Johnson Foundation, 1985.

553. Annas, G. J., "Back to the future: The IOM report reconsidered." *American Journal of Public Health* 81 (1991): 835–837.

554. Pickett, G., "The future of health departments: The governmental presence." *Annual Review of Public Health* 1 (1980): 297–321. Roper, W. L., Baker, E. L., Dyal, W. W., et al., "Strengthening the public health system." *Public Health Reports* 107 (1992): 609–615.

555. The report noted the following goals that were set in *Healthy People 1990,* versus what had actually been achieved by that date:

Life Stage	1990 Goal	Actual 1990
Infants	35% lower death rate	28% lower death rate
Children	20% lower death rate	21% lower death rate
Teens/Young Adults	20% lower death rate	13% lower death rate
Adults	25% lower death rate	21% lower death rate
Seniors	20% fewer days of restricted activity	17% fewer days of restricted activity

See U.S. Public Health Service, *Healthy People 2000*. Washington, D.C.: U.S. Department of Health and Human Services, 1990.

556. His remarks were later published. See McBeath, W. H., "Health For All: A public health vision." *American Journal of Public Health* 81 (1990): 1560–1565.

557. Navarro, V., "The future of public health in health care reform." *American Journal of Public Health* 84 (1994): 729–730.

558. Baker, E. L., Melton, R. J., Stange, P. V., et al., "Health reform and the health of the public." *Journal of the American Medical Association* 272 (1994): 1276–1282; and Roper, W. L., Baker, E. L., Dyal, W. W., et al., "Strengthening the public health system." *Public Health Reports* 107 (1992): 609–616.

559. DALYs analysis revealed to the World Bank that the poorer a country was, the greater its financial burden due to disease and, conversely, the more dramatic would be the expected economic impact of public health interventions that reduced the disease's incidence. Sub-Saharan Africa, the world's poorest region, was calculated by the World Bank in 1990 to suffer nearly 600 DALYs lost per 1,000 people each year, representing a dramatic loss in productivity due to disease. In India the annual toll was about 320 DALYs per 1,000 people, and in the wealthy industrialized nations it was just over 100 DALYs.

World Bank, *Investing in Health*. New York: Oxford University Press, 1993; World Health Organization, *Global Burden of Disease and Injury*. Geneva: World Health Organization, several volumes released since 1988 (with more to be released after 2000); World Health Organization, *Implementation of the Global Strategy for Health For All By the Year 2000, Second Evaluation; and Eighth Report on the World Health Situation*. Geneva: World Health Organization, March 6, 1992; and World Health Organization, *Investing in Health Research and Development*. TDR; shGen/96.1. Geneva: World Health Organization, 1996.

The WHO's *Global Burden of Disease and Injury* series is a monumental cost analysis executed by the Harvard School of Public Health's Christopher Murray, WHO's Alan D. Lopez, and the World Bank's Dean Jamison. The series seeks to assess the present and future (to 2020) costs of all possible illnesses and injuries, of their prevention efforts, of their treatments, of productivity losses to society, and of comparative disease rates. It is the most massive effort of its kind ever undertaken and, almost by definition, highly controversial. After all, such studies begin with available data and assumptions, all of which are less than perfect and subject to interpretation.

"Publication of the *Global Burden of Disease and Injury* series marks the transition to a new era of health outcome accounting—an era for which these volumes establish vastly higher standards for rigor, comprehensiveness and internal consistency," Jamison wrote in Volume III of the series. See Murray, C. J. L. and Lopez, A. D., editors, *Health Dimensions of Sex and Reproduction*. Geneva: World Health Organization, 1998.

560. The World Bank calculated, for example, that eradication of polio in the United States through mass immunization at a total cost of $220 million between 1975 and 1990 had spared 220,000 children from the disease, saving the nation up to $1.3 billion in medical costs and even more in DALYs.

561. Johnson, H., *Divided We Fall: Gambling with History in the Nineties*. New York: W. W. Norton, 1994.

562. Ibid. See also Castro, J., "Condition: Critical." *Time* magazine (November 25, 1991): 34–42; Easterbrook, G., "The revolution in medicine." *Newsweek* (July 26, 1987): 40–74; Friedman, E., "Problems plaguing public hospitals: Uninsured patient transfers, tight funds, mismanagement, and misperception." *Journal of the American Medical Association* 257 (1987): 1850–1857; "The healthy option." *The Economist* (February 8, 1992): 14–15; Walton, S. "For-profit health care facilities: Higher costs, comparable care." *News Report* XXXVI (1986): 4–10; and Watt, J. M., Derzon, R. A., Renn, S. C., et al., "The comparative economic performance of investor-owned chain and not-for-profit hospitals." *New England Journal of Medicine* 314 (1986): 89–96.

563. Imershein, A. W., Rond, P. C., and Mathis, M. P., "Restructuring patterns of elite dominance and the formation of state policy in health care." *American Journal of Sociology* 97 (1992): 970–993.

564. U.S. Bureau of the Census, *Census Brief: Children Without Health Insurance*. CENBR/98–1. Washington, D.C.: U.S. Bureau of the Census, March 1998; Davis, K., Rowland, D., Altman, D., et al., "Health insurance: The size and shape of the problem." *Inquiry* 32 (1995): 196–203; Lewis, K., Ellwood, M., and Czajka, J. L., *Counting the Uninsured: A Review of the Literature*. Washington, D.C.: The Urban Institute, 1998; and Swartz, K., Marcotte, J., and McBride, T. D., "Personal characteristics and spells without health insurance." *Inquiry* 30 (1993): 64–76.

565. Evans, R. G. and Stoddart, G. L., "Producing health, consuming health care." In Evans, R. G., et al., 1994, op. cit.

566. Further, the burden of the uninsured was not spread evenly across the society. See Kaiser Commission on the Future of Medicaid. *Health Needs and Medicaid Financing: State Facts*. Menlo Park: Kaiser Foundation, 1993; and Erdman, K. and Wolfe, S. M., *Poor Health Care for Poor Americans: A Ranking of State Medicaid Programs*. Washington, D.C.: Public Health Research Group, 1988.

567. Hay, J. W., Osmond, D. H., and Jacobson, M. A., "Projecting the medical costs of AIDS and ARC in the United States." *Journal of Acquired Immune Deficiency Syndrome* 1 (1988): 466–485.

This represented a modest increment compared to the $16 billion as forecast by the CDC. See U.S. Department of Health and Human Services, "Coolfont Report: APHS plan for prevention and control of AIDS and the AIDS virus." *Public Health Report* 101 (1986): 341–348.

By 1999 HIV-related medical spending in the United States would total $6.9 billion in federal dollars meted out through Medicaid, the Ryan White AIDS Fund, Social Security, and Medicare. The federal government would also spend the following in FY 1999:

HIV Research	$1.8 billion
HIV Prevention	$0.77 billion
International Aid	$0.14 billion
Treatment and patient support	$6.9 billion
TOTAL	$9.717 billion

That was up from total federal HIV/AIDS spending levels as follows:

FY 1995	$6.718 billion
FY 1996	$7.265 billion
FY 1997	$8.144 billion
FY 1998	$8.727 billion

These figures do *not* include private or state subsidized spending (insured or otherwise) for treatment, research, drug development, patient assistance, hospitalization, etc. See Foster, S., Gregory, A., Niederhausen, P., et al., *Federal HIV/AIDS Spending: A Budget Chartbook*. Menlo Park: Kaiser Family Foundation, 1999.

568. Franks, P., Clancy, C. M., and Gold, M. R., "Health insurance and mortality." *Journal of the American Medical Association* 270 (1993): 737–741.

Yet of the top twenty-four industrialized nations, only Turkey's government contributed a smaller percentage than the United States to the cost of health for its people. Ninety-five percent of all health costs in Norway were borne by government and Norwegians had the lowest infant mortality rate in the world (4 per 1,000 babies in 1994) and one of the highest life expectancies (78 years for babies born in 1993). Though the government spent heavily on health, Norwegians still enjoyed excellent standards of living with a per-capita GNP of $26,390 annually. Comparable U.S. figures were an infant mortality of 8 per 1,000; life expectancy of seventy-seven years; per-capita GNP of $25,880. These are World Bank estimates from the bank's annual *World Development Reports*. New York: Oxford University Press, 1995.

In 1990 just over 40 percent of America's health care tab was picked up by government. See Schieber, G. J., Poullier, J. P., and Greenwald, L. M., "U.S. health expenditure performance." *Health Care Financing Review* 13 (1992): 4.

569. Evans, R. G., "Health care as a threat to our health." *Daedalus* (Fall 1994): 21–42.

570. Lavis, J. N. and Stoddart, G. L., "Can we have too much health care?" *Daedalus* (Fall 1994): 43–60.

571. Reagan, M. D., *The Accidental System: Health Care Policy in America*. Boulder: Westview Press, 1999.

572. Though polls showed that by 1991 68 percent of U.S. voters said that they "prefer the Canadian system" over that in the United States. Louis Harris and Associates conducted a poll with these results in November 1991.

573. Jacobs, L. R., Shapiro, R. Y., and Schulman, E. C., "The polls—poll trends: Medical care in the United States—an update." *Public Opinion Quarterly* 57 (1993): 394–427.

574. Ibid.

575. Ibid.

576. Blendon, R. J., Altman, D. E., Benson, J. M., et al., "The implications of the 1992 presidential election for health care reform." *Journal of the American Medical Association* 268 (1992): 3371–3375.

577. Ginzberg, E., 1996, op. cit.

578. Sen, A., *Development as Freedom*. New York: Alfred A. Knopf, 1999.

579. Jones, S., Cohodes, D. M., and Scheil, B., "The risks of ignoring insurance risk management." *Health Affairs* (Spring 1994): 108–122; Oliver, T. R. and Dowell, E. B., "Interest groups and health reform: Lessons from California." *Health Affairs* (Spring 1994): 120–130; and Rubin, A. J., "Reinvention of health care is key to Clinton overhaul." *Congressional Quarterly* (March 13, 1993): 595–600.

580. Freeman, P. and Robbins A., "National health care reform minus public health: A formula for failure." *Journal of Public Health Policy* 15 (1994): 261–282.

581. "Warning: Doctors can damage your wealth." *The Economist* (October 20, 1990): 19–20.

582. Aaron, H. J. and Schwartz, W. B., "The painful prescription: Rationing health care." *The Brookings Institute, Studies in Social Economics Series*. Washington, D.C.: Brookings Institute, 1984; Feldstein, P. J., *Health Care Economics*. Fourth edition. Albany: Delmar Publishing, 1993.

583. Gordon, L., "Public health is more important than health care." *Journal of Public Health Policy* 14 (1993): 261–264.

584. Gordon, R. L., Gerzoff, R. B., and Richards, T. B., "Determinants of U.S. local health department expenditures, 1992 through 1993." *American Journal of Public Health* 87 (1997): 91–95; Halverson, P. K., Miller, C. A., Fried, B. J., et al., "Performing public health functions: The perceived contribution of public health and other community agencies." *Journal of Health and Human Services Administration* (Winter 1996): 288–303; Mays, G. P., Halverson, P. K., and Miller, C. A., "Assessing the performance of local public health systems: A survey of state health agency efforts." *Journal of Public Health Management Practice* 4 (1998): 63–78; Miller, C. A., Moore, K. S., and Richards, T. B., "The impact of critical events of the 1980s on core functioning for a select group of local health departments. *Public Health Reports* 108 (1993): 695–701; and Miller, C. A., Moore, K. S., Richards, T. B., et al., "Longitudinal observations on a selected group of local health departments: A preliminary report." *Journal of Public Health Policy* 14 (1993): 34–50.

585. Osterholm, M. T., "A survey of public health infectious disease surveillance in the United States, 1992," unpublished data provided by the author.

586. Dowdle, W. R., "The future of the public health laboratory." *Annual Review of Public Health* 14 (1993): 649–664.

587. Holland, E. J., Mahanti, R. L., Belongia, E. A., et al., "Ocular involvement in an outbreak of *Herpes gladiatorum.*" *American Journal of Ophthalmology* 114 (1992): 680–684.

588. Hedberg, C. W., David, M. J. White, K. E., et al., "Role of egg consumption in sporadic *Salmonella enteriditis* and *Salmonella typhirium* infections in Minnesota." *Journal of Infectious Diseases* 167 (1993): 107–111; Hedberg, C. W., White, K. E., Johnson, J. A., et al., "An outbreak of *Salmonella enteritidis* infection at a fast-food restaurant: Implications for foodhandler-associated transmission." *Journal of Infectious Diseases* 164 (1991): 1135–1140; and Hedberg, C. W., Korlath, J. A., D'Aoust, J. Y., et al., "A multistate outbreak of *Salmonella javiana* and *Salmonella oranienburg* infections due to consumption of contaminated cheese." *Journal of the American Medical Association* 268 (1992): 3203–3207.

589. Hedberg, C. W., Levine, W. C., White, K. E., et al., "An international foodborne outbreak of shigellosis associated with a commercial airline." *Journal of the American Medical Association* 268 (1992): 3203–3212; and Wood, R. C., MacDonald, K. L., Osterholm, M. T., "*Campylobacter* enteritis outbreaks associated with drinking raw milk during youth activities." *Journal of the American Medical Association* 268 (1992): 3228–3230.

590. MacDonald, K. L., Mills, W. A., Wood R. C., et al., "Evolution of clinical and laboratory aspects of antibody tests for detection of hepatitis C virus infection in blood donors and recipients from a low-risk population." *Transfusion* 34 (1994): 202–208; and Wood, R. C., MacDonald, K. L., White, K. E., et al., "Risk factors for lack of detectable antibody following hepatitis B vaccination of Minnesota health care workers." *Journal of the American Medical Association* 270 (1993): 2935–2939.

591. Ehresmann, K. R., Hedberg, C. W., Grimm, M. B., et al., "An outbreak of measles at an international sporting event with airborne transmission in a domed stadium." *Journal of Infectious Diseases* 171 (1995): 679–683.

592. Institute of Medicine, *Emerging Infections: Microbial Threats to Health in the United States.* Washington, D.C.: National Academy Press, 1992.

593. Centers for Disease Control and Prevention, *Addressing Emerging Infectious Disease Threats: A Prevention Strategy for the United States.* Washington, D.C.: U.S. Department of Health and Human Services, 1994. This report was updated in 1998 as Centers for Disease Control Prevention, "Preventing emerging infectious diseases: A strategy for the twenty-first century." *Morbidity and Mortality Weekly Report* 47 (RR-15) (September 11, 1998): 1–14.

594. See Chapter 5 of this book.

595. Homer-Dixon, T. F., "Environmental scarcities and violent conflict: Evidence from cases." *International Security* 19 (1994): 5–40; Homer-Dixon, T. F., "On the threshold: Environmental changes as causes of acute conflict." *International Security* 16 (1991): 76–116; Huntington, S. P., *The Clash of Civilizations and Remaking of World Order*. New York: Simon & Schuster, 1996; Kennedy, P., *Preparing for the Twenty-First Century*. New York: Vintage, 1994.

See also Fiedler, D. P., "Microbialpolitik: Infectious diseases and international relations." *International Law Review* 14 (1998): 2–21; Garrett, L., "The return of infectious diseases." *Foreign Affairs* 75 (1996): 66–79; Hammond, A., *Which New World? Scenarios for the 21st Century*. Washington, D.C.: Shearwater, 1998; Institute of Medicine, *Vital Interests in Global Health*. Washington, D.C., National Academy Press, 1997; Kegley, C. W. and Wittkopf, E. R., *The Global Agenda: Issues and Perspectives*. Fifth edition. New York: McGraw Hill, 1998; O'Brien, E., "The diplomatic implications of emerging diseases." In Cahill, K. M., editor, *Preventive Diplomacy*. New York: Basic Books, 1996; and World Bank, *World Development Report 1997: The State in a Changing World*. New York: Oxford University Press, 1997.

596. Many biologists found a *direct* correlation between environmental concerns and disease emergence, the linking being climate change as a result of ozone layer weakening. Shifts in climates, they said, favored disease-causing insects and algae.

See Epstein, P. R., "Climate and health." *Science* 285 (1999): 347–348; Garfield, R., "Malaria control in Nicaragua: Social and political influences on disease transmission and control activities." *Lancet* 354 (1999): 414–418; Linthicum, K. J., Anyamba, A., Tucker, C. J., et al., "Climate and satellite indicators to forecast Rift Valley Fever epidemics in Kenya." *Science* 285 (1999): 397–398; and Wilson, M. E., Levins, R., and Spielman, A., editors, *Disease in Evolution*. Part I: "Water related diseases." New York: New York Academy of Sciences, 1994.

597. "Disease fights back." *The Economist* (May 20, 1995): 79–81; and MacKenzie, D., "Can we afford not to track deadly viruses?" *New Scientist* (May 20, 1995): 4.

598. Working Group on Emerging and Re-emerging Infectious Diseases, *Global Microbial Threats in the 1990s*. Washington, D.C.: NSTC Committee on International Science, Engineering and Technology (CISET), 1995.

599. Garrett, L., "A call to arms against new infectious diseases." *Newsday* (July 26, 1995): A25.

600. Ibid.

601. Skocpol, T., *Boomerang*. New York: W. W. Norton, 1996.

602. The plan's basic strategy was to require that all U.S. employers provide health insurance for their workers. Small businesses, unemployed, and self-employed workers would receive federal subsidies to offset their insurance costs. Insurance would be purchased from regional health alliances, formed of medical care providers, HMOs, physicians, and the like. These alliances would be community-based and run by boards on which would sit representatives of government, the citizenry, and the employers. The alliances would negotiate reimbursement rates for hospitals and physicians, as well as set local standards of quality expected for those funds.

603. See: "Got it? An OMB version of a new health-care system." *Medical World News* (September, 1993): 21; "Health-care debate takes off." *Congressional Quarterly Almanac* (1993): 335–347; Johnson, H., 1994, op. cit.; and Peterson, M. A., "How health policy information is used in Congress." In Mann, J. E. and Ornstein, N. J., editors, *How Congress Shapes Health Policy*. Washington, D.C.: Brookings Institute Press, 1995.

604. "Appropriations process tough on public health." *The Nation's Health* (August 1995): 1; Centers for Disease Control and Prevention, "CDC's national profile of local boards of health, September 1997." *Morbidity and Mortality Weekly Report* 47 (1997): 573–574; Gordon, R. L., Baker, E. L., Roper, W. L., et al., "Prevention and the reforming U.S. health care system: Changing roles of responsibilities for public health." *Annual Review of Public Health* 17 (1996): 489–509; Iglehart, J. K., "Politics and public health." *New England Journal of Medicine* 334 (1996): 203–207; Levy, B. S., "Creating the future of public health: Values, vision, and leadership." *American Journal of Public Health* 88 (1998): 188–192; Schwab, M. and Syme, S. L., "On paradigms, community participation, and the future of public health." *American Journal of Public Health* 87 (1997): 2049–2052; Wellever, A., Hill G., and Casey, M., "Commentary: Medicaid reform issues affecting the Indian health care system." *American Journal of Public Health* 88 (1998): 193–195; and "Who's putting the pinch on public health?" *Columbia Public Health* (Fall 1996): 23–26.

605. Carlson, M., "Another dose of Harry and Louise." *Time* magazine (November 4, 1997): 34; and Ellis, D. "Band-aids to patch up health care." *Time* magazine (February 17, 1992): 20–22.

606. Derthick, M., "Whither federalism?" *The Future of the Public Sector* 2 (June 1996): 1–4. Published by the Urban Institute, Washington, D.C.

607. Meacham J., "Defiance in the Sun Belt." *Newsweek* (April 24, 1995): 33.

608. Callahan, D., 1998, op. cit.

609. Blumenthal, D., "Health care reform at the close of the twentieth century." *New England Journal of Medicine* 340 (1999): 1916–1920.

610. A 1994 survey of Oklahomans showed that only those citizens with strong health needs were inclined to reject the prevailing view that universal health equaled Big Government, which was bad. The poorer Oklahomans, those lacking health insurance, favored universal health care. The majority, however, found their own health needs met decently enough in 1994 that they saw no need to support Big Government. Goldsteen, R. L., Goldsteen, K., Kronenfeld, J. J., et al., "Antigovernment sentiment and support for universal access to care: Are they incompatible?" *American Journal of Public Health* 87 (1997): 25–28.

See also Donelan, K., Blendon, R. J., Hill, C. A., et al., "Whatever happened to the health insurance crisis in the United States?" *Journal of the American Medical Association* 276 (1996): 1346–1350.

611. Budetti, P. P., "Health reform for the 21st century?" *Journal of the American Medical Association* 277 (1997): 193–198; and Skolnick, A. A., "Democrats drop universal coverage." *Journal of the American Medical Association* 276 (1996): 931.

612. Mullan, F., "Federal public health, semi-reinvented." *American Journal of Public Health* 87 (1997): 21–24.

613. Pear, R., "More Americans were uninsured in 1998, U.S. says." *New York Times* (October 4, 1999): A1.

614. Kuttner, R., "The American health care system." *New England Journal of Medicine* 340 (1999): 248–252.

615. Marquis, M. S. and Long, S. H., "Federalism and health system reform." *Journal of the American Medical Association* 278 (1997): 514–517.

616. Gordon, R. L., Baker, E. L., Roper, W. L., et al., "Prevention and the reforming U.S. health care system: Changing roles and responsibilities for public health." *Annual Review of Public Health* 17 (1996): 489–509; Lasker, R. D., *Medicine and Public Health: The Power of Collaboration*. New York: Academy of Medicine, 1997; Lasker R. D., Abramson, D. M., and Freedman, G. R., *Pocket Guide to Cases of Medicine and Public Health Collaboration*. New

York: Academy of Medicine, 1998; Loeppke, R. R., "Prevention and managed care: The next generation." *Journal of Occupational and Environmental Medicine* 37 (1995): 558–562; Reisner, S. J., "Medicine and public health: Pursuing a common destiny." *Journal of the American Medical Association* 276 (1996): 1429–1430; and Schauffler, H. H. and Rodriguez, T., "Managed care for preventive services: A review of policy options." *Medical Care Review* 50 (1993): 153–198.

617. Johnson, H., 1994, op. cit.

618. Ibid.

619. For renditions of these events, see Ayers, B. D., "In California uncertainty chills illegal aliens." *New York Times* (November 21, 1994): A10; Cheevers, J., "County seeks private takeover of clinics." *Los Angeles Times* (August 18, 1995): B1; Church, G. J., "Teaching hospitals in crisis." *Time* magazine (July 17, 1995): 40–43; Clark, F., "Maybe, the county's sky is falling." *LACMA Physician* (August 14, 1995): 16–24; Garrett, L., "L.A. hemorrhage." *Newsday* (September 12, 1995): A12; Garrett, L., "L.A.'s poor see a bleak future without clinics." *Newsday* (September 12, 1995): Discovery B21; Garrett, L., "The prognosis isn't pretty." *Newsday* (September 12, 1995): B28; Meyerson, H., "Death of a county." *LA Weekly* (August 18, 1995): A1; Moffat, S., "Clinic's grim prospect: Turning away the desperate." *Los Angeles Times* (August 22, 1995): A1; Rabin, J. L. and Williams T., "Health czar says county could lose 4 hospitals." *Los Angeles Times* (September 6, 1995): A1; Rabin, J. S., Meyer, J., and Cheevers, J., "How public health care got sick." *Los Angeles Times* (October 29, 1995): A1; Sack, K., "Public hospitals around country cut basic service." *New York Times* (August 20, 1995): A1; Shuit, D. P., "Cuts pose threat to AIDS programs, county workers say." *Los Angeles Times* (August 19, 1995): B3; Sterngold, J., "Budget slashes could close hospital." *New York Times* (July 17, 1995): A21; and Yaroslavsky, Z., "The buck stops in Sacramento." *Los Angeles Times* (August 23, 1995): Op-ed.

620. Reed, S. R., Chief Administrative Officer, *1995–96 Proposed County Budget.* Memo to the Board of Supervisors of the County of Los Angeles, June 20, 1995.

621. UCLA Center for Health Policy Research. *At Risk: Los Angeles County, the Health of its People and its Health System.* A briefing document prepared for the Health and Mental Health Advocacy Coalition, October 21, 1994.

A further problem was that fewer employers were offering health insurance to their workers in Los Angeles during the nineties—less than half did so. Indeed, 87 percent of all medically uninsured Los Angelenos were fully employed.

See Cornwell, E. E., Berne, T. V., Belzberg, H., et al., "Health care crisis from a trauma center perspective: The LA story." *Journal of the American Medical Association* 276 (1996): 940–944.

622. UCLA Center for Health Policy Research, 1994, op. cit.

623. Interview with the author, September 1995. All quotations in this Los Angeles section, except when specifically cited, were derived from author interviews.

624. Indeed, LAC-USC Medical Center had already suffered considerable damage during the recent Los Angeles earthquake, and repairs were expected to cost millions of dollars.

625. That sentiment was echoed by USC professor of medicine Dr. Steven Asch. Writing in the *LA Weekly*, Asch, S., 1995, op. cit compared Los Angeles County's health care situation to what he had experienced working as a physician in Ecuador: "Like the IMF [International Monetary Fund], Wall Street says that the government—in this case, L.A. County—must balance its budget. As in Ecuador, public health care will take the brunt of the cuts. The federal and state governments, like the international donors of the 1980s, preach tough love and seem unlikely to come to the rescue."

626. According to county budget reports, Reed, S. R. and Sasaki, A. T., *County of Los*

Angeles 1995–96 Proposed Budget, Health Services Addendum. Los Angeles County Board of Supervisors, June, 1995. Department of Health Services revenues for 1990 broke down as follows: 13.1 percent from county taxes; 14.0 percent from special grants from a variety of sources; 23.9 percent from the federal government; and 48.9 percent from the state. But by 1994–95 that had changed dramatically: county taxes contributed only 6.25 percent and outside grants 7.65 percent; state contributions fell to 21.5 percent; and federal dollars represented 64.5 percent of health department revenues. The dramatic drop in state and county contributions was largely the result of the severe recession spurred by the nearly complete collapse of Southern California's aerospace industry. The county's hospitals took an additional hit because they lost a heavy percentage of their Medi-Cal clients and public facilities after 1991. Because the state reimbursed providers so poorly before 1991, private physicians and hospitals refused to care for Medi-Cal patients. After 1991, however, California raised its reimbursement rates sufficiently that private hospitals and HMOs actively recruited the state-subsidized patients. Prior to 1991 about half of the patients treated at LAC-USC Medical Center and other public hospitals were Medi-Cal reimbursed—it wasn't great compensation, but it was something. By 1995 most of those patients had moved to the private sector, and LAC-USC's patient population was overwhelmingly uninsured.

See Friedman, E, "California public hospitals: The buck has stopped." *Journal of the American Medical Association* 277 (1997): 577–581.

627. But Yaroslavsky reserved special contempt for the second target of his blame: Governor Wilson and the Republican-controlled state legislature. Together, they had continuously blocked all attempts to save the county through either liquor and tobacco taxes or diversion of $75 million from the L.A. subway construction funds.

Most members of Yaroslavsky's party, however, including fellow liberal supervisor Gloria Molina, opposed both of these avenues for garnering revenue. Los Angeles, with the worst metropolitan mass transit system in the nation, was desperate to complete its multibillion-dollar subway system. And the powerful wine and tobacco industries had lobbied hard and successfully to keep California's so-called sin taxes among the lowest in the nation.

There was no unanimity within the California Democratic party on the question of what to do with L.A. County's public health crisis. Some in the state legislature wanted a Felix Rohatyn–type business executive to head a Board of Control, similar to the one that had saved New York City during the Koch administration, to wrest control of all county finances from the supervisors.

See Seeley, J., "The state withers away." *LA Weekly* (August 18, 1995): 31.

628. Genetic analysis of TB strains found in L.A. patients from 1994 to 1996 revealed that most cases involved new infections spreading among the county's homeless people, particularly Skid Row men.

See Barnes, P. F., Yang, Z., Preston-Martin, S., et al., "Patterns of tuberculosis transmission in central Los Angeles." *Journal of the Medical Association* 278 (1997): 1159–1163.

629. Disease Control Programs, *1992 Communicable Disease Morbidity Report.* County of Los Angeles Department of Health Services, 1993; and Fanin, S., *Report: Toward the Future of Disease Control in Los Angeles County.* Memo to Mark Finucane, Department of Health Services, Los Angeles County, April 10, 1996.

630. Data obtained from Beth Zachary, chief executive officer of White Memorial Hospital, 1995.

631. Halfon, N., Wood, D. L., Valdez, B., et al., "Medicaid enrollment and health services access by Latino children in inner-city Los Angeles." *Journal of the American Medical Association* 277 (1997): 636–641.

632. Commonwealth Fund. *U.S. Minority Health: A Chartbook*. New York: Commonwealth Fund, 1999.

The Fund noted the following:

- 46 percent of all Hispanics in the United States over eighteen years of age were without a regular doctor (compared to 39 percent of blacks and 26 percent of whites).
- 53 percent of Hispanics used public hospital ERs as their primary source of health care (versus 47 percent of blacks and 30 percent of whites).
- 56 percent of Hispanics lacked any form of health insurance (as did 48 percent of Asians, 38 percent of blacks, and 35 percent of whites).
- Among uninsured Hispanics, 44 percent were noncitizens and 16 percent were born in the United States.

633. Task force on the Future of Health Insurance for Working Americans, "Working without benefits: The health insurance crisis confronting Hispanic Americans." New York: The Commonwealth Fund, 2000.

634. In 1998, when Sweeney became the head of America's largest labor consortium, the AFL-CIO, Clinton was no doubt relieved that in 1995 he had listened to the then-leader of SEIU.

635. Department of Health Services, *Medicaid Demonstration Project for Los Angeles County*. Los Angeles: Department of Health Services, 1996.

636. On July 29, 1999, California's newly elected governor, Democrat Gray Davis, brokered a deal with the U.S. Court of Appeals that nullified most provisions of Proposition 187.

637. During the first months of the Demonstration Project, heads rolled. The county's top health leadership resigned. Thousands of employees were either laid off, quit out of fear of layoffs, or down-shifted to lower status, lower-paying positions. By December 1995 the Department of Health Services had lost 6 percent of its employees, downsized another 15 to 20 percent, and reduced its annual payroll by $138 million. Morale collapsed. Patient care suffered.

638. New York City Mayor Giuliani was trying to sell off the city's public hospitals, turning care for the poor over to the private sector. By 2000 he would still, unsuccessfully, be trying to find buyers for the aging, rundown facilities.

639. Reed, S. R., *1996–97 Proposed County Budget*. Report for the Los Angeles County Board of Supervisors, April 25, 1996.

All of Reed's radical recommendations were implemented before the Demonstration Project's first birthday on October 1, 1996. And they represented just one painful rung on the ladder to long-term solvency. By the middle of 1997, another sixteen community health clinics had been sold off, leaving the huge county with just twenty-two clinics and five hospitals.

Reed's 1996–97 proposed budget made the future look ominous. Even with the White House bailout and so many massive cuts, Los Angeles still faced continued debt crises due to what economists called a "structural gap"—the difference between inflation-adjusted costs and actual property tax revenues. California's gap was caused by the permanent revenue shortfalls that were the legacy of Prop. 13, and the budget office estimated for 1996 it exceeded $1 billion.

"Once again, our recommendations . . . represent what can best be described as a compromise between what is most fiscally advisable and what is operationally and practically feasible," Reed warned. "Our projections indicate little, if any, increase in general County revenues over the next few years and there is a strong likelihood that we will experience revenue decreases, particularly at the federal level." Ibid.

640. Twenty years previously, for example, when the county had only seven million residents, one hundred physicians were on staff, functioning as local public health officers responsible for spotting disease problems in their districts. In 1996 the by-then far more populous county had only fourteen such district health officers.

And after October 1995, according to DHS documents [See: Fannin, S., 1996, op. cit.], the repercussions for the public's health grew more serious in other areas as well. Among the greatest concerns were that when compared to January 1995 the number of people visiting sexually transmitted diseases clinics had plummeted 55.8 percent, TB clinic visits had fallen 68 percent, and visits for child vaccinations had dropped 58.2 percent. "The immunization program estimates that we declined from capturing about 25 percent of the annual birth cohort in our immunization clinics to a low of 10 percent," said a May 13 DHS memo.

In addition, the memo continued, "the number of new cases of TB reported this year has declined by 44 percent. This is unlikely to be due to actual decline of new cases of TB, but probably reflects delayed diagnosis, lag time in confirmation of cases, or delay in symptomatic persons coming to attention. The long term effect will be more infection and more disease."

641. Cornwell, E. E., et al, 1996, op. cit.

642. Ginzberg, E., 1996, op. cit.; Glied, S., Sparer, M., and Brown, L., "Comment: Containing state health care expenditures—the competition vs. regulation debate." *American Journal of Public Health* 85 (1995): 1347–1349; and Reagan, M. D., 1999, op. cit.

643. The largest government health provider in L.A. County, aside from the county hospitals, was the huge Veterans' Administration facility in West Los Angeles. The VA complex dwarfed all other buildings in Westwood and was a major teaching and research resource for nearly adjacent UCLA. In 1999 the U.S. Department of Health and Human Services revoked more than one thousand clinical research projects funded by the NIH at the VA complex in Los Angeles—systemic ethics violations and improprieties in the use of human research subjects had been uncovered. It was a severe blow to the county, to UCLA, and to the VA.

See Cohen, J., "Research shutdown roils Los Angeles VA." *Science* 284 (1999): 18–21.

644. Here are some examples of the mysterious infectious diseases deaths Osterholm's team uncovered, as detailed in the Minnesota Department of Health's November 13, 1998 "Request for noncompeting continuation funding for the emerging infections program," which was submitted to the CDC and provided to the author:

Case 070: 4-year-old-E.D. on 11/10 with symptoms of viral gastroenteritis. Returned to E.D. on 11/21 with lethargy, vomiting, dehydration, sore throat and headache. Sent home on antibiotics. Mother found her unresponsive next morning. Dead on arrival at E.D. Death attributed to airway obstruction due to aspiration of stomach contents.

Case 073: 37-year-old male with evidence of immune suppression over last year with no known cause. Died of apparent infection—no cause identified.

Case 088: 9-year-old female found dead at home one day after returning from camp. Complained of fatigue on day before death but no other symptoms. Cerebral edema noted on autopsy, suspected meningioencephalitis but all cultures, viral studies negative. Probable viral myocarditis identified by cardiac pathologist.

Case 018: 28-year-old female collapsed in store. Cardiac arrest; unable to resuscitate and died in emergency room. Ill with gastrointestinal symptoms following trip to Mexico a few weeks prior to death. Per autopsy, death due to acute lymphocytic myocarditis.

Case 050: 30-year-old female found dead. Presented in ER one day before death with difficulty breathing, nausea, and vomiting. Death due to staphylococcal pneumonia and toxic shock syndrome per autopsy.

These were five of eighty-nine such cases detailed in the report, all of which occurred in 1995, 1996, or 1997.

645. Minnesota Department of Health, "Distribution of insurance coverage in Minnesota." *Issue Brief* 96–07 (1997) (www.health.state.mm).

646. "Minnesota's job market: Land of 1,000 opportunities." *The Economist* (May 29, 1999): 24–25.

647. This and other Minnesota interviews were conducted by the author in Minneapolis and St. Paul during January, 1999.

648. Osterholm, M., Speech before the Infectious Disease Society of America, San Francisco, September 13, 1997.

649. In 1999 the CDC listed the following foodborne microbes as those that had been newly discovered in the U.S. food supply during the previous decade:

> *Campylobacter coli*
> *Campylobacter jejuni*
> *Campylobacter fetus ssp.*
> *Cryptosporidium paryum*
> *Cyclospora cayetanenis*
> *Escherichia coli* 0157: H7
> *Listeria monocytogenes*
> Norwalk-like viruses
> *Nitschia pungens*
> *Salmonella* Enteritidis
> *Salmonella* Typhimurium DT 104
> *Vibrio cholerae* Non-01
> *Vibrio vulnificus*
> *Vibrio parahaemolyticus*
> *Yersina enterocolitica*

See Centers for Disease Control and Prevention, "Safer and healthier foods." *Morbidity and Mortality Weekly Report* 48 (1999): 905–913.

650. Here is some of what they found:

PERCENT OF STRAINS THAT WERE DRUG RESISTANT

ANTIBIOTIC	*1995* *(N=148)*	*1996* *(N=139)*	*1997* *(N=128)*	*Jan–June, 1998* *(N=68)*
	Salmonella			
Ampicillin	11	21	21	14
Chloramphenicol	7	9	12	9
Ciprofloxacin	0	0	0	0
Tetracycline	16	20	22	31
TMP/SMX	3	2	3	12
Two or more drugs	11	14	17	24
	Shigella			
Ampicillin	81	75	69	89
Chloramphenicol	15	16	19	17

ANTIBIOTIC	1995 (N=148)	1996 (N=139)	1997 (N=128)	Jan–June, 1998 (N=68)
Ciprofloxacin	0	0	0	0
Tetracycline	38	47	59	72
TMP/SMX	42	47	44	83
Two or more drugs	48	47	59	93

(*Source*: Osterholm, September 13, 1997 speech, op. cit.)

Drug-resistant *E. coli* 0157: H7 was still almost nonexistent (3 percent of 1997 strains were not suspectable to tetracycline), but that wasn't clinically relevant as antibiotic therapy wasn't wise for that bacterium—stress caused the microorganism to release its toxin, thus exacerbating the illness and potentiating patient death.

651. Ventura drew the ire of his Reform Party, but admiration from many Americans, for his remarkably frank, if not always tactful, comments (including, "Organized religion is a sham and a crutch for weak-minded people who need strength in numbers"), his open support of gays in the military and legalization of prostitution and all illicit drugs (including heroin), and his abhorrence of "fat people."

652.

SHIFTING MINNESOTA DEMOGRAPHICS
1990–1997

AGE GROUP	PERCENTAGE CHANGE BETWEEN 1990–1997			
	TOTAL	WHITE	BLACK	ALL MINORITIES, COMBINED
Under 5 years	−7.6	−9.3	5.0	14.3
5 to 9 years	−0.2	−3.1	45.4	35.1
10 to 14 years	15.9	13.0	46.0	49.9
15 to 19 years	20.0	19.8	14.6	22.8
20 to 24 years	−7.6	−9.4	−0.7	17.0
25 to 29 years	−18.6	−21.0	0.2	18.2
30 to 34 years	−9.0	−10.4	7.8	19.9
35 to 39 years	15.8	14.4	51.4	46.5
40 to 44 years	24.9	23.5	67.7	56.1
45 to 49 years	39.0	37.6	85.9	78.0
50 to 54 years	34.1	33.4	50.0	55.6
55 to 59 years	16.4	15.6	33.6	38.8
60 to 64 years	−2.8	−3.5	3.3	25.7
65 to 69 years	−3.1	−3.7	9.5	22.8
70 to 74 years	3.1	2.8	−2.2	23.3
75 to 79 years	7.8	7.8	−24.2	7.9
80 to 84 years	15.8	16.5	−50.9	−17.7
85+ years	15.2	16.5	−63.4	−34.7
TOTAL	6.8	5.5	22.1	30.3

Source: Minnesota State Demographic Center, 1997.

653. Liska, D. W., Brennan, N. J., and Brueu, B. K., *State-Level Databook on Health Care Access and Financing*. Third edition. Washington, D.C.: Urban Institute, 1998. In the United States, only Wisconsin had a wider chasm between African-American and white infant death rates than did its neighbor Minnesota.

654. According to the Minnesota Department of Health the differentials were as follows:

FIVE-YEAR AGE-ADJUSTED PREMATURE MORTALITY RATES
PER 100,000 1989–1993

Cause	African-American	American Indian	White
Injury, unintended	n/a	85.6	26.5
Homicide	35.7	30.2	1.9
Suicide	n/a	19.6	11.2
Stoke	44.7	n/a	25.1
Diabetes	80.3	129.2	33.0
Cirrhosis	11.0	35.5	5.3

(*Source: Healthy Minnesotans: Public Health Improvement Goals 2004.* Minneapolis: Minnesota Department of Health, 1998.)

655. Heithoff, K. B., Berne, E. Q., Christenson, R., et al., *Minnesota Policy Blueprint: Health*. St. Paul: Center of the American Experiment, 1998.

656. Centers for Disease Control and Prevention, "CDC data provides most complete estimate to date on food-borne disease in the United States." Press Release, Department of Health and Human Services, September 16, 1999 (www.hhs.gov).

657. "Government and private sectors join forces for food safety." *Prevention Report* 12 (issue 4) (1998): 1–5.

658. The U.S. Department of Agriculture offered the *New York Times* the following breakdown:

Food	Millions of Pounds Imported Annually	Percentage of U.S. Market Foreign Grown
Cucumbers	700	41.0
Watermelons	500	8.8
Grapefruit	30	1.4
Kiwi	50	54.8
Papayas	35	63.7
Strawberries	34	5.3
Mangos	300	97.4
Onions	600	6.2
Bell peppers	375	19.4
Asparagus	100	40.0
Grapes	750	30.7
Cantaloupes	700	23.2

See Gerth, J. and Weiner, T., "Imports swamp U.S. food-safety efforts." *New York Times* (September 29, 1997): A1.

659. Details on *Cyclospora* come from multiple sources, including Layton, M., Speech

to the Infectious Diseases Society of America, San Francisco, September 15, 1997; and Sterling, C. R. and Ortega, Y. R., "*Cyclospora*: An enigma worth unraveling." *Emerging Infectious Diseases* 5 (1999): 48–53.

660. In 1997 Osterholm's group reported on an outbreak of cryptosporidiosis in children who visited the Minnesota Zoo during warm July days. The ailing kids had played in or around a new decorative fountain that, it turned out, contained contaminated water. The source of contamination was never confirmed. See Centers for Disease Control and Prevention, "Outbreak of cryptosporidiosis associated with a water sprinkler fountain—Minnesota, 1997." *Morbidity and Mortality Weekly Report* 47 (1998): 856–860.

661. Ford, T. E. and Colwell, R. R., *A Global Decline in Microbiological Safety of Water: A Call for Action*. Washington, D.C.: American Academy of Microbiology, 1996.

662. Ibid.

663. Centers for Disease Control and Prevention, "Surveillance for waterborne-disease outbreaks—U.S., 1995-96." *Morbidity and Mortality Weekly Report* 47 (No. SS-5) (December 11, 1998): 1–34.

664. See also Meinhardt, P. L., Casemore, D. P., and Miller, K. B., "Epidemiological aspects of human cryptosporidiosis and the role of waterborne transmission." *Epidemiologic Reviews* 18 (1996): 118–136.

665. Cole, W., "Do water filters work?" *Time* magazine (June 10, 1996): 70.

666. Natural Resources Defense Council, *Think Before You Drink*. Washington, D.C.: Natural Resources Defense Council, 1993.

667. Abelson, P. H., "Chlorine and organochlorine compounds." *Science* 265 (1994): 1155; Amato, I. "The crusade to ban chlorine." *Garbage* (Summer 1994): 30–39; Cantor, K. P., Lynch, C. F., Hildesheim M. E., et al., "Drinking water source and chlorination byproducts in Iowa. III. Risk of brain cancer." *American Journal of Epidemiology* 150 (1999): 552–560; Cantor, K. P., "Water chlorination, mutagenicity, and cancer epidemiology." *American Journal of Public Health* 84 (1994): 1121–1123; Komulainen, H., Kosma, V. M., Vaittinen, S. L., et al., "Carcinogenicity of the drinking water mutagen 3-chloro-4-(dichloromethyl)-5-hydroxy-2(5H)-furonone (MX) in the rat." *Journal of the National Cancer Institute* 89 (1997): 848–856; Melnick, R. L., Boorman, G. A., Dellarco, V., "Water chlorination, 3-chloro-4-(dichloromethyl)-5-hydroxy-2(5H)-furonone (MX), and potential cancer risk." *Journal of the National Cancer Institute* 89 (1997): 832–833; and Tao, X., Zhu, H., Matanoski, G. M., "Mutagenic drinking water and risk of male esophageal cancer: A population based case-control study." *American Journal of Epidemiology* 150 (1999): 443–452.

668. See Garrett, L., 1994, op. cit.; and Levy, S. B., *The Antibiotic Paradox: How Miracle Drugs are Destroying the Miracle*. New York: Plenum, 1992.

669. Cheevers, J., "Drug-resistant bacteria pose an increasing threat." *Los Angeles Times* (March 25, 1999): A1; Leslie, J., "Unsanitary behavior." *Mother Jones* (July 1997): 28–30; and Woodward, T. E., "Will antibiotics become obsolete?" *American Journal of Medicine* 65 (1978): 397–398.

670. Amábile, C. F., Cárdenas-García, M., Ludgar, M., "Antibiotic resistance." *American Scientist* (July 1995); Craig, L. F. and Hughes, J. M., "Trends in antimicrobial drug prescribing among office-based physicians in the United States." *Journal of the American Medical Association* 273 (1995): 214–219; Westh, H., "Influence of erythromycin consumption on erythromycin resistance in *Staphylococcus aureus* in Denmark." *Alliance for the Prudent Use of Antibiotics (APUA) Newsletter* (Spring 1995) (Boston); and Wise, R., "Global paradox." *Lancet* 348 (1996): 282.

671. *Report of Joint Committee on the Use of Antibiotics in Animal Husbandry and*

Veterinary Medicine (Swann Committee). London: Her Majesty's Stationery Office, September 1969.

672. For example, some antibiotic use rates in livestock versus humans during the nineties were as follows:

ANTIBIOTIC USE

YEAR	COUNTRY	ANTIBIOTIC/TARGET (Human or Livestock)	AMOUNT USED
1994	Denmark	Vancomycin/Human	24 kg
		Avoparcin*/Livestock	24,000 kg
1992–96	Australia	Vancomycin/Human	582 kg
		Avoparcin/Livestock	62,642 kg
1990–99	United States	Various Antibiotics Pesticides/Fruit Trees	3 million pounds
1990–99	United States	Various Antibiotics/Livestock	200 million pounds
1990–99	Netherlands	Various Antibiotics/Livestock	6 million kg

*Vancomycin is a last-ditch drug used when all others fail to cure human cases of enterococcal, streptococcal, or staphylococcal infections. Avoparcin is its clinical sister, used as a livestock growth promoter. Resistance to avoparcin is the same as vancomycin resistance.

Sources: Grady, D. "A move to limit antibiotic use in animal feed." *New York Times* (March 18, 1999): A1; Institute of Medicine, *Antimicrobial Resistance: Issues and Options*. Washington, D.C.: National Academy of Science, 1998; van den Bogaard, A. E. and Stobberingh, E. E., "Time to ban all antibiotics as animal growth-promoting agents?" *Lancet* 348 (1996): 619; and Witte, W., 1998, op. cit.

673. Even wild animals never treated directly with antibiotic-laced feeds had acquired drug-resistant bacteria by 1999. See Gilliver, M. A., Bennett, M., Begon, M., et al., "Antibiotic resistance found in wild rodents." *Nature* 401 (1999): 233.

674. See, for example, Das, I., Fraise, A., and Wise, R., "Are glycopeptide-resistant enterococci in animals a threat to human beings?" *Lancet* 349 (1997): 997–998; Ike, Y., Tanimoto, K., Ozawa, Y., et al., "Vancomycin-resistant enterococci in imported chickens in Japan." *Lancet* 353 (1999): 1854; van den Bogaard, A. E. and Stobberingh, E. E., "Contamination of animal feed by multiresistant enterococci." *Lancet* 354 (1999): 163; and van den Bogaard, A. E., Jensen, L. B., and Stobberingh, E. E., "Vancomycin-resistant enterococci in turkeys and farmers." *New England Journal of Medicine* 337 (1997): 1558–1559.

675. For example, the crucial human-use antibiotic vancomycin attacked by inhibiting cell wall synthesis for bacteria such as *Enterococcus faecium* and *Streptococcus pneumoniae*. A livestock growth promoter, avoparcin, had precisely the same effect on bacterial cells. So if a *Streptococcus* bacterium in an avoparcin-fed cow mutated, becoming able to make its cell wall despite the chemical's action, it would also be able to maintain its cell wall integrity in the face of vancomycin.

676. For a much longer discussion of these points, see "Revenge of the Germs," in Garrett, L., 1994, op. cit.

677. Institute of Medicine, *Antimicrobial Resistance: Issues and Options*, 1998, op. cit.

678. The IOM report estimated that U.S. hospitals used 190 million doses of antibiotics per year, and doctors prescribed an additional 145 million full courses (enough for several days) of antibiotic therapy annually. Veterinary and livestock use of the drugs was also enormous, with four million pounds of antibiotics used annually in the United States to treat illnesses in animals, and at least sixteen million pounds given as growth promoters.

679. Unless noted otherwise, this and other quotes in this section were taken from interviews done with the author in May 1998.

680. American Society for Microbiology, *Report of the ASM Task Force on Antibiotic Resistance.* Washington, D.C.: American Society for Microbiology, 1995; *Report of the WHO Meeting on the Medical Impact of the Use of Antimicrobial Drugs in Food Animals, Berlin, 13–17 October 1997.* Geneva: World Health Organization, 1998.

681. Pantosti, A., Del Grosso, M., Tagliabue, W., et al., "Decrease of vancomycin-resistant enterococci in poultry meat after avoparcin ban." *Lancet* 354 (1999): 741–742.

682. Grady, D., 1999, op. cit.

683. And in 1997, as a result of a citywide campaign Hamburg had initiated, the city reported a dramatic decline in infant mortality, averaging 7.1 per 1,000 live births. Even traditionally high infant mortality neighborhoods such as Harlem and eastern Brooklyn showed radical improvements, reaching levels ranging from 6.6 per 1,000 in central Harlem to 8.6 in Mott Haven. Key to the success was a city-funded insurance outreach program for children and pregnant women.

Even more astounding was Hamburg's achievement with child vaccination rates—by 1997 New York City ranked second-best in the nation, having fully immunized 81 percent of its five-year-olds. The key, again, was vigorous outreach coupled with city-subsidized child insurance.

684. Miller, J., "With crisis in mind, center opens." *New York Times* (June 8, 1999): B3.

685. Thorpe, K. E., *Current Population Survey.* Tabulations prepared for the United Hospital Fund, New York City, 1997.

686. Uninsured New York City residents were three times more likely to be denied health care, compared to their privately insured counterparts. Seventy-five percent of uninsured middle-aged men had never had a prostate exam; 58 percent of their counterpart women hadn't had a mammogram. Louis Harris and Associates Inc., *The Commonwealth Fund Survey of Health Care in New York City, 1997.* New York: Louis Harris and Associates, 1997.

The Urban Institute reviewed available demographic data in New York State, versus the overall United States, for 1994–96 and sized it up as follows:

	New York	U.S.A.
Percent Hispanic	13.3	10.7
Percent black (non-Hispanic)	15.2	12.5
Percent noncitizen immigrant	17.5	9.3
Per-capita income	$27,678	$23,208
Unemployment rate (percent)	6.2	5.4
Percent below poverty line	15.9	14.3
Percent uninsured	16.8	15.5
Percent Medicaid	14.7	12.2
Infant mortality rate (per 1,000 births)	7.8	7.6
Premature death rate (years lost per 1,000)	60.3	54.4
Violent crimes per 100,000 (1995)	841.9	684.6
AIDS cases per 100,000 (1995)	68.4	27.8

Source: Holahan, J., Evans, A., Liu, K., et al., *Health Policy for Low-Income People in New York.* Washington, D.C.: Urban Institute, 1997.

687. Markon, J., "Medicaid cutbacks criticized." *Newsday* (January 28, 1999): A42.

688. Cantor, J., Haslanger, K., Tassi, A., et al., *Health Care in New York City: Service Providers' Response to an Emerging Market.* Washington, D.C.: Urban Institute, 1998.

NOTES

689. Lagnado, L., "New York study could stoke hospital debate." *Wall Street Journal* (January 25, 1999): B1.

690. Lonks, J. R., Durkin, M. R., Meyerhoff, A. N., et al., "Meningitis due to ceftriaxone-resistant *Streptococcus pneumoniae.*" *New England Journal of Medicine* 332 (1995): 893–894.

691. Centers for Disease Control and Prevention, "Surveillance for penicillin-nonsusceptible *Streptococcus pneumoniae*—New York City, 1995." *Mortality and Morbidity Weekly Report* 46 (1997): 297–299.

Nationally, the CDC found it impossible to replicate such surveillance—only a handful of communities in the United States had the wherewithal to monitor penicillin-resistant strep, as New York City did. The CDC roughly estimated that each year in the United States strep was causing three thousand cases of meningitis, fifty thousand blood poisonings, half a million pneumonia cases, and seven million child ear infections. The pneumonias were very dangerous to people over sixty-five years of age: 40 percent died of their infections. And meningitis infections were lethal to 6 percent of the infected children and a third of the adults who developed central nervous system infections.

See Centers for Disease Control and Prevention, "Assessment of national reporting of drug-resistant *Streptococcus pneumoniae* in United States, 1995–96." *Mortality and Morbidity Weekly Report* 45 (1996): 947–949.

692. Ploy, M. C., Grélaud, C., Martin, C., et al., "First clinical isolate of vancomycin-intermediate *Staphylococcus aureus* in a French hospital." *Lancet* 351 (1998): 1212.

693. Centers for Disease Control and Prevention, "Reduced susceptibility of *Staphylococcus aureus* to vancomycin—Japan, 1996." *Mortality and Morbidity Weekly Report* 46 (1997): 624–635; Hiramatsu, K., "The emergence of *Staphylococcus aureus* with reduced susceptibility to vancomycin in Japan." *American Journal of Medicine* 104 (1998): 7S–10S; and Hiramatsu, K., Hanaki, H., Ino, K., et al. "Methicillin-resistant *Staphylococcus aureus* clinical strain with reduced vancomycin susceptibility." *Journal of Antimicrobial Chemotherapy* 40 (1997): 135–136.

694. Centers for Disease Control and Prevention, "Update: *Staphylococcus aureus* with reduced susceptibility to vancomycin—United States, 1997." *Mortality and Morbidity Weekly Report* 46 (1997): 813–815; Gorman, C., "Germ Warfare." *Time* magazine (September 1, 1997): 65; Smith, T. L., Pearson, M. L., Wilcox, K. R., et al., "Emergence of vancomycin resistance in *Staphylococcus aureus.*" *New England Journal of Medicine* 340 (1999): 493–501; and Waldvogel, F. A., "New resistance in *Staphylococcus aureus.*" *New England Journal of Medicine* 340 (1999): 556–557.

695. Rotun, S. S., McMath, V., Schoonmaker, D. J., et al., "*Staphylococcus aureus* with reduced susceptibility to vancomycin isolated from a patient with fatal bacteremia." *Emerging Infectious Diseases* 5 (1999): 147–149.

696. Chuard, C., Vaudaux, P., Waldvogel, F. A, et al., "Susceptibility of *Staphylococcus aureus* growing on fibronectin-coated surfaces to bactericidal antibiotics." *Antimicrobial Agents and Chemotherapy* 37 (1993): 625–632.

697. Sieradzki, K., Roberts, R. B., Haber, S. W., et al., "The development of vancomycin resistance in a patient with methicillin-resistant *Staphylococcus aureus* infection." *New England Journal of Medicine* 340 (1999): 517–523.

698. Waldvogel, F. A., 1999, op. cit.

699. See also Ariza, J., Pujol, M., Cabo, J., et al., "Vancomycin in surgical infections due to methicillin-resistant *Staphylococcus aureus* with heterogenous resistance to vancomycin." *Lancet* 353 (1999): 1587–1588; Collignon, P., Gosbell, I., Vickery, A., et al., "Community-acquired methicillin-resistant *Staphylococcus aureus* in Australia." *Lancet* 352 (1998): 145; Howe, R. A., Bowker, K. E., Walsh, T. R., et al., and Lessing, M. P. A. and Rafferty,

M. J., Letters. *Lancet* 351 (1998): 601–602; and Morris, K., "Antibiotic resistance hogs the limelight." *Lancet* 349 (1997): 1674.

700. Cefai, C., Ashurst, S., and Owens, C., "Human carriage of methicillin-resistant *Staphylococcus aureus* linked with pet dog." *Lancet* 344 (1994): 539–540; Pate, K. R., Nolan, R. L., Bannerman, T. L., et al., "Methicillin-resistant *Staphylococcus aureus* in the community." *Lancet* 346 (1995): 978; Rosenberg, J., "Methicillin-resistant *Staphylococcus aureus* (MRSA) in the community: Who's watching?" *Lancet* 346 (1995): 132–133; and Rossi, T., Laine, J., Eerola, E., et al., "Denture carriage of methicillin-resistant *Staphylococcus aureus*." *Lancet* 345 (1995): 1577.

701. Centers for Disease Control and Prevention, "Four pediatric deaths from community-acquired methicillin-resistant *Staphylococcus aureus*—Minnesota and North Dakota, 1997–1999." *Mortality and Morbidity Weekly Report* 48 (1999): 707–710.

702. "CDC reports on drug-resistant staph." *Associated Press* (August 20, 1999); and Stolberg, S. G., "After 4 deaths, scientists fear germ's threat." *New York Times* (August 20, 1999): A17.

703. Brown, P. and Lerner, S., "Community-acquired pneumonia." *Lancet* 352 (1998): 1295–1302; and Holmes, A., Jacklin, A., Impallomeni, M., et al., "Community-acquired pneumonia." *Lancet* 353 (1999): 1528–1529.

704. Novak, R., Henriques, B., Charpentier, E., et al., "Emergence of vancomycin tolerance in *Streptococcus pneumoniae*." *Nature* 399 (1999): 590–593.

705. The other nosocomial infection that became a disastrous community public health problem was hepatitis C, which readily spread via nonsterile needles, blood transfusions, and nonhygenic medical procedures. By 1999 the CDC estimated that more than four million Americans were infected with the virus, putting them at serious risk of dying of cirrhosis or liver cancer.

See Cohen, J. "The scientific challenge of hepatitis C." *Science* 285 (1999): 26–30; El-Serag, H. B. and Mason, A. C., "Rising incidence of hepatocellular carcinoma in the United States." *New England Journal of Medicine* 340 (1999): 745–750; Hager, M. and Reibstein, L., "Do you have hepatitis C?" *Newsweek* (May 4, 1998): 83; MacDonald, M., Crofts, N., and Kaldor, J., "Transmission of hepatitis C virus: Rates, routes and cofactors." *Epidemiological Reviews* 18 (1996): 137–148; "Making sense of hepatitis C." *Lancet* 352 (1998): 1485; Moss, A. and Hahn, J. A., "Needle exchange—no help for hepatitis?" *American Journal of Epidemiology* 149 (1999): 214–218; and Talen, J., "A grave threat." *Newsday* (July 28, 1998): C6.

706. Centers for Disease Control and Prevention, National Center for HIV, STD, and TB Prevention, *HIV/AIDS Surveillance Report*. Year-end edition. Vol. 10 (No. 2) (December 1998).

707. Data presented by the CDC at the National HIV Prevention Conference, Atlanta, Georgia, August 30, 1999.

708. Data from the U.S. National Vital Statistics Web site (www.hhs.gov). The improvements were not, of course, uniform. In 1998 whites infected with HIV were ten times more likely to survive the year compared to African-Americans, and blacks accounted for half of all AIDS deaths that year. While AIDS deaths declined by 73 percent among whites from 1996 through 1998, the drop was just 52 percent among blacks. Hispanic AIDS death rates fell 63 percent over those years. Ibid.

In New York City the overall AIDS death rate declined 88 percent from 1995 through 1998. But in 1998 in New York City HIV-positive women remained 34 percent more likely, and African-Americans were 150 percent more likely, to die of the virus compared with HIV-positive white males. Chiasson, M. A., Heffess, J., Li, W., et al., "Differential decline in AIDS mortality by gender and race/ethnicity in New York City." Presentation to the National HIV

Prevention Conference. Atlanta, Georgia, August 30, 1999. Among New York's injecting drug users, HIV seroprevalence plummeted from a 1990 high of 27.2 percent to just 4.3 percent in 1998, largely because pure heroin became so cheap and readily available during the late 1990s that users could snort, rather than inject, the drug. And needle exchange programs had gained popularity among injecting drug users, so fewer needles were shared. Rothman, J., Presentation to the National HIV Prevention Conference. Atlanta, Georgia, August 30, 1999.

709. Centers for Disease Control and Prevention, "Primary and secondary syphilis." *Morbidity and Mortality Weekly Report* 48 (1999): 873–878.

710. Comments at a press conference, National HIV Prevention Conference, Atlanta, Georgia, August 30, 1999.

711. These figures come from the 1998 and 1999 annual reports of the United Nations AIDS Programme, based in Geneva, Switzerland.

By the close of 1998, according to UNAIDS, the pandemic broke down as follows:

People living with HIV/AIDS	33.4 million
Newly HIV-infected in 1998	5.8 million
Deaths due to HIV/AIDS in 1998	2.5 million
Cumulative HIV/AIDS death toll since 1979	13.9 million

712. Gao, F., Bailes, E., Robertson, D. L., et al., "Origin of HIV-1 in the chimpanzee *Pan troglodytes troglodytes*." *Nature* 397 (1999): 436–441; and Weiss, R. A. and Wrangham, R. W., "From *Pan* to pandemic." *Nature* 397 (1999): 385–386.

713. Cowley, G., "Is AIDS forever?" *Newsweek* (July 6, 1998): 60–61; DeCock, K., Presentation to the Human Retrovirus Conference. Chicago, Illinois, February 1, 1998; and Garrett, L. "Staggering trend: HIV pandemic worsening among Africa, Asia youth." *Newsday* (November 24, 1998): A7.

714. Baltimore, Miami, New Orleans, Houston, Denver, and Los Angeles.

715. Baltimore, Dallas, Los Angeles, Miami, New York City, San Francisco, and Seattle.

716. These studies were presented by the CDC at the National HIV Prevention Conference. Atlanta, Georgia, August 30, 1999.

717. Garrett, L., "The uncounted: New estimates show tens of thousands of New Yorkers may be unknowingly infected with HIV." *Newsday* (August 18, 1998): C1.

718. Portions of this section appeared in the March 1999 issue of *Esquire* magazine. At the family's request, the last name has been withheld.

719. Brown, D., "Triple-drug therapies are changing patterns, costs of AIDS treatment." *Washington Post* (January 27, 1997): A4; Dunlap, D. W., "Hype, hope and hurt on the AIDS front lines." *New York Times* (February 2, 1997): E3; Garrett, L., "A home run: Detectable traces of HIV gone from patients' bodies in short-term clinical trials." *Newsday* (January 30, 1996): A5; and Martone, W. J. and Phair, J. P., "HIV protease inhibitors: When and how they should be used." *Infections in Medicine* Supplement. 1996.

720. Garrett, L., "Miracle Backlash." *Newsday* (December 17, 1996): B19; and Garrett, L., "New AIDS cocktails: What we fear—experts say resistance could develop." *Newsday* (July 2, 1996): B19.

Obviously the revolution also passed by the millions of HIV-positive individuals who lived in poor countries where the $10,000 to $60,000 annual HAART price tag was utterly out of reach. Per-capita health care spending was less than $5 a year in each of Africa's hardest-hit countries—nations in which 20 to 26 percent of all men and women aged fifteen to forty-nine were HIV positive. Indeed, it would prove an ironic turn of events in the summer of 1998 that representatives of developing countries would, at the International Conference on

AIDS in Geneva, demand affordable access to HAART just as the first doubts about its long-term efficacy and safety began to percolate among Western researchers.

In the United States by the close of 1996 direct treatment costs for HIV topped $5.1 billion. By mid-1997, in just six months of that year, spending exceeded $6.7 billion, averaging $20,000 per patient. See Bozette, S. A., Berry, S. R., Duan, N., et al., "The care of HIV-infected adults in the United States." *New England Journal of Medicine* 339 (1998): 1897–1904.

721. Garrett, L., "AIDS drugs fading: New prevention approach sought." *Newsday* (August 31, 1999): A4; and Wainberg, M. A. and Friedland, G., "Public health implications of antiretroviral therapy and HIV drug resistance." *Journal of the American Medical Association* 279 (1998): 1977–1983.

722. For example, in New York City in 1994 nearly seven thousand people died of AIDS. By the end of 1996 that number had fallen to five thousand and rough data for 1998 looked like James's death may have been one of only 3,500. Similar trends were seen in most major U.S. cities. And nationally AIDS death rates between 1996–97 fell a breathtaking 47 percent. See Holmes, S. A., "AIDS deaths in U.S. drop by nearly half as infections go on." *New York Times* (October 8, 1998): A1.

Europeans had seen an even more dramatic trend: between 1994 and 1998 death rates for HIV patients fell an astonishing 80 percent. The greater successes in Europe may be functions of both wider access to health care (there were more than forty-three million uninsured Americans, Western Europe had near-universal health care), and greater initial conservatism there in use of experimental anti-HIV drugs during the period 1980–1995. (The latter could explain the relatively lower rates of multidrug-resistance seen in European, versus American, HIV patients.)

723. Interview with the author, November 1998.

724. These and other comments regarding HAART, unless otherwise noted, were gleaned in interviews during 1998 and 1999.

725. Barr, M., "Now what? Maverick researcher Dr. Steven Miles explains why the next great drug isn't coming and what we can do to redeem the dream of a cure." *POZ* (October 1999): 60–63; Cooper, D. A. and Emery, S., "Therapeutic strategies for HIV infection—time to think hard." *New England Journal of Medicine* 339 (1998): 1319–1320; and Garrett, L., "AIDS after the 'cure': Amid setbacks search for new hope." *Newsday* (June 14, 1998): A7.

726. Interview with the author, October 1998.

727. Finzi, D., Harmankova, M., Pierson, T., et al., "Identification of a reservoir for HIV-1 in patients on highly active antiretroviral therapy." *Science* 278 (1997): 1295–1300; Grossman, Z., Feinberg, M. B., and Paul, W. E., "Multiple modes of cellular activation and virus transmission in HIV infection: A role for chronically and latently infected cells in sustaining viral replication." *Proceedings of the National Academy of Sciences* 95 (1998): 1–6; Paul, W. E. and Grossman, Z., "Ongoing HIV dissemination during HAART." *Nature Medicine* 5 (1999): 1099–1104; and Stafford, M. A., Cao, Y., Ho, D., et al., *Modeling plasma virus concentration and CD4+ T cell kinetics during primary HIV infection.* Santa Fe Institute publication # 99-05-036, 1999.

728. "Abnormal fat distribution and use of protease inhibitors." Various letters in *Lancet* 351 (1998): 1735–1737; Carr, A., Sarnaras, K., Thorisdotter, A., et al., "Diagnosis, prediction, and natural course of HIV-1 protease-inhibitor-associated lipodistrophy, hyperlipidaemia, and diabetes mellitus: a cohort study." *Lancet* 353 (1999): 2093–2099; Carr, A., Sarnaras, K., Chisholm, D. J., et al., "Pathogenesis of HIV-1-protease inhibitor-associated peripheral lipodystrophy, hyperlipidaemia, and insulin resistance." *Lancet* 351 (1998): 1881–1883; Colebunders, R., Smets, E., Verdonck, K., et al., "Sexual dysfunction with protease inhibitors." *Lancet* 353 (1999): 1802; Martinez, E., Collazos, J., Mayo, J., et al., "Sexual dys-

function with protease inhibitors." *Lancet* 353 (1999): 810–811; Various letters in *Lancet* 351 (1998): 1958–1959.

729. Carr, A. and Cooper, D. A., "Gap between biology and reality in AIDS." *Lancet* 352 (1998): siv16–siv17; Gazzard, B. and Moyle, G., "1998 revision to the British HIV Association guidelines for antiretroviral treatment of HIV seropositive individuals." *Lancet* 352 (1998): 314–316; Goldstein, R., "Climb every mountain: The art of selling HIV drugs." *POZ* (October 1998): 64–67; Louis Harris and Associates, Inc., *National HIV/AIDS Treatment Survey*. Washington, D.C.: Johns Hopkins University and UCSF, June 13, 1998. Office of AIDS Research, *Adherence to New HIV Therapies: A Research Conference*. Washington, D.C., November 21–21, 1997; and Veugelers, P. J., Cornelisse, P. G. A., Craib, K. J. P., et al., "Models of survival in HIV infection and their use in the quantification of treatment benefits." *American Journal of Epidemiology* 148 (1998): 487–496.

Worse yet, HAART failure appeared to be an unpredictable, stochastic event in terms of timing in individual patients. But over the long haul, it was an inevitable event. See Balter, M., "HIV survives drug onslaught by hiding out in T cells." *Science* 278 (1997): 1227; Grant, R. M. and Abrams, D. I., "Not all is dead in HIV-1 graveyard." *Lancet* 351 (1998): 308–309; Havlir, D. V., Marschner, I. C., Hirsch, M., et al., "Maintenance antiretroviral therapies in HIV-infected subjects with undetectable plasma HIV RNA after triple-drug therapy." *New England Journal of Medicine* 339 (1998): 1261–1268; Levy, J., "Caution: Should we be treating HIV infection early?" *Lancet* 352 (1998):982–983; Markham, R. B., Wang, W. C., Weisstein, A. E., et al., "Patterns of HIV-1 evolution in individuals with differing rates of CD4 T cell decline." *Proceedings of the National Academy of Sciences* 95 (1998): 12568–12573; Pomerantz, R. J., "Residual HIV-1 disease in the era of highly active antiretroviral therapy." *New England Journal of Medicine* 340 (1999): 1672–1674; and Wong, J. K., Hezareh, M., Günthard, H. F., et al., "Recovery of replication-competent HIV despite prolonged suppression of plasma viremia." *Science* 278 (1997): 1291–1295.

730. The need for prophylactic drugs eased in 1999 as physicians found that patients who responded well to HAART tended to have strong enough immune systems to keep those bugs in check. See Macdonald, J. C., Torriani, F. J., Morse, L. S., et al., "Lack of reactivation of cytomegalovirus (CMV) retinitis after stopping CMV maintenance therapy in AIDS patients with sustained elevations in CD4 T cells in response to highly active antiretroviral therapy." *Journal of Infectious Diseases* 177 (1998): 1182–1187; and Weverling, G. J., Mocroft, A., Ledergerber, B., et al., "Discontinuation of *Pneumocystis carinii* pneumonia prophylaxis after start of highly active antiretroviral therapy in HIV-1 infection." *Lancet* 353 (1999): 1293–1298.

731. Condra, J. H., "Resisting resistance: Maximizing the durability of antiretroviral therapy." *Annals of Internal Medicine* 128 (1998): 951–954; Durant, J., Clevenbergh, P., Halfon, P., et al., "Drug-resistance genotyping in HIV-1 therapy: The VIRADAPT randomized controlled trial." *Lancet* 353 (1999): 2195–2199; Hirsch, M. S., Conway, B., D'Aguilla, R. T., et al., "Antiretroviral drug resistance testing in adults with HIV infection." *Journal of the American Medical Association* 279 (1998): 1984–1991; Kalb, D., "Now, a scary strain of drug-resistant HIV." *Newsweek* (July 13, 1998): 63; Levy, J. A., "Pathogenesis of human immunodeficiency virus infection." *Microbiology Reviews* 57 (1993): 183–289; Mayers, D. L., "Drug-resistant HIV-1: The virus strikes back." *Journal of the American Medical Association* 279 (1998): 2000–2002; and Montaner, J. and Mellors, J., "Better salvage therapy for HIV-1 infection still needed." *Lancet* 353 (1999): 1857.

732. One explanation for the seemingly mysterious tendency of HAART drugs to lose their effectiveness over time was simple human physiology. Anybody who took five to ten even mildly toxic drugs a day was giving his liver, kidneys, intestinal tract, and bowel a real beating. Over time, these vital organs became less able to absorb and process the medicines,

so the antiviral agents never got to their targets. The patients might be compliant with doctors' orders, but the liver or duodenum was not.

733. Coombs, R. W., Speck, C. E., Hughes, J. P., et al., "Association between culturable human immunodeficiency virus type 1 (HIV-1) in semen and HIV-1 RNA levels in semen and blood: Evidence for compartmentalization of HIV-1 between semen and blood." *Journal of Infectious Diseases* 177 (1998): 320–330; Dyer, J. R., Kazembe, P., Vernazza, P. L., et al., "High levels of human immunodeficiency virus type 1 in blood and semen of seropositive men in sub-Saharan Africa." *Journal of Infectious Diseases* 177 (1998): 1742–1746; Goulston, C., McFarland, W., Katzenstein, D., "Human immunodeficiency virus type 1 RNA shedding in the female genital tract." *Journal of Infectious Diseases* 177 (1998): 1100–1103; and Zhang, H., Dornadula, G., Beaumont, M., et al., "Human immunodeficiency virus type 1 in the semen of men receiving highly active antiretroviral therapy." *New England Journal of Medicine* 339 (1998): 1803–1809.

734. Interview with the author, January 1999.

735. Invented in 1998, the detuned ELISA technology was put into use in a handful of health departments in the United States in 1999, for the first time giving the agencies glimpses of their HIV epidemics as they unfolded. And what they saw often belied long-held assumptions about who was getting HIV and revealed terrible deficiencies in HIV prevention strategies.

See McFarland, W., "Monitoring the leading edge of the HIV epidemic." Presentation to the National HIV Prevention Conference, Atlanta, Georgia, August 29–September 1, 1999; and Garrett, L., "Another crisis in gay communities?" *Newsday* (August 19, 1999): A1.

736. Standard HIV ELISA tests measured the presence in the blood of antibodies against the virus. Refined, highly tuned ELISAs could pick up even minute numbers of antibodies present in the first days of infection, before the immune system mounted a full response to the virus. Detuned ELISAs did the reverse, picking up only the large antibody presences that typically appeared three to five months after infection. By administering both the standard and detuned ELISAs, laboratory technicians could tell in which stage of infection an individual might be.

737. McFarland, W., 1999, op. cit.

738. Altman, L. K., "New York study finds gay men using safer sex." *New York Times* (August 28, 1999): A1.

739. Centers for Disease Control and Prevention, "Increases in unsafe sex and rectal gonorrhea among men who have sex with men—San Francisco, California, 1994–1997." *Morbidity and Mortality Weekly Report* 48 (1999): 45–48; Centers for Disease Control and Prevention, "New data show decline in AIDS deaths slowing down." Press release. Atlanta, Georgia, August 30, 1999; Handsfield, H. H., "Resurgence of syphilis and gonorrhea in men who have sex with men, Seattle-King County, Washington." *Morbidity and Mortality Weekly Report* 48 (1999): 773–777; and San Francisco Department of Public Health. *San Francisco Monthly STD Report.* June 1999.

740. New York City Department of Health. "Increased rates of hepatitis A among men who have sex with men." Memo. New York City: Bureau of Communicable Disease, July 13, 1998.

741. Osmond, D., Charlebois, E., Page-Shafer, K., et al., "Increasing risk behavior has not led to higher HIV incidence rates in the San Francisco Young Men's Health Study: 1993–1998." Twelfth International Conference on AIDS, Geneva, June 28–July 3, 1998.

742. Ekstrand, M. L., Stall, R. D., Paul, J. P., et al., "Gay men report high rates of unprotected anal sex with partners of unknown or discordant HIV status." *AIDS* 13 (1999): 1525–1533.

743. Elovich, R. "Beyond Condoms." *POZ* (June 1999): 86–91; Gendin, S., "They shoot barebackers, don't they?" *POZ* (February 1999): 48–71; Rotello, G., *Sexual Ecology: AIDS and the Destiny of Gay Men.* New York: Dutton, 1996; Rotello, G., "The Twilight of AIDS?" *The Nation* (1996) (www.thenation.com); Scarce, M., "Life after latex." *POZ* (June 1999): 92–93; Sheon, N. and Plant, A., "Protease dis-inhibitors? The gay bareback phenomenon." *HIV InSite* (1997) (www.hivinsite.ucsf.edu); and Vittingoff, E., Douglas, J., Judson, F., et al., "Pre-contact risk of human immunodeficiency virus transmission between male sexual partners." *American Journal of Epidemiology* 150 (1999): 306–311.

744. Nieves, E., "Privacy questions raised in cases of syphilis linked to chat room." *New York Times* (August 25, 1999): A1. One controversial old approach was also revisited: In 1999 the question of reopening San Francisco's bathhouses was revived by the gay community. Coates, T. J., Acree, M., Stall, R., et al., "Men who have sex with men in public places are more likely to have unprotected anal intercourse." Abstract # Mo.D.492. Eleventh International Conference on AIDS, Vancouver, July 1996; Elwood, W. N. and Williams, M. L., "Strategic Silence: Gay men and the use of bathhouse communication rules for unprotected anal sex." *AIDS Weekly Plus* (February 8, 1999); Richwald, G. A., Morisky, D. E., Kyle, G. R., et al., "Sexual activities in bathhouses in Los Angeles County: Implications for AIDS prevention education." *Journal of Sexual Research* 25 (1988): 169–180.

745. Boden, D., Hurley, A., Zhang, L., et al., "HIV-1 drug resistance in newly infected individuals." *Journal of the American Medical Association* 282 (1999): 1135–1141; Cohen, O. J. and Fauci, A. S., "Transmission of drug-resistant strains of HIV-1: Unfortunate, but inevitable." *Lancet* 354 (1999): 697–698; Garrett, L., "New, deadly HIV?" *Newsday* (September 22, 1999): A3; Little, S. J., Daar, E. S., D'Aquila, R. T., et al., "Reduced antiretroviral drug susceptibility among patients with primary HIV infection." *Journal of the American Medical Association* 282 (1999): 1142–1149; Pomerantz, R. J., "Primary HIV-1 resistance: A new phase in the epidemic?" *Journal of the American Medical Association* 282 (1999): 1177–1179; and Yerly, S., Kaiser, L., Race, E., et al., "Transmission of antiretroviral-drug-resistant HIV-1 variants." *Lancet* 354 (1999): 729–733.

746. Dr. Martin Markowitz of the Aaron Diamond AIDS Research Center in Manhattan led a team of New York City and Los Angeles researchers who analyzed HIVs found in seventy-seven men and three women who had been infected, on average, for less than two months. This meant that the scientists were able to recover from the patients' blood the same virus strains in their bodies that carried known mutations that conferred resistance to HAART drugs. Even more of the patients—26.8 percent—had viruses that were able to grow in test tubes filled with various anti-HIV drugs. That meant that there were more genetic types of resistance in HIV than scientists had so far been able to pin down. Most critically, 3.8 percent of the individuals had multidrug-resistance—one person's strain was more than a thousand times less sensitive than normal to an entire class of HAART drugs.

"The transmission of drug resistance should not be considered insignificant," Markowitz insisted. "Sixteen percent resistance in any organism is very significant."

Another research team presented analysis of viruses taken from 129 men and 10 women within twelve months of their infection. These individuals were infected from 1989–1998 in San Diego, Los Angeles, Denver, Dallas, or Boston. In this group, 26 percent of the individuals carried drug resistant viruses and 2 percent had highly multidrug-resistant strains.

Geneva University Hospital researcher Dr. Luc Perrin published similar findings based on a study of eighty-two newly infected French and Swiss patients. Keeping in mind that HAART had been in widespread use in those countries for about a year less than in the United States, it was interesting that Perrin's drug-resistant pool was just 11 percent of those patients. But 4.3 percent of them were infected with HIVs that were resistant to the newest class of drugs—protease inhibitors—compared to 9 percent resistant to the oldest drug, AZT. And the one patient who had highly multidrug-resistant HIV was infected in 1998.

Perrin wrote that this finding presented "a serious threat to the management of anti-retroviral therapy," and he advocated resistance testing of *all* HIV patients as a matter of routing.

747. Centers for Disease Control and Prevention, "Monitoring Hospital-Acquired Infections to Promote Patient Safety—United States, 1990–1999." *Morbidity and Mortality Weekly Report* 49 (2000): 149–153.

748. Murray, B., "Vancomycin-Resistant Enterococcal Infections." *New England Journal of Medicine.* 342 (2000): 710–721.

749. Centers for Disease Control and Prevention, "*Staphylococcus aureus* with reduced susceptibility to vancomycin—Illinois, 1999." *Morbidity and Mortality Weekly Report.* 48 (2000): 1165–1167.

750. National Intelligence Council. "The global infections disease threat and implications for the United States." Released on the Internet in January, 2000, at http://www.cia.gov/cia/publications/nie/report/nie99-17d.html.

751. Chemical and Biological Arms Control Institute and CSIS International Security Program, "Contagion and conflict: Health as a global security challenge." Center for Strategic and International Studies. Washington D.C., 2000.

752. The Commonwealth Fund, "U.S. minority health: A chartbook." New York: The Commonwealth Fund, 1999.

753. The differences were really striking: citywide the 1998 death rate was 8.3 per 1,000 residents. In central Harlem it was 12.3 per 1,000. The city heart diseases death rate was 348 per 1,000—in Harlem it was 359.4. The cancer death rate was wider: 197.4 per 1,000 citywide versus 280.6 in Harlem. Harlem had an HIV rate three times the city average (72.7 per 1,000 versus 27 citywide). Pneumonia deaths were almost double in Harlem (61.5 per 1,000 vs. 36.6 citywide). Diabetes deaths were double (42.4 per 1,000 Harlemites vs. 21.1 citywide). See Office of Vital Statistics, "Summary of Vital Statistics 1998 The City of New York." New York: New York City Department of Health, 2000.

754. Senior, K., "Worrying trend in hypertension described for USA." *Lancet* 354 (1999): 747.

755. Reuters, "U.S. health care can kill, study says." *San Francisco Chronicle* (October 21, 1997): A3.

756. Edmonson, M. B., Stoddard, J. L., Owens, L. M., "Hospital readmission with feeding-related problems after early postpartum discharge of normal newborns." *Journal of the American Medical Association.* 278 (1997): 299–303.

757. Mays, G. P., Miller, C. A., Halverson, P. K., et al., "Performing essential public health services in the nation's most populous communities: Who contributes?" In press, 2000.

CHAPTER FIVE

1. Fenn, E. A., "Biological warfare, circa 1750." *New York Times* (April 11, 1998): A11.

2. Part of the problem Osterholm and others faced was a lack of scientific expertise inside the agencies. For example, the Department of State had virtually no one on staff with genuine expertise in science and technology. See: Solomon, A. K., "The science and technology-bereft Department of State." *Science* 282 (1998): 1649–50.

In 1998 President Clinton appointed Dr. Kenneth Bernard to the National Security Council, marking the first time that an individual with science and medical expertise sat on that crucial advisory group. John Gannon, chair of the National Intelligence Council, openly sought such expertise from university scientists. In a 1998 speech at Stanford University, for example, he said, "When I look at this distinguished audience, I can spot just the kind of talent we need to attract . . . to contribute to the defense of our country against the mounting biowarfare threat." See: Gannon, J., Speech, Stanford University, November 16, 1998.

3. The meeting, and Henderson's speech, took place at the IDSA meeting in San Francisco, September 13, 1997.

4. A brilliant account of these events can be found in Remnick, D., *Resurrection: The Struggle for a New Russia*. New York: Random House, 1997.

5. Much of Henderson's thesis later appeared in print: Henderson, D. A., "Bioterrorism as a public health threat." *Emerging Infectious Diseases* 4 (1998): 488–94.

6. Henderson, D. A., "Biological terrorism." International Conference on Emerging and Infectious Diseases. Centers for Disease Control and Prevention, Atlanta, Georgia, March 10, 1998.

7. Lederberg, J., Speech to the International Conference on Emerging and Infectious Diseases, Atlanta, Georgia, March 8, 1998.

8. Lillibridge, S., "Public health preparedness and response roles for CDC related to bioterrorism." International Conference on Emerging and Infectious Diseases, Atlanta, Georgia, March 10, 1998.

9. This account was drawn from a multitude of interviews and printed sources. For further details the reader is referred to: Falkenrath, R. A., Newmann, R. D., and Thayer, B. A., *America's Achilles' Heel: Nuclear, Biological and Chemical Terrorism and Covert Attack*. Boston: Massachusetts Institute of Technology Press, 1998; Hoffman, B., *Inside Terrorism*. New York: Columbia University Press, 1998; Schweitzer, G. E., and Dorsch, C. C., *Superterrorism: Assassins, Mobsters, and Weapons of Mass Destruction*. New York: Kluwer Academic, 1998; Stern, J., *The Ultimate Terrorists*. Cambridge, Mass.: Harvard University Press, 1999; and Taylor, R., "All fall down." *New Scientist* (May 11, 1996). New York psychiatrist Robert Jay Lifton offers a chilling account of how the Aum Shinrikyo cult members saw their mission and rationalized their deeds. From 1995 to 1997 Lifton interviewed dozens of cult members, obtaining further details not only of their actions but also of their collective psychology. See Lifton, R. J., *Destroying the World to Save It: Aum Shinrikyo, Apocalyptic Violence, and the New Global Terrorism*. Metropolitan Books, New York, 1999.

10. There are many sources for the details presented on the Aum Shinrikyo cult and its activities. In addition to interviews, the following sources were used: "Congress probes Japanese cult." Military Newswire, 1996; Henderson, D. A., 1998, op. cit.; NSTC Committee on International Science and (CISET) Working Group on Emerging and Re-Emerging Infectious Diseases. "Global microbial threats in the 1990s." The White House, 1996; "Japanese cult member gets life." Associated Press, May 26, 1998; "Japanese guru will hear litany of nerve-gas victims." Associated Press (April 20, 1996); Lewthwaite, G. A., "Terrorist attacks in US expected." *Baltimore Sun* (November 1, 1995): A1; Morita, H., Yanagisawa, N., Nakajima, T., et al., "Sarin poisoning in Matsumoto, Japan." *The Lancet* 346 (1995): 290–93; Neifert, A., "Case study: Sarin poisoning of subway passengers in Tokyo, Japan, in March 1995." Camber Corporation, 1998; White House Office of Science and Technology Policy. "The role of science and technology in promoting national security and global stability." White House Forum, March 29–30, 1995; WuDunn, S., Miller, J., and Broad, W., "How Japan germ terror alerted world." *New York Times* (May 26, 1998): A1; and Zajtchuk, R., ed. *Textbook of Military Medicine. Part 1: Chemical and Biological Warfare*. Office of the Surgeon General, United States Army, Bethesda, MD, 1997.

11. Some authorities in 1998 were convinced that Aum Shinrikyo not only continued

to exist, but was at that time also actively recruiting new members. See Miller, J., "Some in Japan fear authors of subway attack are regaining ground." *New York Times* (October 11, 1998): A12.

12. A year previously, on June 27, 1994, Aum Shinrikyo had conducted their first successful attack, releasing sarin gas in the central Japan city of Matsumoto. This time the cultists released their weapon in the evening, when most Matsumotans were at home. The calls for ambulances started pouring in at eleven that night—some two hours after the gas release. Within the first hours seven people died and fifty-eight were hospitalized—a total of six hundred people sought treatment. Among the injured were many rescue workers and firefighters who reached the scene within four hours. Three weeks after the attack most surviving people who were exposed to the gas were still ill and had abnormal brain scan readings that indicated epileptic-type disorders months afterward.

Despite the sophisticated efforts of Japanese authorities, it took more than three months to determine the chemical cause of these deaths and injuries. And it was only after the Tokyo subway attacks that Aum Shinrikyo was retrospectively credited with the Matsumoto homicides.

13. John Sopko, an advisor to the U.S. Senate, told *New Scientist's* Robert Taylor that "the actions of the Aum . . . create a terrifying picture of a deadly mix of the religious zealotry of groups such as the Branch Davidians, the anti-government agenda of the U.S. militia movements, and the technical know-how of a Doctor Strangelove."

14. Office of Technology Assessment. *Technology Against Terrorism: The Federal Effort.* Washington, D.C., 1993.

15. Excellent reviews of the limitations inherent in the Biological Toxins and Weapons Convention can be found in: Johnson, S. E., editor. *The Niche Threat: Deterring the Use of Chemical and Biological Weapons.* Washington, D.C.: National Defense University Press, 1997; Kadlec, R. P., Zelicoff, A. P., and Vrtis, A. M., "Biological weapons control: Prospects and implications for the future." *Journal of the American Medical Association* 278 (1977): 351–56; MacKenzie, D., "Biological weapons treaty needs teeth." *Los Angeles Times* (March 23, 1998): A11; Pearson, G. S., "The complementary role of environmental and security biological control regimes in the 21st century." *Journal of the American Medical Association* 278 (1997): 369–72; Roberts, R., editor. *Biological Weapons: Weapons of the Future?* The Center for Strategic and International Studies, Washington, D.C., 1993; Roberts, B. and Moodie, M., *Combating NBC Terrorism: An Agenda for Enhancing International Cooperation.* Center for Global Security Research, Livermore, Cal., 1996; Rosenberg, B. H., "North vs. South: Politics and the biological weapons convention." *Politics and Life Sciences,* February (1993): 69–77; Titball, R. W., "BWC verification measures: Technologies for the identification of biological warfare agents." *Politics and the Life Sciences* (August 1993): 255–63; Watson, R., et al., "The wings of death." *Newsweek* (January 16, 1989): 22; "Ban the bug bomb." *The Economist,* American edition (November 23, 1996): 19; and "The desperate efforts to block the road to doomsday." *The Economist,* American edition (June 6, 1998): 23–25.

16. I covered the Persian Gulf war for *Newsday,* along with *Newsday* reporters Tim Phelps, Susan Sachs, David Firestone, Ron Howell, Josh Friedman, and Pat Sloyan. Sloyan, who garnered a Pulitzer Prize for his efforts, disclosed the downsides of Allied military action. Some of the details herein are derived from the reportage of my *Newsday* colleagues. In addition: "Memopack: The gulf crisis." Nicosia, Cyprus: Memopacks Publishing Company, 1991; and Matar, F., *Saddam Hussein: A Biography.* London: Highlight, 1990.

17. Matar, F., 1990, ibid (English-language edition), 59.

18. The Iran/Iraq war began with diplomatic tensions between the two countries in 1980. Hussein, then president of Iraq, announced he was unilaterally ending the Algiers

accord, which had kept the peace between Iran and Iraq. Referring to Iran's leader, the Ayatollah Khomeini, Hussein announced that the Iranian "is under the illusion that he can occupy the country that gave him hospitality for fourteen years. He can conquer it if he wishes to by ties of brotherliness, but he cannot extend his racism over one iota of this country's soil. Khomeini knows that he can only cross the Arab Gulf over the dead bodies of Iraqi martyrs." See: Matar, F., 1990, ibid, 135.

19. No one really knows how many people were wounded or died in the Iran/Iraq war. Neither government felt it in their interests to release real numbers. The figures cited in the text come from U.S. intelligence estimates. But these are surely conservative. One estimate puts Irani deaths, alone, as high as one million, including elimination of 20 percent of all eighteen to thirty-year-old men. Another estimates 250,000 Irani dead and 100,000 Iraqi. The Iraqi Ministry of Defense claimed one million Iranians were killed; three million injured and maimed. Whatever the case, the carnage was horrendous. And it was reified in Teheran with the famous fountain of martyrs, flowing with human blood.

20. United Nations. "Report of the mission dispatched by the Secretary-General to investigate allegations of the use of chemical weapons in the conflict between the Islamic republics of Iran and Iraq." New York: UN Security Council, March 12, 1986; and Dingeman, J. and Jupa, R., "Chemical warfare in the Iran-Iraq conflict." *Strategy and Tactics* 113 (1987): 51–52.

21. Sidell, F. R. and Franz, D. R., "Overview: Defense against the effects of chemical and biological warfare agents." In Zajtchuk, R., op. cit.

22. Manngold, T. and Goldberg, J., *Plague Wars: The Terrifying Reality of Biological Warfare.* New York, St. Martin's Press, 1999.

23. Two events seem to have propelled Iraq in the CBW (chemical/biological warfare) direction. In 1981 the Israeli Air Force had bombed and destroyed Iraq's Osirak nuclear reactor—a gift from the French government. Israel claimed Hussein's government was obtaining weapons-grade nuclear material and making atomic bombs at the site. Israel's credibility in such matters was tainted by its own 1990 admission that it had a chemical weapons program—details of which were not forthcoming.

Interestingly, there is no evidence in the public record that the United Nations demanded right of inspection of the acknowledged Israeli chemical weapons, despite the fact that their use would violate at least two international treaties to which Israel is party. Further, intelligence sources agree that Israel has bioweapons capabilities and may have stockpiled some offensive biological agents. But Israel has never been compelled by the UN or any Western government to provide an accounting of its CBW efforts or submit to a UNSCOM inspection.

Though Western military experts were certain that Israel's claim was exaggerated, they had no doubt at the time that Hussein was, indeed, trying to make Iraq a nuclear nation.

McKay, S. and Baker, J., "Weapons proliferation after the storm: What implications should the United States draw from the Iraqi experience?" Conference on Arms Control and Verification, Williamsburg, Virginia, June 1–4, 1992.

24. George, A., "Saddam bought germ warfare chemicals in UK." *Evening Standard* (London) (July 11, 1995): 23; Butcher, T., "Iraq crisis: Germ warfare 'jelly' sold to Iraq until 1996." *The Daily Telegraph* (London) (February 19, 1998): 19; Beal, C., "How to spot a killer cloud." *New Scientist* (April 8, 1995): 24; and Bone, J., "Chemical agents." *The Times* (London) (December 13, 1997), Features.

25. Tucker, J. B., "Hide-and-seek, Iraqi style." *New York Times*, Op Ed page (November 22, 1997).

26. Zilinskas, R. A., "Iraq's biological weapons: The past as future?" *Journal of the American Medical Association* 278 (1997): 418–24.

27. Regis, E., *The Biology of Doom: The History of America's Secret Germ Warfare Project*. New York, Henry Holt and Company, 1999.

28. Scientific and Technical Advisory Section, U.S. Armed Forces, Pacific, "Biological warfare." Vol. 5 (1945).

29. Smart, J. K., "History of chemical and biological warfare: An American perspective." In Zajtchuk, R., op. cit., 9–86.

30. Cole, L. A., "The worry: Germ warfare. The target: Us." *New York Times* (January 25, 1994): A19; and Hersh, S. M., *Chemical and Biological Warfare: America's Hidden Arsenal.* New York: Doubleday and Company, 1969. Regis, E., 1999, op. cit.

31. For an exhaustive, hair-raising account of U.S. chemical-biological weapons use in Korea see: Endicott, S. and Hagerman, E., *The United States and Biological Warfare: Secrets from the Early Cold War and Korea.* Bloomington, Indiana: Indiana University Press, 1998.

The following is particularly illuminating: the U.S. role in Korea "reveals a military culture that allowed an army to resort to scorched-earth tactics, to incendiarism, to a strategy of total warfare within the confines of Korea, even the condoning of war crimes. Prominent among the factors promoting such a culture was a brand of moral certitude exemplified in General Ridgway's message to his troops . . . in which he implied that the Almighty was on the side of the U.S. Army. This certitude encouraged ethical blindness and required the utmost secrecy and deception to prevent the American people—with their deeply ingrained democratic culture—from learning about questionable activities that violated the moral consensus."

32. For a litany see Broad, W. J. and Miller, J., "Once he devised germ weapons; now he defends against them." *New York Times* (November 3, 1998): F1.

33. Nixon, R. M., Speech to the Nation, November 1969.

34. Though there have been allegations to the contrary, I can find no evidence that the United States used biological weapons in Indochina during the U.S./Vietnam War. For details on yellow rain and Soviet use of mycotoxins in Laos and Afghanistan, see: Cole, L. A., *The Eleventh Plague: The Politics of Biological and Chemical Warfare.* New York: W. H. Freeman & Company, 1997, 179–81; Ember, L. R., "Yellow Rain." *Chemical and Engineering News* 62 (1984): 8–34; Marshall, E., "The apology of yellow rain." *Science* 221 (1983): 242; Marshall, E., "Yellow rain evidence slowly whittled away." *Science* 233 (1986): 18–19; Mirocha, C. J., "Hazards of scientific investigation: Analysis of samples implicated in biological warfare." *Journal of Toxicology—Toxin Reviews* 1 (1982): 199–203; Nowicke, J. W. and Meselson, M., "Yellow rain—a palynological analysis." *Nature* 309 (1984): 205–07; Rosen, R. T. and Rosen, J. D., "Pressure of four *Fusarium* mycotoxins and synthetic material in 'yellow rain': Evidence for the use of chemical weapons in Laos." *Biomed. Mass Spectrum* 10 (1982): 443–50; Seagrave, S., *Yellow Rain: A Journey Through the Terror of American Warfare.* New York: Evans, 1981; and Seeley, T. D., Norvicke, J. W., Meselson, M., et al., "Yellow Rain." *Scientific American* 253 (1985): 128–37.

35. Zilinskas, R., op. cit.

36. *Transparency* is a classic term used in national security circles. It refers to the willingness of a nation to leave its weapons programs "transparent" to outsiders concerned with treaty verification or international security issues. Any weapons treaty must allow outsiders to verify claims a participating nation makes—a process that can only be completed if the given country makes its programs "transparent." For example, no nuclear arms treaty can possibly be enforced if one of the parties lies, hides its weapons, refuses inspection, or

otherwise obfuscates. The lack of Iraqi transparency, alone, constituted a treaty violation even if the country wasn't hiding anything.

It should be noted, however, that neither Iraq nor Libya had signed the Biological Weapons Convention.

37. Bodansk, Y., "The Iraqi WMD challenge—Myths and reality." Task Force on Terrorism and Unconventional Warfare. U.S. House of Representatives, February 10, 1998.

38. A month later British Prime Minister Tony Blair ordered all his nation's air and sea ports placed on full alert following word that Iraqi agents were smuggling into the United Kingdom various disguised products containing anthrax. No such contaminants were found, but, as in Washington, a new mood of bioweapons concern took hold in London. The British alert followed on the heels of Baghdad's arrest of microbiologist Nassir al-Hindawi, considered the mastermind of Iraq's biological weapons program. UNSCOM inspectors speculated that Hindawi's arrest was intended to keep the scientist sequestered from inquiring investigators.

39. Sloyan, P., "The attack on Iraq." *Newsday* (December 17, 1998): A3.

40. Crossette, B., "Iraq still trying to conceal arms programs, report says." *New York Times* (January 27, 1999): A8; and Broad, W. J. and Miller, J., "The hunt for germs and poisons." *New York Times* (December 20, 1998): Section 4, 1.

41. Crossette, B., "Iraq suspected of secret germ war effort." *New York Times* (February 8, 2000): A14.

42. Monath, T. P. and Gordon, L. K., "Strengthening the Biological Weapons Convention." *Science* 282 (1998): 1423–24; Roberts, B., "New challenges and new policy priorities for the 1990s." In Roberts, B., 1993, op. cit.; and "Bioweapon threat seen rising but treaty talks far from results." Daniel J. Denoon's Insider Newsfile, December 28, 1998.

43. Roberts, B., "Between panic and complacency: Calibrating the chemical and biological warfare problem." In Johnson, S. E., 1997, op. cit.

44. Mangold, T. and Goldberg, J., 1999, op. cit.

45. Schweitzer, G. E. and Dorsch, C. G., 1998, op. cit.

46. There are many press accounts of Volkov's statements and corroboration. The most to the point is Englund, W., "New questions raised about '79 Russian anthrax outbreak." *Baltimore Sun* (February 20, 1998): A8.

47. Untreated pneumonic anthrax normally has a 90 percent kill rate. Even if diagnosis is swiftly made antibiotic therapy is tricky and death rates of 10 to 20 percent can occur.

48. Abramova, F. A., Grinberg, L. V., Yampolskaya, O. V., et al., "Pathology of inhalation anthrax in 42 cases from the Svendlovsk outbreak of 1979." *Proceedings of the National Academy of Sciences* 90 (1993): 2291–94. Please note that Yekaterinburg was in Soviet times called Sverdlovsk. References may be coded under that name. See also Guillemin, J., *Anthrax: The Investigation of a Deadly Outbreak*. Berkeley, University of California Press (1999).

49. Colonel Arthur Friedlander of the U.S. Army Medical Research Institute on Infectious Diseases, located at Fort Detrick, Maryland.

50. During World War II the British military had performed anthrax experiments on Gruinard Island, Henderson noted. Fifty-five years later the soils of Gruinard were still toxic, loaded with potentially lethal anthrax spores.

51. But significant debate over destruction of the remaining smallpox stocks persisted. For key components of that debate see: National Academy of Sciences, *Assessment of Future Scientific Needs for Live Variola Virus*. Washington, D.C.: National Academy Press, March 15, 1999; and Garrett, L., "Smallpox as tool adds to destruction debate," *Newsday* (March 16, 1999); A18; Shalala, D. E., "Smallpox: Setting the research agenda," *Science* (1999) 285: 1011.

52. Commission to Assess the Organization of the Federal Government to Combat the Proliferation of Weapons of Mass Destruction, *Combating Proliferation of Weapons of Mass Destruction* (1999), 104th Congress, Washington, D.C., Government Printing Office.

53. Broad, W. I. and Miller J., "Government report says 3 nations hide stocks of smallpox," *New York Times* (June 13, 1999): A1.

54. Wirth, T., Speech to the CISET Conference on Emerging Diseases, U.S. State Department, Washington, D.C., July 25, 1995.

55. Downie, A. W., "Smallpox," in Mudd, S., (edit.) *Infectious Agents and Host Reactions*. New York, W. B. Saunders, 1970.

56. Information about VECTOR and Biopreparat was obtained during an on-site visit in March 1997. And see: Adams, J., "Iran: Russia helps Iran's bio-warfare." Reuters (August 27, 1995); Adams, J., "Russia: Scientists make doomsday toxin." Reuters (October 1, 1995); Adams, J., "Russia: Yeltsin clones plague plants." Reuters (April 10, 1994); Alibek, K., "Russia's deadly expertise." *New York Times* (March 27, 1998): A19; Bases, D., "Russian doctors set aside pride to learn in U.S." Reuters (March 17, 1998); Broad, W. J., "Gene-engineered anthrax: Is it a weapon?" *New York Times* (February 14 1998): A4; Caudle, L. C., "The biological warfare threat." In Zajtchuk, 1997, op. cit.: 451–66; Cole, L. A., 1997, op. cit.; Crossette, B., "A Russian scientist cautions chemical arms safety is lax." *New York Times* (October 1, 1995): A1, Duesbery, N. S., Webb, C. P., et al., "Proteolytic inactivation of MAP-kinase-kinase by anthrax lethal factor." *Science* 280 (1998): 734–38; Erlanger, S., "Russians deny report of '95 deal with Iraq." *New York Times* (February 13, 1998): A8; Feshbach, M., *Ecological Disaster: Cleaning Up the Hidden Legacy of the Soviet Regime*. A Twentieth Century Fund Report, New York, 1995; Garrett, L., "Concern over Russia's anthrax." *Newsday* (February 19, 1998): A4; Garrett, L., "Inside Russia's germ warfare labs." *Newsday* (August 10, 1997): A1; Gates, R. M., "Weapons proliferation in the new world order." Senate Hearing 102–720, Congress, 2nd Session, January 15, 1992; Gordon, M. R., "Russia's stake in Iraq bolsters anti-war cry." *New York Times* (February 14, 1998): A1; Korchagina, V., "Corruption in army rampant." *St. Petersburg Times* (May 30, 1997): 5; Morris, K., "US anthrax-vaccine producer saved for now." *The Lancet* 351 (1998): 657; National Academy of Sciences. *Controlling dangerous pathogens: A blueprint for U.S.-Russian cooperation*. Washington, D.C.: National Academy Press, October 27, 1997; Pomerantsev, A. P., Staritsin, N. A., et al., "Expression of cereolysine AB genes in *Bacillus anthracis* vaccine strain ensures protection against experimental hemolytic anthrax infection." *Vaccine* 15 (1997): 1846–50; Preston, R., "The bioweaponeers." *The New Yorker* (March 9, 1998): 52–65; Smith, R. J., "Document indicates illicit Russia-Iraq deal." *Washington Post* (February 12, 1998): A1; Stone, R., "U.S. blacklists Russian institutes." *Science* 280 (1998): 513; Strasser, S., et al., "A cloud of terror—and suspicion." *Newsweek* (April 3, 1995): 36; Strauss, E., "New clue to how anthrax kills." *Science* 280 (1998): 1671–73; Wade, N., "Anthrax findings fuel worry on vaccine." *New York Times* (February 3, 1998): A6; Watson, R., et al., "No more lies—ever." *Newsweek* (June 29, 1992): 26 Weiner, T., "Soviet defector warns of biological weapons." *New York Times* (February 25, 1998): A19; Russia's in-the-red Army." *The Economist*, U.S. edition (August 2, 1997): 37–38; "Anthrax warning." *Moscow Times* (April 5, 1997); "Russia: Revealed—Russia's secret weapons for germ warfare." Reuters (March 27, 1994); "Technical aspects of biological weapons proliferation." In National Technical Information Service. "Technologies underlying weapons of mass destruction." U.S. Department of Commerce, Washington, D.C., 1994; and "Proliferation of weapons of mass destruction: Assessing the risks." Office of Technology Assessment, Washington, D.C., 1993.

57. Yergin, D. and Gustafson, T., *Russia 2010 and What It Means for the World*. New York: Vintage Books, 1995.

58. In 1998 Alexander Lebed was elected governor of Russia's Krasnoyarsk State,

which includes numerous former bioweapons facilities. Krasnoyarsk is potentially the richest of all Russian states, as within its borders are among the world's greatest reserves of gold, silver, high-grade coal, oil, diamonds, and precious minerals.

59. Office of Technology Assessment, 1993, op. cit.

60. Soviet health expert Murray Feshbach, of Georgetown University, considers Vozrozhdeniya Island one of the most dangerous places on earth. Once controlled by the Soviet military, the island now straddles the Aral Sea territories of Kazakhstan and Uzbekistan, neither of which have armed forces capable of defending Vozrozhdeniya. Further, the Aral Sea, as a result of inane Soviet water policies and pollution, is rapidly shrinking. Twenty years ago, Vozrozhdeniya was easily defended, as it took several hours to reach the island by boat. Today it is possible to get within spitting distance of the "island" by driving a high-chassis vehicle across the "lake." Feshbach says several mass die-offs of wild fish and animal populations near the island since 1976 were probably the result of exposure to bioweapons. See: Feshbach, M., 1995, op. cit.

61. Personal interviews with the author, 1998 and 1999.

62. Alibek's chilling autobiography, rich in details of the Biopreparat and Soviet military bioweapons programs, was published in 1999. See Alibek, K. and Handelman, S., *Biohazard*. New York, Random House, 1999.

63. And Pasechnik's information jibed nicely with evidence obtained ten years earlier by British intelligence following the assassination of Bulgarian defector Georgi Makrov. The Bulgarian stood at a London street corner awaiting a bus when an unseen man approached, carrying a most unusual umbrella. The man, a KGB operative, had a tiny canister filled with high-pressure gas, attached to a pellet of the deadly biotoxin ricin hidden inside the umbrella. That canister was connected at one end to a spring lock system triggered by tapping a button located near the umbrella's handle. At the opposite end of the umbrella the tip was bored, creating a barrel through which the lethal pellet was propelled. The KGB agent simply strolled up to Markov, tapped the naive Bulgarian with his umbrella, and disappeared in a British crowd. Markov died, but another Bulgarian defector, Vladimir Kostov, survived being assaulted by a similar device. Kostov came out of a Paris metro station on a cold winter day. He felt a sudden pain and saw a man, carrying an umbrella, run away. French physicians successfully removed the pellet from Kostov's back, and he survived, probably because his heavy winter clothing slowed the pellet's entry into his body, preventing ricin from getting into his bloodstream. U.S. intelligence claims there were at least six other ricin assassination incidents of this kind, including one in a shopping mall in Virgina. Eitzen, E. M. and Takafuji, E. T., "Historical overview of biological warfare." In Zajtchuk, R., 1997, op. cit.

64. Kudoyarova-Zubavichene, N. M., Chepurnov, A. A., Sergeyev, N. N., et al., "Preparation and use of Hyperimmune serum for therapy of filoviruses"; and Ryabchikova, E., Kolesnikova, L., Netesov, S. Y., et al., "An analysis of filovirus pathogenesis on animal models"; both were presentations at the International Colloquium on Ebola Virus Research, Antwerp, Belgium, September 4–7, 1996.

65. As described in chapter 3, VECTOR's Elena Ryabchikova had also done studies comparing responses to Ebola infection in various animal species, including rhesus monkeys, baboons, African green monkeys, and guinea pigs. By passaging the virus through successive generations of guinea pigs she successfully increased the virus's virulence, eventually making a form of Ebola that was, after eight generations, 100 percent lethal to guinea pigs. Besides being an interesting piece of virology this study could have indicated that Biopreparat was trying to determine how to make Ebola more deadly to human beings.

66. Alibek insists that some elements of the old Biopreparat and military bioweapons programs continue today. And he claims that his former bosses continue to conduct genetic

engineering of pathogens. He even claims that these Russian scientists have attempted his assassination on at least one occasion in Virginia. See Alibek, K. and Handlemas, S., op. cit., 1999.

67. The careful reader will note that the personnel estimates for Biopreparat and the Russian Ministry of Health's bioweapons program are variously reported over a range of some 10,000. It appears that even those Russians who were in leadership positions in those programs cannot recall precisely how many people were in the biowar machine.

68. According to a disputed *New York Times* account some top Biopreparat scientists have turned up in Iran. See: Miller, J. and Broad, W. J., "Bio-weapons in mind, Iranians lure needy ex-Soviet scientists. *New York Times* (December 8, 1998): A1; Broad, W. J., "Iranian denies seeking biological arms in Russian." *New York Times* (December 12, 1998): A3; and Miller, J., "Russian biologist denies work in Iran on germ weapons." *New York Times* (January 19, 1997): A7.

69. Miller, J., "Bombs-to-plowshares program criticized." *New York Times* (February 22, 1999): A8; Stout, D., "U.S. imposes sanctions on tech labs in Russia." *New York Times* (January 13, 1999): A7; and Miller, J. and Broad, W. J., "Germ weapons: In Soviet past or in the new Russia's future?" *New York Times* (December 28, 1998): A1.

70. Pomerantsev, A. P., Staritsin, N. A., et al., 1997, op. cit.

71. As the paper's authors wrote: "acquisition of hemolytic properties by *B. anthracis* strains can allow them to escape host immunity by means of penetrating [human] host cells." This, the authors continued, constituted "an evolutionary leap."

72. An august team of anthrax experts wrote in 1999: "Whether our medical system would be able to provide appropriate prophylaxis and therapy in the event of a large-scale exposure to pathogenic endospores remains uncertain, even doubtful." See Dixon, T. C., Meselson, M., Guillemin, J., and Hanna, P. C., "Anthrax," *The New England Journal of Medicine* (1999) 341: 815–26.

73. Bielecki, J., Youngman, P., Conelly, P., and Portnoy, D. A., "*Bacillus subtilis* expressing a haemolysin gene from *Listeria monocytogenes* can grow in mammalian cells." *Nature* (1990) 345: 175–76.

74. For a discussion of possible ways to limit such access versus its deleterious impact on science, see: Roberts, B., "Export controls and biological weapons: New roles, new challenges." *Critical Reviews in Microbiology* 24 (1998): 235–54.

75. Based on author interview of Dr. Sue Bailey, assistant defense secretary for Health Affairs, March 1999.

76. Author interview of Todd Ensign, March 1999.

77. Some Gulf War veterans insisted that squalene had been in the anthrax vaccines they were given during the Persian Gulf conflict and was the basis of Gulf War Syndrome. Retired Army General Philip Russell, who had been in charge of vaccine development during the war, adamantly denied that squalene had been used. Tulane University virologist Robert Garry claimed that he could, indeed, measure antisqualene antibody responses in Gulf War Syndrome sufferers. This was viewed with incredulity by most immunologists because squalene is a fat, and the immune system does not make antibodies against pure fat molecules.

78. Author interview of David Rothman, March 1999.

79. The only precedent for such disbelief was the Vietnam War use of Agent Orange, an herbicide later implicated in a wide range of health defects in Vietnam veterans, Vietnamese civilians, and their children. In the Agent Orange case, however, government and the medical community were divided in their interpretation of data, and those who doubted official DOD safety claims had widespread support in establishment circles. Such was not the case with protest over the anthrax vaccine.

80. Inglesby, T. V., Stephenson G., et al, "Medical response to anthrax attack," *Journal of the American Medical Association* (1999) 281: 1735–45.

81. This list has appeared numerous places, cited from a variety of sources. See in particular, Office of Technology Assessment, August 1993, op. cit.

82. Complex BW alliances formed in the 1990s. North Korea's most lucrative export was the SCUD missile, in some cases adapted for delivery of chemical or biological weapons. Among North Korea's buyers were Egypt, Cuba, Iran, Syria, Iraq, and Libya. (See: Grubb, J., "Nonproliferation 'progress' in Korea: Next steps." Conference on Arms Control and Verification Technology, Williamsburg, Virginia, June 1–4, 1992.) Any doubts about North Korea's missile sophistication dissipated on August 31, 1998, when Pyongyang successfully launched a ballistic missile that flew from North Korea, over northern Japan, and into the Pacific Ocean—a distance of nearly 1,500 miles. Western and Japanese military experts believed that North Korea's National Defense Research Institute and Medical Academy had in various stages of development weapons based on a veritable hit parade of horror: anthrax, cholera, plague, smallpox, and yellow fever. If allegations that North Korea had been working on smallpox weapons since the 1960s were true, the government had executed an enormous deception, having reported complete elimination of all samples of the virus at about that time.

NATO concluded in 1997 that Libya possessed medium-range ballistic missiles capable of carrying bioweapons. Further, the agency surmised that Libya and Iraq signed a defense pact in May, 1997 of biological warfare technology. Code named Ibn Hayan, the program allegedly included a large laboratory outside Tripoli, operated by the Libyan Ministry of Defense. (These allegations were made in testimony before the Task Force on Terrorism and Unconventional Warfare, February 10, 1998, op. cit.) These claims could not be independently confirmed or denied—at least, not publicly. Both Iraq and Libya repudiated the NATO claims.

And the roster was expected to grow.

83. Typically the evidence publicly offered for allegations that international terrorists were already in 1999 in the business of making biobombs is strategic, rather than concrete. The groups of concern have steadily escalated both their weaponry and kill rates. In the 1990s the World Trade Center in New York City and U.S. Embassies in Nairobi and Dar es Salaam were bombed, signaling, intelligence sources say, just this sort of escalation.

The other factor they point to is a general proliferation in the number of international groups that are willing to resort to terrorist tactics. The Rand Corporation estimates, for example, that there were eleven such organizations in the world in 1968; fifty-five in 1978, and steady growth thereafter. (See Hoffman, B., 1998, op. cit.). An even more startling estimate for 1997 was offered by Glenn Schoen: one thousand terrorist organizations worldwide. (See Schoen, G., "Understanding contemporary terrorism." Georgetown University, 1997, and Schweitzer, G. E. and Dorsch, C. G., 1998, op. cit.) The specter of organizations not under the control of any government gaining weaponized microbes was the driving force of concern in most policy circles, despite the lack of publicly available, concrete evidence that any such organization was, indeed, contemplating such a horrific tactic to meet its political ends. Given the sudden urgency bioterrorism attracted in the White House, U.S. DOD, and counterparts in Europe in 1998 it must be assumed that secret information gathered by intelligence agencies did, indeed, then point to such activities and intentions in terrorist circles.

84. Office of Technology Assessment, August 1993, op. cit., 40.

85. Landau, M., "How the cholera bacterium got its virulence." *Focus*, Harvard Medical School, July 19, 1996, 1.

86. Valdivia, R. H. and Falkow, S., "Fluorescence-based isolation of bacterial genes expressed within host cells." *Science* 277 (1997): 2007–11.

87. Some further examples of work in the genetics of virulence include: Cotter, P. A. and Miler, J. F., "Triggering bacterial virulence." *Science* 273 (1996): 1183–84; Grady. D., "Quick-change pathogens gain an evolutionary edge." *Science* 274 (1996): 1081; George, K. M., Chatterjee, D., Gunawardana, G., et al., "Mycolactone: A polyketide toxin from *Mycobacterium ulcerans* required for virulence." *Science* 283 (1999): 854–57; Hensel, M., Shea, J. E., Gleeson, C., et al., "Simultaneous identification of bacterial virulence genes by negative selection." *Science* 269 (1995): 400–03; Le Clere, J. E., Li., B., Payne, W. L., et al., "High mutation frequencies among *Esherichia coli* and Salmonella pathogens." *Science* 274 (1996): 1208–11; Mecsas, J. and Strauss, E. J., "Molecular mechanisms of bacterial virulence: Type III secretion and pathogenicity islands." *Emerging Infectious Diseases* 2 (1996): 27–85; Petersson, J., Wordfelth, R., Dubinina, E., et al., "Modulation of virulence factor expression by pathogen target cell contact." *Science* 273 (1996): 1231–33; Rahme, L. G., Stevens, E. J., Wolfort, S. F., et al., "Common virulence factors for bacterial pathogenicity in plants and animals." *Science* 268 (1995): 1899–1902; Senkevich, T. G., Bugert, J. J., Sisler, J. R., et al., "Genome sequence of a tumorigenic poxvirus: prediction of specific host response—evasion genes." *Science* 273 (1996): 813–16; and Wuethrich, B. "Bacterial virulence genes lead double life." *Science* 268 (1995): 1850.

88. Duesberg, N. S., Webb, C. P., Leppla, S. H., et al., "Proteolytic inactivation of MAP-kinase-kinase by anthrax lethal factor." *Science* 280 (1998): 734.

89. From 1975 to 1991 the numbers of people who got Ph.D.s in the United States in biology increased by 30 percent, reaching 5,700 per year. Some 60,000 biologists were by the 1990s employed in the United States. And the number of biotechnology companies went from zero in 1975 to more than 1,800 in the United States and Europe in 1992. See: Taylor, R., "All fall down," op. cit.

90. By the late 1990s scientific tools were developed that might allow for genetic targeting of microbes against specific human races, and finding ways to turn a contact-transmissable agent (such as HIV) into an airborne one (e.g., influenza). See: Eickoff, T., "Airborne disease: Including chemical and biological warfare." *American Journal of Epidemiology* 144 (1996): S39–S46; and Reany, P., "Ethnically targeted weapons may not be far off." Reuters (January 21, 1999).

91. Note Nass, M., "Biological warfare." *Lancet* 352 (1998): 491.

92. Also "Such strategies appear increasingly likely at a time when some states seek to enforce norms through collective security operations. For the former, biological weapons may be deemed useful in blunting the front edge of an invasion, when interventionary forces are at their most vulnerable, or in creating a political backlash against intervention within the major powers. In circumstances short of war, biological weapons may be deemed less useful; nuclear weapons continue to operate more fundamentally on perceptions than do biological weapons, especially given the outlaw status of the latter. But a state brandishing biological weapons as an instrument of last resort or threatening to unleash them in terrorist strikes would gain important leverage in times of crisis. The leaders of such states may also reckon that the threat or actual use of biological weapons would be less likely to incite a powerful counter response by the stronger adversary than would nuclear use." See: Roberts, B., "Controlling the proliferation of biological weapons." *The Nonproliferation Review*, ISSN 1073–6700, Monetary Institute of International Studies, 1994, 55–60.

93. Wright, R., "Be very afraid." *The New Republic* (May 1, 1995): 19–27.

Nuclear weapons production required access to enriched plutonium, which was heavily guarded internationally, and to multimillion-dollar plants staffed with highly skilled personnel. Such an H-bomb production capacity cost from $2 billion to $20 billion and was extremely difficult to conceal. It was known for years, for example, that India and Pakistan had developed such weapons, but was not internationally acknowledged until both publicly tested their weapons of mass destruction in 1998. Once put into use nuclear weapons would release a killing power that lasted for millions of years, long after the initial blast. The global impact of multiple nuclear weapons use was considered so horrific that their employment seemed apocalyptic.

Like nuclear weapons, biologicals could have an impact on a scale that far exceeded the size of the population in the initial exposure site. One millionth of a microgram of some organisms was sufficient to kill a human being. A cleverly released quantity weighing no more than a handful of paper clips could kill thousands. And the killing would continue for weeks, perhaps months, as the contagion spread.

Biologicals are far cheaper and easier to develop than are their chemical or nuclear counterparts. A large killer arsenal could be manufactured and stockpiled for less than $10 million, having been produced in apparently normal medical laboratories. See: Estimate from the Office of Technology Assessment, 1993, op. cit.

94. The targets of such rogue attacks, also in Nunn's parlance, were likely to be civilian: national landmark symbols, dense centers of economic activity, crossroads of vehicular or mass transport, commercial jets, national parades, sporting events that drew international audiences. In the 1990s the following examples of Nunn's thesis were targeted by domestic or foreign terrorists: the World Trade Center in New York City, the Tokyo subway system, Pan Am flight 103, the Oklahoma Federal Building, numerous sites in Israel, several civilian locales in England and Ireland hit by the IRA, the Olympics pavilion during the Atlanta competition, Buddhist sanctuaries attacked by Tamil nationalists in Sri Lanka, abortion clinics throughout the United States, a Jewish cultural center in Argentina, the training headquarters of the Saudi National Guard in Riyadh, American consulate officials in Pakistan, and opponents of the Bhagwan Shree Rajineesh cult in Oregon. See also Hoffman, B., "Terrorism today and tomorrow." In *Inside Terrorism*, 1998, op. cit.

95. Mayer, T. N., "The biological weapon: A poor nation's weapon of mass destruction." At www.cdsar.af.mil/battle/chp8.html.

96. Henderson, D. A., "The looming threat of bioterrorism," *Science* (1999) 283: 1279–82.

97. Although twelve million doses are stored in CDC freezers—as of 1998—the quality of several lots is considered highly suspect. It is possible that less than five million doses remain of viable immunogenicity. See Breman, J. G. and Henderson, D. A., "Poxvirus dilemmas—Monkeypox, smallpox, and biological terrorism." *Lancet* (August 20, 1998): 556–59.

98. Garret, L., "Smallpox vaccine tainted," *Newsday* (April 13, 1999) A6; Altman, L. K., Broad, W. J., and Miller J., "Smallpox: the once and future scourge?" *New York Times* (June 15, 1999): F1.

99. Though Henderson thought it wise for the United States and other nations likely to be targeted by biobombers to rebuild vaccine stockpiles, his primary position was that "all known stocks of variola [smallpox] virus should be destroyed as soon as possible," including identified samples at VECTOR and the CDC. See Breman, J. G. and Henderson, D. A., 1998, ibid.

100. For an excellent description of the politics behind this American decision, see Broad, W. J. and Miller, J., "Germ defense plan in peril as its flaws are revealed." *New York Times* (August 7, 1998): A1.

101. Appropriations Hearing on Epidemics and Bioterrorism, U.S. Senate Committee on Appropriations, Subcommittee on Labor, Health and Human Services, June 2, 1998.

102. Kaufman, A. F., Meltzer, M. I., and Schmid, G. P., "The economic impact of a bioterrorist attack: Are prevention and postattack intervention programs justifiable?" *Emerging Infectious Diseases* 3 (1997): 83–94.

103. In 1984 a European revolutionary organization called the Red Army Faction established a safehouse in Paris. The kitchen and bathroom of the apartment were full of lab equipment; flasks contained *C. botulinum.* Despite a massive surveillance and infiltration effort spanning several police and intelligence agencies in Europe, authorities had no idea the Red Army Faction was moving into bioterrorism—and never would had known until masses of Parisians showed up in local hospitals. Fortunately, a coincident arrest prevented what would have been the first modern biobombing in Europe. See: Douglas, J. D., *America the Vulnerable: The Threat of Chemical/Biological Warfare.* Lexington, Mass: Lexington Books, 1987.

104. Staten's organization and database may be accessed at www.emergency.com.

105. Layton, M., "Bioterrorism preparedness: The local public health perspective." International Conference on Emerging and Infectious Diseases, Atlanta, March 10, 1998.

106. Williams, A., "As the war with terrorists heats up, many experts believe Manhattan could be Ground Zero for bioweapons attack." *New York* (November 16, 1998): 29–35.

107. See: Hauer, J., Comments at the National Symposium on Medical and Public Health Response to Bioterrorism, Crystal Gateway Marriott, February 16–17, 1999.

108. United States Senate Committee on Appropriations, 1998, op. cit.

109. In the fall of 1998 Secretary of Defense William S. Cohen announced plans to simplify the chain of command for responding to a bioterrorist attack. Under the plan the FBI would carry the lead role in domestic attacks. See: Miller, J., "U.S. to reduce bureaucracy in responding to terrorism." *New York Times* (October 18, 1998): A26.

110. Thomas-Lester, A. and Wilgoren, D., "In the B'nai B'rith building, some waited in fear, others prayed." *Washington Post* (April 25, 1997): A20; "Doomsday scene as chemical bomb alert hits Washington." *Daily Mail* (London) (April 25, 1997): 7: and "FBI probes 'terrorist matter' at B'nai B'rith headquarters." *The Patriot Ledger* (Quincy, Mass.) (April 25, 1997): 3.

111. Garrett, L., "Germ terror: Is U.S. ready?" *Newsday* (April 6, 1998): 1.

112. For a startling look at the federal response scenario, see the "Timeline for response to incidents involving weapons of mass destruction," in Fincher, L. L., "Strengthening the local response to domestic terrorism." United States Senate Committee on Appropriations, Subcommittee on Labor, Health and Human Services, Education and Related Agencies, June 2, 1998.

113. Skeels, M., "Firsthand experience and perspective of a state health department." International Conference on Emerging Infectious Diseases, March 10, 1998, Atlanta; and Torok, T. J., Tauxe, R. V., Wire, R. P., et al., "Large community outbreak of salmonellosis caused by intentional contamination of restaurant salad bars." *Journal of the American Medical Association* 278 (1997): 379–95.

114. Fester, U., *Silent Death.* 2nd Edition. Port Townsend, Wash.: Loompanics Unlimited, 1989.

115. Interview with the author, 1998.

116. Saxon, K., *Poor Man's James Bond,* Vols. 1 and 2. El Dorado, Ariz.: Desert Publications, 1992.

117. Southern Poverty Law Center. "Intelligence Report." Montgomery, Alabama, 1998.

118. For more details see Hoffman, B., 1998, op. cit.

119. Hutchkinson, M., *The Poisoner's Handbook*. Port Townsend, Wash.: Loompanics Unlimited, 1988.

120. Vinch, C. "Services Complete Chemical Suit Check." *European Stars and Stripes* (April 6, 2000): 4.

121. See also Alper J., "From the bioweapons trenches, new tools for battling microbes," *Science* (1999) 284: 1754–55; and Belgrader, P., Bennett, W., Hadley, D., et al, "PCR detection of bacteria in seven minutes." *Science* (1999) 284: 449–50.

122. Graham, B., "Approval sought for permanent task force to coordinate military's response to chemical or biological attack." *Washington Post* (February 2, 1999): A1.

123. Clinton, B., "Remarks by the president on keeping America secure for the 21st century." National Academy of Sciences, January 22, 1998, distributed by the Office of the Press Secretary.

124. Garrett, L., "Plan to fight new terrorism." *Newsday* (January 23, 1998): A4.

125. White House Office of the Press Secretary. "Interview of the President by the *New York Times*," January 21, 1999.

126. Stern, J., "Anthrax incidents: Hoaxes and threats." National Symposium on Medical and Public Response to Bioterrorism, February 16, 1999.

127. Centers for Disease Control and Prevention. "Bioterrorism alleging use of anthrax and interim guidelines for management—United States, 1998." *Morbidity and Mortality Weekly Report* 48 (1999): 69–74. Sanchez, R., "Calif. anthrax threats spawn costly wave of fear." *Washington Post* (January 11, 1999): A1.

128. Danzig, R., "The next superweapon: Panic." *New York Times* (November 15, 1998): WK15.

129. See FBI agent Randall Murch's remarks at the International Conference on Emerging and Infectious Diseases, Centers for Disease Control and Prevention, Atlanta, Ga., March 10, 1998.

130. At the Crystal City role-playing session in February 1999 a clear example of this arose in the smallpox scenario. Once the cause of illnesses in a hospital was discerned the FBI wanted the entire hospital placed under quarantine and all patients and personnel detained for questioning. But Osterholm, playing the role of a state health officer, said that this would spark citywide panic, bring in national TV coverage, and cause an exodus of people from the area—some of whom would no doubt be infected and carry the disease to their destinations.

131. The National Research Council wrestled with this dilemma in its December 1998 report, *Chemical and Biological Terrorism: Research and Development to Improve Civilian Medical Response*. Washington, D.C.: National Academy of Sciences, 1998.

132. Cohen, H. W., Gould, R. M., and Sidel, V. W., "Bioterrorism initiatives: Public health in reverse?" *American Journal of Public Health* (1999) 89: 1629–30.

133. See Malakoff, D., "DOE lab exchanges targeted in wake of espionage claims." (1999) *Science* 283: 1986–87; and National Academy of Sciences, *Finding the Balance: National Security and Scientific Openness* (1999), National Academy Press, Washington, D.C.; and Garrett, L., "For biologists, a big chill?" *Newsday* (August 2, 1999): A8; and *Arms Control Today*, special section on the Cox Report (April/May 1999); 29: 17–37.

CHAPTER SIX

1. Sen, A. *Development as Freedom.* New York: Knopf, 1999.

2. Farmer, P., *Infections and Inequalities: The Modern Plague.* Berkeley: University of California Press, 1999.

3. Evans, R. G., Hodge, M., and Pless, I. B., "If not genetics, then what?" In Evans, R. G., Barrer, M. L., and Marmor, T. R., *Why Are Some People Healthy and Others Not?* New York: Aldine De Gruyter, 1994.

4. Consider the arguments and forecasts for twenty-first-century economics in: Kennedy, P., *Preparing for the Twenty-First Century.* New York: Vintage, 1993; Kegley, C. W. and Wittkopf, E. R., *The Global Agenda,* Chapter 3, "Politics and Markets." New York: McGraw Hill, 1998; and Soros, G., *The Crisis of Global Capitalism.* New York: Public Affairs, 1998.

5. World Health Organization. "World Health Report: 1998." World Health Organization, Geneva, 1999.

6. United Nations Children's Fund. *The State of the World's Children 2000.* New York: UNICEF, 2000.

7. Hale, S., Howden-Chapman, P., Salmond, C., et al., "National infant mortality rates in relation to gross national product and distribution of income." *Lancet* 354 (1999): 2047. And Bloom, D. E. and Canning D., "The health and wealth of nations." *Science* 287 (2000): 1207–09. And Sen, A., "Economics and health." *Lancet* 354 (2000): siv 20.

8. U.S. Bureau of the Census. "Health insurance coverage, 1997." Washington, D.C.: Government Printing Office, September 1998: 60–202˚d Pear, R., "Government lags in steps to widen health coverage." *New York Times* (August 9, 1998): A1.

9. Pear, R., "More Americans were uninsured in 1998, U.S. says." *New York Times* (October 4, 1999): A1.

10. Lashoff, J. C., "A new public health—or a return to our roots." Commencement Address, School of Public Health, University of California, Los Angeles, 1991.

11. Rowland, D., Feder, J., and Keenan, P. S., "Uninsured in America: The causes and consequences." In *The Future U.S. Healthcare System: Who Will Care for the Poor and Uninsured?* S. H. Altman et al., eds. Chicago: Health Administration Press, 1998.

12. Kaiser/Commonwealth Health Insurance Survey, 1997.

13. Even among insured families out-of-pocket costs rose dramatically, as Medicare cut back on $115 billion worth of coverage, pharmaceutical costs increased a breathtaking 17 percent in a single year (1997–1998), and employers sought ever-cheaper managed care plans. For an excellent summary of these issues, see Ginzberg, E. "The uncertain future of managed care." *New England Journal of Medicine* 340 (1999): 163–68.

14. Blendon, R. J., and Donelan, K. "1998 Commonwealth Fund International Health Policy Survey." Commonwealth Fund, New York, October 1998.

15. Anderson, G. F. "Multinational comparisons of health care: Expenditures, coverage, and outcomes." New York: The Commonwealth Fund, October 1998.

The findings were:

Country	Percentage of Population insured by govt.	Per capita spending in 1997	Cost as percentage of GDP		Percentage change
			1960	1997	
USA	32.9	$4,090	5.2	13.6	8.4
Germany	92.2	$2,339	4.8	10.4	5.6
France	99.5	$2,051	4.2	9.6	5.4
Japan	100	$1,741	3.0	7.3	4.3
Canada	100	$2,095	5.5	9.3	3.8

Country	Percentage of Population insured by govt.	Per capita spending in 1997	Cost as percentage of GDP		Percentage change
			1960	1997	
OECD median	100	$1,747	3.9	7.6	3.7
Australia	100	$1,805	4.9	8.3	3.4
New Zealand	100	$1,352	4.3	7.6	3.3
United Kingdom	100	$1,347	3.9	6.7	2.8

OECD = Organization for Economic Cooperation and Development, a twenty-nine nation association of industrialized states. U.S. per capita spending on health was 134 percent of the OECD median.

16. Anderson, G. F., ibid. Life expectancy was as follows:

Country	1960	1996	Change (years)
Japan	67.8	80.3	12.6
Canada	71.4	78.5	7.1
Australia	70.9	78.2	7.3
France	70.3	78.1	7.8
OECD median	70.1	77.2	7.1
New Zealand	71.3	77.1	5.7
United Kingdom	71.3	76.9	5.6
Germany	69.9	76.8	6.9
USA	69.7	76.1	6.4

17. Evans, R. G., and Stoddart, G. L. "Producing health, consuming health care." In Evans, R. G., Barrer, M. L., and Marmor, T. R., 1994, op. cit.

18. McCarthy, M. "U.S. maternal death rates are on the rise." *Lancet* 348 (1996): 394.

19. UNICEF. *The State of the World's Children, 1998.* Oxford University Press: New York, 1998.

20. Children's Defense Fund. *The State of America's Children.* Yearbook 1998. Beacon Press: Boston, 1998.

21. "Too many or too few." *The Economist* (September 25, 1999): 19.

22. Dissenters differed, forecasting far greater population growth in the twentieth century. See: Bongaarts, J. "Demographic consequences of declining fertility." *Science* 282 (1998): 419–20; Cohen, J. E. "Population growth and Earth's human carrying capacity." *Science* 269 (1995): 341–46; Crossette, B. "World less crowded than expected, the U.N. reports." *New York Times* (November 17, 1996): A3; Haer, M. "How 'Demographic Fatigue' will defuse the population bomb." *Newsweek* (November 2, 1998): 2; National Research Council. *Our Common Journey: A Transition Toward Sustainability.* Washington, D.C.: National Academy of Sciences, 1999; Pimentel, D. "How many people can the Earth support?" Annual Meeting of the American Association of the Advancement of Science, Baltimore, February 8–13, 1996; Rees, W. E. "The footprints of consumption: Tracking ecospheric decline." Annual Meeting of the American Association of the Advancement of Science, Baltimore, February 8–13, 1996; and Various authors. *Population,* special issue of *National Geographic,* October 1998.

23. Iglehart, J. K. "The American health care system." *New England Journal of Medicine* 340 (1999): 327–32.

24. In 1998 Medicare was already eating up 2.7 percent of the U.S. GDP: by 2025 it would devour at least 5.3 percent of the GDP. Moon, M. *Growth in Medicare Spending: What Will Beneficiaries Pay?* New York: The Commonwealth Fund, 1999.

25. World Health Organization. "Population aging—a public health challenge." Fact Sheet No. 135. World Health Organization, Geneva, September 1998.

26. The World Health Organization forecast the following:

- One out of every four Europeans by 2020 would be elders.
- Nearly one out of three Japanese and Swiss would be elders in 2020.
- Twenty-three percent of North Americans and 12 percent of Latin Americans would be elders.
- Elder populations in key developing countries would include 230 million in China; 142 million in India; 29 million in Indonesia; 18 million in Pakistan; and 27 million in Brazil.
- By 2020 the percentage of populations that reach their elder years in much of Africa and Asia would increase 768-fold.

(*Source:* ibid.)

27. Population Health and Nutrition Department. *Population in Developing Countries.* The World Bank, Washington, D.C., 1998.

28. U.S. Department of Health and Human services. "BBA expected to restrain public-sector health spending while private sector health spending increases." U.S. Health Care Financing Agency, Office of the Actuary, September 14, 1998.

29. Even Americans covered by their employers witnessed 4 to 9 percent increases in their premiums in *one year* (1998–1999), and the costs skyrocketed. See KPMG Peat Marwick. *The 1999 Annual Employer Health Benefits Survey.* Menlo Park, Calif.: Kaiser Family Foundation, 1999.

30. Uchitelle, L. "Devising new math to define poverty." *New York Times* (October 18, 1999): A1.

31. Stevenson, R. W., "Fed reports family gains from economy," *New York Times* (January 19, 1999): C1,

32. Children's Defense Fund, 1998, op. cit.

The wealth gap, as it was called, had widened since 1980. That year the top fifth wealthiest Americans consumed 42.7 percent of the nation's aggregate wealth. By 1990 the top 20 percent consumed 44.3 percent of U.S. wealth. And by 1999 they devoured 50.4 percent, versus just 4.2 percent consumed by the poorest fifth of America's population. (These figures come from Danziger, S., Sandefur, G., and Wenberg, D., eds. *Confronting Poverty: Prescriptions for Change.* Congressional Budget Office. Washington, D.C.: Government Printing Office, 1994.

The breakdown is as follows:

PERCENTAGE OF AGGREGATE U.S. INCOME CONSUMED

Year	Top 20%: Wealthiest U.S. Population	Bottom 20%: Poorest U.S. Population
1950	42.7	4.5
1960	41.3	4.8
1970	40.9	5.4
1977	44.2	5.7
1980	41.6	5.1
1990	44.3	4.6
1999	50.4	4.2

In starker terms, in 1999 the top 1 percent of wealthiest Americans had more money to burn than the combined wealth of the bottom 100 million. And that ratio had more than doubled since 1977. (See Johston, D. C. "Gap between rich and poor found substantially wider." *New York Times* (September 5, 1999): A16.) Yes, America was a phenomenally rich country in 2000, ranking number two behind Luxembourg in per capita GDP. But that was an *average*, which failed to note the widening wealth gap. For most Americans life didn't *feel* on top of the fiscal world.

New York City, for example, transformed in the late 1990s into a boomtown full of family-friendly entertainment and entire neighborhoods composed of chic, mall-like shopping. In 1998 it ranked as the metropolis with the seventh highest cost of living in the world, and the Gotham real estate market was among the most rapidly inflating on earth. (According to *The Economist* (June 20, 1998: 122), the cost-of-living index was, in order from costliest to cheapest: Tokyo, Hong Kong, London, Moscow, Tel Aviv, Beijing, New York City, Singapore, Taipei, Buenos Aires, Sâo Paulo, Athens.)

But such numbers disguised the underclass reality of New York, which in 1999 had the largest population percentage living below the poverty line in urban United States. One out of four New Yorkers earned less than $16,665 a year for a family of four. And the city had a 6.9 percent unemployment rate, compared to a national rate of 4.5 percent. Further, changes in federal and local welfare and Medicaid access laws had forced more of New York's poor out of government services: from 1996 to 1998 there was a 14 percent decline in the number of Gotham poor who received Medicaid and a 16.6 percent fall in food stamps recipients.

From whence did these swelling ranks of poor come? The middle class, which in New York City shrank from 1989 to 1998 from representing 35 percent of the population to just 29 percent. (See Bernstein, N. "Poverty rate persists in city despite boom." *New York Times* (October 7, 1999): B1.)

33. From Wolfe, A. "The politics of inequality." *New York Times* (September 22, 1999): A27.

"Once upon an Arabian night, sultans were paid their weight in gold," wrote *The Economist* in the summer of 1999. "Today, such an approach to pay would leave the typical boss of a large American company sorely disappointed. Bosses now prefer to be paid in share options, which are far more valuable than mere metal. Tipping the scales—let's be kind, and ignore those boardroom lunches—at around two hundred pounds, and with gold now at about $258 a tray ounce, the average chief executive officer of America's top two hundred firms would take home just over $750,000 in gold. In fact, in 1998 he made a pre-tax profit of $8.3 million by exercising executive share options, which give the right to buy a fixed number of his company's shares at a fixed price in what is now a risky market. At the end of last year, he also had total unrealized profits on stock options of nearly $50 million." (See "Share and share unalike." *The Economist* (August 7, 1999): 18.)

Half of the CEOs of the top two hundred U.S. corporations earned through such stock options *more than $31 million*—each—in 1998, or nearly 350 times the average U.S. per capita income. Some executives took in more than $200 million in personal income annually, often for managing companies that were actually losing money, sinking into debt, and performing poorly on the stock market.

34. Miringoff, M. L. *The Index of Social Health*. Fordham University, New York, 1995.

35. World Bank. *World Development Report 1999*. The World Bank, Washington, D.C., 1999.

WORLD GROSS DOMESTIC PRODUCT

Country	Percentile
1. Asia	26.5
2. United States	20.4
3. European Union	19.8
4. Latin America	8.8
5. Other Devoloping Economies	8.0
6. Japan	7.7
7. Ex-USSR	4.8
8. Other Developed Economies	4.0

36. The World Bank's 1997 *World Development Report* offered these estimates:

WEALTH GAP—DISTRIBUTION OF INCOME

COUNTRY (ranked by economy)	YEAR DATA COLLECTED	PERCENT (%) SHARE OF NATION'S INCOME			TOP 10% CONTROLS MORE THAN 30% OF NATION'S WEALTH
		POOREST 10% OF SOCIETY	POOREST 20% OF SOCIETY	RICHEST 10% OF SOCIETY	
Mozambique	1993	2.9	6.9	30.2	√
Ethiopia	1993	2.9	6.9	30.2	√
Tanzania	1993	2.9	6.9	30.2	√
Burundi	1993	2.9	6.9	30.2	√
Malawi	1993	2.9	6.9	30.2	√
Rwanda	1985	4.2	9.7	24.2	
Nepal	1996	3.2	7.6	29.8	
Niger	1992	3.0	7.5	29.3	
Madagascar	1993	2.3	5.8	34.9	√
Vietnam	1993	3.5	7.8	29.0	
Bangladesh	1992	4.1	9.4	23.7	
Uganda	1993	3.0	6.8	33.4	√
Guinea-Bissau	1991	0.1	2.1	42.4	√
Nigeria	1993	1.3	4.0	31.3	√
Kenya	1992	1.2	3.4	37.7	√
India	1992	3.7	8.5	28.4	
Laos	1992	4.2	9.6	26.4	
Nicaragua	1993	1.6	4.2	39.8	√
Ghana	1992	3.4	7.9	27.3	

COUNTRY (ranked by economy)	YEAR DATA COLLECTED	PERCENT (%) SHARE OF NATION'S INCOME			TOP 10% CONTROLS MORE THAN 30% OF NATION'S WEALTH
		POOREST 10% OF SOCIETY	POOREST 20% OF SOCIETY	RICHEST 10% OF SOCIETY	
Zambia	1993	1.5	3.9	31.3	√
Pakistan	1991	3.4	8.4	25.2	
Mauritania	1988	0.7	3.6	30.4	√
Zimbabwe	1990	1.8	4.0	46.9	√
Guinea	1991	0.9	3.0	31.7	√
Honduras	1992	1.5	3.8	41.9	√
Senegal	1991	1.4	3.5	42.8	√
China	1995	2.2	5.5	30.9	√
Côte d'Ivoire	1988	2.8	6.8	28.5	
Sri Lanka	1990	3.8	8.9	25.2	
Lesotho	1987	0.9	2.8	43.4	√
Egypt	1991	3.9	8.7	26.7	
Bolivia	1990	2.3	5.6	31.7	√
*Moldova	1992	2.7	6.9	25.8	
Indonesia	1993	3.9	8.7	25.6	
Philippines	1988	2.8	6.5	32.1	√
Morocco	1991	2.8	6.6	30.5	√
*Bulgaria	1992	3.3	8.3	24.7	
*Kazakhstan	1993	3.1	7.5	24.9	
Guatemala	1989	0.6	2.1	46.6	√
Ecuador	1994	2.3	5.4	37.6	√
Dominican Republic	1989	1.6	4.2	39.6	√
*Romania	1992	3.8	9.2	20.2	
Jordan	1991	2.4	5.9	34.7	√
Jamaica	1991	2.4	5.8	31.9	√
Algeria	1988	2.8	6.9	31.5	√
*Ukraine	1992	4.1	9.5	20.8	
Tunisia	1990	2.3	5.9	30.7	√
*Lithuania	1993	3.4	8.1	28.0	
Colombia	1991	1.3	3.6	39.5	√
*Belarus	1993	4.9	11.1	19.4	
*Russia	1993	1.2	3.7	38.7	√

COUNTRY (ranked by economy)	YEAR DATA COLLECTED	PERCENT (%) SHARE OF NATION'S INCOME			TOP 10% CONTROLS MORE THAN 30% OF NATION'S WEALTH
		POOREST 10% OF SOCIETY	POOREST 20% OF SOCIETY	RICHEST 10% OF SOCIETY	
*Latvia	1993	4.3	9.6	22.1	
Peru	1994	1.9	4.9	34.3	√
Costa Rica	1989	1.2	4.0	34.1	√
Thailand	1992	2.5	5.6	37.1	√
Panama	1989	0.5	2.0	42.2	√
*Poland	1992	4.0	9.3	22.1	
*Estonia	1993	2.4	6.6	31.3	√
*Slovak Republic	1992	5.1	11.9	18.2	
Venezuela	1990	1.4	3.6	42.7	√
South Africa	1993	1.4	3.3	47.3	√
Mexico	1992	1.6	4.1	39.2	√
Brazil	1989	0.7	2.1	51.3	√
Czech Republic	1993	4.6	10.5	23.5	
Malaysia	1989	1.9	4.6	37.9	√
*Hungary	1993	4.0	9.5	22.6	
Chile	1994	1.4	3.5	46.1	√
Slovenia	1993	4.1	9.5	23.8	
Spain	1988	8.3	13.7	21.8	
New Zealand	1982	—	5.1	28.7	
Israel	1979	—	6.0	23.5	
United Kingdom	1988	—	4.6	27.8	
Australia	1985	—	4.4	25.8	
Italy	1986	—	6.8	25.3	
Canada	1987	—	5.7	24.1	
Finland	1981	—	6.3	21.7	
Sweden	1981	—	8.0	20.8	
Netherlands	1988	—	8.2	21.9	
Belgium	1979	—	7.9	21.5	
France	1979	—	5.6	26.1	
Singapore	1983	—	5.1	33.5	√
United States	1985	—	4.7	25.0	
*Germany	1988	—	7.0	24.4	

COUNTRY (ranked by economy)	YEAR DATA COLLECTED	PERCENT (%) SHARE OF NATION'S INCOME			TOP 10% CONTROLS MORE THAN 30% OF NATION'S WEALTH
		POOREST 10% OF SOCIETY	POOREST 20% OF SOCIETY	RICHEST 10% OF SOCIETY	
Denmark	1981	—	5.4	22.3	
Norway	1979	—	6.2	21.2	
Japan	1979	—	8.7	22.4	
Switzerland	1982	—	5.2	29.8	
**United States	1977	5.7	17.2	44.2	√
**United States	1999	4.2	13.9	50.4	√

* NOTE: Most of these figures do not reflect the impact of the fall of Soviet and Warsaw Pact communism. Generally, since 1991 the region's post-Communist wealth gap widened considerably.
** SOURCE: U.S. Congressional Budget Office, 1999. According to the Congressional Budget Office in 1999 the top 1 percent income earners in the United States controlled 12.9 percent of the nation's wealth.

37. Keegan, V. "Highway robbery by the super-rich." *The Guardian* (July 22, 1996): 16.

38. "Numbers." *Time* (July 26, 1999): 17.

39. See, for example, Bauman, Z. *Globalization: The Human Consequences*. New York: Columbia University Press, 1998.

40. For example, see The World Bank. *From Plan to Market, World Development Report 1996*. The World Bank, Washington, D.C., 1996; and "A global war against bribery." *The Economist* (January 16, 1999): 22–24.

41. *The Economist* expressed the difference by asking how many minutes an average worker would have to toil to earn enough to buy a Big Mac hamburger. In 1997 a Tokyo, Hong Kong, or New York City worker could grab a Big Mac with the least stress, having to toil less than twenty minutes to make enough to pay for the burger; at the other end of its list of thirty sample cities were Manila (eighty minutes), Budapest (ninety minutes), Jakarta and Moscow (one hundred minutes), and Caracas (nearly two hours). Obviously for those living in nations where average workers made less than one dollar a day it would take several days to earn enough to dine on the patties of meat sandwiched between buns, vegetables, and cheese. (See: "Purchasing power." *The Economist* [October 11, 1997]: 126.)

42. Miller, J. "Globalization widening rich-poor gap, U.N. report says." *New York Times* (July 13, 1999): A8.

43. For an excellent summary, see *The Economist* special supplement section, "The world economy: On the edge." (September 5, 1998). Using J. P. Morgan estimates *The Economist* presented the following pie chart of world gross domestic product:

Ramonet, I. "The politics of hunger." *World Press Review* (February 1999): 47; E. M. "Research 'must aid fight against poverty.' " *Nature* 400 (1999): 9; Kristoff, N. D. "Asia feels strain at society's margins." *New York Times* (June 8, 1999): A1; Kristoff, N. D. "With Asia's economies shrinking, women are being squeezed out." *New York Times* (June 11, 1998): A12; "Poverty and inequality—The other side of Asia's miracle." *World Bank News* XVI (1997): 1–2; and Landes, D. *The Wealth and Poverty of Nations: Why Some Are So Rich and Some Are So Poor*. New York and London: Little Brown, 1998.

44. See Table: "The Global Picture: A Sampler" on pages 611–617.

45. Nobel Prize–winning economist Amartya Sen argued that literacy—particularly that of mothers—was the key to social well-being. And UNICEF agreed, having for decades found links between the educational level of mothers and the health of their children. Thus,

as horrible as the post-Communist crisis was for families of the Steppes, Siberia, or Eastern Europe, their greater than 95 percent male and female literacy rates put them in better positions to protect the health of their youngsters than counterparts in, for example, India. Indeed, Sen argued that India, with only half its adults literate—only a third of its mothers—was worse off than most sub-Saharan African countries. And the proof of that principle was the Indian state of Kerala, a largely Christian area with better than 90 percent literacy in both genders. There, life expectancy was seventy-two years, compared to a dismal sixty-two years for the average Indian.

46. Health expenditures (as a percent of GNP) correlated closely with infant mortality up to a point—after spending tops 8 percent of GNP the link gets statistically fuzzy. But countries that spent heavily on weapons or highways rather than health, suffered, with children paying with their lives. It appeared infant mortality declines correlated with spending in excess of 4 percent of GNP.

47. Public Health Service. *Healthy People 2000: National Health Promotion and Disease Prevention Objectives*. Conference edition. Department of Health and Human Services, Washington, D.C., 1990.

48. The most telling table, on page 4 of the report, was as follows:

PROGRESS TOWARD 1990 LIFE STAGE GOALS—1987

Life Stage	*1990 Target*	*Actual 1987 Status*
Infant	35% lower death rate	28% lower
Children	20% lower death rate	21% lower
Adolescents	20% lower death rate	13% lower
Adults	25% lower death rate	21% lower
Older Adults	20% fewer days of restricted activity	17% lower

49. The report states:

A health strategy for the 1990s, however, must put particular emphasis on the arena where health professionals in both the private and public sectors have most responsibility, namely the arena of preventive services. These services, made available to all Americans, can provide the foundation for achievement of other parts of our health strategy. . . . Access to preventive services involves more than just availability of services. Preventive services cannot, and should not, be separated from basic primary health care. Approximately 18 percent of all Americans and 31 percent of those without either private or public health insurance have no source of primary health care. Thus, tracking of progress to achieve access to preventive services over the coming decade must focus on increases in the number of people who have a source of primary health care and those who have adequate insurance coverage, with particular attention to the extension of health insurance and managed health care systems to cover preventive services such as immunization, screening, and patient education and counseling.

50. Public Health Service. *Healthy People 2010 Objectives*. Department of Health and Human Services, Washington, D.C., 1998.

51. For biting comments on this matter, see Haerlin, B., and Parr, D. "How to restore public trust in science." *Nature* 400 (1999): 499.

52. Centers for Disease Control and Prevention. "Public opinion about public health—United States, 1999." *Morbidity and Mortality Weekly Report* 49 (2000): 258–60.

53. "Between 1970 and 1980 the social regulatory agencies of the federal government grew from twelve to eighteen and their budgets increased from $1.4 billion to $7.5 billion. During the same decade the *Code of Federal Regulations* almost doubled, from 54,000 pages to nearly 100,000 pages," wrote Lou Canon. See Cannon, L. *President Reagan: The Role of a Lifetime.* New York: Simon and Schuster, 1991: 820.

54. "The future of the state: A survey of the world economy." *The Economist* (September 20, 1997): 5–48.

55. Bodenheimer, T. "The American health care system: Physicians and the changing marketplace." *New England Journal of Medicine* 340 (1999): 584–88; Lewis, C. E., Prout, D. M., Chalmers, E. P., et al. "How satisfying is the practice of internal medicine? A national survey." *Annals of Internal Medicine* 114 (1991): 1–22; Louis Harris and Associates. *Survey of Physician Experiences with Managed Care.* Conducted for The Commonwealth Fund, New York, 1996; and Zuger, A. "A bad year for A.M.A., doctors debate its prognosis." *New York Times* (December 2, 1997): B11.

56. Task Force on the Future of Health Insurance for Working Americans. *Can't Afford to Get Sick: A Reality for Millions of Working Americans.* The Commonwealth Fund, New York, 1999.

57. Interview with the author, December 1998.

58. Heart disease deaths had already declined markedly during the second half of the twentieth century, thanks not to *Star Trek* interventions but to classic public health measures related to smoking, exercise, and diet. In 1950 heart disease killed 307.4 of every 100,000 Americans annually. By 1996 the death rate was down to 134.6 per 100,000 (age-adjusted figures). See Centers for Disease Control and Prevention. "Decline in deaths from heart disease and stroke—United States, 1900–1999." *Morbidity and Mortality Weekly Report* 48 (1999): 649–56.

Cancer death rates first began a downward dip in 1992, largely due to lower tobacco smoking rates in the United States and associated declines in lung cancer deaths. In 1998 about half a million Americans died of cancers, primarily of the lung (160,000); colon (55,000); breast (44,000); and prostate (39,000).

59. Service, R. F. "Borrowing from biology to power the petite." *Science* 283 (1999): 27–28.

60. See, for example, Dickson, D. "Ventner's *Drosophila* 'success' set to boost human genome efforts." *Nature* 401 (1999): 729; "Genome prospecting." Special issue. *Science* 286 (1999): 443–31; Normille, D., and Pennisi, E. "Team wrapping up sequence of first human chromosome." *Science* 285 (1999): 2038–39; "Special issue: The future of medicine." *Time* (January 11, 1999); and Tang, Y. P., Shimizu, É., Dube, G. R., et al. "Genetic enhancement of learning and memory in mice." *Nature* 401 (1999): 63–69.

61. Strauss, E. "New ways to probe the molecules of life." *Science* 282 (1998): 1406–07; and Friedmann, T. *The Development of Human Gene Therapy.* Cold Spring Harbor, N.Y.: Cold Spring Harbor Press, 1999.

62. Interview with the author, December 1998.

63. Editorial, "The promise of proteomics." *Nature* 402 (1999): 703. And Abbott, A., "A post-genomic challenge: Learning to read patterns of protein synthesis." *Nature* 402 (1999): 715–20. And Sander, C. "Genomic medicine and the future of health care." *Science* 287 (2000): 1977–78.

64. Interview with the author, December 1998.

65. A large array of technical and ethical issues need to be confronted before the

genomic/protemic revolution could become reality. These are beyond the scope of this book. See, for example, Wingerson, L. *Unnatural Selection*. New York: Bantam Books, 1998; Etzioni, A. *The Limits of Privacy*. New York: Basic Books, 1999; Holtzman, N. A. "Are genetic tests adequately regulated?" *Science* 286 (1999): 409; Nelson, D., and Weiss, R. "NIH not told of deaths in gene studies." *Washington Post* (November 3, 1999): A1; Committee on Genetic Diversity. "Human rights and human genetic variation research." In Mann, J. M., Gruskin, S., Grodin, M. A., et al. 1999, op. cit.

66. Interview with the author, November 1998.

67. Fisher, L. M. "The race to cash in on the genetic code." *New York Times* (August 29, 1999): BU-1.

68. Fisher, L. M. "The science of holding the stake." *New York Times* (February 13, 1999): B8; and Wade, N. "10 drug makers join in drive to find diseases' genetic roots." *New York Times* (April 15, 1999): A27.

69. The National Cancer Institute's Klausner, like Tobias, predicted an end to cancer surgery. Surgery might even lose its preeminence in treatment of other disorders, such as burns, spinal cord trauma, and brain damage. In 1998 scientists successfully brewed batches of healthy cells by cloning a normal adult cell, or stem cell. And researchers also proved that, contrary to prior dogma, neurons could grow and reproduce in the brains of adults.

So in the future, optimists forecast, burns and spinal cord injuries might be treated with direct growth of appropriate stem cells on the injured site.

Getting even further away from surgery, economist Juan Enriquez, who at Harvard University studied the future of health care, saw nutraceuticals on the horizon. "We will build a bridge between medicine and foods," Enriquez opined. "When you go to the grocery stores you see that the pharmacy lines are getting longer and bigger. And when you go to the drugstores you see the food sections are getting bigger. And we're going to see those businesses merge. Nutraceuticals is the merger between nutrition and pharmaceutics."

Already scientists had by 1999 developed a potato that contained a hepatitis B vaccine and bananas that carried pieces of a potential malaria vaccine. In the future, Enriquez insisted, consumers would punch their gene cards into supermarket computers and get a readout on suggested foods they should consume. It was high-tech preventive medicine, he claimed, that would complement other interventions to virtually eliminate cancer, heart disease, and vaccine-preventable infections.

70. "The new alchemy." *The Economist* (January 22, 2000): 61–62.

71. Langreth, R., and Lipin, S. "AHP, Warner-Lambert discuss merger." *Wall Street Journal* (November 3, 1999): A3.

72. Zeisel, S. H. "Regulation of 'Nutraceuticals.' " *Science* 285 (1999): 1853–55.

73. Interview with the author, November 1998.

74. Tanouye, E. "Hard to swallow, America's soaring drug costs." *Wall Street Journal* (November 16, 1998): A1.

75. Those who hope to reform the pharmaceutical market are well advised to take note of the large stake many Americans, Canadians, and Western Europeans have in the continued profitable expansion of these companies. It is supremely ironic that by 2000 many financial advisors were pushing individuals in their forties and fifties to buy drug company stocks as a hedge against future shrinkage or collapse of government services for senior citizens, such as Medicare and national health systems in Canada and Europe. Given that pharmaceutical inflation was a key factor driving collapse of cost containment in the health industry, middle-class investors were essentially being advised to bank on their own collective ill health when planning for their retirement dollars.

76. From annual statements released by the National Institute for Health Care Management, Washington, D.C.

77. During 1997 to 1998 global pharmaceutics sales broke down as:

USA	$99.5 billion
Japan	38.8 billion
Germany	18.2 billion

In terms of company sales in the world market the breakdown was:

Rank	Company	Country Base	Sales ($ billions)
1	Novartis A.G.	Switzerland	10.64
2	Merck & Co.	USA	10.63
3	Glaxo Wellcome	UK	10.54
4	Pfizer Inc.	USA	9.91
5	Bristol-Myers Squibb	USA	9.79
6	Johnson & Johnson	USA	9.02
7	American Home Products	USA	7.81
8	Roche Holding, A.G.	Switzerland	7.62
9	Eli Lilly & Co.	USA	7.36
10	SmithKline Beecham	UK	7.35

See: Morrow, D. J. "Worldwide drug sales up 7% in '98." *New York Times* (March 23, 1999): C5.

78. Tanouye, E., 1998, op. cit. In this excellent *Wall Street Journal* analysis the reporter notes that the U.S. market was driving not only profits but also *all* industry research and development plans.

79. Health insurance providers and HMOs reported at the close of the decade that pharmaceutic costs had outstripped total expenditures on inpatient care. Health Care Financing Administration. "Growth in national health care spending stable in 1997." U.S. Health and Human Services, Washington, D.C., November 11, 1998; Iglehart, J. K. "The American health care system: Expenditures." *New England Journal of Medicine* 340 (1999): 70–76; Soumerai, S. B., and Ross-Degnan, D. "Inadequate prescription-drug coverage for Medicare enrollees—A call to action." *New England Journal of Medicine* 340 (1999): 722–28; Steinhauer, J. "Rising costs of medications take bigger share of insurance outlays." *New York Times* (October 29, 1999): A1; and Zagorin, A. "Who's really raising drug prices?" *Time* (March 8, 1999): 46–48. The average citizen of a Western European or North American country spent $234 on pharmaceutical drugs in 1996 (Anderson, G. F., and Pouillier, J. P. "Health spending, access, and outcomes: Trends in industrialized countries." *Health Affairs* (May/June 1999): 178–92), and the figure was projected to rise radically during the first decade of the twenty-first century. In the United States, for example, the government estimated that total public expenditures on pharmaceuticals would jump from $74.3 billion in 1998 to $171.1 billion by 2007. And as a percentage of overall health spending drugs had accounted for just 4.9 percent in 1980, 6.5 percent in 1998, and would amount to 8 percent by 2007. Iglehart, J. K., 1999, op. cit.

80. Armstrong, K., Schwartz, J. S., and Asch, D. A. "Direct sale of Sildenafil (Viagra) to consumers over the Internet." *New England Journal of Medicine* 341 (1999): 1389–92; Ostrom, C. M. "Internet medicine opens can of worms: Tremendous potential good—and

harm." *Seattle Times* (May 12, 1999): A1; and Stolberg, S. G. "The boom in medications brings rise in fatal risks." *New York Times* (June 3, 1999): A1.

81. Murray, C. J., and Lopez, A. D. *The Global Burden of Disease*. Geneva: World Health Organization, 1996.

82. See: Murray, C. J. L., and Lopez, A. D. "Global mortality, disability, and the contribution of risk factors: Global Burden of Disease study." *Lancet* 349 (1997): 1436–42; and "Spirit of the age." *The Economist* (December 19, 1999): 113–17.

83. Tanouye, E., 1998, op. cit.

84. Trouiller, P. "R & D drug development trends." Conference on Drugs for Communicable Disease, Paris, October 14–15, 1999; and Silverstein, K. "Millions for Viagra, pennies for diseases of the poor." *The Nation* (July 19, 1999): 13–19.

85. Ibid.

86. Bale, H., and Kettler, H. E. "Industry's role in meeting the need for CDC-specific medicines." Conference on Drugs for Communicable Diseases, Paris, October 14–15, 1999.

87. Given by the pharmaceutical Research and Manufacturers of America.

88. Love, J. "Call for more reliable costs on clinical trials." *Marketletter* (January 13, 1997). Comaner, W. S. "The pharmaceutical research and development process, and its costs." Conference on Drugs for Communicable Disease, Paris, October 14–15, 1999.

89. Wunsch, H. "Expert warns of possible poliomyclitis vaccine shortfall in 2000." *The Lancet* 355 (2000): 728. And Associated Press. "Vaccine price prompts shift." *New York Times* (February 17, 2000): A23. And Pécoul, B., Chirac, P., Trouiller, P., and Pinel J. "Access to essential drugs in poor countries: A lost battle?" *Journal of the American Medical Association* 281 (1999): 361–67. And Yudkin, J. S. "Insulin for the world's poorest countries." *Lancet* 355 (2000): 919–21. And Silverstein, K. "Millions for Viagra, pennies for diseases of the poor." *The Nation* (July 19, 1999): 13–19.

90. Interview with the author, January 1999.

91. Aventin, L. "Trade agreements and public health: Role of WHO." *Lancet* 355 (2000): 580.

92. Price, D., Pollock, A. M., and Shaoul, J. "How the World Trade Organization is shaping domestic policies in health care." *Lancet* 354 (1999): 1889–92.

93. Defense spending fell after 1991, according to the Stockholm International Peace Research Institute, and the overall decline from 1988 to 1998 was 30 percent. More than a third of all defense expenditures were in the United States ($259 billion in 1997). In second place, spending just $50 billion, was Japan. The only developing countries that ranked in the top-twenty club of military spenders were Saudi Arabia ($19 billion), South Korea ($18 billion), Brazil ($16 billion), and India ($11 billion). See: "Defense spending." *The Economist* (June 20, 1998): 120.

94. The record on this point was mixed, but the general consensus among world health experts was that drug donations did not work over the long haul. The cases in point involved river blindness, schistosomiasis, malaria, trachoma, and filariasis. In each of these cases between 1974 and 1999 drug manufacturers provided a product that was either curative or prophylactic to the World Health Organization, either gratis or at a greatly reduced price. The task of distributing the drugs to people in need was left to WHO and the pertinent local governments. The results were decidedly mixed, with the river blindness effort proving most successful. In that case the Merck pharmaceutical company developed a veterinary drug called ivermectin during the early 1970s. When it was shown that the drug completely cured the parasitic disease onchocerciasis, WHO in 1974 negotiated a landmark arrangement with Merck. The profits from veterinary use of ivermectin were sufficient to more than offset the costs of Merck donating the drug, gratis, to WHO for human use. In 1999 West African

countries had nearly eradicated river blindness, following twenty-five years of toil funded by the World Bank, getting the medicine to the remote rural villages in the region most heavily afflicted. But it took twenty-five years. And the job wasn't yet over in 2000.

Far less successful were the other programs. Failure was due to many factors, invariably all linked to the poor quality of local public health and primary medical care in the affected areas. Donations of drugs could not affect the fundamental underpinnings of disease. For example, donated praziquantel couldn't eliminate schistosomiasis from Egypt unless the parasites' life cycle in the Nile and its tributaries was also disrupted, eliminating environmental schistosomes. Other drug donations lowered disease incidences for a brief time, but when treatment costs or public health infrastructural exigencies proved insurmountable the programs became unsustainable. And disease returned. See: Ahmad, K. "Global onchocerciasis programme under threat." *Lancet* 354 (1999): 1455; Govindaraj, R. "The case of praziquantel and its lessons." Conference on Drugs for Communicable diseases, Paris, October 14–15, 1999; Kale, O. O. "Review of disease-specific corporate drug donation programmes for the control of communicable diseases." Conference on Drugs for Communicable Diseases, Paris, October 14–15, 1999; Reich, M. R., ed. *International Strategies for Tropical Disease Treatments: Experiences with Praziquantel.* Division of Control of Tropical Diseases/WHO/DAP/CTD/98.5, Geneva, 1998; and World Health Organization. "River blindness: Its impending elimination signals a landmark in public/private sector collaboration." Press Release WHO/53 (October 6, 1999).

Finally, not all drug company charity was a matter of enlightened generosity. The World Health Organization found, for example, that of the 108 stocks of drug supplies donated to the Albanian Ministry of Health during the Kosovo refugee crisis of 1999, "some 50 percent of these lists only mentioned trade names, many of which were unfamiliar to local health professionals; only 56 percent included information on shelf life, of which about 41 percent of the drugs had a remaining shelf life of less than one year; and 18 percent of the donations contained small packs of free samples or drugs returned to pharmacies." See: World Health Organization. "WHO calls for good drug donation practice during emergencies as it issues new 'guidelines.' " Press Release WHO/45 (September 2, 1999).

Further, more than half of all drugs donated for Bosnian relief from 1993 to 1998 were deemed inappropriate, as were drug donations during crises in Rwanda, Somalia, Turkey, and Honduras. "Unwanted drug donations are bad enough, but if accumulated can become a major chemical waste problem," WHO said. "It will cost U.S. $2 to $4 million to ship one thousand metric tons of inappropriate pharmaceuticals and medical supplies from Croatia for appropriate disposal." See: World Health Organization. "WHO calls for good drug donation practice during emergencies as it issues new 'guidelines.' " Press Release WHO/45 (September 2, 1999).

95. Zuger, A. "Type of penicillin is in critical supply." *New York Times* (October 29, 1999): A20.

96. Rosamond, J. and Allsop, A. "Harnessing the power of the genome in the search for new antibiotics." *Science* 287 (2000): 1973–76.

97. World Health Organization. "Removing obstacles to health development." World Health Organization, Geneva, June 17, 1999.

98. UNAIDS. "UN leaders call AIDS in Africa a massive development catastrophe." Lusaka, Zambia, September 13, 1999.

99. Interview with the author, January 1999.

100. Interview with the author, January 1999.

101. National Intelligence Council. "The global infectious disease threat and its implications for the United States." Central Intelligence Agency (January 2000): NIE-99-17D.

102. Balter, M. "French-led therapy fund kicks off in Africa." *Science* 284 (1999): 1101; Dowell, W. "Ethics and AIDS drugs." *Time* (July 12, 1999): 49; and Mabry, M. "No money, no meds." *Newsweek* (July 12, 1999): 32–33. Many developing countries did, however, have adequate infrastructures to appropriately distribute life-extending drugs for treatment of opportunistic infections in AIDS patients, such as TB, pneumocystis pneumonia, and cryptococcal meningitis. But here, too, they came up squarely against TRIPS, patent laws, and pricing inequities. See Wilson, D., Cawthorne, P., Ford, N., and Aongsonwang, S. "Global trade and access to medicines: AIDS treatments in Thailand." *Lancet* 354 (1999): 1893–95.

103. Fisher, I. "Malaria, a swamp dweller finds a hidden home." *New York Times* (July 21, 1999): A4; White, N. J., Nosten, F., Looareesuwan, S., et al. "Averting a malaria disaster" and Letters in response. *Lancet* 353 (1999): 1965–67 and 354 (1999): 1389–90.

104. Attaran, A. "Respective public and private sector contributions to the development of new drugs." Drugs for Communicable Diseases Conference, Paris, October 14–15, 1999; Helenport, J. P. "The development and registration of artemisinin derivatives, a triangular development." Drugs for Communicable Diseases Conference, Paris, October 14–15, 1999; Jomaa, H., Wiesner, J., Sanderbrand, S., et al. "Inhibitors of the nonelevating pathway of Isoprenoid Isoprenoid biosynthesis as antimalarial drugs." *Science* 285 (1999): 1573–76; and Ridley, R. G. "Planting the seeds of new antimalarial drugs." *Science* 285 (1999): 1502–04.

105. Centers for Disease Control and Prevention. "Primary multidrug-resistant tuberculosis—Ivanovo Oblast, Russia, 1999." *Morbidity and Mortality Weekly Report* 48 (1999): 661–64.

106. Kim, J. Y., Farmer, P., and Dahl, O. Letter to Partners in Health, September 18, 1997.

107. Rifampicin, isoniazid, pyrazinamide, and either ethambutol. or streptomycin. Either rifampicin or ethambutol combined with isoniazid. Murray, C. J. L. "Results of directly observed short-course chemotherapy in 112,842 Chinese patients with smear-positive tuberculosis." *Lancet* 347 (1996): 358–62.

108. Blanc, D. C. "Incentives and disincentives for new anti-tuberculosis drug development." World Health Organization, Geneva, November 1998.

109. World Health Organization. *The World Health Report 1998*. World Health Organization, Geneva, 1998.

110. Centers for Disease Control and Prevention. "Tuberculosis elimination revisited: Obstacles, opportunities, and a renewed commitment." *Morbidity and Mortality Weekly Report* 48 (Supplement) (1999):RR-9.

111. Program in Infectious Disease and Social Change. *The Global Impact of Drug-Resistant Tuberculosis*. Open Society, New York, 1999. (Available in full on-line at www.opensociety.com.)

112. MRSA: methicillin-resistant *Staphylococcus aureus*; VRE: vancomycin-resistant *Enterococcus*; VISA: vancomycin-insensitive *Staphylococcus aureus*. See Chapter 4 for details on these organisms.

113. Interview with the author, 1998, op. cit.

114. Bloom, B. R., Bloom, D. E., Cohen, J. E., et al. "Investing in the World Health Organization." *Science* 284 (1999): 911; "Smokescreens." *The Economist* (March 14, 1998): 91–92; "WHO steps closer to its responsibilities." *Nature* 398 (1999): 175; and "WHO: Where there is no vision, the people perish." *Lancet* 350 (1997): 749.

115. Brundtland, G. H. "WHO—The road ahead." Speech to the World Health Organization Executive Board, Geneva, January 24, 1999; and World Health Organization. *The World Health Report 1999*. World Health Organization, Geneva, 1999.

116. Interview with the author, September 1996.

117. See previously cited Murray, C. J. L., references and Garrett, L. "The future of death." *Newsday* (October 8, 1996): B21.

118. See also: "From what will we die in 2020?" *Lancet* 349 (1997): 1263; Husten, L. "Global epidemic of cardiovascular disease predicted." *Lancet* 352 (1998); 1530; Lee, W. C. "Quantifying the future impact of disease on society: Life table-based measures of potential life lost." *American Journal of Public Health* 87 (1997): 1456–60; Murray, C. J. L., and Lopez, A. D. "Alternative projections of mortality and disability by cause 1990–2020: Global Burden of Disease Study." *Lancet* 349 (1997): 1498–1504; Murray, C. J. L., and Lopez, A. D. "Evidence-based health policy—Lessons from the Global Burden of Disease Study." *Science* 274 (1996): 740–43; Murray, C. J. L, and Lopez, A. D. "Mortality by cause for eight regions of the world: Global Burden of Disease Study." *Lancet* 239 (1997): 1269–76; and Schneider, E. L. "Aging in the Third Millennium." *Science* 283 (1999): 796–97.

119. Armstrong, G. L., Conn, L. A., and Pinner, R. W. "Trends in infectious disease mortality in the United States during the 20th century." *Journal of the American Medical Association* 281 (1999): 61–66. See also McGinnis, J. M., and Foege, W. H. "Actual causes of death in the United States." *Journal of the American Medical Association* 170 (1993): 2207–12.

120. National Intelligence Council, op. cit, 2000.

121. World Health Organization. *Removing Obstacles to Healthy Development.* World Health Organization, Geneva, June 17, 1999.

122. De Kruif, P., 1936, op. cit.

123. Nadis, S. "U.S. concern grows over secrecy clauses." *Nature* 398 (1999): 359; and Cimons, M., and Jacobs, P. "Biotech battlefield: Profits vs. public." *Los Angeles Times* (February 21, 1999): A1

124. Reich, M. R., "The global drug gap." *Science* 287 (2000): 1979–81. And Enserink, M. "Group urges action on Third World drugs." *Science* 287 (2000): 1571. And Kasper, T. "Global patent police block cost-reduction efforts." *Treatment Issues* 13 (1999): 1–2. And Orbinski, J. "Speech on acceptance of the 1999 Nobel Peace Prize." Médecins Sans Frontières, Oslo, December 14, 1999.

INDEX